HEALTH INFORMATICS
AN INTERPROFESSIONAL APPROACH

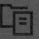

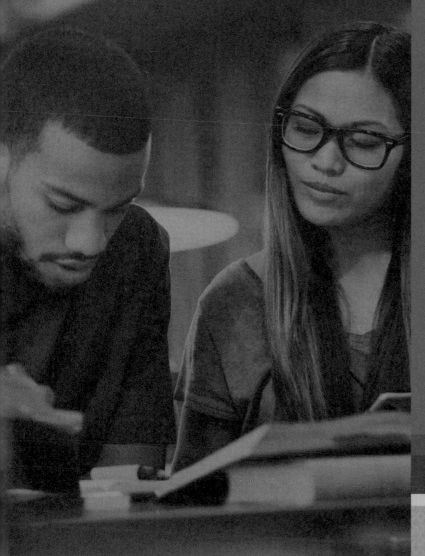
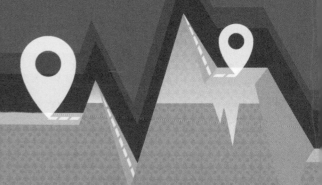

THIRD EDITION

HEALTH INFORMATICS

AN INTERPROFESSIONAL APPROACH

Lynda R. Hardy, PhD, RN, FAAN
Wake Forest University School of Medicine
Master of Clinical Research
Management Program
Winston-Salem, North Carolina

Elsevier
3251 Riverport Lane
St. Louis, Missouri 63043

HEALTH INFORMATICS: AN INTERPROFESSIONAL APPROACH, THIRD EDITION

ISBN: 978-0-323-71196-8

Notice

Practitioners and researchers must always rely on their own experience and knowledge in evaluating and using any information, methods, compounds or experiments described herein. Because of rapid advances in the medical sciences, in particular, independent verification of diagnoses and drug dosages should be made. To the fullest extent of the law, no responsibility is assumed by Elsevier, authors, editors or contributors for any injury and/or damage to persons or property as a matter of products liability, negligence or otherwise, or from any use or operation of any methods, products, instructions, or ideas contained in the material herein.

Previous editions copyrighted 2018, 2014.

Content Strategist: Heather Bays-Petrovic
Content Development Manager: Laura Schmidt
Content Development Specialist: Kristen Helm
Publishing Services Manager: Julie Eddy
Senior Project Manager: Cindy Thoms
Design Direction: Ryan Cook

Printed in Canada

Last digit is the print number: 9 8 7 6 5 4 3 2 1

Working together
to grow libraries in
developing countries

www.elsevier.com • www.bookaid.org

Lynda R. Hardy holds a baccalaureate degree in nursing from the State University of New York at New Paltz, a master's degree in administration from George Mason University in Fairfax, Virginia, and a PhD in Nursing from the University of North Carolina – Chapel Hill.

She held positions as an Associate Professor of Nursing and Director of Data Science and Discovery at The Ohio State University where she taught health informatics to doctoral nursing students. Lyn also held positions as the Associate Dean of Research at the University of Tennessee Knoxville and health science administrator at the National Institutes of Health. Currently, Lyn is faculty at the Wake Forest University School of Medicine where she teaches in the Master of Clinical Research Management program. Her primary areas of interest include all things 'data' specifically informatics education for health professionals, data science and maximization of currently held data, data standardization, empowering and educating patients about their health-related data, and the application of data science analytics to advance precision medicine.

Her publications include a health informatics primer textbook, book chapters, journal articles, abstracts, scientific policies and procedures. She was named as a fellow in the American Academy of Nursing in 2016. She was awarded the 2022 American Medical Informatics Association Leadership award for her work in the health informatics certification coursework.

Madeline Araya, MS, RN
Systems Analyst IV
Information Technology Services
University of Utah Health
Salt Lake City, Utah

Vickie Bennett, DNP, RN-BC
eLearning Nurse Educator
Professional Development
Nationwide Children's Hospital
Columbus, Ohio

Lisa M. Blair, PhD, RN
Assistant Professor
College of Nursing
Wayne State University
Detroit, Michigan

Michele Bosworth, MD, FAAFP, LSSGB
Principal Consultant
Health Management Associates
Austin, Texas

Nancy C. Brazelton, RN, MS
Senior Director
Information Technology Services
University of Utah Health
Salt Lake City, Utah

Juliana J. Brixey, PhD, MPH, MSN, RN
Associate Professor
School of Biomedical Informatics
Cizik School of Nursing
University of Texas Health Science Center at
    Houston
Houston, Texas

Zach Burningham, PhD, MPH
Research Health Scientist
HSR&D IDEAS COIN
VA Salt Lake City Health Care System;
Assistant Professor
Division of Epidemiology
Department of Internal Medicine
University of Utah
Salt Lake City, Utah

Heather Carter-Templeton, PhD, RN-BC
Chairperson, Adult Health Department
Associate Professor
School of Nursing
West Virginia University
Morgantown, West Virginia

Guilherme Del Fiol, MD, PhD
Professor and Vice-Chair for Research
Department of Biomedical Informatics
University of Utah School of Medicine
Salt Lake City, Utah

Paul DeMuro, PhD, JD, MBA, CPA
Nossaman LLP
Austin, Texas

Teresa Gore, PhD, DNP, APRN, FNP-BC
CHSE-A, FSSH, FAAN
Professor, Director of Teaching and Learning
Ron and Kathy Assaf College of Nursing
Nova Southeastern University
Clearwater, Florida

Aaron Zachary Hettinger, MD
Assistant Professor
Georgetown University School of Medicine;
Director and Chief Research Information
    Officer
MedStar Health Research Institute
Washington, District of Columbia

Maia Hightower, MD, MPH, MBA
Chief Executive Officer
Equality AI
Park City, Utah;
Senior Director Health Equity, Diversity, and
    Inclusion
University of Utah Health
Salt Lake City, Utah

Sarah J. Iribarren, PhD, RN
Associate Professor
Biobehavioral Nursing and Health
    Informatics
University of Washington
Seattle, Washington

Jonathan M. Ishee, JD, MPH, MS, LLM,
CIPP/US
Assistant Professor
School of Biomedical Informatics
University of Texas Health Science Center
Houston, Texas;
Partner, Troutman Pepper Hamilton Sanders,
    LLP
Washington, District of Columbia

Ashish Joshi, PhD, MBBS, MPH
Dean and Distinguished University Professor
School of Public Health
The University of Memphis
Memphis, Tennessee

Kensaku Kawamoto, MD, PhD, MHS
Associate Chief Medical Information Officer
University of Utah
Professor
Department of Biomedical Informatics
University of Utah;
Salt Lake City, Utah

Sadaf Kazi, PhD
Research Scientist
National Center for Human Factors in
    Healthcare
MedStar Health Research Institute;
Assistant Professor
Emergency Medicine
Georgetown University School of Medicine
Washington, District of Columbia

Tiffany Kelley, PhD, MBA, RN
Frederick A. DeLuca Foundation Visiting
    Professor for Innovation and New
    Knowledge
Director, Healthcare Innovation Certificate
    Program
School of Nursing
University of Connecticut
Storrs, Connecticut;
Founder and CEO
iCarc Nursing Solutions and Nightingale Apps
Boston, Massachusetts

Michael H. Kennedy, PhD, MHA, FACHE
Associate Professor and Chair
Department of Healthcare Policy, Economics,
    and Management
University of Texas at Tyler
Tyler, Texas

Polina V. Kukhareva, PhD, MPH
Research Assistant Professor
Department of Biomedical Informatics
University of Utah School of Medicine
Salt Lake City, Utah

Gerald R. Ledlow, PhD, MHA, FACHE
Professor
Department of Healthcare Policy, Economics,
    and Management
University of Texas at Tyler
Tyler, Texas

Jim Livingston, MBA
Chief Technology Officer
Information Technology Services
University of Utah Health
Salt Lake City, Utah

Louis Luangkesorn, PhD
Senior Data Scientist
Highmark Health
Pittsburgh, Pennsylvania

Ann M. Lyons, PhD, RN
Medical Informaticist
Data Science Services
University of Utah Health
Salt Lake City, Utah

John D. Manning, MD, FAMIA, FACEP
Assistant Professor
Department of Emergency Medicine
Atrium Health
Charlotte, North Carolina

Karen S. Martin, RN, MSN, FHIMSS, FAAN
Health Care Consultant
Martin Associates
Omaha, Nebraska

Michele Mills, MBA PM, PMP, CPHIMS, FHIMSS
Director
Information Technology Services
University of Utah Health Care
Salt Lake City, Utah

Craig B. Monsen, MD, MS
Chief Medical Information Officer
Clinical Systems
Atrius Health
Auburndale, Massachusetts

Michael Morris, PhD, CHFP
Associate Professor
Department of Healthcare Policy, Economics, and Management
The University of Texas at Tyler
Tyler, Texas

Ramona Nelson, PhD, RN-BC
President
Ramona Nelson Consulting
Allison Park, Pennsylvania;
Professor Emerita, Nursing
Slippery Rock University
Slippery Rock, Pennsylvania

Henry Norwood, JD
Attorney at Law
The Herman Law Firm
Brookline, Massachusetts

Sally Okun, BSN, MMHS
Executive Director
Clinical Trials Transformation Initiative
Durham, North Carolina

Jeanette M. Olsen, PhD, RN, CNE
Associate Professor
Director of Assessment and Evaluation
College of Nursing and Health Sciences
University of Wisconsin – Eau Claire
Eau Claire, Wisconsin

Elizabeth G. Olson, MD
Pediatric Emergency Medicine Fellow and Emergency Medicine Junior Faculty
Department of Emergency Medicine
Atrium Health
Charlotte, North Carolina

Michael J. Paluzzi, JD
Associate
Troutman Pepper Hamilton Sanders, LLP
Chicago, Illinois

Thomas H. Payne, MD, FACP, FRCP (Edin), FACMI
Professor of Medicine
Professor of Biomedical Informatics and Medical Education
University of Washington School of Medicine;
Adjunct Professor
Department of Health Systems and Population Health
University of Washington School of Public Health
Seattle, Washington

David A. Pearson, MD, MS, MBA
Department of Emergency Medicine
Carolina Medical Center, Atrium Health
Charlotte, North Carolina

Amanda Ray, JD, Esq.
Associate
McGuireWoods, LLP
Chicago, Illinois

Donna Roach, MS, CHCIO, FCHIME, FHIMSS
Chief Information Officer
Health Sciences Center Utah
South Salt Lake, Utah;
Hospital Administration
University of Utah Health
Salt Lake City, Utah

Jessica M. Ruff, MD, MA, MSPH
Department of Wellness and Peventive Medicine
Cleveland Clinic Foundation
Cleveland, Ohio

Matthew Sakumoto, MD
Department of Medicine
University of California, San Francisco
San Francisco, California

Rebecca Schnall, PhD, MPH, RN-BC
Mary Dickey Lindsay Professor of Disease Prevention and Health Promotion (in Nursing);
Associate Dean for Faculty Development (Nursing);
Professor of Population and Family Health (Public Health)
Columbia University
New York, New York

Charlotte A. Seckman, PhD, RN-BC, CNE, FAAN
Associate Professor, Nursing Informatics Specialist
School of Nursing, Organizational Systems and Adult Health
University of Maryland, School of Nursing
Baltimore, Maryland

Sarah C. Shuffelton, DNP, RN-BC
Assistant Professor of Clinical Practice
College of Nursing
The Ohio State University
Columbus, Ohio

Meera Subash, MD
Assistant Professor
UTHealth School of Biomedical Informatics McGovern Medical School
Department of Internal Medicine
Division of Rheumatology
University of Texas Health Science Center at Houston
Houston, Texas

Todd B. Taylor, MD, FACEP
Emergency Physician and Clinical Informaticist
Phoenix, Arizona;
Vice-Chair
Health Innovation & Technology Committee
American College of Emergency Physicians
Dallas, Texas

Timothy Tsai, DO, MMCi
Clinical Informatics
Duke Health Technology Solutions
Duke University Health System
Durham, North Carolina

Michael Wang, MD
Assistant Professor
Division of Hospital Medicine
University of California, San Francisco
San Francisco, California

Charlene R. Weir, PhD
Professor Emeritus
Department of Biomedical Informatics
University of Utah School of Medicine
Salt Lake City, Utah

Marisa L. Wilson, DNSc, MHSc, MHSc, RN-BC, CPHIMS, FAMIA, FIAHSI, FAAN
Director, Nursing Health Services Leadership Graduate Pathways;
Specialty Track Coordinator, MSN Nursing Informatics
The University of Alabama at Birmingham School of Nursing
Birmingham, Alabama

Kathy H. Wood, PhD, MBA, BSBA
Program Director MHA/MHS
University of St. Augustine for Health Sciences
St. Augustine, Florida

Nathan Yung, MD, MS
Clinical Informatics Fellow
Emergency Department
University of California, San Diego
San Diego, California

Deborah Ariosto, PhD, RN
Vanderbilt University Medical Center (Retired)
Nashville, Tennessee;
Adjunct Professor
University of Maryland School of Nursing
Baltimore, Maryland

Ashley Hunsucker, MSN, RN
Nursing Informatics Advisor
Patient Physician Network
Nova Southeastern University
Corinth, Texas

ACKNOWLEDGMENTS

First, I would like to acknowledge Heather Bays-Petrovic, Content Strategist, whose overview and coordination of this third edition is greatly appreciated. We also thank Kristen Helm, Content Development Specialist, who was responsible for providing support during the process of writing and editing; and especially Cindy Thoms, Senior Project Manager, whose attention to detail was invaluable during the editing process. Finally, we would like to acknowledge Ryan Cook, the Designer. His expertise was imperative for developing a polished and professional product.

Each chapter of this book is supported with Evolve resources. We also wish to acknowledge the support of Umarani Natarajan, Senior Project Manager, and Hariprasad Maniyaan, Multimedia Producer, for the Evolve resources, as well as the ancillary writers, Deborah Ariosto and Ashley Hunsucker, for their development of these resources.

Finally, we would like to acknowledge the reviewers from the previous edition. Their many suggestions, tips, and comments were invaluable in creating this book.

Lynda R. Hardy

Health informatics and information technology (IT) have been brought to center stage by a global pandemic; they have become powerful tools for a challenged healthcare system. Our healthcare system is comprised of resolute professionals aimed at improving health. This concerted effort underscores the interprofessional requirement ensuring a comprehensive understanding and use of health informatics, its practices, and its use in research. Through experiential work in health informatics I saw, firsthand, the impact data, data science, and informatics made on the opioid epidemic, precision medicine, and a never-ending pandemic. Considering the impact health informatics has on understanding, managing, and communicating health-related issues, the authors and content of this book were updated and applied to our new world order, providing a robust overview of the field from an interdisciplinary approach. The contributors to this book are leaders in facets of health informatics representing multiple disciplines, settings, areas of expertise, and positions.

Health Informatics: An Interprofessional Approach provides a comprehensive understanding of health informatics, its practice, and relevant research on health informatics topics. Each chapter opens with key terms, learning objectives and an abstract and chapter outline covering chapter topics. Chapter headings give readers a conceptual framework for understanding the content in the chapter. Each chapter ends with conclusions that include thoughts about future directions for the topic. Every chapter includes a set of discussion questions to encourage critical thinking and to encourage the reader to consider how the content in the chapter can be applied in the ever-changing world of healthcare. Case studies with analytic questions demonstrate how informatics applies in real-life practice.

USES OF THE BOOK

This textbook is an excellent resource for use within and across various health disciplines. Every attempt has been made to be culturally sensitive to the various disciplines within healthcare while encouraging readers to recognize themselves as key members of an interprofessional team. This book is written to be used for both intradisciplinary and interdisciplinary informatics courses. The text can span levels of education depending on the program of study, depth of informatics material needed, and faculty and student needs. This book is targeted to all students needing introductory health informatics knowledge. As with the second edition, it is useful at several levels: for upper division or advanced undergraduate courses, for health-related programs, for introductory health informatics content or courses in master's programs and, particularly, for clinical care students.

VENDORS, APPLICATIONS, FOUNDATIONS, AND INSTITUTIONS

Vendors, health IT applications, commercial products, and organizations and institutions are discussed throughout the textbook. They are included for information purposes and to provide readers with examples of the variety of resources available. No endorsement of a specific company, product, or organization is intended.

ORGANIZATION OF THE BOOK

The book is organized into seven units. The first unit is *Foundational Knowledge in Health Informatics* and focuses on material basic to understanding the discipline. Content includes the definition and significance of the field, theories and models, health systems and information flow, informatics standards, and program evaluation for health IT.

The second unit is *Health Information Systems and Applications*. This unit begins with an introduction into the technical infrastructure of health informatics. It proceeds with discussion of the electronic health record, precision care, and administrative applications in healthcare. This unit culminates with discussions related to community health systems and public health informatics. This unit provides the nuts and bolts of health informatics and their importance in managing our community and public health systems.

The third unit, *Decision-Making, and the Digitally Engaged Patient*, recognizes the need for and evidence supporting accurate decision-making and the increased shift toward patient engagement. Patients have become partners in their own healthcare and are equipped with health IT applications. Topics in this unit include evidence-based informatics, clinical decision support, the digitally engaged patient, mHealth (mobile health), personal health records, and social media tools for advancing health informatics. Readers are introduced to the impact of health informatics on patients, providers, and the patient-provider partnership. It also provides an association between components required for appropriate and health IT solutions for informed decision-making.

The fourth unit is entitled *Life Cycle Management*, addressing key nuances of planning, management, and implementing health care systems. The reader is introduced to salient topics that include project management, strategic planning, contract negotiations, implementing and upgrading a system, and downtime and disaster recovery. This material provides the knowledge and skills to lead and participate in health informatics systems projects through every phase of the systems life cycle.

The fifth unit, *Usability, Analytics, and Education*, explains the user experience, introducing data science and analytics into decisions, data safety and quality initiatives, informatics in the curriculum, and distance education. An emphasis is placed on the educational needs of users noting new requirements for nursing education. This unit introduces concepts and practical uses for data science and analytics, representing a major focus of health organizational leaders, health professionals, and informatics specialists today.

The sixth unit, *Data Governance, Legal, and Regulatory Issues*, addresses local and national structures, laws, and regulations important to health informatics and data privacy. Locally, the contributors discuss how organizations develop support structures for managing health IT. Nationally, federal programs and regulations incorporating HITECH, MU, MACRA, MIPS, and ACO are carefully explained. Other chapters outline privacy, security, and governance concerns and health policy issues. This unit provides the reader with directions for professional involvement in these activities.

The seventh unit, *Global and Future Perspectives in Health Informatics*, provides an overview of international approaches and effects of health informatics. It presents ideas on future directions and future research needed in the field of health informatics and postulates what is next. Health informatics is a growing field, and the future will be made by this book's readers.

TEACHING AND LEARNING PACKAGE

Health informatics is a fast-changing field. Educational needs, as noted in the Institute of Medicine reports, has been noted in college and university settings with an uptick in the initiation of informatics courses and programs. This book continues to be focused on encouraging learning related to informatics in general and specifically health informatics. Medical facilities and disciplines require informatics knowledge encouraging its use to provide better healthcare decision-making.

Each chapter includes discussion questions and a case study. These questions and case studies are carefully designed to represent the reality of health informatics, including the typical ill-defined problems common in informatics practice. Approaches are available to manage these challenges. The discussion questions and case studies can stimulate discussion, and faculty and students can explore how the material in the chapters can be applied for developing approaches for practice situations.

NEW TO THIS EDITION

The third edition updates the changing world of informatics adding new information, policies, and regulations in healthcare. Regulations, like the Cures Act, accentuate the need for informatics implementation from various fronts, e.g., practice and cost. The book accentuates new regulations allowing access to the most up-to-date information. It provides multilayered information for understanding informatics essentials, bringing current needs to the forefront.

It also elevates the learning experience by providing a novel approach to self-learning. First, content has been streamlined into shorter, "digestible" bits. This is in recognition of the demands on students' time and attention. We have revised the material to reduce students' cognitive load by minimizing distractions and extraneous material. This allows space for information to be absorbed into students' long-term memory and apply that knowledge. Second, the new edition is aligned to Bloom's Revised Taxonomy that enables objectives to be measurable and appropriate to the level of cognition required of students. Lastly, every objective has been revised to provide measurable goals for the reader, students, and instructors. Those reading this book will understand what they are being asked to do and what they will be asked to demonstrate, and instructors can clearly see what students can and cannot do after completing each lesson. The focused objectives can be used by the student/reader as self-learning modalities or can be used by faculty as question/answer discussions. The electronic (eBook) version of the text links these objectives to the corresponding content, making it easier for students to easily absorb information.

We continue to recommend that students be encouraged to consider how these materials apply to their own experiences and situations.

For the Instructor

- **TEACH Lesson Plans** contain measurable objectives and key terms from the text. Topics from the book are mapped to American Health Information Management Association (AHIMA) competencies, Quality and Safety Education for Nurses (QSEN) standards, and American Association of Colleges of Nursing (AACN) Essentials Series. Lesson plans connect chapter resources for effective material presentation and include highlights and learning activities tied to content within the chapters. Lessons and chapters use current professional organization and association guidance and policy to provide appropriate and accurate information. Materials are further supported by The American Association of Medical Colleges (AAMC), the American Association of Colleges of Nursing (AACN), the National Advisory Council on Nursing Education and Practice (NAC-NEP), and the Medical Library Association (MLA) Task Force for Knowledge and Skills and the International Medical Informatics Association (IMIA) Group on Health and Medical Informatics Education. Digital Activities for each chapter provide additional assignments to deepen students' understanding of the content of the text.
- **Microsoft PowerPoint® Presentations** are available to accompany the TEACH Lesson Plans. The PowerPoint® slides provide students with chapter highlights and provide instructors with additional relevant topics of conversation by extracting and imbedding content and figures from the text.
- A **Test Bank** containing more than 300 questions is compliant with the NCLEX® standards and provides text page references and cognitive levels. The ExamView software allows instructors to create new tests; edit, add, and delete text questions; sort questions; and administer and grade online tests.
- The **Image Collection** contains all the art from the text for use in lectures or to supplement the PowerPoint presentations.

For the Student

- **Student Review Questions** provide additional practice for students trying to master the content presented within the text.
- Chapters may include **Additional Readings** and **Digital Links (URLs)** to provide sources of additional research on the subject.

CONTENTS

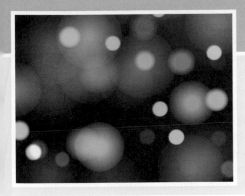

An Introduction to Health Informatics

Lynda R. Hardy

The goal of health informatics is to empower populations, communities, families, and individuals with the opportunity to improve the quality and increase the quantity of their days by maximizing the use of technology in healthcare.

OBJECTIVES

At the completion of this chapter, the reader will be prepared to:
1. Describe the sources of medical errors.
2. Summarize health informatics.
3. Summarize the seven major book units.

KEY TERMS

data, 1	health informaticians, 3	medical error, 2
data science, 8	health informatics, 3	usability, 8

ABSTRACT ❖

Health informatics is changing at warp speed. Managing this changing ecosystem requires keen attention and a large eraser! This chapter introduces updates and thoughtful consideration to the current state of health informatics as a discipline and a profession. It begins by addressing the nature, history, and definition of health informatics. Next, the chapter provides an overview of the topics inherent in the discipline and profession of health informatics. These topics are organized around the book's seven units.

INTRODUCTION

The Institute of Medicine (IOM), now the National Academies of Sciences, Engineering, and Medicine, supported the development of a book series surrounding the need to improve healthcare. Early books thoughtfully criticized healthcare, including patient safety and care quality. One early publication, *To Err is Human* (Institute of Medicine, 2000), provided an in-depth discussion of medical errors, rationale for error occurrence, and recommendations that included the need to use of technology to understand data that described why errors occurred and how they could be reduced. This book was followed by *Crossing the Quality Chasm,* (Institute of Medicine US, 2001) providing unmistakable evidence supporting the need for "information technology" to improve patient care and safety. Emphasis is placed on electronic health records (EHRs), clinical and decision support systems, use of computers and computer analytics, and automation. These publications and those that followed provided a path and set the standards for *health informatics*. Information and updates of these topics, and others, are discussed throughout this book.

Nearly 20 years after the IOM report *To Err Is Human* was released, John T. James published a seminal article on patient safety in *The Journal of Patient Safety*. Using a carefully designed methodology, he analyzed data published from 2008 to 2011 to estimate the number of preventable adverse events occurring in American hospitals. James found that each year, an estimated 440,000 hospitalized Americans experience a preventable adverse event that contributed to their death. In addition, serious harm is estimated to be 10- to 20-fold more common than lethal harm (James, 2013). These findings were reinforced in 2016 when Martin Makary and Michael Daniel published a study in *The BMJ* entitled "Medical Error—The Third Leading Cause of Death in the US." (Makary & Daniel, 2016) Dr. James continues his work in support of patient safety through his website.

The numbers of medical errors are astounding, but the personal consequences are even greater for the people and the families who suffer such "preventable events." Today, questions arise related to how preventable events are determined, measured, and analyzed, but they continue to exist with attributed rationale. The precision and power of health informatics contribute to an understanding of the magnitude of preventable events, predictive capabilities, and solutions and benefit our ability to reduce or control these events. Currently, health informatics have provided near real-time COVID-19 pandemic information reporting case reports, vaccination rates, length of stay, and contact tracing. Informatics plays a key role in managing and reporting on this pandemic, crucial to patients, populations, and providers (Dixon & Holmes, 2021 Aug).

The World Health Organization (WHO), the Centers for Medicare and Medicaid Services (CMS), and other national and international organizations are placing global efforts on the need for patient safety and quality of care. The WHO placed patient safety as a high priority for healthcare providers, noting that adverse events are among the top 10 causes of death (https://www.who.int/news-room/fact-sheets/detail/patient-safety). The CMS launched efforts to better understand and improve patient safety through improving hospital-acquired conditions and partnering with the Agency for Healthcare Research and Quality (AHRQ) in the use of a healthcare scorecard. CMS has also made data available for health informaticians and organizations to better understand causality and predictability.

CONSIDERING MEDICAL ERRORS

Defining Medical Error

Medical error, otherwise known as an *adverse event*, connotes a vulnerability in healthcare. It is well published that medical errors result in death, but the associated mortality rate is not firmly established. James Reason suggests that each complex organization has a system of *defenses* that protect persons from adverse outcomes or medical errors. Fig. 1.1 provides Reason's Swiss cheese model indicating holes within the organizational defenses that result in medical errors (Grober & Bohnen, 2005). However, quality assurance metrics with clearly define measurements can assist in determining what holes there are in the defenses and how to steer around them (Reason, 1997).

Reason defines medical error as "*the failure of a planned action to be completed as intended (an error of execution) or the use of a wrong plan to achieve an aim (an error of planning)*" (Reason, 1990), where he elaborates noting that medical error is a result of planning, mental/judgmental, and physical/technical failures but fails to include the error of omission. Reviewing Reason's determinants of error suggests that health informatics is a prime process to model the determinants for error reduction methods.

Common Sources of Medical Errors

Medical errors are preventable. A medical error, as described by Carver, Gupta and Hipskind, is a "preventable adverse effect of medical care, whether or not it is evident or harmful to the patient." (Carver et al., 2021) Initial medical error studies suggested that, in 1999, 98,000 deaths were caused by medical errors, making it the sixth leading cause of death (Institute of Medicine, 2000). Discussions about the validity of this number and the rising estimates suggest the medical error mortality is as high as 250,000 annually in one report to nearly 400,000 in another. The discrepancy in methodologies, variables, and analytics serves to muddy the water. However, the reason for medical errors is a valuable lesson. The most common reasons for medical errors are adverse drug events, catheter-associated urinary tract infections, central line infections, fall injuries, pressure ulcers (decubiti), ventilator-associated pneumonia, wrong site/wrong procedure, deep vein thrombosis, and misdiagnosis (Carver et al., 2021). Another important reason for medical errors was the intersection of health and medical

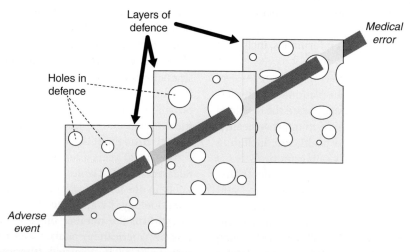

Fig. 1.1 James Reason's "Swiss cheese" model of error causation in complex organizations. (From: Reason, J. T. [2001]. Understanding adverse events: the human factor. In C. Vincent [Ed.], *Clinical risk management: Enhancing patient safety* [pp. 9–30]. London: BMJ Publishing Group.)

errors. A study by Melnyk and colleagues found that suboptimal physical and mental health resulted in higher likelihood of medical errors and a diminished patient care quality (Melnyk et al., 2018).

Patient Safety—An Example

Dr. James continues to investigate patient safety noting that, in 2016, 3 years after publication of his article, the same journal published another research study focusing on adoption rates and occurrence of adverse events with the use of health information technology (IIIT) (Furukawa et al., 2020). Key points from this research note that analysis of the Medicare Patient Safety Monitoring System (MPSMS) patient medical record data for 1351 hospitals from the years 2012 and 2013 found:

- 347,281 exposures to adverse events. Of these exposures, 7820 adverse events resulting in a 2.25% occurrence rate.
- Thirteen percent (5876) of these patients received care captured by an EHR.
- Cardiovascular, surgery, and pneumonia patients whose complete treatment was captured in an EHR were between 17% and 30% less likely to experience in-hospital adverse events.

The studies taken together suggest that if EHRs were in use in American hospitals, somewhere between 74,800 and 132,000 preventable fatal hospital-based events each year might never occur.

Best practices are taking an interprofessional approach to system design where health informaticians and other healthcare professionals are fully involved in the design, selection, and implementation of health information systems (HISs). Educators and practitioners realize the need for a common language used by all team members to provide a holistic view of patient needs to ensure the best outcomes. Patients are being introduced to the system as participants with the ability to aid in decision-making. There is an urgent need for healthcare systems to incorporate an interprofessional approach by including all disciplines in the discussion of how the EHR provides essential information to inform a learning health system aimed at patient safety, quality of care, healthcare cost reduction, and provider burden relief. These are reasons why the study of health informatics is imperative for all healthcare professionals. This book provides a real-world approach to health informatics, including all team members and supplies vital reasons why this approach is necessary. Competent, compassionate healthcare depends on healthcare providers who understand and can maximize their use of health IT and informatics knowledge in providing care to patients. This book provides the foundation required to develop that competence.

DEFINITION OF HEALTH INFORMATICS

Multiple Approaches to Defining Health Informatics

Currently, health informatics is a well-established field with an associated certification process. It is recognized as both a discipline and a profession. As a discipline, health informatics provides an overarching umbrella that houses subcategories such as nursing, clinical, public health, and pharmacy informatics. It focusses on it as a field of study like medicine, sociology, and pharmacy. Disciplines are mandating the inclusion of informatics that address specific learning outcomes associated with required competencies. Learning outcomes include the skills, knowledge, and professional aptitudes expected of all graduates within the profession. In 2003, the IOM identified five core competences that should be achieved by all healthcare professionals:

- Delivering patient-centered care
- Working as part of interdisciplinary teams
- Practicing evidence-based medicine
- Focusing on quality improvement
- Using informatics (Institute of Medicine US, Greiner, & Knebel, 2003)

Other professional groups and accrediting agencies are including an informatics-related requirement. For example, the American Association of Colleges of Nursing (AACN) developed a group of documents titled the Essentials Series (American Association of Colleges of Nursing [AACN], 2021). The Essentials outline the necessary curriculum content and expected competencies for all levels of nursing education (baccalaureate to doctoral). Early and advanced competency levels are identified, including Domain 8: Informatics and Healthcare Technologies that focus on the need to capture and analyze data for decision-making and efficient healthcare. The Healthcare Information and Management Systems Society (HIMMS) provides multidisciplinary health informatics core competencies in the areas of applied computer science, fiscal management, and medical technology based on the IOM's five core competency recommendation noted earlier (HIMMS—available at https://www.himss.org/resources/health-informatics).

Health information, as previously noted, continues to expand its knowledge base, incorporating a vast infrastructure that includes all healthcare disciplines. Health informatics is understood as both a discipline and as a profession, but it is noted that an accepted name or standard definition has yet to be agreed upon. Current titles for members of this profession include health informatics specialist, informaticist, or informatician (sometimes spelled *informaticien*). Table 1.1 lists accepted definitions and the source of those definitions. Fig. 1.2 is a word cloud incorporating all definitions in Table 1.1 to provide a visual depiction of *health informatics*.

Common Themes in Defining Health Informatics

Health informatics, in this book, is defined as an interdisciplinary professional specialty and scientific discipline that integrates the health sciences, computer science, and information science, as well as other analytic sciences, with the goal of managing and communicating data, information, knowledge, and wisdom in the provision of healthcare for individuals, families, groups, and communities. A review of this definition as well as the definitions in Table 1.1 demonstrates three common themes within these definitions, noting health informatics is:

- An interdisciplinary professional specialty:
- Tied to the use of IT in healthcare

- Focused on assisting healthcare providers with tasks related to collecting data, processing information, and applying that information to processes such as problem solving, knowledge development, and decision-making

Health IT affects every aspect of healthcare and has been shown to improve healthcare quality (Pinsonneault et al., 2017). Research done by Pinsonneault, and colleagues examined the interdisciplinary use of HIT's effect on the fragmentation of healthcare noting that patients treated by providers using a more digitally integrated system had better quality of care than those less HIT involvement. There was less fragmentation of care and greater integration of information

TABLE 1.1	**Common Definitions of Health Informatics**
Source	**Definition**
AHIMA	• A scientific discipline that is concerned with the cognitive, information-processing, and communication tasks of healthcare practice, education, and research, including the information science and technology to support these tasks (AHIMA, 2014) • A field of information science concerned with the management of all aspects of health data and information through the application of computers and computer technology (Fenton & Biedermann, 2014)
HIMSS	Health informatics is the interdisciplinary study of the design, development, adoption, and application of information technology (IT)-based innovations in healthcare services delivery, management, and planning (defined by the US National Library of Medicine [NLM]) (HIMSS TIGER Interprofessional Community).
AMIA	*Biomedical informatics* is the interdisciplinary field that studies and pursues the effective uses of biomedical data, information, and knowledge for scientific inquiry, problem solving and decision-making, motivated by efforts to improve human health (Kulikowski et al., 2012).
US NLM	*Health informatics* is "the interdisciplinary study of the design, development, adoption, and application of IT-based innovations in healthcare services delivery, management, and planning." (National Library of Medicine website, 2020)

that reduced medication issues and redundant procedures (Pinsonneault et al., 2017). A digital healthcare ecosystem is a patient-centric approach to increasing care quality and decreasing care costs. HIT affects all levels of patient care with novel approaches in imaging technology such as holographic camera's that provide a higher resolution that allows images with the ability to look around corners and x-ray imaging with capability of increased visual acuity. Technology has also increased research abilities such as the National Institutes of Health (NIH) Human Connectome Project, with the ability to visually navigate the brain's pathways. Modern technology related to telehealth has increased patient access to care, robotics increase surgical precision, and an emphasis is being placed on the use of healthcare data within a learning health system environment or to support new predictive and prescriptive algorithms.

TOPICS AND AREAS OF STUDY IN INFORMATICS

This book is divided into seven units outlining key topics and areas of study within health informatics. Each subsection presented here focuses on one of the seven units beginning with a thematic description of the unit. Consider the application of health informatics and how health informaticians, using health informatics, could improve healthcare quality and safety while decreasing costs.

Unit 1: Fundamental Knowledge in Health Informatics

The five chapters within Unit 1 of this book provide a foundation for health informatics that include theoretical frameworks, a conceptual discussion of data and information flow, standards, and programmatic evaluation. It provides a framework that introduces the reader to common threads found throughout the book, such as systems approaches and theories, the learning health system, background, and rationale related to interoperability, and the definitions of health informatics.

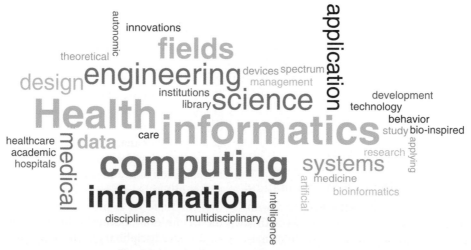

Fig. 1.2 Health informatics definition word cloud.

The Need for Health Informatics

Data, data everywhere—but who will make sense of it? The recognition of the importance of patient care data and information was clearly documented in *To Err is Human* and *Crossing the Quality Chasm* and the focus of the American Recovery and Reinvestment Act (ARRA) that provided the impetus and initial funding to stand up EHRs.

This unit reviews foundational issues in health informatics such as seminal IOM publications noting paucities in healthcare provision, theoretical approaches to support the use of informatics in improving healthcare, essential standardized nomenclature to facilitate data collection, and evaluation tools to determine if improvements have been made. These important foundational perspectives assist in determining how the quadruple healthcare aims (patient safety, quality of care, healthcare cost reduction, and provider burden) (Bodenheimer & Sinsky, 2014) are being met.

Data fragmentation impeded the ability to make appropriate healthcare decisions. Multiple disciplines provide essential healthcare documentation in patient care. The language each discipline uses is the basis for healthcare decisions. Imagine if each discipline used an alternate language, where one was French, another was German, and a third was Italian; how would a unified decision be made for patient care? Pieces of patient information are collected from diverse sources, such as admission and discharge summaries, laboratory and imagine sources, healthcare provider notes, and medical insurance information. Data fragmentation is a source of security, privacy, and ethical issues. Healthcare professions were charged with developing a standardize language that would assist instead of impede healthcare decision-making (Olaronke & Oluwaseun, 2016). Big data in healthcare are necessary but required standardization.

Standardization of the data within the EHR began to show pathways leading to knowledge about patient care within a system, paving the way for the learning health system. It was well known that medical errors were increasing, becoming one of the top 10 causes of death in the United States. Issues arose regarding how to collect, aggregate, and analyze for application to healthcare practice.

The weblog GeriPal, an online community of interdisciplinary providers interested in geriatrics or palliative care, published a 2013 research study, "Transfers from a hospital to nursing home: an F-grade for quality" (Covinsky, 2013) that assigned a failing grade to US healthcare, stating: a *Journal of the American Geriatrics Society* article (King et al., 2013) is "suggests the quality of communication between the hospital and the nursing home is horrendous" (Covinsky, 2013). A 2015 report by the Kaiser Family Foundation noted that nursing home star ratings (the method now used to evaluate nursing home care) found that more than one third of the 15,500 nursing homes received low star ratings (1 or 2 stars) and for-profit nursing homes had lower star ratings than nonprofits (Boccuti et al., 2015). More recently, Britton et al. noted that one in four or 23% of Medicare patients discharged from a skilled nursing facility were readmitted within 30 days, a metric followed by the CMS (Britton et al., 2017). Both instances noted missing or inaccurate information, poor communication, and overall disruptive transitions from skilled facilities. Access and analyses of data could identify key disruptive issues, provide key identifiers, and provide predictive algorithms to prevent future disruptions.

The analysis, a necessary component for a learning health system, can mitigate disruptive events. Enter the health informaticist. The time had come to harness *big data* and leverage it for interoperability allowing for data reusability and high-level analyses.

Unit 2: Health Information Systems and Applications

HISs are the work horses of health information storage and solutions. Unit 2 is a hierarchical approach to system types and their importance to health informatics. Fig. 1.3, Health System Hierarchy, provides a visualization of how HISs intersect. Every system requires administrative applications to support healthcare delivery. These applications are designed to facilitate healthcare delivery, such as financial, supplies, human

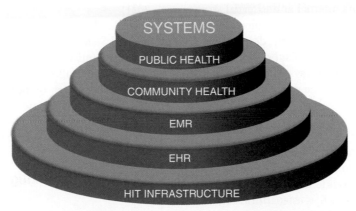

Fig. 1.3 Health system hierarchy. *EHR,* Electronic health record; *EMR,* electronic medical record. (Created by Lynda R. Hardy.)

and material resources, and business intelligence. They provide essential data and information to inform system leadership of the system's health.

System Types

The technical infrastructure or architecture supports a system's ability to capture, store, and retrieve institutional and patient related data. They are foundational to an institutions ability make decisions on how to manage institutional resources and the patient's ability to review their personal data for better decision-making. Health informaticists play a vital role in managing the infrastructure and assisting in data analyses. These analyses provide essential knowledge supporting a learning health system. The infrastructure supports clinical decision-making, research, and data access and allows for analyses for enhancing patient safety and improving care quality. A component of the HIS is the EHR or electronic medical record (EMR) for community use. The EHR is one of the most significant healthcare innovations in past decades, making it possible for patients and clinicians to monitor their data within a healthcare system. A primary goal of the EHR was the digitization of patient health records and the hope that these records would be allowed to be shared across systems. The health information exchange (HIE), the means of sharing patient data or interoperability, is the methods initiated to provide a mechanism to digitally share appropriate patient data to minimize redundancy and therefore patient care costs. It was a method of providing the right information to the right person and the right time, thereby minimizing error and maximizing efficiency. A key role of the EHR in precision medicine is to allow for translation of evidence into practice.

System Requirements

Each health information management system is composed of multiple internal systems that interface to provide patient-related data. The Health Information Management Systems Society (HIMSS) provides a searchable website for applications used in healthcare. Their focus is to provide information and insight into digital health transformations to inform and assist health systems to maximize performance. System selection and use require a response to three questions: (1) what is the purpose of the system or application (e.g., staffing, medication administration)? (2) What is the system or application's function (e.g., assigning schedules, identifying, and describing medication use and dosage)? And (3) what is the system's internal and external structure, where *internal structure* determines how efficiently and effectively the application functions (a poorly designed user interface can increase user errors) and *external structure* determines how it fits into the environment (system interoperability). Fig. 1.4 provides a visualization of the intersection between individual, community, and public health.

Health Informatics Improving Healthcare: An Exemplar

Health informatics delivers a multifaceted approach to bettering healthcare. Healthcare applications have increased patient-provider communication and provide a foundation for self-management of chronic conditions such as osteoarthritis, (Barber et al., 2019) whereas others have used informatics for predictive modeling. One study, published in 2021, "Predicting Vaccine

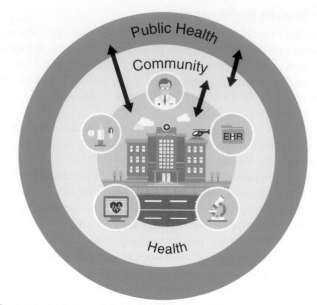

Fig. 1.4 Individual, community, and public health intersection. (Created by Lynda R. Hardy.)

Hesitancy From Area-level Indicators: A Machine Learning Approach," used analytical approach to better understand vaccine hesitancy (VH) in Italy during the COVID-19 pandemic (Carrieri et al., 2021). The authors suggest that VH is not unique to a single country and attempted to determine methods to mitigate VH. The COVID-19 pandemic has seen the emergence of multiple virus variants, thereby increasing its virulence. This novel study showed an effective method of using a machine learning approach to administrative data. Researchers identified "hot spots" for VH based on municipality-level data indicators and applied an machine learning (ML) approach to (1) minimize the use of incomplete data for immunization coverage and (2) predict areas of high VH from previous immunization data. They noted that an association could be made related to VH and fake (inaccurate) news on the internet and political endorsements or antivaccine campaign promises. This was borne out by data analyses on measle vaccination data. Study results, using ML, predicted that rural areas had a higher potential for VH due to waste recycling and employment rates. They suggest that ML use of administrative data can be a key predictor of VH areas, thus providing keys to encouraging vaccine use (Carrieri et al., 2021).

Consider this, how would a similar approach affect VH within the United States? Are there data sets that could be aggregated with administrative data and an element of clinical data for validity, which would allow us to determine how to address VH? Consider the impact of health informaticians coupled with bioinformaticists to review publicly available databases to help increase vaccine acceptance and potentially reduce illness that could be prevented by vaccine use.

Unit 3: Decision-Making and the Digitally Engaged Patient

Unit 3 continues with the exploration of changing relationships between decision-making, the digitally engaged patient, and health informatics. This unit focuses on the patient as an informed, participative member of the healthcare team. Technology has taken a front seat in healthcare. Advances have been made to advance clinical decision support, electronic records, telehealth, and wearable sensors. Patient registries combine geographically or nationwide patient data related to a specific disease or condition, allowing analyses by health and bioinformaticians to improve practice and disease management. Currently, healthcare is a patient-centric team approach often using real-time data.

Recognition of the increased use of data to support decision-making emphasizes that healthcare practice is evidence based, and the evidence is generated by system interoperability and health informatics. System interoperability led to the development of critical decision support systems (CDSSs) that inform best practices and incorporate knowledge management capabilities. The use of CDSSs provides actionable information essential to patient care but are not without challenges as we consider issues such as alarm fatigue and provider burden. Consideration should be given to determining if the alarms are accurate or due to missing data. The use of CDSSs continues to grow, but the efficiency is sometimes called in question. The Centers for Disease Control and Prevention (CDC) suggests that the impact of CDSS use has led to increased cardiovascular screening such as blood pressure and lipids but also finds that, conversely, the impact evidence is not as supportive as providers would like to see. Fig. 1.5 provides impact evidence being hampered in areas of health disparities and economics (CDC, https://www.cdc.gov/dhdsp/pubs/guides/best-practices/clinical-decision-support.htm [accessed December 1, 2021]).

The patient as a member of the healthcare team is growing as we see increased use of technology, such as electronic tablets, being used at the bedside, providing patient access to healthcare results often before their providers.

Patient and Patient Care Tools

Technology has spawned tools that assist in patient care. mHealth and the use of digital technologies have transformed how healthcare providers and patients interact and how care is provided. These advances have empowered to patients to participate in their care, to ask questions, and to provide their views. mHealth provides patient education and the potential to monitor patient activities. Apps (applications) have been developed for mobile phones to function as digital coaches for patients to self-manage

chronic conditions. A study conducted by Bruce and colleagues compared the effectiveness of mHealth intervention in 2059 orthopedic patients in the treatment arm and 2554 in the non-intervention mHealth group to determine patient satisfaction, length of stay, and readmission rates. Results provided evidence that, in the 2059 orthopedic patients, improvement was seen in patient length of stay, readmission rates, and overall patient satisfaction. Thirty-day readmission rates for the nonintervention group were 1.36% higher (p .001); 60-day readmission rates showed a 3.21% increase in readmissions in the nonintervention group (p .001). The patient length of stay was also higher in the nonintervention group (Bruce et al., 2020).

The advancement of personal health records and the use of social media for patient education and research are advancing our understanding and need for patient inclusion and the use of multimodal education and health-related devices.

Unit 4: Health Information System Lifecycle Management

Unit 4 focuses on the life cycle of an HIS. The basic concept of life cycle management (design, implementation, maintenance, planning, and analysis) is a cyclical process for continual improvement. It is a continual project management process of an organism from conception through its life allowing for growth/maturity, evaluation, and revisions. Fig. 18.2 provides a methodological approach to project management phases that can be applied to IT applications. The systems life cycle (SLC) model remains a widely used method for selecting/tailoring or building, implementing, and evaluating IT applications. Life cycle management continues to evolve, using innovative approaches providing integrative approaches to the rapid growth of IT needs. The system needs to be flexible and adaptable to maintain its integrity and ensure even the weakest link is protected. Current IT approaches use new software applications, including modeling approaches, to achieve solutions. Applied Lifecycle Management, a wider approach to SLC, defines the stages after development by harmonizing the constructs during the development phase. Newer and more adaptive types of life cycle management continue to grow (Kozma et al., 2021).

Healthcare providers and health informaticians play a significant role in the life cycle of healthcare information systems. Acquiring new systems is a complicated process affecting the entire healthcare system. Previously, selection of a healthcare system lacked input from providers. Currently, system selection is made through a systematic, multidisciplinary team approach with clear definition of the system's needs, and full cooperation from organizational leadership. Everyone is on the same page.

System Life Cycle Approaches

This unit approaches life cycle management by first looking at the project management principles. This acts as a preliminary or preplanning approach to the project. It continues describing the content of the strategic planning process and methods for system selection. This requires and understanding of the vendor and vendor systems. Contract negotiations, under the purview of experienced and knowledgeable individuals, constructs the legal requirements for the acquisition and software licensing.

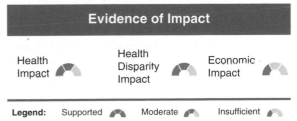

Fig. 1.5 Critical decision support system evidence of impact. (Centers for Disease Control and Prevention, https://www.cdc.gov/dhdsp/pubs/guides/best-practices/clinical-decision-support.htm)

This component is essential to ensure organizational protections. The unit culminates with descriptions of the implementation and evaluation processes and describes implications of what to do if the system is disrupted and disaster recovery is necessary.

Unit 5: Usability, Analytics, and Education

This unit is focused on discovering and using information and knowledge to improve healthcare delivery. The system will not survive unless it is usable, with the ability to analyze the data within it for application to a learning health system, and an understanding of the education of those tasked with using and managing it. This is a broad-brush approach to what the system needs and how to meet it.

Usability and Education

Usability. System usability is a requirement for the success of the system and patient satisfaction. There was a time when patient records were paper based and computers were not an everyday occurrence. Introduction of an HIS was a foreign concept that alarmed those charged with using it, primarily because of the lack of personnel input, education, and training. Healthcare professionals and those who use and maintain the system require system knowledge and skills. Healthcare providers are required to understand what the system provides (what organizational systems interact with the EHR and how are they accessed). Informaticians are required to know how to access the organizational components for data analysis and dissemination. Health IT, from the EHR to mobile devices, are a worldwide concern that require skills and understanding to manage the ever-changing data, algorithms, and uses of healthcare information.

Education. Managing the knowledge-base for HIT requires a multidisciplinary approach to education. Major developments accentuated by a pandemic have increased distance and more virtual forms of education. These methods may be confusing, but they provide a greater ability to reach more individuals and to integrate the type of individuals accessing the education. Providing an interdisciplinary approach to informatics education allows a more diverse conversation that discusses health informatics through multiple lenses. Developing a curriculum that provides essential information related to systems, data, theory, and analytics decreases the "alarmness" of users and increases a more facile system where positive patient outcomes are the result of data and information incorporation into a learning health system.

Using Data Analytics: A Real-Life Example for Human Immunodeficiency Virus Care

Human immunodeficiency virus (HIV) infection, another pandemic, has been collecting surveillance data since the 1980s. Data from health departments, public health systems, and other data types have been aggregated to determine if "Data to Care," a public health strategy, can improve continuity of care in person with HIV (PWH) individuals. This new strategy reported improved surveillance data and successfully linked or reengaged PWHs to care. The authors suggest that the strategy will help public health systems to move closer to a uniform national strategy for care for PWHs (Sweeney et al., 2019).

Unit 6: Data Governance, Legal and Regulatory Issues

Unit 6 provides an overview of federal regulations impacting health informatics, policy, and governance. The US government and related legal systems have established processes for achieving justice, defense, promotion of the general welfare of citizens, and security. Unit 6 is built around these concepts. The first chapter describes an overview of the US legal system's understanding of health informatics regulation, providing selected laws and regulations impacting health informatics. It further describes the organizational accreditation related to informatics, and the insight of technology within healthcare.

The unit continues with a review of privacy and security constructs and how they impact patient information. Major legislation is reviewed noting the Health Insurance Portability and Accountability Act (HIPAA), the Health Information Technology for Economic Clinical Health (HITECH) Act, and the Medicare and CHIP Reauthorization Act (MACRA). Healthcare leaders, informaticians, and health IT users play active roles in developing these and other policies and enforcing them within the healthcare ecosystem.

Health Policy in Operation: An Example

- The HITECH Act, providing financial incentives for the adoption of EHRs, was implemented in 2009 with the goal to modernize the IT infrastructure of the US healthcare system (DesRoches, 2015). As of 2015, 84% of hospitals have adopted a basic EHR system (Office of the National Coordinator for Health Information Technology, 2017).
- The HITECH Act created eligibility criteria related to the application for EHR funding, noting only short-term acute care hospitals were eligible for the incentive program; those eligible facilities increased EHR adoption rates from 3.2% to 14.2% (Adler-Milstein & Jha, 2017).
- Results of HITECH's incentive program suggested that use of EHRs reduced mortality rates over time (Lin et al., 2018).

This unit provides foundational policies and concepts that govern the use of patient related data, especially within the EHR. It reinforces the need for an interdisciplinary team approach to understand the issues of patient data, data governance, and data use to better inform decision-making and a learning health system.

Unit 7: Global and Future Perspectives in Health Informatics

We have seen significant advances in the advancement of data science in healthcare, noting proliferation of the EHR and informatics approaches to bettering patient care quality and safety. The continued progress of technology in healthcare provides clues to decision-making, advancing preventive and predictive approaches to illness, and algorithmic methods for providing healthcare that reduce patient and provider burden. The proliferation and application of health informatics is creating a pathway for patient care and learning health systems. There is no certainty to this pathway, but, based on current information, there is significant improvement.

As we consider the future of health informatics, consideration must be given to societal needs—if we have learned nothing from the COVID-19 pandemic, it is that informatics can provide real-time data to manage public health approaches to healthcare. The pandemic has also provided insight into the safety and security of health data and cybersecurity issues. Future needs suggest that novel approaches to technical needs and approaches such as analytics, data visualization, and user experiences are and will continue to be issues requiring continued evaluation and revision.

Lastly, the pandemic has also provided fodder for a deep dive into the societal and public health impact of health informatics on healthcare.

CONCLUSION AND FUTURE DIRECTIONS

Health informatics, although still a young discipline, is growing exponentially. It is the responsibility of all healthcare personnel to have a basic understanding of the power of data to benefit patient care. Our abilities to predict and prevent illness, thereby providing needed interventions to ensure wellness for everyone, will help drive a continued understanding of health informatics and data science. As a society, we also need to recognize human variation and strive for an interdisciplinary approach to understanding and using data to inform health decision.

Data assists in an increase in patient/provider discussion empowering the patient as a member of the healthcare team. Continuation of this dialogue is paramount in the need for education across the healthcare continuum. A solid foundation in the concepts, principles, methods, and science of health informatics will provide both future and current providers with the knowledge and skills needed to maximize the benefits of technology, while managing the challenges it presents. The goal of this book is to provide that foundation.

ACKNOWLEDGEMENT

The author acknowledges the contributions of Ramona Nelson and Nancy Staggers to the previous edition of this chapter.

■ DISCUSSION QUESTIONS

1. Health informatics is both a discipline and a profession. Describe how health informatics as a discipline influences health informatics as a profession, as well as how the profession influences the discipline.
2. Describe how health informatics content and related courses fit within the curriculum for your discipline. For example, if you are a nurse or student of nursing, explain how health informatics is integrated into the curriculum for your profession.
3. Develop a definition of *health informatics* that might be used to describe and explain it to a patient with limited literacy.
4. Select three units in the book. Read the abstract for each chapter in each of the three units. Now write a paragraph summarizing each unit. At the end of the three paragraphs, write a fourth paragraph describing the interrelationships you can identify among these units.

■ CASE STUDY

You are currently employed as a healthcare provider in a local community hospital. The science department of a regional high school is designing a learning unit for sophomores with an expressed an interest in technology, including computers and data analytics as a potential future career. The teacher overseeing this educational unit asked you to attend one of the classes as a guest speaker to discuss how data science and technology are used in healthcare. Design a 20- to 30-minute presentation that you might use in meeting the teacher's request.

■ DISCUSSION QUESTIONS

1. What questions might you ask the teacher to assess the literacy levels of the students?
2. The first 2 minutes of the presentation should be designed to grab the student's interest. What content would you include in these first 2 minutes?
3. What are the 3 to 5 key points you would want to include in this presentation?
4. What questions do you anticipate the students might ask, and how would you prepare to answer their questions?

REFERENCES

Adler-Milstein, J., & Jha, A. K. (2017 Aug 1). HITECH Act drove large gains in hospital electronic health record adoption. *Health Affairs (Millwood), 36*(8), 1416–1422. https://doi.org/10.1377/hlthaff.2016.1651. PMID: 28784734.

AHIMA, (2014). *Pocket glossary of health information management and technology* (4th ed.). Chicago, IL: AHIMA Press,.

American Association of Colleges of Nursing (AACN). The Essentials: Core Competencies for Professional Nursing Education; 2021.

Barber, T., Sharif, B., Teare, S., Miller, J., Shewchuk, B., Green, L. A., et al. (2019). Qualitative study to elicit patients' and primary care physicians' perspectives on the use of a self-management mobile health application for knee osteoarthritis. *BMJ Open*, 9(1). e024016–e024016. Web.

Boccuti, C., Casillas, G., Neuman, T. (2015). *Reading the stars: Nursing home quality star ratings, nationally and by state*. Kaiser Family Foundation issue brief.

Bodenheimer, T., & Sinsky, C. (2014). From triple to quadruple aim: care of the patient requires care of the provider. *Annals of Family Medicine*, 12(6), 573–576. https://doi.org/10.1370/afm.1713.

Britton, M. C., Ouellet, G. M., Minges, K. E., Gawel, M., Hodshon, B., & Chaudhry, S. I. (2017). Care transitions between hospitals and skilled nursing facilities: perspectives of sending and receiving providers. *Joint Commission Journal on Quality and Patient Safety*, 43(11), 565–572. https://doi.org/10.1016/j.jcjq.2017. 06.004.

Bruce, C. R., Harrison, P., Nisar, T., Giammattei, C., Tan, N. M., Bliven, C., et al. (2020). Assessing the impact of patient-facing mobile health technology on patient outcomes: retrospective observational cohort study. *JMIR Mhealth Uhealth*, 8(6), e19333. https://doi.org/10.2196/19333.

Carrieri, V., Lagravinese, R., & Resce, G. (2021). Predicting vaccine hesitancy from area-level indicators: a machine learning approach. *Health Economics*, 30(12), 3248–3256.

Carver N, Gupta V, Hipskind JE. Medical error. [Updated July 9, 2021]. In: StatPearls [Internet]. Treasure Island (FL): StatPearls Publishing; January 2021. Available from: https://www.ncbi.nlm. nih.gov/books/NBK430763/

Covinsky K. *Transfers from the hospital to nursing home: An F-grade for quality*; 2013. http://www.geripal.org/2013/08/transfers-from-hospital-to-nursing-home.html.

DesRoches, C. (2015). Progress and challenges in electronic health record adoption: findings from a national survey of physicians. *Annals of Internal Medicine*, 162(5), 396.

Dixon, B. E., & Holmes, J. H. (2021 Aug). Section editors for the IMIA Yearbook Section on managing pandemics with health informatics. *Yearbook of Medical Informatics*, 30(1), 69–74. https://doi.org/10.1055/s-0041-1726504.

Fenton, S., & Biedermann, S. (2014). *Introduction to healthcare informatics*. Chicago, IL: AHIMA Press.

Furukawa, M. F., Eldridge, N., Wang, Y., & Metersky, M. (2020 Jun). Electronic health record adoption and rates of in-hospital adverse events. *Journal of Patient Safety*, 16(2), 137–142. https://doi. org/10.1097/PTS.0000000000000257. PMID: 26854418.

Grober, E. D., & Bohnen, J. M. (2005). Defining medical error. *Canadian Journal of Surgery. Journal canadien de chirurgie*, 48(1), 39–44.

HIMSS TIGER Interprofessional Community—Global Informatics Definitions. https://www.himss.org/sites/hde/files/media/file/2021/10/18/tiger-definitions.pdf

Institute of Medicine (US), (2001). *Committee on Quality of Health Care in America. Crossing the quality chasm: A new health system for the 21st century*. Washington, DC: National Academies Press (US). PMID: 25057539.

Institute of Medicine (US), (2003). Committee on the Health Professions Education Summit. In A. C. Greiner & E. Knebel (Eds.), *Health professions education: A bridge to quality*. Washington, DC: National Academies Press (US). PMID: 25057657.

Institute of Medicine, (2000). *To err is human: building a safer health system*. Washington, DC: The National Academies Press. https://doi.org/10.17226/9728.

James, J. T. (2013). A new, evidence-based estimate of patient harms associated with hospital care. *Journal of Patient Safety*, 9(3), 122–128.

King, B. J., Gilmore-Bykovskyi, A. L., Roiland, R. A., Polnaszek, B. E., Bowers, B. J., & Kind, A. J. (2013). The consequences of poor communication during transitions from hospital to skilled nursing facility: A qualitative study. *Journal of the American Geriatrics Society*, 61(7), 1095–1102.

Kozma, D., Varga, P., & Larrinaga, F. (2021). System of systems lifecycle management—a new concept based on process engineering methodologies. *Applied Sciences*, 11, 3386. https://www.mdpi.com/2076-3417/11/8/3386.

Kulikowski, C. A., Shortliffe, E. H., Currie, L. M., Elkin, P. L., Hunter, L. E., Johnson, T. R., et al. (2012). AMIA board white paper: definition of biomedical informatics and specification of core competencies for graduate education in the discipline. *Journal of the American Medical Informatics Association*, 19(6), 931–938.

Lin, S. C., Jha, A. K., & Adler-Milstein, J. (2018 Jull). Electronic health records associated with lower hospital mortality after systems have time to mature. *Health Affairs (Millwood)*, 37(7), 1128–1135. https://doi.org/10.1377/hlthaff.2017.1658. PMID: 29985687.

Makary, M. A., & Daniel, M. (2016). Medical error—the third leading cause of death in the US. *BMJ.*, 353, i2139.

Melnyk, B. M., Orsolini, L., Tan, A., Arslanian-Engoren, C., Melkus, G. D., Dunbar-Jacob, J., et al. (2018). A national study links nurses' physical and mental health to medical errors and perceived worksite wellness. *Journal of Occupational and Environmental Medicine*, 60(2), 126–131. https://doi.org/10.1097/JOM.0000000000001198.

National Library of Medicine. 2020. Accessed May 20, 2020. https://hsric.nlm.nih.gov/hsric_public/topic/informatics.

Office of the National Coordinator for Health Information Technology. Non-federal acute care hospital electronic health record adoption, health it quick-stat #47. https://www.healthit.gov/data/quickstats/non-federal-acute-care-hospital-electronic-health-record-adoption. September 2017.

Olaronke, I., & Oluwaseun, O. (2016). Big data in healthcare: prospects, challenges and resolutions. *2016 Future Technologies Conference (FTC)*, 1152–1157. https://doi.org/10.1109/FTC.2016.7821747.

Pinsonneault, A., Addas, S., Qian, C., Dakshinamoorthy, V., & Tamblyn, R. (2017). Integrated health information technology and the quality of patient care: a natural experiment. *Journal of Management Information Systems*, 34(2), 457–486. https://doi.org/10.1080/07421222.2017.1334477.

Reason, J. (1990). *Human error*. Cambridge: Cambridge University Press.

Reason, J. (1997). *Managing the risks of organizational accidents*. Abingdon: Taylor & Francis Group. ProQuest Ebook Central. https://ebookcentral.proquest.com/lib/WFU/detail.action?docID=4387688.

Sweeney, P., DiNenno, E., Flores, S., Dooley, S., Shouse, R., Muckleroy, S., et al. (2019). HIV data to care-using public health data to improve HIV care and prevention. *JAIDS Journal of Acquired Immune Deficiency Syndromes*, 82, S1–S5. https://doi.org/10.1097/QAI.0000000000002059.

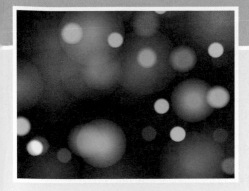

2

Theoretical Frameworks

Ramona Nelson

Whether designing effective and innovative technology-based solutions, implementing these approaches, or evaluating them, truly nothing is as useful as a good theory to guide the process.

Judith Effken

OBJECTIVES

At the completion of this chapter, the reader will be prepared to:

1. Explain the technology-related literacies and their relationship to health informatics.
2. Differentiate between the roles theories and models play in informatics.
3. Describe key components of systems theory.
4. Explain various forms of information theory.
5. Determine the role of planned change in health informatics.
6. Discuss the evolution of systems life-cycle models.

KEY TERMS

attributes, 19	entropy, 20	personal health literacy, 15
automated system, 26	equifinality, 20	phenomenon, 15
basic literacy, 12	FIT persons, 13	receiver, 24
boundary, 19	fractal-type patterns, 20	reiterative feedback loop, 20
change theory, 27	health literacy, 15	reverberation, 20
channel, 24	information, 25	sender, 23
chaos theory, 20	information literacy, 13	subsystem, 18
closed systems, 16	information theory, 23	supersystem, 18
Complex Adaptive System (CAS), 21	knowledge, 25	systems life cycle (SLC), 31
complexity theory, 20	lead part, 18	target system, 18
conceptual framework, 16	negentropy, 20	theoretical model, 16
data, 24	noise, 24	theory, 15
digital literacy, 13	open systems, 16	wisdom, 25
dynamic homeostasis, 20	organizational health literacy, 15	

ABSTRACT ❖

This chapter provides an overview of technology-related literacies, theories, and models useful for guiding practice in health informatics. For both providers and patients, developing knowledge and related skills in health informatics first requires a foundation in technology-related literacies. The chapter begins by exploring these literacies and their relationship to health informatics. Next, the chapter defines and explains components of grand, middle-range, and micro theories. Whether designing effective and innovative technology-based solutions, implementing these approaches, or evaluating them, truly nothing is as useful as a good theory to guide the process. Specific theories relevant to informatics are outlined. Systems and complexity adaptation theory provide the foundation for understanding each of the theories presented. Information models from Blum, Graves, and Nelson outline the data, information, knowledge, and wisdom continuum. The next section presents change theories, including the diffusion of innovation theory. In the chapter's final section, the Staggers and Nelson model of the systems life cycle is described and its application outlined.

INTRODUCTION

Health informatics is a profession. In turn, the individuals who practice this profession function as professionals. These statements may seem obvious, but there are important implications in these statements that can be easily overlooked. The professionals who practice a profession possess a body of knowledge, as well as values and skills unique to that profession. The body of knowledge, values, and skills guide the profession, as well as the individual professional, in decisions related directly or indirectly to the services provided to society by that profession. Professional practice is not solely based on a set of rules that can be carefully followed. Rather, the profession, through its professional organizations, and the professional, as an individual, make decisions by applying their knowledge, values, and skills to the specific situation. The profession and the professional within that profession have a high degree of autonomy and are therefore responsible for the practice and the decision made within that practice.

This chapter provides an overview of the primary technology-related literacies, theories, and models useful for guiding professional practices in health informatics. It focuses on basic literacy and technology-related literacies that relate directly to the work of patients and health care providers. Successful use of technology depends on basic, computer or technology, information, digital, and health literacies. These specific literacies both overlap and interrelate, as illustrated in Fig. 2.1.

FOUNDATIONAL LITERACIES FOR HEALTH INFORMATICS

Developing knowledge and related skills in health informatics requires a foundation in technology-related literacies for providers and patients.

Definition of Basic Literacy

As illustrated in Fig. 2.1, basic literacy is a foundational skill. Without a basic level of literacy, other types of literacy become impossible and irrelevant. The United Nations Educational, Scientific and Cultural Organization (UNESCO) offers one of the first definitions of *literacy*: "A literate person is one who can, with understanding, both read and write a short simple statement on his or her everyday life" (UNESCO, Education section, p.12). This definition is still used today. In 2003, UNESCO proposed an operational definition that attempted to encompass several

different dimensions of literacy: "Literacy is the ability to identify, understand, interpret, create, communicate, and compute, using printed and written materials associated with varying contexts. Literacy involves a continuum of learning in enabling individuals to achieve their goals, to develop their knowledge and potential, and to participate fully in their community and wider society" (UNESCO, Education section, p.13). The current definition is built on this definition.

Literacy is the ability to identify, understand, interpret, create, communicate, and compute, using printed and written materials associated with varying contexts.

Literacy involves a continuum of learning in enabling individuals to achieve their goals, develop their knowledge and potential, and participate fully in their community and wider society (UNESCO, 2018, p.1).

The U.S. Department of Education, Institute of Education Sciences, National Center for Education Statistics conducts the (National Assessment of Adult Literacy [NAAL], 2003) in the United States. The NAAL definition of *literacy* includes both knowledge and skills. NAAL assesses three types of literacy: prose, document, and quantitative.

Prose literacy: The knowledge and skills needed to search, comprehend, and use continuous texts such as editorials, news stories, brochures, and instructional materials.

Document literacy: The document-related knowledge and skills needed to perform a search, comprehend, and use noncontinuous texts in various formats such as job applications, payroll forms, transportation schedules, maps, tables, and drug or food labels.

Quantitative literacy: The quantitative knowledge and skills required for identifying and performing computations, either alone or sequentially, using numbers embedded in printed materials such as balancing a checkbook, figuring out a tip, completing an order form, or determining an amount (NAAL, 2003).

The focus of the national and international definitions is the ability to understand and use information in printed or written format. This includes the ability to understand both text and numeric information. Many people assume that if one can read and understand information in printed format, presumably that individual can also read and understand the same information on a computer screen. However, this assumption is frequently

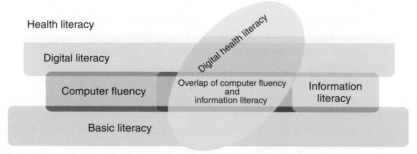

Fig. 2.1 Overlapping relationships of technology-related literacies and basic literacy. (Printed with Permission of Ramona Nelson. All rights reserved.)

incorrect because the presentation and flow of information on a website is often different from the same information in hard-copy form. Recognizing this, the concept of computer literacy begin to develop in the 1970s. However, computer literacy involves much more than the ability to read information on a computer screen. In fact, the term *computer literacy*, with its limited scope, is outdated.

Definition of Computer Literacy/Fluency

The term "computer literacy" was coined by Andrew R. Molnar in 1978. While the term experienced widespread uptake in the 1980s to early 2000s, its definition remained vague (Etherington, 2018). A consistent definition of the concept faces two major challenges. First, the functionality expands both in terms of what the technology can do and how this expanded technology is being used in society. Second, personal information technology (IT) is constantly evolving as demonstrated by the evolution from a basic PC or computer to include tablets, smartphone, and other devices.

However, over 15 years ago, the National Academy of Science coined the term FIT persons to describe people who are fluent in IT. By focusing on the types of knowledge needed for computer literacy and not on the specific technology or functionality, the concepts in this definition remain current today. FIT persons possess three types of knowledge:

Contemporary skills comprise the ability to use current computer applications, such as word processors, spreadsheets, or an internet search engine—in other words, the correct tool for the job (e.g., spreadsheets when manipulating numbers and word processors when manipulating text).

Foundational concepts entail understanding the how and why of IT. This knowledge provides insight into the opportunities and limitations of social media and other information technologies.

Intellectual capabilities refer to the ability to apply IT to the problems and challenges of everyday life—for example, the ability to think critically when evaluating health information on a social media site (Committee on Information Technology Literacy NRC 1999).

Definition of Information Literacy

The Association of College and Research Libraries (ACRL), a division of the American Library Association (ALA), initially defined information literacy and has led the development of information literacy standards since the 1980s. As part of this effort, the ACRL established standards of information literacy for higher education, high schools, and even elementary education. The ALA defines *information literacy* as a set of abilities requiring individuals to recognize when information is needed and locate, evaluate, and effectively use that information (American Library Association, 2000). This definition has gained wide acceptance. However, because of the extensive growth of new technologies, including different internet-based information sources, calls to revise the definition and the established standards developed several decades ago have increased. "Social media environments and online communities are innovative collaborative technologies that challenge the traditional definitions of information literacy … information is not a static object that is simply accessed and retrieved. It is a dynamic entity that is produced and shared collaboratively with such innovative Web 2.0 technologies as Facebook, Twitter, Delicious, Second Life, and YouTube" (Mackey & Jacobson, 2011, p. 62).

For example, different types of knowledge and skills are required to evaluate dissimilar sources of information, such as Facebook posts; Wikipedia articles; online peer-reviewed, pre-published articles; and peer-reviewed published articles. Professional students need different writing skills when participating in an online dialogue as opposed to preparing a term paper. There are standards that apply to text messaging, especially if the message is between healthcare colleagues or is being sent to a patient. Developing appropriate policies, procedures, and standards are the challenges facing healthcare leaders in the world of evidence-based practice, social media, and engaged patients. Recognizing the changing world of information creation, access, and use, the ACRL has expanded the definition of *information literacy*:

Information literacy is the set of integrated abilities encompassing the reflective discovery of information, the understanding of how information is produced and valued, and the use of information in creating new knowledge and participating ethically in communities of learning (Association of College and Research Libraries [ACRL], 2016).

The ACRL, in line with the expanded definition, developed a Framework for Information Literacy for Higher Education (Framework) (ACRL, 2016). The Framework grows out of their belief that information literacy as an educational reform movement will realize its potential only through a richer, more complex set of core ideas. While the Framework does not replace the standards previously developed, it does provide a less prescriptive approach for incorporating information literacy, knowledge, and skills into education, including the education of health professionals. Using this framework, one group of researchers completed a review of the literature related to information literacy and nursing education. Based on this review they concluded there is a need for librarians to liaise with faculty in nursing programs to facilitate the development of curriculum-related activities that support information literacy and, in turn, evidence-based practice (Cantwell, et al. 2021).

Table 2.1 lists and gives a brief description of the six frames in the Framework. As can be seen from the changing definition of *information literacy* the internet and related apps, as well as technologies, are changing the concept of information literacy. Arising from this change is the concept of digital literacy.

Definition of Digital Literacy

The term digital literacy first appears in the literature in the 1990s; however, to date, there is no generally accepted definition. Conceptual notions or definitions of digital literacy are slippery, as defining what is meant by digital literacy has become more complicated over time (Pangrazio & Sefton-Green, 2021). No generally accepted definition exists, but there are several activities demonstrating significant interest in this concept.

TABLE 2.1   Framework for Information Literacy for Higher Education

Frames	Description
Authority is constructed and contextual	Information resources reflect their creators' expertise and credibility and are evaluated based on the information need and the context in which the information will be used.
Information creation as a process	The iterative processes of researching, creating, revising, and disseminating information vary, and the resulting product reflects these differences.
Information has value	Information possesses several dimensions of value, including as a commodity, as a means of education, as a means to influence, and as a means of negotiating and understanding the world.
Research as inquiry	Research is iterative and depends on asking increasingly complex or new questions whose answers in turn produce additional questions or lines of inquiry in any field.
Scholarship as conversation	Communities of scholars, researchers, or professionals engage in sustained discourse with new insights and discoveries occurring over time as a result of varied perspectives and interpretations
Searching as strategic exploration	Searching for information is often nonlinear and iterative, requiring the evaluation of a range of information sources and the mental flexibility to pursue alternate avenues as new understanding develops.

Association of College and Research Libraries (ACRL). (2016). *Framework for Information Literacy for Higher Education.* http://www.ala.org/acrl/standards/ilframework.

For example, there are several national and international digital literacy centers supporting digital literacy development. Some examples include:

- Syracuse University's Center for Digital Literacy at http://digital-literacy.syr.edu/
- The University of British Columbia's Digital Literacy Centre at http://dlc.lled.educ.ubc.ca/
- Microsoft Digital Literacy Curriculum at www.microsoft.com/en-us/DigitalLiteracy
- University of South Florida Libraries at https://lib.usf.edu/dmc/

There are also several books published about digital literacy. A search done in October 2021 of books at Amazon using the term "digital literacy" returned over 10,000 results.

There are three recognized definitions are published even though there is no generally accepted definition. The earliest of these is provided in a 2010 white paper commissioned by the Aspen Institute Communications and Society Program and the John S. and James L. Knight Foundation: "Digital and media literacy are defined as life skills that are necessary for participation in our media-saturated, information-rich society." These skills include:

- Making responsible choices and accessing information by locating and sharing materials and comprehending information and ideas

- Analyzing messages in a variety of forms by identifying the author, purpose, and point of view, and evaluating the quality and credibility of the content
- Creating content in a variety of forms, making use of language, images, sound, and new digital tools and technologies
- Reflecting on one's own conduct and communication behavior by applying social responsibility and ethical principles
- Taking social action by working individually and collaboratively to share knowledge and solve problems in the family, workplace, and community, and by participating as a member of a community (Hobbs, 2010).

The second and most recognized definition, provided by the ALA's Digital Literacy Task Force, describes digital literacy as "the ability to use information and communication technologies to find, understand, evaluate, create, and communicate digital information, an ability that requires both cognitive and technical skills" (The American Library Association [ALA], 2013, p.2). A digitally literate person:

- Possesses a variety of skills—cognitive and technical—required to find, understand, evaluate, create, and communicate digital information in a wide variety of formats
- Uses diverse technologies appropriately and effectively to search for and retrieve information, interpret search results, and judge the quality of the information retrieved
- Understands the relationships among technology, lifelong learning, personal privacy, and appropriate stewardship of information
- Uses these skills and the appropriate technologies to communicate and collaborate with peers, colleagues, family, and, on occasion, the public
- Uses these skills to participate actively in society and contribute to a vibrant, informed, and engaged community.

The third definition, published by Springer in a book focused on social media for nurses, states that digital literacy includes:

- Competency with digital devices of all types, including cameras, e-readers, smartphones, computers, tablets, and video games boards. This does not mean that one can pick up a new device and use it without orientation. Rather, one can use trial and error, as well as a manufacturer's manual, to determine how to use a device effectively.
- The technical skills to operate these devices, as well as the conceptual knowledge to understand their functionality.
- The ability to use these devices creatively and critically to access, manipulate, evaluate, and apply data, information, knowledge, and wisdom in activities of daily living.
- The ability to apply basic emotional intelligence in collaborating and communicating with others.
- The ethical values and sense of community responsibility to use digital devices for the enjoyment and benefit of society (Nelson & Joos, 2013).

These three definitions have much in common, and together they demonstrate that digital literacy is a more comprehensive concept than computer or information literacy. The definition goes beyond the comfortable use of technology demonstrated by the digital native. Digital literacy is about understanding the implications of digital technology and the impact it has, and will continue to have, on every aspect of our lives. As the importance of understanding this impact has become more obvious in the last decade, the reality of the following quote made over a decade ago remains true today: "The truth is, though most people think kids these days *get* the digital world, we are actually breeding a generation of digital illiterates. How? We are not teaching them how to really understand and use the tools. *We are only teaching them how to click buttons.* We need to be teaching our students, at all levels, not just how to click and poke, but how to communicate, and interact, and build relationships in a connected world" (Murphy 2011).

Definition of Health Literacy

Although health literacy is concerned with the ability to access, evaluate, and apply information to health-related decisions, the definition of this term has been evolving. In 2011, a published systematic review of the literature in Medline, PubMed, and Web of Science identified 17 definitions of health literacy and 12 conceptual models. The most frequently cited definitions of health literacy were from the American Medical Association, the Institute of Medicine, and World Health Organization (WHO) (Sorensen, et al., 2012). These definitions from the Institute of Medicine and the WHO include: The Institution of Medicine uses the definition of health literacy developed by Ratzan and Parker and cited in Healthy *People 2010 and again in Healthy People 2020.* Health literacy is "the degree to which individuals have the capacity to obtain, process, and understand basic health information and services needed to make appropriate health decisions" (The IOM Committee on Health Literacy Medicine, 2004).

The focus in these definitions is on an individual's skill in obtaining and using the health information and services necessary to make appropriate health decisions. However, there are two limitations with these definitions.

First, they do not fully address the networked world of the internet. Recognizing this deficiency, Norman and Skinner introduced the concept of eHealth as "the ability to seek, find, understand, and appraise health information from electronic sources and apply the knowledge gained to addressing or solving a health problem", (Norma & Skinner, 2006). This definition acknowledges the need for computer fluency and the use of information skills to obtain an effective level of health literacy. However, this definition is not especially sensitive to the impact of social media. For example, it does not address the individual as a patient/consumer collaboratively creating health-related information that others could use in making health-related decisions. There is increasing evidence that patients bring to the dialog a unique knowledge base for addressing health-related problems (Hartzler & Pratt, 2011). Creating a comprehensive definition and model for assessing of health literacy levels that includes the social media literacy skills needed for today's communication processes remains a challenge for healthcare professionals.

Second, these definitions do not recognize the context or the role of the healthcare community. Recognizing this limitation,

Healthy People 2030 addresses both personal health literacy and organizational health literacy in its definition:

- Personal health literacy is the degree to which individuals can find, understand, and use information and services to inform health-related decisions and actions for themselves and others.
- Organizational health literacy is the degree to which organizations equitably enable individuals to find, understand, and use information and services to inform health-related decisions and actions for themselves and others (DHHS Office of Disease Prevention and Health Promotion, 2021).

A key resource in meeting health literacy needs in the clinical setting and the community can be found at https://www.cdc.gov/healthliteracy/learn/index.html

Overlapping Relationships of Technology-Related Literacies

While each of the technology-related communication literacies presented here focuses on a different aspect of literacy and has a different definition, they all overlap and are interrelated. Fig. 2.1 demonstrates those interrelationships. In this figure, basic literacy is depicted as foundational to all other literacies. Digital literacy includes computer and information literacy as well as other social media–related knowledge and skills that were not initially included in the definitions of computer and information literacy. For example, playing online games is not usually considered part of information or computer literacy, but it clearly requires digital literacy. Health literacy now requires both digital literacy and a basic knowledge of health unrelated to automation. The misinformation crisis related to Covid-19 has clearly demonstrated that all literacies require the ability to evaluate online information and especially to pay attention to information generated on social media sites. Understanding these technology-related communication literacies and integrating them into current policies and procedures is the challenge all healthcare providers and informaticians face.

ROLE OF THEORIES AND MODELS IN INFORMATICS

THEORIES AND MODELS

A theory explains the process by which certain phenomena occur (Hawking, 1988). Theories vary in scope depending on the extent and complexity of the phenomenon of interest. Grand theories are wide in scope and attempt to explain a complex phenomenon within the human experience. For example, a learning theory that attempted to explain all aspects of human learning would be considered a grand theory. Because of the complexity of the theory and the number of variables interacting in dependent, independent, and interdependent ways, these theories are difficult to test. However, grand theories can be foundational within a discipline or subdiscipline. For example, learning and teaching theories are foundational theories within the discipline of education.

Middle-range theories are used to explain specific defined phenomena. They begin with an observation of the specific phenomena. For example, one might note how people react to change and then ask why and how this phenomenon occurs. A theory focused on the phenomenon of change would explain the process that occurs when people experience change and predict when and how they will respond in adjusting to the change.

Micro theories are limited in scope and specific to a situation. For example, one might describe the introduction of a new electronic health record (EHR) in a large ambulatory practice and even measure the variables in that situation that could be influencing the acceptance and use of the new system. In the past, micro theories, with their limited scope, have rarely been used to test theory. However, this is changing with the development of Web 2.0 and the application of meta-analysis techniques to automatized natural language processing.

The development of a theory occurs in a recursive process, moving on a continuum from the initial observation of the phenomenon to developing a theory to explain that phenomenon. The process of moving on this continuum can be divided into several stages, including the following:

- A specific phenomenon is observed and noted.
- An idea is proposed to explain the phenomenon.
- Key concepts used to explain the phenomenon are identified, and the processes by which the concepts interact are described.
- A conceptual framework is developed to clarify the concepts and their relationships and interactions. Conceptual frameworks can be used to propose theories and generate research questions. The conceptual framework can also be used to develop a conceptual model. A conceptual model is a visual representation of the concepts and their relationships.
- A theory and related hypothesis are proposed and tested.
- Evidence accumulates, and the theory is modified, rejected, or replaced or gains general acceptance.

Many of the models used to guide the practice of health informatics discussed in this chapter can be considered theoretical models or frameworks. Because theoretical frameworks explain a combination of related theories and concepts, they can be used to guide practice and generate additional research questions. With this definition, one can argue that the concept of a theoretical framework can be conceived as a bridge between a middle-range theory and a grand theory. A theoretical model is a visual representation of a theoretical framework. Many of the models in healthcare and health informatics use a combination of theories to explain phenomena of interest within these disciplines and fit the definition of a theoretical framework.

Even though the terms *theory* and *concept* are consistently defined and used in the literature, the terms *conceptual* and *theoretical framework*, as well as the terms *conceptual* and *theoretical models*, are not. No set of consistent criteria can be applied to determine whether a model is conceptual or theoretical. As a result, researchers and informaticians will often publish models without clarifying that the proposed model is either conceptual or theoretical. In turn, it is possible for one reference to refer to a model as a conceptual framework whereas another uses the term *theory* when it refers to a model as a theoretical framework.

Theories and Models Underlying Health Informatics

Health informatics is an applied field of study incorporating theories from information science; computer science; the science for the specific discipline, such as medicine, nursing, or pharmacy; and the wide range of sciences used in healthcare delivery. Therefore, health professionals and health informatics specialists draw on a wide range of theories, models, and frameworks to guide their practice. In addition, there are several theories, models, and frameworks that focus on specific aspects of health informatics. For example, one research team conducting a systematic review of the literature identified 23 frameworks for evaluating health information technologies (Neame, et al., 2020). Table 2.2 provides some examples of theories, models, and frameworks that focus on specific aspects of health informatics. This book also incorporates several models, frameworks, and theories that are incorporated into various chapters as appropriate to that chapter.

This chapter focuses on selected theories that are of major importance across all fields or specialties in of health informatics. and those that are most directly applicable. These theories are vital to understanding and managing the challenges and decisions faced by healthcare professionals and informatics specialists. In analyzing the selected theories, the reader will discover that understanding these theories presents certain challenges. Some of the theories overlap, different theories are used to explain the same phenomena, and sometimes, different theories have the same name. The theories of information are an example of each of these challenges.

The one theory that underlies all theories used in health informatics is systems theory. Therefore, this is the first theory discussed in this chapter.

SYSTEMS THEORY

A **system** is a set of related interacting parts enclosed in a boundary (Von Bertalanffy, Ruben, & Kim, 1975). Examples of systems include computer systems, school systems, the healthcare system, and a person. Systems may be living or nonliving (Joos, Nelson, & Lyness, 1985). Systems may be either open or closed. **Closed systems** are enclosed within an impermeable boundary and do not interact with the environment. **Open systems** are enclosed within a semipermeable boundary and do interact with the environment. This chapter focuses on open systems, which can be used to understand technology and the people who interact with it. Fig. 2.2 demonstrates an open system interacting with the environment. Open systems take input (information, matter, and energy) from the environment, process the input, and then return output to the environment. The output then becomes feedback to the system. Concepts from systems theory can be applied in understanding the way people work with computers in a healthcare organization. These concepts can also be used to analyze individual elements such as software or the total picture of what happens when systems interact.

A common expression in computer science is "garbage in, garbage out," or GIGO. GIGO refers to the input-output process. The counter-concept implied by this expression is that quality

TABLE 2.2 Selected Examples of Health Informatics Theories

Name	Focus	Components/ concepts or dimensions	Comments
Socio-technical Model for Studying Health Information Technology in Complex Adaptive Healthcare Systems (Sittig & Singh, 2010)	The socio-technical challenges involved in design, development, implementation, use, and evaluation of health information systems within complex adaptive healthcare system.	• Hardware and software • Clinical content: text and/or numeric data • The human computer Interface • People: users as well as developers • Workflow and communication • Internal organizational features such as culture • External rules and regulations • Measurement and monitoring, both intended and unintended consequences.	The 8 dimensions are not independent, sequential, or hierarchical, but rather are interdependent and interrelated concepts. A diagram of this model can be seen at https://www.ncbi.nlm.nih.gov/pmc/articles/PMC3120130/figure/F1/?report=objectonly
Technology Acceptance Model: TEM (Holden & Karsh, 2010; Ammenwerth, 2019)	Why users accept or reject a given technology and how user acceptance can be improved through technology design.	• Perceived usefulness • Perceived ease of use • Attitude toward using the technology • Behavioral intention to use the technology • Actual use of the technology.	The model published by Fred D. Davis in 1989. It is based on principles from Fishbein and Ajzen's Theory of Reasoned Action. A diagram of this model can be seen at https://www.ncbi.nlm.nih.gov/pmc/articles/PMC2814963/figure/F1/
Unified Theory of Acceptance and Use of Technology (UTAUT) (Holden & Karsh, 2010; Ammenwerth, 2019)	Used to assess the likelihood of success for new technologies and to understand drivers of that acceptance.	• Performance expectancy or usefulness • Effort expectancy or ease of use • Social influence or "peer pressure" • Facilitating conditions such as technical and organizational support • Behavioral intention • Actual use.	UTAUT is based on an analysis of eight technology acceptance models, among them TAM, TAM2, the Theory of Reasoned Action and the Diffusion of Innovation Theory. The goal was to synthesize the 8 models on technology acceptance into one unified model. A diagram of this model can be seen at https://www.ncbi.nlm.nih.gov/pmc/articles/PMC2814963/figure/F1/
Distributed cognition (Hazlehurst, Gorman, & McMullen, 2008)	As opposed to the individual's cognitive process, the unit of analysis for understanding performance is the activity system that comprises a group of human actors, their tools and environment; it is organized by a particular history of goal-directed action and interaction." (Hazlehurst, et al., 2008), p. 226)	• Actors working together • Technologies and artifacts used to achieve a goal • Procedures, rules, and understandings for interactions among the actors that support task at hand.	
Technology, People, Organizations, and Macroenvironmental factors (TPOM) framework (Cresswell, Williams, & Sheikh, 2020)	Supports formative evaluation of HIT implementation and enabled transformation efforts during implementation.	• Technological factors • Social/human factors • Organizational factors • Macroenvironmental factors.	A diagram of this framework can be seen at https://pubmed-ncbi-nlm-nih-gov.pitt.idm.oclc.org/32519968/#&gid=article-figures&pid=figure-1-uid-0
Non-adaption, abandonment, scale-up, spread, and sustainability (NASSS) framework (Greenhalgh & Abimbola, 2019)	Is used to generate a rich narrative of the multiple influences on a complex project, identify parts of the project where complexity might be reduced, and consider how individuals and organizations might be supported to handle the remaining complexities better.	• Illness or condition • Technology • Value proposition, • Individuals intended to adopt the technology • Organization(s) and the wider system • How all these evolve over time.	A diagram is included in a chapter (Greenhalgh & Abimbola, 2019) that can be downloaded from https://ebooks.iospress.nl/volumearticle/51886

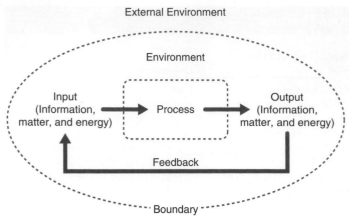

Fig. 2.2 An open system interacting with the environment. (Copyright Ramona Nelson. Reprinted with permission. All rights reserved.)

input is required to achieve quality output. Although GIGO is usually used to refer to computer systems, it can apply to any open system. An example of this concept can be seen when informed active participants provide input for the selection of a healthcare information system. In this example, garbage in can result in garbage out or quality input can support the potential for quality output. Not only is quality input required for quality output, but the system must also have effective procedures for processing those data. Systems theory provides a framework for looking at the inputs to a system, analyzing how the system processes those inputs, and measuring and evaluating the outputs from the system.

Characteristics of Systems

Open systems have three characteristics: purpose, structure, and functions. The purpose is the reason for the system's existence. The purpose of an institution or program is often outlined in its mission statement. Such statements can include more than one purpose. For example, many healthcare institutions have three purposes: (1) provide patient care, (2) provide educational programs for students in the health professions, and (3) conduct health-related research. Computer systems are often referred to or classified by their purpose(s). The purpose of a radiology system is to support the radiology department. A hospital information system can have several purposes, one of which is to maintain a census that can be used to bill for patient care. Another purpose may focus on interdepartmental communication.

One of the first steps in selecting a computer system for use in a healthcare organization is to identify the purposes of that system. Having a succinct purpose answers the question "Why select a system?" Many times, there is a tendency to minimize this step with the assumption that everyone already agrees on the purposes of the system. When a system has several different purposes, it is common for individuals to focus on the purposes most directly related to their area of responsibility. Taking the time to specify and prioritize the purposes helps ensure that representatives from clinical, administration, and technology understand the full scope of the project and agree on the reasons and, in turn, the criteria for selecting a system.

Functions, on the contrary, focus on the question "How will the system achieve its purpose?" Functions are sometimes mistaken for purpose. However, it is important to clarify why a system is needed, and then identify what functions the system will carry out to achieve that purpose. For example, a hospital may maintain patient census data including admissions, discharges, and transfers through a computerized registration system. Each time a department accesses the patient's online record, the name and other identifying information are transmitted from a master file, ensuring consistency throughout the institution. When selecting a computer system, the functions for that system are carefully identified and defined in writing. These are listed as functional specifications. Specifications identify each function and describe how that function will be performed.

Systems are structured to perform their functions. Two different structural models operating concurrently can be used to conceptualize healthcare technical infrastructures. These are hierarchical and web. The hierarchical model is an older architectural model, and the terms, such as *mainframe*, used to describe the model reflect that. Because this is an older architectural model, many people assume that mainframes are being phased out of healthcare. But as healthcare systems have become larger, this level of computer continues to play a key role in designing health information systems (Tozzi, 2021). The location and type of hardware used within a system often follow a hierarchical model; however, as computer systems are becoming more integrated, information flow increasingly follows a web model. The hierarchical model can be used to structure the distribution of computer processing loads at the same time as the web model is used to structure communication of health-related data throughout the institution. The hierarchical model is demonstrated in Fig. 2.3. Each individual computer is part of a local area network (LAN). The LANs combine to form a wide area network (WAN) that is connected to the mainframe computers. In Fig. 2.3, the mainframe is the lead computer or **lead part**. This structure demonstrates a centralized approach to managing the computer structure.

When analyzing the hierarchical model, the term *system* may refer to any level of the structure. In Fig. 2.3, an individual computer may be referred to as a system, or the whole diagram may be considered a system. Three terms are used to indicate the level of reference: **subsystem**, **target system**, and **supersystem**. A subsystem is any system within the target system. For example, if the target system is a LAN, each computer is a subsystem. The supersystem is the overall structure in which the target system exists. If the target system is a LAN, then Fig. 2.3 represents a supersystem.

The second model used to analyze the structure of a system is the web model. The interrelationships between the different LANs function like a web. Laboratory data may be shared with the pharmacy and the clinical units concurrently, just as the data collected by nurses, such as weight and height, may be shared with each department needing the data. The internet is an example of a complex system that demonstrates both hierarchical and web structures interacting as a cohesive unit. As these examples demonstrate, a system includes structural elements from both the web model and the hierarchical model. Complex

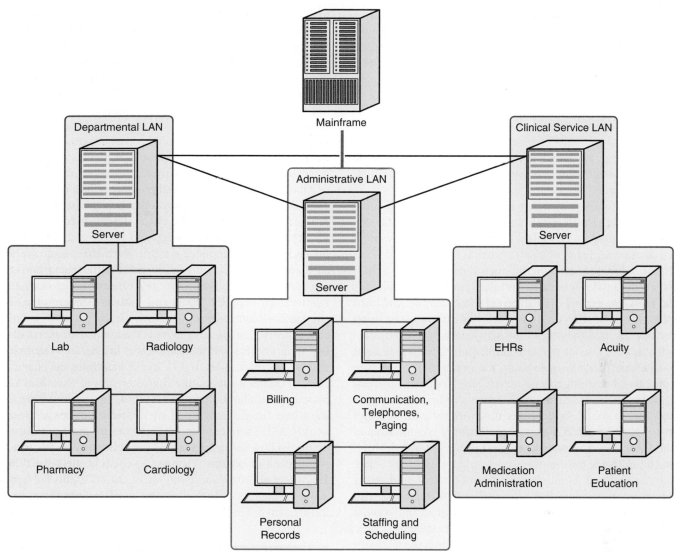

Fig. 2.3 Hierarchical information system model. Departmental information systems; *LAN*, Local area network. (Copyright Ramona Nelson. Reprinted with permission. All rights reserved.)

and complicated systems discussed later in this chapter can include several supersystems organized using both hierarchical and web structures.

Boundary, attributes, and environment are three concepts used to characterize structure. The **boundary** of a system forms the demarcation between the target system and the environment of the system. Input flows into the system by moving across the boundary and output flows into the environment across this boundary. For example, with a web model, information flows across the systems. Thinking in terms of boundaries can help distinguish information flowing into a system from information being processed within a system. Fig. 2.3 can be used to demonstrate how these concepts establish the boundaries of a project. Each computer in the diagram represents a target system for a specific project. For example, a healthcare institution could be planning for a new pharmacy information system. The new pharmacy system becomes the target system. However, as the model demonstrates, the pharmacy system interacts with other systems within the total system. The task group selecting

the new pharmacy system will need to identify the functional specifications needed to automate the pharmacy and the functional specifications needed for the pharmacy system to interact with the other systems in the environment. Clearly, specifying the target system and the other systems in the environment that must interact or interface with the target will assist in defining the scope of the project. Defining the scope of the project makes it possible to focus on the task while planning for the integration of the pharmacy system with other systems in the institution. A key example is planning for the impact of a new pharmacy system in terms of the activities of nurses who are administering medications.

In planning for healthcare information systems, attributes of the system are identified. Attributes are the properties of the parts or components of the system. When discussing computer hardware, these attributes are usually referred to as *specifications*. An example of a list of patient-related attributes can be seen on an intake or patient assessment form in a healthcare setting. Attributes and the expression of those attributes play a major role in the development of databases. Field names are a list of the attributes of interest for a specific system. The datum in each cell is the individual system's expression of that attribute. A record lists the attributes for each individual system. The record can also be seen as a subsystem of the total database system.

Systems and the Change Process

Both living and nonliving systems are constantly in a process of change. Six concepts help clarify the change process: dynamic homeostasis, equifinality, entropy, negentropy, specialization, and reverberation.

Dynamic homeostasis refers to the processes used by a system to maintain a steady state or balance. This same goal of maintaining a steady state can affect how clinical settings respond when changes are made or a new system is implemented.

Equifinality is the tendency of open systems to reach a characteristic final state from different initial conditions and in different ways. For example, two different clinics may be scheduled for the implementation of a new EHR. One unit may be using paper records, and the other unit may have an outdated computer system. A year or two later, both clinical units may be at the same point, comfortably using the new system. However, the process for reaching this point may have been very different.

Entropy is the tendency of all systems to break down into their simplest parts. As it breaks down, the system becomes increasingly disorganized or random. Entropy is demonstrated in the tendency of all systems to wear out. Even with maintenance, a healthcare information system will reach a point where it must be replaced. Healthcare information transferred across many different systems in many different formats can also demonstrate entropy, thereby causing confusion and conflict between different entities within the healthcare system.

Negentropy is the opposite of entropy. This is the tendency of living systems to grow and become more complex. This is demonstrated in the growth and development of an infant as well as in the increased size and complexity of today's healthcare system. With the increased growth and complexity of the healthcare system, there has been an increase in the size and complexity of healthcare information systems. As systems grow and become more complex, they divide into subsystems and then sub-subsystems. This is the process of differentiation and specialization. Note how the human body begins as a single cell and then differentiates into different body systems, each with specialized purposes, structures, and functions. This same process occurs with healthcare. If the mainframe in Fig. 2.3 were to stop functioning, the impact would be much more significant than if an individual computer in one of the LANs were to stop functioning.

Change within any part of the system will be reflected across the total system. This is referred to as reverberation. Reverberation is reflected in the intended and unintended consequences of system change. When planning for a new healthcare system, the team will attempt to identify the intended consequences or expected benefits to be achieved. Although it is often impossible to identify a comprehensive list of unintended consequences, it is important for the team to consider

their reality. The potential for unintended consequences should be discussed during the planning stage; however, these will be more evident during the testing stage that precedes the implementation or "go-live." Many times, unintended consequences are not considered until after go-live, when they become obvious. For example, e-mail may be successfully introduced to improve communication in an organization. However, an unintended consequence can be the increased workload from irrelevant e-mail messages. Unintended consequences are not always negative; they can be either positive or negative.

Unintended consequences are just one example of how difficult it is to describe, explain, and predict events and maybe even control outcomes in complex systems such as a healthcare institutions. Starting in the 1950s, chaos theory, followed by complexity theory, began to develop and was seen as an approach for understanding complex systems. Both chaos and complexity theory involve the study of dynamic nonlinear systems that change with time and demonstrate a variety of cause-and-effect relationships between inputs and outputs because of reiterative feedback loops. "The quantitative study of these systems is chaos theory. Complexity theory is the qualitative aspect drawing upon insights and metaphors that are derived from chaos theory" (Kernick, 2004, p. 14). Box 2.1 outlines the characteristics of chaotic systems. The characteristics of chaotic systems provide a foundation for understanding how complex systems adapt over time. Such systems are termed *complex adaptive systems* (CAS). There are now several examples in healthcare literature of how the concept of CAS is being used to understand phenomena of interest (Holden, 2005; McDaniel, et al., 2009; Holden, et al., 2021; Van Beurden, et al., 2013; Ellis & Herbert, 2011; Rouse, 2008; Chandler, et al., 2016; Sturmberg, et al., 2014; Essen & Lindblad, 2013).

BOX 2.1   Characteristics of Chaotic Systems

- *Chaos* is defined as a physical "mathematical dynamic system which is: (a) deterministic (b) is recurrent and (c) has sensitive dependence on the initial state" (Smith, 2007, p.164). In turn, *chaos theory* can be defined as "the qualitative study of unstable aperiodic behavior in deterministic, nonlinear dynamical systems" (Kellert, 1993, p.2). Chaotic systems demonstrate the following characteristics: They are dynamic systems in a constant state of nonlinear change. In a linear system, the output is consistently proportional to the input. Increase the input, and the output increases at the same rate. In a nonlinear system, the output of the system is not proportional to the input.
- The reiterative feedback loop that exists within these systems has a major effect on how inputs will affect outputs. A minor change in input can create a major change in output. On the contrary, a major change in input can result in minor changes in output.
- Their output is determined by the initial input, reiterative feedback loops, and the dynamic changes that occur over time. "Although it looks disorganized like random behavior, it is **deterministic**-like periodic behavior. However, the smallest difference in any system variable can make a very large difference to the future state of the system" (Kernick, 2004, p. 15).
- Fractal-type patterns begin to emerge from these outputs. Fractals are repeating nonregular geometric shapes such as snowflakes, trees, or seashells. Thus, out of chaos comes order (Walker, 2012).

THE SYSTEMS LIFE CYCLE MODEL

Definition of The Systems Life Cycle Model

The most common change for health professionals and informaticians is the introduction of or upgrade to a health information system. A commonly used model of the stages within this change is the systems life cycle (SLC) model. This model is used in project management to describe stages or phases of an informatics project, and it guides system implementation from initial feasibility through a more completed stage of maintenance and evaluation of the products. Most authors use the title "systems development life cycle" to describe the model. However, the term *development* is too limiting in health informatics because we often purchase systems or applications from vendors and customize them rather than developing them from scratch.

Various iterations of the systems life cycle have been published, and no agreement exists about the numbers and types of stages in the life cycle. The number of stages ranges from three (pre-implementation, implementation, and post-implementation) to at least seven. Project managers may even sort and combine phases to suit their needs according to the complexity and type of project being planned. Deficiencies in past models include:

- The depiction of the life cycle as a circular process, beginning with analysis, cycling through planning, develop/purchase/implement, maintain/evaluate, and returning to analysis. This would indicate a return to the original baseline, which is not the case after implementation. Instead, a new life cycle builds on previous installations and organizational learning.
- The development step does not indicate a choice to purchase a system, a common strategic choice today.
- Evaluation is listed only at the post-implementation phase. Instead, evaluation should be built into the process at the beginning of the cycle, and each phase should include evaluation (Rouse, n.d.)
- Testing is de-emphasized as one aspect of the implementation process. This step is critical in any upgrade or implementation, so it should be a separate step.

An entire life cycle can last many years. The average life cycle is about a decade, but some systems may be in place for longer periods; for example, the original inpatient system in the military is being replaced after two decades. Other systems may evolve continually for several decades with upgrades, module additions, and technology platform changes.

Staggers and Nelson Systems Life Cycle Model

The Staggers and Nelson systems life cycle model (SLCM) depicted in Fig. 2.8 incorporates the steps listed above; combines them with previous work from Thompson, Snyder-Halpern, and Staggers; and expands the steps to include a new, important consideration, the depiction of the cycle as a spiral (Thompson, Snyder-Halpern, & Staggers, 1999). Once an organization completes the SLCM, it does not return in circular fashion to the assessment stage. Instead, reassessment occurs based on the organization's development into a new operating

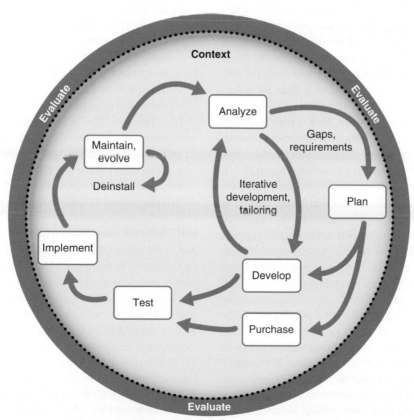

Fig. 2.8 The Staggers and Nelson systems life cycle model.

baseline (see Fig. 2.8). Two notions are used from work first published by Thompson and colleagues outlining an expanded SLC (Thompson, et al. 1999). The first is a step divided into purchase or development. The second is that evaluation occurs at every stage of the SLC versus relegating evaluation to the end of the cycle. The steps of the life cycle are outlined as follows:

1. *Analyze.* The existing environment and systems are evaluated. Major problems and deficiencies are identified using informal or formal methods. A readiness assessment may be done. The feasibility of the system is determined, and system requirements are defined. Analysts or informaticians may interview key system users or potential users and consult with IT personnel. A part of the initial analysis is to understand the organizational culture, learn how the organization handled change in the past, and determine the number of other changes the organization is encountering to understand how a technology change will fit (or not) into their priorities. Formal research projects (e.g., observing users interacting with applications, determining workflow in specialty areas such as the operating room) or formal surveys or focus groups may be conducted to determine needs. Workflow analyses, though time consuming, are important to perform. Deficiencies in the existing system are addressed with specific proposals for improvement. Benefits include engaging staff in the change process, and potential problems in processes can be identified. Gaps are noted, and current capabilities and limitations are outlined. Initial user and system requirements are formulated.

2. *Plan.* The proposed system is comprehensively planned. Planning includes strategic levels, such as whether the system will be developed internally, purchased, and tailored or designed and developed jointly with a vendor. The analysis and planning phases are the most time consuming of any project and are often estimated to require about 70% of a project's time and resources from start to initial implementation. Workflow analyses and process reengineering may be completed as a basis for determining the scope of system functions and the flow of information and activities within care processes. This is time intensive but worth the effort. In this process, the staff becomes involved, and everyone begins to see where the bottlenecks and other issues are. Potential problems can often be avoided through this analysis. Other topics to consider in this step include planning for project governance, key stakeholders, hardware, operating systems, databases, interface engines, programming (if needed), tailoring methods, marketing and communications, support for go-live, support for extensive testing, project maintenance, evaluation and success factors, security and privacy, and systems integration and IT support, such as integration into the call center, on-call support for clinicians, and physical construction.

3. *Develop or purchase.* At this stage, the system is purchased, or new system development begins. New components and programs are obtained and installed. For vendor-supported solutions, extensive tailoring occurs. This step may not be distinct from steps 1 and 2, depending on the type of development and tailoring the organization decides to employ. For instance, the organization may use user-centered techniques that include iterative design and evaluation with actual end users. Training is designed but may be carried out as part of the implementation stage.

4. *Test.* In this stage, extensive testing occurs just before implementation and go or no-go decisions are made about deadlines. The system should be tested intensively before implementation in as close to normal situations as possible. Simulated units are ideal. Ideally, adjustments are made at this stage to correct gaps in the scope of system functions or work processes (Kushniruk, Borycki, Kuwata, & Kannry, 2011). Toward the end of this step, marketing and communication efforts are accelerated to make users aware of the impending change.

5. *Implement or go-live.* The system is implemented using a selected method best suited to the organization and its tolerance for risk. Communication and training plans are executed. Mass user training is completed. The plan for conversion or go-live is implemented. For larger projects, the go-live can include a command center to coordinate activities for a few days or weeks. Users begin to use the system for their activities, such as patient care.

6. *Maintain and evolve.* Once the system has been formally acknowledged as passing user acceptance testing, typically at 90 or 120 days after going live, it enters a maintenance stage. Here, the project is considered routine and is integrated into normal operations in IT, clinical, and business areas. However, the system is not static: it evolves over time. For example, a project in the maintenance stage should have regular upgrades to maintain software currency and have system change requests completed.

7. *Evaluate.* Evaluation occurs at each step of the SLCM, as may be seen in Fig. 2.8. The evaluation stage begins in the planning stage of the project. The system should be tested intensively before implementation in as close to normal situations as possible. A simulated unit is ideal. Ideally, adjustments are made at this stage to correct gaps in the scope of system functions or work processes. Evaluation techniques are discussed in Chapter 5.

8. *Return to analyze.* Unlike the methods depicted in most systems, in life cycle models, the organizational baseline has matured and does not return to the pre-implementation baseline. Thus, the SLCM is typically a spiral of ongoing analysis, refinement with installation of upgrades and enhancements, and new projects building on the initial work. Atypically, a project may have a formal end through deinstallation or replacement with a new system. If that occurs, it would be at this step in the SLCM.

Informatics-Related Models

Although informatics is a new discipline, various models have proven useful to leaders within this field. There is no single comprehensive theoretical or conceptual model of health informatics. Some existing models and frameworks have been adopted and applied to health informatics while other distinct models have been developed and applied. Claude Shannon and Warren Weaver developed a communication model explaining the feedback loop of information from its genesis to reception including method of transmission and reception and effect of systematic noise (Shannon & Weaver, 1963). Graves and Corcoran, discussed earlier, defined an overall model for nursing informatics, whereas Garcia-Smith proposed an integrated model to predict a successful clinical information system (CIS) implementation (Garcia-Smith, n.d.). The

Unified Theory of Acceptance and Use of Technology, comprising eight individual models or theories (Technology Acceptance Model, Theory of Reasoned Action, Diffusion of Innovation) providing information on how age, gender, and experience influence performance and effort expectancy, social influence, facilitating conditions, price value, and habit to determine technology behavior intention and use (Venkatesh, Morris, Davis, & Davis, 2003). Distributed Cognition Theory, developed by Hutchins and Lintern, suggests that cognitive tasks combined with the environment extend the level of cognition. This theory extends the thought that an individual's cognitive processes are impacted by the environment, objects, and social interactions (Hutchins & Lintern, 1995). Additional models are included in Table 2.3.

CONCLUSION AND FUTURE DIRECTIONS

Healthcare is an information-intensive service. Computerization and the use of technology provide an effective and efficient means to manage large volumes of data and information with knowledge and wisdom. However, the move to an electronic healthcare system continues to change every aspect of healthcare. With this degree of change come excitement, anxiety, resistance, and conflict. Health professionals and health informatics specialists function at the very core of this change. They play a major role in implementing, managing, and leading healthcare organizations as they move forward with automation. To fulfil this role, they work directly with the clinical, administrative, and technical

TABLE 2.3 Selected Models of Nursing Informatics

Name	Author	Major Concepts	Reference
The NI Pyramid Model	Patricia M. Schwirian, PhD, RN Professor Emerita School of Nursing The Ohio State University	The four primary concepts are raw nursing information, the technology, the users, and the goal or objective arranged in a pyramid with a triangular base. Although the stated purpose was to describe concepts in NI, the model probably better describes human-computer interaction concepts.	Schwirian, P. M. (1986). The NI pyramid: a model for research in nursing informatics. *Nursing and Computers, 4*(3), 134–136.
Turley's Nursing Informatics Model	James Turley, PhD, RN Associate Professor School of Health Information Sciences University of Texas Health Science Center at Houston	The five primary concepts are cognitive science, information science, computer science, informatics, and nursing science. The concepts of cognitive science, information science, and computer science are depicted as three overlapping circles, with informatics at the junction of all three. Nursing science surrounds and provides a context for the overlapping circles.	Turley, J. (1996). Toward a model for nursing informatics. *IMAGE: The Journal of Nursing Scholarship, 28*(4), 309–313.
Goosen's Framework for Nursing Informatics Research	William T.F. Goosen, RN, PhD Director Results 4 Care Netherlands	Goosen's model builds on and extends the Graves model. The concepts of data, information, knowledge, decision, action, and evaluation are depicted as six boxes, with each of these concepts progressing to the next. Each of these six concepts interacts with the seventh concept in the model: Nursing Management and Processing to Patient Care.	Goosen, W. (2000). Nursing informatics research. *Nurse Researcher, 8*(2), 42–54. Goosen, W. (1996). Nursing information management and processing: a framework and definition for systems analysis, design and evaluation. *International Journal of Bio-medical Computing, 40*(3), 187–195.
IRO Model	Judith Effken, PhD, RN, FACMI, FAAN Associate Professor, Nursing College of Nursing The University of Arizona	This model includes two component models. First is a five-phase systems development life cycle depicted as a circle in the center of the IRO model. This is surrounded by the process of evaluation, which occurs throughout the life cycle. The outer ring includes four constructs that interact with each other and the inner circle. These are (1) the client, (2) NI interventions, (3) outcomes, and (4) the cultural, economic, social, and physical context.	Effken, J. (2003). An organizing framework for nursing informatics research. *CIN: Computers, Informatics, Nursing, 21*(6), 316–323.

IRO, The Informatics Research; *NI*, nursing informatics.

people in the organization. For health professionals and health informatics specialists to provide effective leadership, they must understand the institution's vision and values and the people and processes within these organizations. The theories presented in this chapter provide a foundation for supporting and managing the enormous degree of change experienced by the healthcare system and the people within any healthcare system.

Informatics incorporates several disciplines and, therefore, theories from those disciplines have been effectively used to guide research within the field of informatics. This chapter is an introduction to the use of theory in informatics and not a comprehensive analysis of theories that have or can be used to deal with questions of importance to informatics. Several theoretical and conceptual models used in health informatics are described elsewhere in this book and are not repeated in this section. In the future, one can expect to see additional models developed as the field of informatics continues to mature and as developments in healthcare and technology continue to evolve.

ACKNOWLEDGMENT

The author wishes to acknowledge the contribution of Nancy Staggers to the previous edition of this chapter.

DISCUSSION QUESTIONS

1. Describe the technology-related literacies and explain their relationship to health informatics.
2. Using Shannon and Weaver's model of information as a framework, describe several ways in which miscommunication can occur between healthcare providers working together in a clinical setting. Use this same framework to suggest how technology could be used to decrease this miscommunication.
3. Use Blum's model of information to explain the process used by healthcare providers for diagnosing and managing or treating healthcare problems. Identify the implication of this model for the development of decision support systems to support the patient care process.
4. Some have argued that the data-to-wisdom continuum cannot be used to define the scope of clinical practice because computers cannot process wisdom. Do you agree or disagree? Explain your thinking.
5. The responses of individuals to innovation have been classified into five groups. List and describe the five groups. Now describe how each group should be managed when planning for a major change within a healthcare institution.
6. List and explain the five internal organizational characteristics that can be used to predict how an organization will respond to a change in automation. Now use these same characteristics to predict how the U.S. healthcare system will respond to the automation of healthcare over the next 5 years.

CASE STUDY

A good friend of yours is director of patient services at a 220-bed community hospital. Last year, the hospital merged with a much larger medical center. One of the upsides, as well as one of the challenges, is the rapid introduction of new health information systems. The goal is to bring the hospital up to speed within 3 years. The implementation of the new system will start on the general medical-surgical units and move to the specialty units next.

Before the introduction of the new hospital information system, physicians could either enter their own orders or write the orders out and have the unit secretary enter the orders. The old system was designed to accommodate this option with physicians when it was first installed. The unit secretary would sign in, select the physician, and then select the patient. All other providers, such as NPs or PAs, entered their own orders. The new hospital information system is designed for all providers to enter their own orders. The policies implemented with the new system require that each healthcare provider enter his or her own orders.

Many of the physicians initially complained, but within a short time became more comfortable with the computers and began to integrate the CPOE process into their daily routines. Several physicians are now requesting the ability to enter orders from their offices or even from home. Other providers are also interested in these options.

However, three physicians who did not comment during the implementation of the new system are clearly resisting. For example, after performing rounds and returning to their offices, they called the unit with "emergency" verbal orders. After being counseled on this behavior, they began to write the orders on scraps of paper and put them on the unit secretary's desk or leave them at the nurses' station. When they were informed that these were not "legal orders," they began smuggling in order sheets from the nonactivated units. In addition, they have been coercing the staff nurses on the units to enter the orders for them. This has taken two forms. Sometimes they sign in and then ask the nurses to enter the orders. Other times they ask the nurses to put the orders in verbally, and then they confirm the orders. The nurses feel caught between the hospital's goals and the need to maintain a good working relationship with these physicians.

Open-Ended Discussion Questions

1. How would you use the theories presented in this chapter to diagnose the problems demonstrated in this case? List your diagnoses and explain your analysis.
2. What actions would you recommend to your friend and what reason (theories) would you use as a basis for your recommendations?

REFERENCES

American Library Association. Information Literacy Competency Standards for Higher Education (2000). http://www.ala.org/acrl/standards/informationliteracycompetency.

American Nurses Association, (2008). *Nursing informatics: Scope and standards of practice.* Silver Spring, MD: Nursesbooks.org.

Ammenwerth, E. (2019). Technology acceptance models in health informatics: TAM and UTAUT. In P. Scott & N. de Keizer (Eds.), *Applied interdisciplinary theory in health informatics.* Washington, D.C: A Georgiou. IOS Press. https://ebooks.iospress.nl/ISBN/978-1-61499-990-4.

Association of College and Research Libraries (ACRL). Framework for information literacy for higher education (2016). http://www.ala.org/acrl/standards/ilframework.

Blum, B. (1986). *Clinical information systems.* New York, NY: Springer-Verlag.

Burnes, B. (2018). Kurt Lewin (1890–1947): The practical theorist. In D. Szabla, W. Pasmore, M. Barnes, & A. Gipson (Eds.), *The Palgrave handbook of organizational change thinkers.* Cham: Palgrave Macmillan.

Cantwell, L. P., McGowan, B. S., Wolf, J. P., Slebodnik, M., Conklin, J. L., McCarthy, S., & Raszewski, R. (2021). Building a bridge: A review of information literacy in nursing education. *Journal of Nursing Education, 60*(8), 431–436. 2021.

Chan S. (2001). Complex adaptive systems. ESD.83 Research Seminar in Engineering Systems. <http://web.mit.edu/esd.83/www/notebook/Complex%20Adaptive%20Systems.pdf

Chandler, J., Rycroft-Malone, J., Hawkes, C., & Noyes, J. (2016). Application of simplified complexity theory concepts for healthcare social systems to explain the implementation of evidence into practice. *Journal of Advanced Nursing, 72*(2), 461–480.

Clarke, R. (1999). *Fundamentals of "information systems."* Xamax Consultancy Pty Ltd. http://www.rogerclarke.com/SOS/ISFundas.html.

Committee on Information Technology Literacy NRC, (1999). *Being fluent with information technology.* Washington, DC: National Academy Press.

Conner, D. (2006). *Managing at the speed of change.* New York, NY: Random House.

Cresswell, K., Williams, R., & Sheikh, A. (2020). Developing and applying a formative evaluation framework for health information technology implementations: qualitative investigation. *Journal of Medical Internet Research, 22*(6), e15068. https://doi.org/10.2196/15068. 10.2196/15068.

DHHS Office of Disease Prevention and Health Promotion (2021, August 24) Health literacy in healthy people 2030. https://health.gov/our-work/national-health-initiatives/healthy-people/healthy-people-2030/health-literacy-healthy-people-2030

Ellis, B., & Herbert, S. I. (2011). Complex adaptive systems (CAS): An overview of key elements, characteristics and application to management theory. *The Journal of Innovation in Health Informatics, 19*(1), 33–37.

Essen, A., & Lindblad, S. (2013). Innovation as emergence in healthcare: Unpacking change from within. *Social Science & Medicine, 93*, 203–211.

Etherington, C. (2018, March 12). Computer literacy: What it was and eventually became. eLearningInside.com: Engaging, transformative videos, podcasts, news stories for the e-Learning, https://news.elearninginside.com/computer-literacy-what-it-was-and-eventually-became/.

Garcia-Smith D. (n.d.). Testing a Model to Predict Successful Clinical Information Systems [doctoral dissertation]. The University of Arizona, College of Nursing. https://repository.arizona.edu/handle/10150/195846.

Graves, J., & Corcoran, S. (1989). The study of nursing informatics. *Image, 21*(4), 227–230.

Greenhalgh, T., & Abimbola, S. (2019). The NASSS framework—a synthesis of multiple theories of technology implementation. *Studies in Health Technology and Informatics, 263*, 193–204. https://doi.org/10.3233/SHTI190123. 10.3233/SHTI190123.

Hartzler, A., & Pratt, W. (2011). Managing the personal side of health: how patient expertise differs from the expertise of clinicians. *Journal of Medical Internet Research, 13*(3), e62.

Hasan, H., & Kazlauskas, A. (2014). The Cynefin framework: Putting complexity into perspective. In H. Hasan (Ed.), *Being practical with theory: A window into business research* (pp. 55–57). Wollongong, NSW: THEORI. http://eurekaconnection.files.wordpress.com/2014/02/p-55-57-cynefin-framework-theori-ebook_finaljan2014-v3.pdf. Accessed Oct. 14, 2021.

Hasan, H. M., & Kazlauskas, A. (2009). Making sense of IS the Cynefin framework: *Proceedings of the Pacific Asia conference on information systems (PACIS).* Hyderabad, India: Indian School of Business;. http://aisel.aisnet.org/pacis2009/47/.

Hawking, S. W. (1988). *A brief history of time.* New York, NY: Bantam Books.

Hazlehurst, B., Gorman, P. N., & McMullen, C. K. (2008). Distributed cognition: An alternative model of cognition for medical informatics. *International Journal of Medical Informatics, 77*(4), 226–234. https://doi.org/10.1016/j.ijmedinf.2007.04.008.

Hersh, W. (2009). *Information retrieval: A health care perspective* (3rd ed.). New York, NY: Springer Science.

Hobbs R. Digital and media literacy: A plan of action (2010). https://www.aspeninstitute.org/wp-content/uploads/2010/11/Digital_and_Media_Literacy.pdf

Holden, L. M. (2005). Complex adaptive systems: Concept analysis. *Journal of Advanced Nursing, 52*(6), 651–657.

Holden, R. J., Boustani, M. A., & Azar, J. (2021). Agile Innovation to transform healthcare: innovating in complex adaptive systems is an everyday process, not a light bulb event. *BMJ Innov, 7*, 499–505.

Holden, R., & Karsh, B. (2010). The technology acceptance model: Its past and its future in health care. *Journal of Biomedical Informatics, 43*(1), 159–172. https://www.ncbi.nlm.nih.gov/pmc/articles/PMC2814963/.

Hutchins, E., & Lintern, G. (1995). (Vol. 1). *Cognition in the wild.* Cambridge, MA: MIT Press.

Information. *(2012). Merriam Webster's collegiate dictionary.* http://www.merriam-webster.com/dictionary/information.

Jell-Mann M. (n.d.). Complex adaptive theory. Santa Fe Institute, and Los Alamos National Laboratory < http://authors.library.caltech.edu/60491/1/MGM%20113.pdf >. Accessed October 14, 2021.

Joos, I., Nelson, R., & Lyness, A. (1985). *Man, health and nursing.* Reston, VA: Reston Publishing Company.

Joos, I., Wolf, D., & Nelson, R. (2021). *Introduction to computers for healthcare professional* (7th ed.). Sudbury, Mass: Jones and Bartlett Publisher.

Kellert, S. (1993). *In the wake of chaos: Unpredictable order in dynamical systems.* Chicago, IL: University of Chicago Press.

Kernick, D. (2004). *Complexity and healthcare organizations: A view from the street.* Oxon, United Kingdom: Radcliffe-Medical Press Ltd;.

Kotter, J. P. (2012). *Leading change.* Boston, MA: Harvard Business School Press.

Kushniruk, A. W. 1, Borycki, E. M., Kuwata, S., & Kannry, J. (2011). Emerging approaches to usability evaluation of health information systems: towards in-situ analysis of complex healthcare systems and environments. *Studies in Health Technology and Informatics, 169,* 915–919.

LaMorte, W. (2019a) The transtheoretical model (stages of change). Boston University School of Public Health. https://sphweb. bumc.bu.edu/otlt/mph-modules/sb/behavioralchangetheories/ behavioralchangetheories6.html

LaMorte, W. (2019b) The theory of planned behavior. Boston University School of Public Health. Located at https://sphweb. bumc.bu.edu/otlt/mph-modules/sb/behavioralchangetheories/ BehavioralChangeTheories3.html

Lippitt, R., Watson, J., & Westley, B. (1958). In Willard B. Spalding (Ed.), *The dynamics of planned change.* New York: Harcourt, Brace & Company.

Mackey, T. P., & Jacobson, T. E. (2011). Reframing information literacy as a metaliteracy. *College & Research Libraries, 72*(1), 62–78.

Matney, S. A., Avant, K., Clark, L., & Staggers, N. (2020). Development of a theory of 2766 wisdom-in-action for clinical nursing. *Advances in Nursing Science, 43*(1), 28–41.

McDaniel, R. R., Lanham, H. J., & Anderson, R. A. (2009). Implications of complex adaptive systems theory for the design of research on health care organizations. *Health Care Management Review, 34*(2), 191–199. http://www.ncbi.nlm.nih.gov/pmc/ articles/PMC3667498/pdf/nihms107789.pdf.

Murphy S. (2011) Digital literacy is in crisis. *Social Media Today.* https://www.socialmediatoday.com/content/digital-literacy-crisis

National Assessment of Adult Literacy (NAAL). (2003). Three types of literacy. https://nces.ed.gov/NAAL/literacytypes.asp

Neame, M. T., Sefton, G., Roberts, M., Harkness, D., Sinha, I. P., & Hawcutt, D. B. (2020). Evaluating health information technologies: A systematic review of framework recommendations. *International Journal of Medical Informatics, 142,* 104247. https://doi.org/10.1016/j.ijmedinf.2020.104247. 10.1016/j. ijmedinf.2020.104247.

Nelson, R., & Joos, I. (2013). An introduction: social media and the transforming roles and relationships in health care. In R. Nelson, I. Joos, & D. M. Wolf (Eds.), *Social media for nurses: Educating practitioners and patients in a networked world.* New York, NY: Springer Publishing Company.

Nelson, R., & Joos, I. (1989). On language in nursing: from data to wisdom. *PLN Vis, 6*(Fall).

Nelson, R. (2002). Major theories supporting health care informatics. In S. Englebardt & R. Nelson (Eds.), *Health care informatics: An interdisciplinary approach* (pp. 3–27). St. Louis: Mosby.

Nelson, R. (2020, July 21). Informatics: evolution of the Nelson data, information, knowledge and wisdom model: Part 2. *OJIN: The Online Journal of Issues in Nursing, 25*(3).

Norman, C. D., & Skinner, H. A. (2006). eHealth literacy: essential skills for consumer health in a networked world. *Journal of Medical Internet Research, 8*(2), e9.

Pangrazio, L., & Sefton-Green, J. (2021). Digital rights, digital citizenship and digital literacy: What's the difference? *Journal of New Approaches in Educational Research, 10*(1), 15–27. e-ISSN: 2254-7339. https://files.eric.ed.gov/fulltext/EJ1282919.pdf.

Robertson J. (2004). The fundamentals of information science: An online overview. http://jamescrobertson.com/infosci/.

Rogers E.M., & Scott K.L. (1997). The Diffusion of Innovations Model and outreach from the National Network of Libraries of Medicine to Native American communities. *National Network of Libraries of Medicine.* http://www.au.af.mil/au/awc/awcgate/documents/ diffusion/rogers.htm.

Rogers, E. M. (1995). *Diffusion of innovation* (4th ed.). New York, NY: The Free Press.

Rogers, E. M. (2003). *Diffusion of innovation* (5th ed.). New York, NY: The Free Press.

Rouse M. (n.d.). Systems development life cycle (SDLC). http://www. pld.ttu.ee/IAF0320/14/lec4-1.pdf

Rouse, W. (2008). Health care as a complex adaptive system: Implication design and management. *Bridge, 38*(1), 7–25. https:// www.nae.edu/7704/HealthCareasaComplexAdaptiveSystemImplic ationsforDesignandManagement.

Sapp, S. (2012). Diffusion of innovation: Part 1 and part 2. Iowa State University, Department of Sociology. http://www.soc.iastate.edu/ sapp/soc415read.html.

Schein, E. (1995). *Kurt Lewin's change theory in the field and in the classroom.* Purdue University, College of Technology. http://dspace. mit.edu/bitstream/handle/1721.1/2576/SWP-3821-32871445.pdf.

Shannon, C., & Weaver, W. (1948). The mathematical theory of communication. *The Bell System Technical Journal, 27,* 379–423. https://people.math.harvard.edu/~ctm/home/text/others/ shannon/entropy/entropy.pdf Accessed October 15, 2021.

Sittig, D. F., & Singh, F. (2010). A new sociotechnical model for studying health information technology in complex adaptive healthcare systems. *Quality & Safety in Health Care, 19*(Suppl 3), i68–i74. https://www.ncbi.nlm.nih.gov/pmc/articles/ PMC3120130/pdf/nihms297306.pdf.

Smith, L. (2007). *Chaos: A very short introduction.* New York, NY: Oxford University Press.

Snowden, D. J., & Boone, M. E. (2007). A leader's framework for decision making. *Harvard Business Review, 85*(11), 68–76. 149.

Snowden, D. J. (2011). Good fences make good neighbors. *Information Knowledge Systems Management, 10,* 135–150.

Snowden, D.J. (2014). Managing under conditions of uncertainty state of the net 2014. YouTube. https://www.youtube.com/ watch?v=APB_mhpsQp8.

Snowden D.J. The Cynefin Framework YouTube (2010). https://www. youtube.com/watch?v=N7oz366X0-8.

Sorensen, K., Van den Broucke, S., Fullam, J., et al. (2012). Health literacy and public health: a systematic review and integration of definitions and models. *BMC Public Health, 12,* 80.

Sturmberg, J. P., Martin, C. M., & Katerndahl, D. C. (2014). Systems and complexity thinking in the general practice literature: An integrative, historical narrative. *Annals of Family Medicine, 12*(1), 66–74.

The American Library Association (ALA). Office for Information Technology Policy (OITP). (2013). Digital literacy, libraries and public policy. https://alair.ala.org/bitstream/ handle/11213/16261/2012_OITP_digilitreport_1_22_13_ Marijke%20Visser.pdf?sequence=1&isAllowed=y

The IOM Committee on Health Literacy Medicine. (2004). Health literacy: A prescription to end confusion. https://www.nap.edu/ catalog/10883/health-literacy-a-prescription-to-end-confusion

Thompson, C., Synder-Halpern, R., & Staggers, N. (1999). Analysis, processes, and techniques: case study. *CIN: Computers, Informatics, Nursing, 17*(5), 203–206.

Tozzi, C. (2021, Jan 29) 6 Industries where mainframes are still king. Precisely https://www.precisely.com/blog/mainframe/6-industries- mainframes-king

Trujillo, M.F. (2000). Diffusion of ICT Innovations for Sustainable Human Development: Problem Definition. Tulane University Law School, Payson Center for International Development. http://payson.tulane.edu/research/E-DiffInnova/ diff-prob.html.

4. Compare open and closed systems as they related to healthcare. Discuss how both system types benefit or detract from data communication and patient care benefits.

5. Interoperability is key to decision-making; informaticians are key to interoperability. Identify why interoperability is important and how informaticists can help to improve it.

CASE STUDY

You are an informaticist at a large metropolitan healthcare system. There has been an outbreak of the COVID-19 omicron variant in your city. Your healthcare system has collected data on patients with or exposed to COVID within the system's electronic health record.

DISCUSSION QUESTIONS

1. What are key steps that you should take to determine if the COVID data are standardized?
2. How can you determine the best method of storing these data for further evaluation?
3. What data synthesizing strategies could you employ to improve knowledge production and transfer to system leadership so that appropriate actions can be taken to prepare for an increase in hospitalizations?
4. How could these data, coupled with unstructured symptom data, be used to forecast health system resource needs in the next 30 days?

REFERENCES

American Medical Informatics Association (AMIA). (2021b). *What is informatics?* https://amia.org/about-amia/why-informatics/informatics-research-and-practice

Anderson, G. F., Frogner, B. K., Johns, R. A., & Reinhardt, U. E. (2006). Health care spending and use of information technology in OECD countries. *Health Affairs (Project Hope), 25*(3), 819–831.

Boulding, K. E. (1956). General systems theory-the skeleton of science. *Management Science, 2*(3), 197–208. http://www.jstor.org/stable/2627132.

Bourke, A., Bate, A., Sauer, B. C., Brown, J. S., & Hall, G. C. (2016). Evidence generation from healthcare databases: recommendations for managing change. *Pharmacoepidemiology and Drug Safety, 25*(7), 749–754.

Brigham, T. J. (2016). Feast for the eyes: an introduction to data visualization. *Medical Reference Services Quarterly, 35*(2), 215–223. https://doi.org/10.1080/02763869.2016.1152146.

Burningham, Z., Jackson, G. L., Kelleher, J., Stevens, M., Morris, I., Cohen, J., Maloney, G., & Vaughan, C. P. (2020). The enhancing quality of prescribing practices for older veterans discharged from the emergency department (EQUIPPED) potentially inappropriate medication dashboard: A suitable alternative to the in-person academic detailing and standardized feedback reports of traditional EQUIPPED. *Clinical Therapeutics, 42*(4), 573–582. https://doi.org/10.1016/j.clinthera.2020.02.013.

Chassin, M. (2019, November 18). *To err is human: The next 20 years.* https://www.jointcommission.org/resources/news-and-multimedia/blogs/high-reliability-healthcare/2019/11/to-err-is-human-the-next-20-years/

Danese, M. D., Halperin, M., Duryea, J., & Duryea, R. (2019). The generalized data model for clinical research. *BMC Medical Informatics and Decision Making, 19*(1), 117.

Federer, L. M., Lu, Y. L., & Joubert, D. J. (2016). Data literacy training needs of biomedical researchers. *Journal of the Medical Library Association: JMLA, 104*(1), 52–57. https://doi.org/10.3163/1536-5050.104.1.008.

Gamal, A., Barakat, S., & Rezk, A. (2021). Standardized electronic health record data modeling and persistence: A comparative review. *Journal of Biomedical Informatics, 114*, 103670. https://doi.org/10.1016/j.jbi.2020.103670.

Genes, N., Violante, S., Cetrangol, C., Rogers, L., Schadt, E. E., & Chan, Y. Y. (2018). From smartphone to EHR: A case report on integrating patient-generated health data. *NPJ Digital Medicine, 1*, 23. https://doi.org/10.1038/s41746-018-0030-8.

Institute of Medicine. (2000). *To err is human: Building a safer health system.* Washington, DC: The National Academies Press. https://doi.org/10.17226/9728.

Institute of Medicine. (2001). *Crossing the quality chasm: A new health system for the 21st century.* Washington, DC: The National Academies Press. https://doi.org/10.17226/10027.

Ivers, N., Jamtvedt, G., Flottorp, S., Young, J. M., Odgaard-Jensen, J., French, S. D., O'Brien, M. A., Johansen, M., Grimshaw, J., & Oxman, A. D. (2012). Audit and feedback: Effects on professional practice and healthcare outcomes. *The Cochrane Database of Systematic Reviews*(6), CD000259. https://doi.org/10.1002/14651858.CD000259.pub3.

Johnson, O. (2019). General system theory and the use of process mining to improve care pathways. *Studies in Health Technology And Informatics, 263*, 11–22.

Khairat, S. S., Dukkipati, A., Lauria, H. A., Bice, T., Travers, D., & Carson, S. S. (2018). The impact of visualization dashboards on quality of care and clinician satisfaction: Integrative literature review. *JMIR Human Factors, 5*(2), e22. https://doi.org/10.2196/humanfactors.9328.

Kimia, A. A., Savova, G., Landschaft, A., & Harper, M. B. (2015). An introduction to natural language processing: How you can get more from those electronic notes you are generating. *Pediatric Emergency Care, 31*(7), 536–541. https://doi.org/10.1097/PEC.0000000000000484.

Klann, J. G., Joss, M. A. H., Embree, K., & Murphy, S. N. (2019). Data model harmonization for the All Of Us Research Program: Transforming i2b2 data into the OMOP common data model. *PloS One, 14*(2), e0212463.

Koleck, T. A., Dreisbach, C., Bourne, P. E., & Bakken, S. (2019). Natural language processing of symptoms documented in free-text narratives of electronic health records: A systematic review. *Journal of the American Medical Informatics Association, 26*(4), 364–379.

Martin, K., Bégaud, B., Latry, P., Miremont-Salamé, G., Fourrier, A., & Moore, N. (2004). Differences between clinical trials and postmarketing use. *British Journal of Clinical Pharmacology, 57*(1), 86–92. https://doi.org/10.1046/j.1365-2125.2003.01953.x.

Moore, G.E. (2021). Moore's law or how overall processing power for computers will double every two years. http://moreslaw.org

Naughton, J. (2021). *2017: What scientific term or concept ought to be more widely known?*. Edge. https://www.edge.org/response-detail/27150

Parmanto, B., Scotch, M., & Ahmad, S. (2005). A framework for designing a healthcare outcome data warehouse. *Perspectives in Health Information Management, 2*, 3.

Pathak, J., Kho, A. N., & Denny, J. C. (2013). Electronic health records-driven phenotyping: challenges, recent advances, and perspectives. *J Am Med Inform Assoc, 20*(e2), e206–e211. 2013.

Reinsel, D., Gantz, J., & Rydning, J. (2018, November). *The digitization of the world from edge to core.* IDC White Pate #US44413318

Senge, Peter, M. (1990). *The fifth discipline: The art and practice of the learning organization.* New York: Doubleday/Currency.

Shannon, C. E. (1948). *Bell System Technical Journal, 27*, 379–423.

Smith, M., Saunders, R., Stuckhardt, L., & McGinnis, J. M. (Eds.). (2012). *Committee on the Learning Health Care System in America, Institute of Medicine.* Washington, DC: National Academies Press. ISBN: 9780309260732.

Techopedia. (2017). *Access control: What does access control mean?* https://www.techopedia.com/definition/5831/access-control Retrieved December 12, 2021.

Thorell, L., Molin, J. D., Fyfe, J., Hone, S., & Lwin, S. M. (2019). Working towards a master patient index and unique identifiers to improve health systems: the example of Myanmar. *WHO South-East Asia Journal of Public Health, 8*(2), 83–86. https://doi.org/10.4103/2224-3151.264851.

Thye, J. Understanding Health Informatics Core Competencies. Health Informatics, HIMSS. https://www.himss.org/resources/health-informatics#:~:text=Core%20competencies%20can%20be%20understood%20as%20a%20broadly,knowledge%2C%20but%20also%20about%20abilities%2C%20skills%20and%20behaviour.

Von Bertalanffy, L. (1972). The history and status of general systems theory. *Academy of Management Journal, 15*(4), 407–426. Web.

Watson, R. T. (2020). *Data management: Databases and organizations* (6th ed.). Project Press.

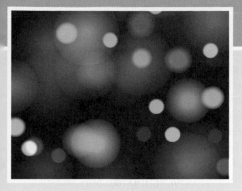

4

Informatics-Related Standards and Standard Setting

Juliana J. Brixey and Zach Burningham

The use of standardized clinical terminology can allow patient data to be available across the full spectrum of healthcare settings.

OBJECTIVES

At the completion of this chapter, the reader will be prepared to:

1. Examine key concepts surrounding how standardization of data and terminology in health information exchanges improves interoperability.
2. Discuss key multidisciplinary standardizations.
3. Discuss key nursing terminologies that assist in managing patient care.
4. Outline how harmonization of key system-related standards benefits healthcare.
5. Summarize the role of standardized terminologies in the development process of data exchange.

KEY TERMS

classification, 50
data exchange, 59
data standards, 60
interface terminology, 50
interoperability, 60

ontology, 50
reference terminology, 50
standardized terminology, 50
standards development organizations
  (SDO), 48

standards-setting organizations
  (SSO), 48
terminology cross-mapping, 60
terminology harmonization, 60

ABSTRACT ❖

Shaping a cost-effective, quality healthcare system based on best practices is only possible if interoperability within and between all aspects of the healthcare delivery system has been achieved. Achieving interoperability requires a system-wide consensus concerning the standards for the operating of that system.

This chapter begins with an explanation of standards and the standard development process in health informatics, including the relationship between standards and interoperability as these concepts relate to health informatics. The chapter then focuses on standardized terminologies, one of the fundamental components of standards and interoperability. These terminologies facilitate coherent communication as well as the collection and aggregation of healthcare data across settings. The advantages of adopting standard terminologies in practice include (1) an enhanced user interface in electronic health records (EHRs), (2) effective data retrieval and exchange, (3) improved monitoring of the quality of care, and (4) discovered knowledge through clinical research. The role of standardized terminologies in the process of exchanging healthcare data across systems is discussed. The chapter concludes with a discussion of topics for future research and development, including data summarization and mining, knowledge management and decision support, linkage of professional vocabulary and consumer vocabulary, and clinical translational and comparative effectiveness research.

INTRODUCTION

The Institute of Medicine (IOM), now the National Academies of Sciences, Engineering, and Medicine, identified Health Information Technology (HIT) as critical to closing the quality chasm, and shaping a better healthcare delivery system in the 21st century (Institute of Medicine, 2001). Achieving this goal is only possible if interoperability within and between all aspects of the healthcare delivery system has been achieved. Interoperability, defined as the extent that healthcare systems and devices can exchange data, can interpret shared data (Healthcare Information and Management Systems Society

[HIMSS], n.d.). Thus, interoperability is essential to developing a nationwide Learning Health System (LHS) that utilizes electronic health record (EHR) data generated from routine clinical care to serve as a source of clinical intelligence with the goal of improving the delivery of healthcare at a reduced cost (Friedman et al., 2010). Unfortunately, poor interoperability remains a significant barrier to implementing a nationwide LHS model. The near universal adoption of EHRs has provided large volumes of data available for advancing the LHS model, but much of these data remain in siloed environments, unable to leverage today's data analytics. Poor interoperability results in reduced generalizability of the knowledge byproduct the LHS model is attempting to achieve, and impedes sharing of such knowledge across health systems (Morain et al., 2016). Standards are imperative for the achievement of interoperability. A standard is defined as an established specification, guideline, or characteristic that describes the measurement, material, product, processes, and/or services required for a specific purpose (International Organization for Standardization [ISO], n.d.). Standards can be as straightforward as the distance between the prongs on a plug for a household appliance or as complex as the standards of practice for the treatment of a disease or medical condition.

The household plug provides an example of the relationship between standards and interoperability. There are very few rooms within any home in North America that do not have a wall outlet. Plugged into those outlets are a variety of electrical devices produced by companies across the world. All devices have the same size plug, thereby meeting the specific standards required to connect to the electrical grid for all of North America.

Achieving this level of standardization involves both a process for establishing and maintaining the standards and an organizational infrastructure for implementing that process. For example, in the case of the electrical grid for North America, the North American Electric Reliability Corporation (NERC) develops and enforces reliability standards (North American Electric Reliability Corporation [NERC], n.d.).

In health informatics, similar organizations exist, referred to as either **standards development organizations (SDO)** or **standards-setting organizations (SSO)**.[1a] There are several standards developed by these organizations. The SSOs and the standards evolve from three primary sources: (1) standards related to the technology used in health informatics, (2) standards related to healthcare, and (3) standards specific to health informatics. In most cases, these standards have evolved when the need for a specific standard has been identified and refined. For example, the Digital Imaging and Communications in Medicine (DICOM) standard was developed in 1985 when the National Electrical Manufacturers Association identified the need for a nonproprietary data interchange protocol, digital image format, and file structure for biomedical images and image-related information. This example demonstrates that groups identifying the need for standards are usually focused on

a specific need. This results in diverse needs and fragmentation of the standard development process. SDOs have focused on consensus building and coordination in healthcare standards. For example, the American National Standards Institute (ANSI) has emerged as "the accreditor and coordinator of the US private sector voluntary standardization system, ensuring that its guiding principles—consensus, due process, and openness—are followed by the entities accredited by this organization." (HIMSS, n.d.) Not all standards are established by an accredited SSO. Standards are established primarily through one of two different processes:

Dominant vendors. With this process, the standard becomes the de facto established standard due to market dominance of the vendor. Examples of this process for establishing standards are demonstrated by both the Microsoft and Apple operating systems. Several companies unrelated to either Microsoft or Apple have designed their applications to run on top of one or both operating systems. While there are other computer operating systems, most applications for personal computing use one or both of these operating systems.

Official SSO. These organizations are founded with the mission of developing or coordinating specific standards. Official SSOs use a formal process that stresses the building of consensus through open communication. Standards established by an official SSO are referred to as *de jure* standards. Table 4.1 includes several examples of SSOs of importance in health informatics.

There are many existing standards to choose from in healthcare. Given this reality, learning about and understanding standards related to health informatics cannot be done by studying lists of standards. Such an approach would be the equivalent of reading a textbook on diagnostic tests, such as a laboratory manual, with no background or understanding of the disorders being diagnosed. Likewise, developing an understanding of standards in health informatics is best done by learning individual standards in the context of their specific purpose. The remainder of the chapter will focus on standard languages and their purpose in communicating health-related data, especially across EHRs.

HEALTHCARE DATA STANDARDIZATION

Standardized Use of Electronic Health Record Systems

The use of health IT, including EHRs, has become a component of a funded national agenda in the United States and is considered a core requirement needed to support the LHS model and patient-centered care. It has been shown to improve the quality and safety of treatments during the last decade (Colicchio et al., 2019). EHRs are lauded for collecting longitudinal data, providing the best evidence for practice, supporting efficient care delivery, and promoting electronic access by authorized users for quality care, research, and policy development (Institute of Medicine, 2012). Data standardization and data exchange are needed as fundamental components to make EHRs optimally beneficial. EHRs facilitate clear, concise communication,

---

[1a] The terms *standards development organizations (SDO)* or *standards-setting organizations (SSO)* are used interchangeably in the literature and this chapter.

TABLE 4.1   Select Standards-Setting Organizations Impacting Health Information Technology

Name	Description	Health IT Standards	Website
Accredited Standards Committee (ASC) X12N Insurance subcommittee	Develops electronic data interchange (EDI) standards that facilitate electronic interchange relating to business transactions.	X12N Insurance Subcommittee: Develops components of the ASC X12 Standards related to the insurance industry's business activities, including those related to healthcare insurance.	http://www.x12.org/x12org/subcommittees/sc_home.cfm?strSC=N
American National Standards Institute (ANSI) NOTE: ANSI is the US representative to International Organisation for Standardization (ISO).	Promotes the use of US standards internationally; advocates for US policy and technical positions in international and regional standards organizations; encourages the adoption of international standards as national standards where these meet the needs of the user community, and provides a process for the accreditation of standards development organizations.	Primarily focused on health IT for establishing communications among standards development organizations concerned with health IT.	https://www.ansi.org/
American Society for Testing and Materials (ASTM) International	Provides a forum for the development of international standards for materials, products, systems, and services.	E31 Healthcare Informatics develops standards related to the architecture, content, storage, security, confidentiality, functionality, and communication of information used within healthcare.	http://www.astm.org/COMMIT/SCOPES/E31.htm
Clinical Data Interchange Standards Consortium (CDISC)	Establishes standards to support the acquisition, exchange, submission, and archiving of clinical research data and metadata.	—	http://www.cdisc.org
Digital Imaging and Communications in Medicine (DICOM)	Provides the international standard for the electronic exchange of medical images and related information.	—	http://dicom.nema.org
Health Level Seven (HL7) International	Provides a framework and related standards for the exchange, integration, sharing, and retrieval of electronic health information that supports clinical practice, and management, delivery, and evaluation of health services.	Clinical Document Architecture Release 2 (CDA) Fast Health Interoperability Resources (FHIR)	http://www.hl7.org/index.cfm
Institute of Electrical and Electronics Engineers (IEEE) Standards Association	Develops industry standards in a broad range of technologies.	IEEE Engineering in Medicine and Biology Society Technical Committee on Biomedical and Health Informatics focuses on standards for medical devices (http://tc-bhi.embs.org).	http://standards.ieee.org
Integrating the Healthcare Enterprise (IHE) International	Promotes the coordinated use of established standards in health IT.	—	http://www.ihe.net
International Organization for Standardization (ISO)	Develops international standards by working with their 162 national standards bodies.	ISO Technical Committee (TC) 215 on Health Informatics has published over 154 standards (http://www.iso.org/iso/iso_technical_committee?commid=54960)	http://www.iso.org/iso/home.htm
MedBiquitous Consortium	Develops information technology standards for healthcare education and quality improvement.	—	http://www.medbiq.org
National Council for Prescription Drug Programs (NCPDP)	Develops standards supporting the information exchange of prescribing, dispensing, monitoring, managing, and paying for medications and pharmacy services.	—	https://www.ncpdp.org
Working Group for Electronic Data Interchange (WEDI)	Supports the development of transaction standards with the goal of enhancing the quality of care, improving efficiency, and reducing costs of the American healthcare system.	—	http://www.wedi.org/home

including the collection and aggregation of healthcare data across settings.

The Centers for Medicare and Medicaid Services (CMS) established an incentive program for the use of a certified EHR system to meet the standards and criteria of Meaningful Use (currently termed promoting interoperability) (Blumenthal & Tavenner, 2010; The Office of the National Coordinator for Health Information Technology [ONC], 2019). Basic functions of EHRs should, for example, support e-prescribing, maintain patient problems and medication lists and care management, and demonstrate interoperability according to the Health Information Technology for Economic and Clinical Health (HITECH) Act (ONC, 2019). HITECH also defines a "comprehensive" EHR which contains the aforementioned functionality but also includes the addition of clinical decision support (CDS) through dynamic visualizations with some data interpretation capabilities. Standards that facilitate data capture and data sharing play a key role in achieving Meaningful Use of healthcare data. This chapter first examines current healthcare data standardization and exchange efforts. Applications of standardized health terminologies are further discussed, along with future directions. Additional information concerning interoperability and HITECH Act regulations is available in Chapter 29.

Standardized Reference Terminology Versus Interface Terminology

Patient records contain words, terms, and concepts that are used in a variety of ways. A *word* is a unit of language while a *term* is a linguistic label used to represent a particular concept (de Keizer et al., 2000). A *concept* is defined as a construct representing the unique meaning for one or multiple terms. For example, *sudden pain in lower back* is composed of five words, and the term *sudden pain* is identical to the term *acute onset pain*, consisting of three words. In this case, both terms can be denoted with the concept *acute pain*. Also, the concept *pressure ulcer* can be represented with diverse terms such as *bedsore*, *decubitus*, *pressure sore*, *decubitus ulcer*, pressure injury, and *pressure ulcer*. These examples indicate that various expressions (including abbreviations) used with identical meanings can be characterized using a representative concept in patient records.

When a list of words or phrases is organized alphabetically, such a collection is called a *vocabulary*. In contrast, a collection of representative concepts in a specified domain of interest is defined as a *terminology*, which is often organized in a hierarchical or tree structure according to semantic relationships among concepts. Continuing with the example, the concept *acute pain* is a type of *pain* and presents a narrower meaning than the parent concept *pain* in a terminology.

Identifying a representative concept for terms with the same meaning is particularly important when communicating healthcare data. With its diverse expressions of terms with equivalent meanings, natural language cannot be used to share information within or across systems in a consistent way. Incongruent descriptions of patient care contribute to poor quality care and hinder the Meaningful Use of EHRs. Accordingly, several healthcare terminologies have been developed by different disciplines and specialties.

When a terminology meets specific requirements established by an SDO, it is referred to as a **standardized terminology**. A **reference terminology** serves as a resource to represent domain knowledge of interest and thus facilitate data collection, processing, and aggregation. However, such a terminology may not be sufficient to design and structure documentation forms used by healthcare providers in daily practice (Rosenbloom

et al., 2006). Task-oriented terms with abundant synonyms can assist documentation by enhancing expressivity and usability of standard concepts. An **interface terminology** is a collection of task-oriented terms considered to support data entry and display in EHRs (Rosenbloom et al., 2006).

A terminology is often called a **classification** when concepts or expressions are organized according to their conceptual similarities rather than semantic (meaning) resemblances. For example, a set of concepts related to the human body could be arranged by physiologic function or body structure. For instance, *chest pain* and *growing pain* are semantically close in that both are considered a type of *pain*. Therefore, both terms can be categorized as a finding of the sensory nervous system. However, they could also be classified by the location of pain (i.e., body structure); *chest pain* can be categorized as a finding of trunk structure, and *growing pain* can be categorized as a finding of limb structure.

Ontology Versus Terminology

A concept refers to a class in an **ontology**, where the meaning of a concept is formally specified using properties and its relationships with other concepts through inheritance (Gruber, 1995). While a terminology often presents only a broad-narrow relationship between two adjacent concepts, an ontology contains multiple subsumptions or subclass relationships of a concept based on its formal definition. A reasoner or classification software can assist in this process by automatically determining logical placements of asserted concepts and creating an inferred hierarchy (Tsarkov & Horrocks, 2006). An example of how an ontology is structured is demonstrated by the BioPortal sponsored by the National Center for Biomedical Ontology, including more than 500 terminologies, classifications, and ontologies maintained by various organizations and individuals (The National Center for Biomedical Ontology, 2021). Fig. 4.1 presents a hierarchical organization of sample concepts (or classes) related to human organ systems and a graphic view of the hierarchy in BioPortal (The National Center for Biomedical Ontology, 2021).

Evaluation of the Quality of Terminology

Healthcare terminologies have a long history of research and development. Currently, the Unified Medical Language System (UMLS) Metathesaurus contains more than 190 source terminologies, classifications, and ontologies used in the healthcare domain (Rewolinski & Wilder, 2021). Regardless of the structure of a source terminology, the UMLS consolidates all source concepts in a unified framework so that it is possible to examine lexical and semantic relations within and across source terminologies (McCray & Nelson, 1995). The UMLS Metathesaurus is distributed by the National Library of Medicine (NLM) every six months and includes more than 4.4 million concepts and 16.1 million unique concept names, available for browsing through UMLS Terminology Services (Rewolinski & Wilder, 2021). Any source concepts with semantically equivalent meanings are assigned to the same concept unique identifier in the UMLS Metathesaurus (McCray & Nelson, 1995). Fig. 4.2 displays a search result

Foundational Model of Anatomy

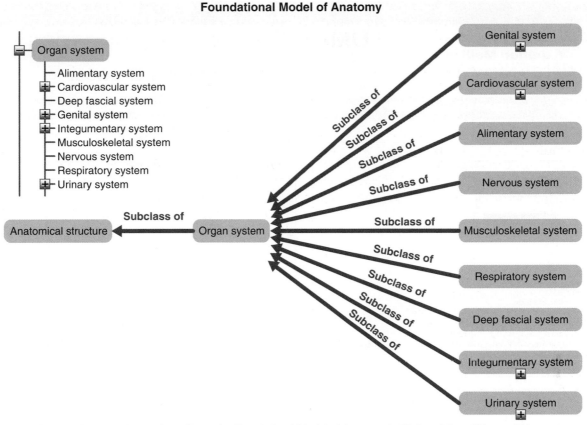

Fig. 4.1 An example ontology. (From the Foundational Model of Anatomy in BioPortal. http://bioportal.bioontology.org/ontologies/FMA.)

for the keyword "comfort alteration" in the UMLS browser. An online resource, "NLM Resource for Standards and Interoperability," developed by the NLM, provides introductions to the terminologies used by nursing and a tutorial on how to find a map between two different terminologies (U.S. National Library of Medicine, 2017).

Given the complexity of the healthcare delivery system in the 21st century, the health IT industry demands a comprehensive solution to promote data standardization and exchange. One terminology is unlikely to meet the needs of the wide range of disciplines within healthcare, yet adopting quality terminologies is crucial for promoting interoperability within EHRs. Assessing the quality of a terminology is not a simple task as each terminology evolves according to its *terminology life cycle* linked to structural and developmental processes (Rogers, 2006; Bakhshi-Raiez et al., 2008; de Coronado et al., 2009; Kim et al., 2010).

A terminology life cycle contains three major phases: change requests, terminology editing, and terminology publication (Kim et al., 2010). A *terminology change request* is a formal mechanism for users to submit requests for any changes or additions with respect to a given terminology (de Coronado et al., 2009; International Health Terminology Standards Development Organisation [IHTSDO], 2021; NANDA International, 2019). *Terminology editing* begins with the activation of a new concept, revision of an existing concept, or inactivation of a concept, and follows formal concept

change and version management guidelines. When terminology editing is completed with subsequent documentation, a series of tasks is performed throughout the *terminology publication* phase to release a new version of terminology for public use. Any products (such as terminologies, cross-maps, translations, subsets, and educational materials) generated through the terminology life cycle should be easily accessible, usable, and interoperable in EHRs (Kim et al., 2010).

Requirements for maintaining healthcare terminology quality address the terminology structure, content, mapping, and process management in alignment with the terminology life cycle (Kim et al., 2010; Cimino et al., 1994; Tuttle et al., 1994; Campbell et al., 1997; Chute et al., 1998; Cimino, 1998; Oliver & Shahar, 2000; Elkin et al., 2002). The International Organization for Standardization (ISO) has developed international terminology standards. Specifically, ISO/TS 17117:2002, Health Informatics—Controlled Health Terminology—Structure and High-Level Indicators describes technical specifications for high-level evaluation of a controlled health terminology. According to the specifications, the terminology's purpose, scope, and content coverage should be explicitly stated for a specified domain of use. Each concept should be clearly defined with a unique identifier, hence there should be no redundancy, ambiguity, or vagueness (International Organization for Standardization, 2002).

Further, ISO/TS 18104:2014, *Categorical Structures for Representation of Nursing Diagnoses and Nursing Actions in Terminological Systems*, provides a framework to promote

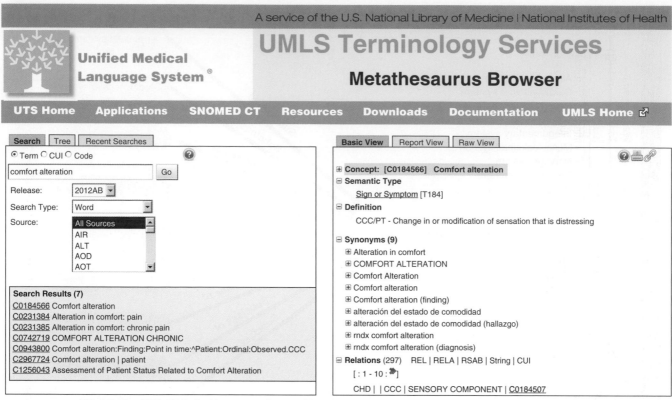

Fig. 4.2 The Unified Medical Language System Metathesaurus Browser. (https://uts.nlm.nih.gov/home.html.)

terminology development and mapping, data analytics, and interoperability of nursing diagnoses and actions across healthcare settings (International Organization for Standardization, 2014). This standard defines categories of healthcare entities for nursing diagnoses, including clinical course, clinical findings, degree, focus, judgment, potential, site, anatomical structure, subject of information, and timing (International Organization for Standardization, 2014; Goossen, 2006). For example, the nursing diagnosis *severe pain* meets this standard, as it consists of the finding concept *pain* and the degree concept *severe*. The ISO standard also requires that a nursing intervention be composed of at least two categories of healthcare entity, including action, means, route, subject of record, and target (International Organization for Standardization, 2014). For example, the nursing intervention *patient education about pain management* comprises a nurse's *education* (action) on *pain management* (target).

Building on these standards, the American Nurses Association (ANA) recognizes 10 healthcare terminologies appropriate for use in nursing (Warren & Bakken, 2002; American Nurses Association, 2018). Of these, seven are explicitly designed for nursing, and the other three are considered multidisciplinary terminologies (Table 4.2). The ANA also recognized two minimum datasets, both now components of LOINC and the Systematized Nomenclature of Medicine—Clinical Terms (SNOMED CT): (1) the Nursing Minimum Data Set (NMDS) as a framework for collecting nursing care data, and (2) the Nursing Management Minimum Data Set (NMMDS) as a framework for collecting nursing service data elements. That is, the NMDS requires patient demographics, nursing process

data (i.e., assessments, diagnoses, interventions, and outcomes), and service elements (e.g., agency and admission and discharge dates) to assess the quality of care (Ryan & Delaney, 1995). The NMMDS focuses on collecting variables associated with the nursing environment, nurse resources, and financial resources to support administrative analysis and decision-making of nurse executives (Huber et al., 1997; Westra et al., 2010; Kunkel et al., 2010).

MULTIDISCIPLINARY TERMINOLOGIES

Terminologies are essential to communicate and document patient care data in alignment with the care process. Various data types are critical to clinical care, such as laboratory results, medications, medical diagnoses and procedures, and billing information. Accordingly, multidisciplinary terminologies, as described in this section, are essential.

Logical Observation Identifiers Names and Codes

Logical Observation Identifiers Names and Codes (LOINC), established in 1994 by the Regenstrief Institute, is a standardized coding system for laboratory and clinical measurements (observations) (Regenstrief Institute, 2021). Each LOINC observation is created using six axes: (1) the name of the observation (or analyte); (2) property (e.g., substance concentration, mass, volume); (3) timing of the measurement; (4) the type of system or sample (e.g., serum, urine, patient, family); (5) scale (e.g., qualitative, quantitative); and (6) the method used to make the observation (optional) (McDonald et al., 2016).

TABLE 4.2 An Overview of Standardized Terminologies Relevant to Nursing Practice

Terminology or Classification[a]	Developer	Discipline or Specialty	Release Time (Current Version)	American Nurses Association (ANA) Recognized	Cross-Maps Available	Web-Based Terminology Browser[b] (Language)
Clinical Care Classification (CCC)	SabaCare	Nursing	As needed (version 2.5)	Yes	ICNP, SNOMED CT, LOINC	https://careclassification.org/ (English)
International Classification for Nursing Practice (ICNP)	International Council of Nurses (ICN)	Nursing	Every 2 years in ICN conference (2015)	Yes	CCC, ICF, SNOMED CT	https://www.icn.ch/what-we-do/projects/ehealth-icnptm/about-icnp (multilingual)
NANDA International (NANDA-I)	NANDA-I	Nursing	Every 2 years (2015–2017)	Yes	Not publicly available (member only)	
Nursing Interventions Classification (NIC)	University of Iowa	Nursing	Every 4 years (2013; 6th ed.)	Yes	Not publicly available (member only)	
Nursing Outcomes Classification (NOC)	University of Iowa	Nursing	Every 4 years (2013; 5th ed.)	Yes	Not publicly available (member only)	
Omaha System	Martin, KS	Nursing	As needed (2005; 2nd ed.)	Yes	SNOMED CT, LOINC	http://www.omahasystem.org (English)
Perioperative Nursing Data Set (PNDS)	Association of Perioperative Registered Nurses (AORN)	Perioperative nursing	As needed (2011; 3rd ed.)	Yes	SNOMED CT	Not publicly available (member only)
Logical Observation Identifiers Names and Codes (LOINC)	Regenstrief Institute Inc.	Multidisciplinary	Biannual (Version 2.56)	Yes	CCC, Omaha System	http://loinc.org/downloads/relma (multilingual; note that it can be browsed after installing RELMA)
Systematized Nomenclature of Medicine—Clinical Terms (SNOMED CT)	International Health Terminology Standards Development Organisation (IHTSDO)	Multidisciplinary	Biannual (July 2016)	Yes	ICD-10, ICD-9-CM, ICNP	http://browser.ihtsdotools.org (multilingual)
ABC Codes	ABC Coding Solutions	Multidisciplinary	Annual (2016)	Yes	Not publicly available (member only)	
Current Procedural Terminology (CPT)	American Medical Association (AMA)	Medicine	Annual (2016)		LOINC	Not publicly available (member only)
International Classification of Diseases (ICD)	World Health Organization (WHO)	Medicine	As needed (10th ed.) (2016)		SNOMED CT	http://apps.who.int/classifications/icd10/browse/2016/en (English)
International Classification of Functioning, Disability and Health (ICF)	WHO	Multidisciplinary	As needed (2008)	—		http://apps.who.int/classifications/icfbrowser/ (multi-lingual)
RxNorm	National Library of Medicine (NLM)	Multidisciplinary (drug)	Monthly (July 2016)	—	—	http://rxnav.nlm.nih.gov/ (English)

[a] All terminologies and classifications are accessible through the Unified Medical Language System (UMLS), released every six months by the National Library of Medicine (NLM). Available at https://uts.nlm.nih.gov/home.html.

[b] All of the web browsers listed are publicly available at no cost. Also, personal digital assistant (PDA) versions of terminology browsers may be available as knowledge resources.

HL7, Health level seven; *RELMA*, Regenstrief LOINC mapping assistant.

TABLE 4.3 Coding Structure and Application of Logical Observation Identifiers Names and Codes

Code	Description
Fully specified name	Length: 3–7 characters The last digit (ranging from 0 to 9) of the LOINC code preceded by a hyphen is required to avoid errors in the transcription of the code. < component/analyte >:<kind of property >:<time aspect >:<system/sample type >:<scale >:<method >
Example coding of laboratory tests	2339-0:Glucose:MCnc:Pt:Bld:Qn This example includes a LOINC code and four attributes: 1. Code = 2339-0 2. Name of component = Glucose 3. Property = Mass concentration (MCnc[a]) 4. Type of system/sample = Patient's blood (Pt:Bld[a]) 5. Measurement scale = Quantitative (Qn[a])	2341-6:Glucose:MCnc:Pt:Bld:Qn:Test strip manual This example includes a LOINC code and five attributes: 1. Code=2341-6 2. Name of component=Glucose 3. Property=Mass concentration (MCnc[a]) 4. Type of system/sample=Patient's blood (Pt:Bld[a]) 5. Measurement scale=Quantitative (Qn[a]) 6. Method=Test strip manual

LOINC, Logical observation identifiers names and codes.

[a]Details on the abbreviations can be found in McDonald, C., Huff, S., Mercer, K., Hernandez, J., & Vreeman, D. J. (Eds.). (2016). *Logical Observation Identifiers Names and Codes (LOINC) users' guide*. Indianapolis, IN: Regenstrief Institute Inc. http://loinc.org/downloads/files/LOINCManual.pdf.

All LOINC names are case-sensitive. Table 4.3 presents an example of blood glucose tests coded using the LOINC system. Actual values of observations need to be documented using numeric values or other standardized terms. LOINC contains more than 80,000 terms (as of 2016) and is widely adopted for ordering and exchanging laboratory and clinical observations in the communication protocol called Health Level Seven International (HL7) (McDonald et al., 2016). The laboratory portion of the LOINC database contains the laboratory categories, such as chemistry, hematology, and microbiology. The domain and scope of clinical LOINC are broad. Some sections include terms for vital signs, obstetric measurements, clinical assessment scales, outcomes from standardized nursing terminologies, and research instruments (Scichilone, 2008). LOINC is also used for document and section names (Hyun et al., 2009). Nursing content is one of the scientific domains with a special focus on clinical LOINC (Matney et al., 2003). Nursing assessments can be structured in LOINC as a "Panel." For example, the Skin Assessment Panel (LOINC ID 72284-3) contains "Skin Color," "Skin Temperature," "Skin Turgor," and "Skin Moisture." Nursing assessment development is an ongoing project for the Nursing Clinical LOINC Subcommittee. Systematized Nomenclature of Medicine—Clinical Terms

SNOMED CT is the most comprehensive clinical terminology and has become an international standard for coding healthcare data (Cornet & de Keizer, 2008; National Library of Medicine (NLM), 2016). The International Health Terminology Standards Development Organization (IHTSDO) has developed a set of principles to guide SNOMED CT development and quality improvement. SNOMED CT is continually updated to meet users' needs. The governments of member countries fund IHTSDO, therefore, healthcare institutions in IHTSDO member countries can use SNOMED CT without additional costs. For example, there are no fees for its use in the United States, whose national release center is responsible for managing concept requests and distributing and supporting IHTSDO products. The NLM, which also maintains and distributes the UMLS, is the US member of the IHTSDO.

SNOMED CT contains preferred terms and the related synonyms (including Spanish translations of preferred terms) organized in a hierarchical tree structure with top-level concepts, such as body structure, clinical finding (e.g., diseases, disorders, drug actions), event, observable entity, procedure (e.g., treatment or therapy, surgical procedure, laboratory procedure), specimen, and substance (SNOMED International, 2021). Concepts lower in the hierarchy are more specific in meaning than those higher in the hierarchy, creating multiple levels of granularity. Defining attribute relationships using description logics further details the meaning of a concept by relating all necessary and sufficient conditions.

In general, clinical questions for assessment and measurable outcomes (e.g., pain level) can be coded using concepts placed under *observable entity*. Most nursing diagnoses and outcomes can be found under *clinical finding* and *event*, while nursing interventions and actions are found under *procedure*. An example of SNOMED CT coding of the clinical question "*ability to manage medication?*" with the answer "*unable to manage medication*" is presented in Fig. 4.3. This set of questions and answers coded using standardized terminologies is ready for data exchange using messaging standards such as HL7.

Classifications Used for Reimbursement

The International Classification of Diseases (ICD), copyrighted by the World Health Organization (WHO), reports mortality and morbidity data worldwide and compares statistics across settings, regions, or countries over time (World Health Organization [WHO], n.d.). Further, ICD is used for billing, reimbursement, and allocation of health service resources for approximately 70% of the world's health expenditures (WHO, n.d.). The current version of ICD-10 (10th edition) was endorsed by the WHO in 1990 and implemented in the United States as of October 1, 2015 (Centers for Medicare & Medicaid Services [CMS], 2021). With the advancement of information technology and EHRs, ICD-11

	Clinical Question	Clinical Answer
Concept with Code	285033005 Ability to manage medication (observable entity)	285035003 Unable to manage medication (finding)
Concept description	Concept Status: **current** ⊟ Descriptions 　⊟ Lang: en-US 　　[F] ability to manage medication (observable entity) 　　[P] ability to manage medication ⊟ Definition: Primitive 　⊟ is a 　　[D] drug therapy observable 　⊟ is a 　　[D] instrumental activity of daily living	Concept Status: **current** ⊟ Descriptions 　⊟ Lang: en-US 　　[F] unable to manage medication (finding) 　　[P] unable to manage medication 　　[S] self-care deficit for medication management ⊟ Definition: Fully Defined as... 　⊟ is a 　　[D] finding related to ability to manage medication 　⊟ Group 　　⊟ Has interpretation 　　　[D] unable 　　⊟ interprets 　　　[D] ability to manage medication
Concept placement in the hierarchy	⊟[C] SNOMED CT Concept 　⊟[C] observable entity 　　⊟[C] clinical history/examination observable 　　　⊟[C] functional observable 　　　　⊟[C] ability to perform function/activity 　　　　　⊟[C] activity of daily living 　　　　　　⊟[C] instrumental activity of daily living 　　　　　　　⊟[→] ability to manage medication 　　　　　　　　[C] ability to administer non-parenteral medication 　　　　　　　　[C] ability to administer parenteral medication 　　　　　　　　[C] ability to store medications	⊟[C] SNOMED CT Concept 　⊟[C] clinical finding 　　⊟[C] clinical history and observation findings 　　　⊟[C] functional finding 　　　　⊟[C] finding of activity of daily living 　　　　　⊟[C] instrumental activity of daily living 　　　　　　⊟[C] finding related to ability to manage medication 　　　　　　　[→] unable to manage medication

Fig 4.3 The Structure and Application of Systematized Nomenclature of Medicine—Clinical Terms (SNOMED CT). (Retrieved from the International Health Terminology Standards Development Organization SNOMED CT browser. http://browser.ihtsdotools.org.)

has been developed and is currently in a revision process, with an anticipated release in January, 2022. ICD-11 provides more detailed information (such as definitions, signs, and symptoms) on disease in a structured way.

Depending on the focus of specialty areas, additional classifications can be used for ordering, billing, and reimbursement of medical procedures and diagnostic services. ICD Clinical Modification (ICD-CM) is a coding system developed to encode medical diagnoses and procedures (such as surgical, diagnostic, and therapeutic procedures) performed in US hospital settings (Centers for Disease Control and Prevention [CDC], 2021). ICD 10 CM, a modified version of ICD-10, is updated annually by the National Center for Health Statistics (NCHS) and CMS. The Current Procedural Terminology (CPT) classification system is used extensively in the United States. CMS mandates its use for reporting outpatient hospital surgical procedures as part of the Omnibus Budget Reconciliation Act (American Medical Association [AMA], 2021). Diagnosis Related Groups (DRG) is a patient classification scheme designed to cluster similar cases using ICD and CPT codes as well as patient characteristics for reimbursement purposes according to the inpatient prospective payment system (IPPS) (Centers for Medicare & Medicaid Services [CMS], 2020a).

Other healthcare providers may use a different coding system for ordering, billing, and reimbursement for care delivered. For example, the *Diagnostic and Statistical Manual of Mental Disorders*, Fourth Edition (DSM-IV), developed by the American Psychiatric Association, has been widely used by clinicians to code mental and behavioral health-related conditions. All DSM-IV diagnostic codes have been integrated into ICD-9-CM (American Psychiatric Association [APA], 2012). Due to differences between the two coding systems, cross-mapping solutions between DSM-IV and ICD-10-CM are available. Effective October 1, 2021, ICD-10-CM will include a limited number of changes in coding DSM-5 behavioral health disorders (APA, 2021). Another example is the ABC Coding Solutions, which provides more than 4,500 codes for integrative healthcare services and products (ABC Coding Solutions, n.d.). In other words, the ABC coding system covers clinical services related to nursing, behavioral health, alternative medicine, ethnic and minority care, midwifery, and spiritual care. An ABC code consists of five characters representing types of services, remedies, supplies, and practitioners (ABC Coding Solutions, n.d.).

RxNorm

RxNorm is a normalized drug-naming system derived from 14 drug terminologies containing drug names, ingredients, strength, and dose form (National Library of Medicine [NLM], 2021). Example source terminologies within RxNorm include Micromedex RED BOOK, the Food and Drug Administration (FDA) National Drug Code Directory, SNOMED CT, and the

Veterans Health Administration National Drug File. Due to different naming systems used in each terminology, the NLM produces normalized generic and brand names of prescription drugs and over-the-counter drugs available in the United States (NLM, 2021). The NLM uses the UMLS framework to maintain and distribute RxNorm, allowing consistent communication among various hospital and pharmacy systems. RxNorm preserves original drug names as synonyms and semantic relationships among drugs. It also serves as a knowledge resource to advance e-prescribing systems with decision support functionality, as RxNorm contains pharmacologic knowledge such as drug interactions (Nelson et al., 2011).

World Health Organization Family of International Classifications

The WHO formed a Family of International Classifications (WHO-FIC), containing a suite of WHO-endorsed classifications, including three reference classifications, five derived classifications, and five related classifications (World Health Organization [WHO], 2021a). ICD and International Classification of Functioning, Disability and Health (ICF) are core reference classification systems in WHO-FIC (WHO, 2021a). While the ICD system provides a set of diagnosis codes to encode causes of death and health conditions, ICF (formerly known as the International Classification of Impairments, Disabilities, and Handicaps) is a classification system that focuses on functional status as a consequence of disease or health conditions (WHO, 2001). Although ICF has been used mainly in physical therapy and rehabilitation professions, previous studies demonstrated the usefulness of ICF in documenting nursing practice in acute care hospitals and early postacute rehabilitation settings (Heerkens et al., 2003; Heinen et al., 2005; Van Achterberg et al., 2005; Mueller et al., 2008). Knowing that these core classifications lack in covering other specialty areas, the WHO recognizes an additional 10 classifications or terminologies in WHO-FIC (WHO, 2021b). For example, ICD-10 Classification of Mental and Behavioral Disorders and ICF Version for Children and Youth are derived from the core classification systems (i.e., ICD and ICF). International Classification of Primary Care and International Classification for Nursing Practice (ICNP) are considered related classifications in WHO-FIC.

NURSING TERMINOLOGIES

As shown in Table 4.2, the ANA recognized seven nursing terminologies or classifications supporting nursing practice as they conform to the terminology development standards (Coenen et al., 2001). All ANA-approved nursing terminologies have been integrated into the UMLS Metathesaurus and widely adopted nationally and internationally. This section succinctly introduces the nursing terminologies and describes their purpose, scope, content coverage, and structure.

Clinical Care Classification

The Clinical Care Classification (CCC) has been used for more than 20 years in nursing across the care continuum since its development as the Home Health Care Classification System in 1991 (Saba, 2002). CCC is a classification system of nursing diagnoses and interventions organized under 21 care components to support documentation of the nursing process (Saba, 2007). In this classification, a nursing care component is a navigation or high-level abstract concept clustering the nursing practice with similar patterns. These care components are further aggregated into four healthcare patterns of patient care: functional, health-behavioral, physiological, and psychological.

CCC Version 2.5 includes 176 nursing diagnoses (60 major categories and 116 subcategories) from which 528 nursing outcomes can be derived using three modifiers: (1) improved, (2) stabilized, and (3) deteriorated (Saba, 2012). As such, 201 nursing interventions (77 major categories and 124 subcategories) can be expanded to as many as 804 nursing actions by combining four action types: (1) monitor/assess/evaluate/observe, (2) perform/direct care/provide/assist, (3) teach/educate/instruct/supervise, and (4) manage/refer/contact/notify. This compositional ability of CCC allows users to express nursing care in any care setting while maintaining a simple classification structure (Table 4.4). Each nursing diagnosis, intervention, and outcome is assigned to a code with alphanumeric characters.

International Classification for Nursing Practice

The ICNP is a nursing terminology designed to represent nursing diagnoses, outcomes, and interventions capturing the delivery of nursing care across settings (International Council of Nurses, 2009). The ICNP is an entity of the International Council of Nurses (ICN) eHealth Programme that was launched to transform nursing through the use of health information and communication technology (International Council of Nurses [ICN], 2021). The ICN is a federation of more than 130 national nurses associations that represents millions of nurses worldwide. Since 1989, the ICNP has evolved from a collection of nursing-related concepts to a logic-based nursing terminology system maintained in an ontology development environment (International Council of Nurses, 2009). The ICNP has been developed using a sophisticated language (i.e., Web Ontology Language or OWL) to ensure the sustainability of the ever-expanding terminology and maintain the quality of the terminology (Hardiker & Coenen, 2007).

In conformance with ISO standards (ISO/TS 18104:2014), nursing diagnosis, outcome, and intervention statements are precoordinated with primitive concepts such as focus, judgment, and action concepts. Each precoordinated concept is assigned a unique identifier, and it is possible for practitioners to postcoordinate primitive concepts to meet their needs (Hardiker & Coenen, 2007). For example, as shown in Box 4.1, the nursing diagnosis *acute pain* is a precoordinated concept with an assigned code (10000454). However, *acute abdomen pain* does not exist in ICNP, meaning that the concept could be post-coordinated with two concepts: *Acute pain* (10000454) in *abdomen* (10000023). All ICNP primitive and precoordinated concepts are organized in a hierarchical tree structure. The 2015 release included 805 nursing diagnoses/outcomes and 1019 intervention statements. A new version of ICNP is released every two years in conjunction with the ICN conference. Due to the size and complexity of ICNP, subsets are created to promote the utility of ICNP in

TABLE 4.4 Structure and Application of Clinical Care Classification in Relation to the Nursing Process for Pressure Ulcer

Nursing Process	CCC Structure	Example Concepts
Assessment	Healthcare patterncare component	Physiologic R. Skin Integrity
Diagnosis	Nursing diagnosis Major category R.46.0 Skin Integrity Alteration Subcategory R.46.2 Skin Integrity Impairment	
Outcome	Expected outcome	R.46.2.1 Skin Integrity Impairment Improved
Planning	Nursing intervention Major category R.51.0 Pressure Ulcer Care Subcategory R.51.1 Pressure Ulcer Stage 1 Care	
Implementation	Nursing action type	R.51.1.2 Perform/Direct Care/Provide/Assist Pressure Ulcer Stage 1 Care
Evaluation	Actual outcome	R.46.2.1 Skin Integrity Impairment Improved

CCC, Clinical care classification.

practice (Coenen & Kim, 2010). That is, ICNP catalogs or subsets with select nursing diagnoses and interventions have been developed and distributed in collaboration with national nurses associations, health ministries and governments, and expert nurses worldwide (International Council of Nurses [ICN], 2008, 2009, 2011, 2012). North American Nursing Diagnosis Association International Nursing Diagnoses

The North American Nursing Diagnosis Association (NANDA) dates back to 1970, and its terminology was the first to be recognized by the ANA (Gordon, 1994). The membership organization was renamed NANDA International (NANDA-I) to reflect worldwide use of the terminology and established network teams in Latin America, Europe, Asia, and Africa (Herdman, 2012). In NANDA-I, a nursing diagnosis is defined as "a clinical judgment about actual or potential individual, family, or community experiences/responses to health problems/life processes." (Herdman, 2012, p. 134). The purpose of NANDA-I is to ensure consistent, accurate documentation of nurses by clinical reasoning judgments and drive nursing interventions and outcome evaluations. As shown in Table 4.5, a three-level structure was adopted to place diagnoses according to conceptual similarities (Herdman, 2012). That is, a nursing diagnosis (Level 3) is in a class (Level 2) according to its definition, defining characteristics and related factors, or risk factors. A class is further clustered into a domain (Level 1). The NANDA-I 2015–2017 release includes 235 nursing diagnoses organized in 47 classes and 13 domains, along with the evidence to support knowledge-based diagnostic decisions.

BOX 4.1 Structure and Application of International Classification for Nursing Practice

ICNP Structure: Asserted Hierarchy	Example Concepts
Article I. Process	The concept *acute pain* is a precoordinated nursing diagnosis composed of the primitive concepts *pain*, *acute*, and *actual*. "10000454 Acute pain" = has focus "10013950 pain" + has onset "10001739 acute" + has potentiality "10000420 actual" The concept *acute abdominal pain* can be post-coordinated if needed by selecting the nursing diagnosis *acute pain* and the body location *abdomen*. Acute abdominal pain = 10000454 Acute pain + 10000023 Abdomen
Article II. Body process	
Article III. Nervous system process	
Article IV. Perception	
Article V. Impaired perception	
Article VI. Pain	
Article VII. Acute pain[a]	
Article VIII. Chronic pain	
Article IX. Labor pain	
Article X. Musculoskeletal pain	

[a]This example shows the placement of the nursing diagnosis "acute pain" in the ICNP asserted hierarchy.
ICNP, International Classification for Nursing Practice.

Regenstrief Institute. (2021). *The international standards for identifying health measurements, observations, and documents.* Regenstrief Institute Inc. http://loinc.org/.

Rewolinski, J., & Wilder, V. (2021). UMLS 2021 AA release available. *NLM Technical Bulletin, 440,* e2. https://www.nlm.nih.gov/pubs/techbull/mj21/mj21_umls_2021aa_release.html.

Rogers, J. E. (2006). Quality assurance of medical ontologies. *Methods of Information in Medicine, 45*(3), 267–274.

Rosenbloom, S. T., Miller, R. A., Johnson, K. B., Elkin, P. L., & Brown, S. H. (2006). Interface terminologies: facilitating direct entry of clinical data into electronic health record systems. *Journal of the American Medical Informatics Association, 13*(3), 277–288.

Ryan, P., & Delaney, C. (1995). Nursing minimum data set. In J. J. Fitzpatrick, & J.S. Stevenson (Eds.) (1995). *Annual Review of Nursing Research* (Vol. 13, pp. 169–194). New York: Springer Publishing Company.

Saba, V. (2007). *Clinical Care Classification (CCC) system manual: A guide to nursing documentation.* New York: Springer Publishing Company.

Saba, V. (2012). *Clinical Care Classification (CCC) system version 2.5 user's guide* (2nd ed.). New York: Springer Publishing Company.

Saba, V. (2002). Nursing classifications: Home health care classification system (HHCC): An overview. *OJIN: The Online Journal of Issues in Nursing, 7*(3). https://tinyurl.com/2xy2r2mh.

Scichilone, R. A. (2008). The benefits of using SNOMED CT and LOINC in assessment instruments. *Journal of AHIMA, 79*(7), 56–57.

SNOMED International. (2021). *SNOMED CT starter guide.* SNOMED International. https://confluence.ihtsdotools.org/display/docstart/snomed+ct+starter+guide.

The National Center for Biomedical Ontology. (2021). BioPortal. http://bioportal.bioontology.org/.

The Office of the National Coordinator for Health Information Technology (ONC). (2019). *What are the differences between Medicare and Medicaid incentive programs?.* tinyurl.com/ev6mpak9.

Tsarkov, D., & Horrocks, I. (2006). FaCT++ description logic reasoner: system description. *Lecture notes in computer science, 4130,* 292–297.

Tuttle, M. S., Olson, N. E., Campbell, K. E., Sherertz, D. D. Nelson, S. J., & Cole, W. G. (1994). Formal properties of the Metathesaurus. *Proceedings Symposium on Computer Applications in Medical Care,* 145–149.

U.S. Department of Health & Human Services. (2015). *A shared nationwide interoperability roadmap.* HealthIT.gov. http://www.healthit.gov/policy-researchers-implementers/interoperability.

U.S. National Library of Medicine. (2017). Nursing Resources for Standards and Interoperability. https://www.nlm.nih.gov/research/umls/Snomed/nursing_terminology_resources.html.

Van Achterberg, T., Holleman, G., Heijnen-Kaales, Y., et al. (2005). Using a multidisciplinary classification in nursing: the International Classification of Functioning Disability and Health. *Journal of Advance Nursing, 49*(4), 432–441.

Warren, J. J., & Bakken, S. (2002). Update on standardized nursing data sets and terminologies. *Journal of AHIMA, 73*(7), 78–83. quiz 85–86.

Watkins, T. J., Haskell, R. E., Lundberg, C. B., Brokel, J. M., Wilson, M. L., & Hardiker, N. (2009). Terminology use in electronic health records: Basic principles. *Urologic Nursing, 29*(5), 321–326. quiz 327.

Westra, B. L., Latimer, G. E., Matney, S. A., et al. (2015). A national action plan for sharable and comparable nursing data to support practice and translational research for transforming health care. *Journal of the American Medical Informatics Association, 22*(3), 600–607.

Westra, B. L., Subramanian, A., Hart, C. M., et al. (2010). Achieving "Meaningful Use" of electronic health records through the integration of the Nursing Management Minimum Data Set. *Journal of Nursing Administration, 40*(7–8), 336–343.

World Health Organization (WHO). *International Classification of Diseases (ICD).* WHO; 20. http://www.who.int/classifications/icd/en/.

World Health Organization (WHO). (2001). *International classification of functioning, disability and health.* Geneva, Switzerland: WHO.

World Health Organization (WHO). (2021a). *WHO Family of International Classifications (FIC).* World Health Organization. https://www.who.int/standards/classifications.

World Health Organization (WHO). (2021b). *WHO Family of International Classifications (FIC).* WHO. https://www.who.int/standards/classifications.

5

Evaluation of Health Information Systems—Purposes, Theories, and Methods

Polina V. Kukhareva and Charlene R. Weir

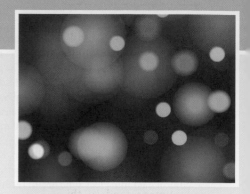

OBJECTIVES

At the completion of this chapter, the reader will be prepared to:
1. Determine the purposes of evaluation throughout the HIS life cycle.
2. Differentiate between social, cognitive, technical and evaluation theoretical perspectives.
3. Discuss the design requirements for a mixed-methods health informatics program evaluation plan.

KEY TERMS

ABSTRACT ❖

Evaluation of social, human, and technical aspects of health information system (HIS) interventions is an essential component in both the science and application of informatics. The full potential of HIS can only be reached if its development has been accompanied by appropriate and rigorous evaluation throughout the entire HIS life cycle. While much of what is done in informatics is cyclical in nature, for the purposes of this chapter, the HIS life cycle is divided into four phases (i.e., planning, development, implementation, and operation) with different evaluation studies recommended for each phase. Knowledge received through evaluation during planning, development and implementation phases could be useful for summative evaluation which is usually performed during the operation phase of HIS life cycle.

In preparation for an evaluation, key questions must be asked regarding the structure of the HIS intervention, phase of the HIS life cycle, and purpose and scope of the evaluation study. These questions, in turn, are best informed by the larger theoretical perspectives and principles of HIS evaluation. The reader of this chapter is expected to gain sufficient background in evaluation to lead or participate in the evaluation of HISs.

There are three sections in this chapter. In the first section, we discuss socio-technical levels of HIS interventions, life cycle of HIS interventions, and the types of evaluation studies that are appropriate at different phases of the HIS life cycle. In the next section, we describe theoretical perspectives that could inform evaluation studies throughout the HIS life cycle. Understanding the theoretical perspectives prepares evaluators for choosing and applying the methodologies that should be implemented when evaluating the HISs. In the third section of this chapter, a review of evaluation methods and designs is presented, including quantitative, qualitative, and mixed methods.

INTRODUCTION

In this chapter, **health information system (HIS) evaluation** is defined as "the act of measuring or exploring properties of an HIS (during planning, development, implementation, or operation), the result of which informs a decision to be made concerning that system in a specific context" (Ammenwerth et al., 2004).

HIS evaluations must take into consideration interactions between sociocultural systems, human behavior, and technology. We begin with introducing a conceptual socio-technical framework which we use through the rest of the chapter (Kukhareva et al., 2022). We chose to organize the discussion around socio-technical levels of the HIS interventions (social, human, and technical) because studies often tend to focus on one level to the detriment of the others. We also organize the presentation in terms of the HIS life cycle. A pitfall that junior evaluators often fall into is not understanding at which phase of the HIS life cycle the evaluation is being conducted. Evaluators should understand whether they were hired to determine how the product should be built, how it should be implemented, or to determine the value of the completed product.

After establishing socio-technical levels of the intervention, the life cycle phases, and the evaluation study types in the first section of this chapter, we delve into theoretical perspectives in the second section. Since evaluators are human, and humans tend to think in concepts, it is important to help evaluators choose appropriate theoretical perspectives to guide their understanding of socio-technical factors and outcomes. We provide examples of technical, cognitive, social, and evaluation process models useful for understanding HIS interventions.

Finally, when the evaluator has developed an understanding of the socio-technical levels of the HIS intervention and has chosen the appropriate theoretical perspectives, it is time to choose appropriate methods for data acquisition and analysis. The third section of this chapter gives examples of the qualitative, quantitative, and mixed methods used in HIS evaluation.

In summary, we recommend that junior investigators use the following approach in planning their evaluation studies: (1) develop an understanding of the HIS intervention, including technical, human and social levels, (2) determine what life cycle phase the HIS is in currently, (3) select an evaluation study type appropriate for the HIS life cycle phase, (4) choose a set of theoretical perspectives appropriate for the evaluation study type, (5) choose methods for data acquisition and analysis, and (6) conduct the study while iteratively refining understandings and choices developed in the previous steps.

First, we need to define some concepts which will be used for the rest of the chapter. HIS is a computer system used to acquire, store, deliver and analyze medical data. HIS intervention is an intervention aiming to develop, introduce into clinical practice, and sustain a new HIS.

HIS Socio-technical Levels: Social, Human, and Technical

Since HIS are usually operated by individuals in a complex societal context, three levels which are especially important for evaluation of HIS are (1) social (e.g., inner and outer context), (2) human, and (3) technical (Kukhareva et al., 2022; Yusof et al., 2008; Cresswell et al., 2020). While HIS represents the technology level, it is nearly always operated by humans (human level) and embedded in the larger programs of care delivery (social level). Human level, also known as human factors, describes the human characteristics, needs and limitations of the users of the HIS. Human factors are important because if users do not use the HIS, then the work has been wasted. The social context level describes the inner context such as organizational culture, workflows, and outer context such as patients and government regulations.

Identification of the unique contribution of the HIS, therefore, is often difficult, and evaluation goals frequently go beyond the technology level alone. In this chapter, the technology level of evaluation is integrated with evaluation of human and the social context levels (Ammenwerth, 2015).

HIS Life Cycle: Planning, Development, Implementation, and Operation

HISs mature through the HIS life cycle, which includes: (1) planning, (2) development, (3) implementation, and (4) operation phases (Fig. 5.1) (Ammenwerth et al., 2004; Kukhareva et al., 2022). The *planning phase* involves HIS intervention idea conception, prioritization, coordination with interested parties, requirements gathering, and project governance review and approval. The *development phase* involves software design, software development, governance review and organizational approval of the clinical implementation. The *implementation phase* involves implementation strategies design, staff communication, education and training, and pilot intervention rollout into clinical practice followed by a wider rollout with iterative innovation improvements as needed. The *operation phase* involves maintaining and monitoring HIS interventions after

IT Life Cycle Phases

I	II	III	IV
PLANNING PHASE	**DEVELOPMENT PHASE**	**IMPLEMENTATION PHASE**	**OPERATION PHASE**
• Software idea conception and prioritization • Software development decision	• Software design • Software development • Software rollout decision	• Software pilot rollout • Software rollout in wider clinical practice	• Software maintenance post-implementation • Software dissemination to other sites

Fig. 5.1 HIS life cycle. (From Kukhareva, P. V., Weir, C., Del Fiol, G., Aarons, G. A., Taft, T. Y., Schlechter, C. R., et al. [2022]. Evaluation in Life Cycle of Information Technology [ELICIT] framework: Supporting the innovation life cycle from business case assessment to summative evaluation. *Journal of Biomedical Informatics, 127,* 104014.)

the changes in the software have stabilized and the intervention may be disseminated to other sites.

Evaluation Study Types

We call a research study conducted for the purpose of evaluation an "evaluation study." Different evaluation study types are appropriate for different HIS life cycle phases (Kukhareva et al., 2022). Fig. 5.2 presents 12 evaluation study types often undertaken at different HIS life cycle phases: (1) business case assessment; (2) stakeholder requirements gathering; (3) technical requirements gathering; (4) technical acceptability assessment; (5) user acceptability assessment; (6) social acceptability assessment; (7) social implementation assessment; (8) initial user satisfaction assessment; (9) technical implementation assessment; (10) technical portability assessment; (11) long-term user satisfaction assessment; and (12) social outcomes assessment. Health informaticists are likely to contribute to all types of studies except for technical requirement gathering and technical validation, which are usually performed by the software developers.

At each life cycle phase, the evaluation questions are different (Table 5.1). A full evaluation study could answer several of these questions. Evaluation activities fall into two types: (1) **formative evaluation** and (2) **summative evaluation**. The difference is in how the information is used, not the type of methods. The results of the formative evaluation are used as feedback to the program for continuous improvement (Ainsworth and Viegut, 2006; Fetterman, 2001). The results of the summative evaluation are used to assess the properties and merit of the program (Brender, 2006). In Table 5.1, the first nine study types are more formative, and the last three study types are more summative. For example, the authors led a summative evaluation study of an interoperable electronic health record (EHR)-integrated app for neonatal bilirubin management that included user satisfaction assessment, summative implementation assessment, and summative effectiveness assessment (Kawamoto et al., 2019).

THEORETICAL PERSPECTIVES IN EVALUATION

Theoretical perspectives are necessary to frame the issues, create generalizable knowledge, and to clarify measurement. Theoretical perspectives clarify the definition and methods of measuring constructs and bring forward an understanding of the mechanisms of action.

For the purposes of this chapter, theoretical perspectives are divided into three levels of scope and complexity: (1) theories, (2) frameworks, and (3) models. At the most complex level with the widest scope are **theories**, which aim to *explain* mechanisms of action. A theory is defined as "a set of interrelated constructs (concepts), definitions, and propositions that present a

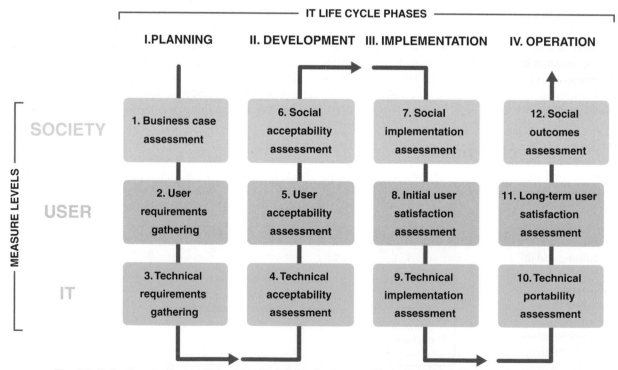

Evaluation in Life Cycle of Information Technology (ELICIT)

Fig. 5.2 Evaluation studies at different health information system life cycle phases. (From Kukhareva, P. V., Weir, C., Del Fiol, G., Aarons, G. A., Taft, T. Y., Schlechter, C. R., et al. [2022]. Evaluation in Life Cycle of Information Technology [ELICIT] framework: Supporting the innovation life cycle from business case assessment to summative evaluation. *Journal of Biomedical Informatics, 127*, 104014.)

TABLE 5.1 Evaluation Study Types Across Socio-technical Levels and Health Information System Life Cycle Phases

HIS Life Cycle Phase	Social Level	Human Level	Technical Level
I. Planning	Business case assessment (What societal needs must be fulfilled for the project to be successful?)	Stakeholder requirements gathering (What human needs must be fulfilled for the project to be successful?)	Technical requirements gathering (What technical needs must be fulfilled for the project to be successful?)
II. Development	Social acceptability assessment (Is it worth deploying this software?)	User acceptability assessment (What designs are optimal to meet needs of interested parties?)	Technical acceptability assessment (Does the software meet technical requirements?)
III. Implementation	Social implementation assessment (Did the system achieve the desired implementation outcomes?)	Initial user satisfaction assessment (Do users find the system enjoyable?)	Technical implementation assessment (Does the software meet technical requirements in the real-world setting?)
IV. Operation	Social outcomes assessment (Did the system have the desired impact on process, clinical, equity, and financial outcomes?)	Long-term user satisfaction assessment (Do users still find the system enjoyable?)	Technical portability assessment (Can the software be deployed across health systems and EHR platforms?)

systematic view of phenomena by specifying relations among variables, with the purpose of explaining and predicting the phenomena" (Kerlinger & Lee, 1999). Because many theories have an empirical foundation based on solid research, the metrics and relationships are usually well-established. At the next level are the **frameworks** which aim to describe the factors influencing the outcomes (determinants) and specify how to measure them. Finally, at the most basic level are **models**, which might be program specific and are intended to represent the goals and processes of a specific project. Models are the most basic and practical level of the theoretical perspectives. They help us to understand HIS interventions at different levels of abstraction. Models make explicit the implicit beliefs of interested parties of the proposed program. With time, models could develop into frameworks and theories as they acquire more empirical evidence and become increasingly generalizable. The descriptions below briefly provide an overview of the possibilities of each level.

Social, Cognitive, Technical, and "Evaluation" Theoretical Perspectives

HIS interventions could be understood on social, human, and technical levels from a variety of theoretical perspectives (i.e., social, cognitive, and technical). We also discuss a fourth type of theoretical perspectives which we call "evaluation" theoretical perspectives.

Social theoretical perspectives describe structures and processes in the social context. These include organizational structures, culture, and the local social context in respect to organization where the HIS is being implemented. The bulk of the theoretical perspectives described in this chapter are social. This chapter discusses social theoretical perspectives that have had significant validation. Like many health informatics theories, they are adapted from several existing social science theories to improve their fit in an applied information technology setting. A sub-type of this domain are implementation science theories. Implementation science is a new scientific domain which was established in the early 2000s with the goal of bridging the gap between research and clinical practice. Implementation science

relies on social science theories concerned with diffusion, dissemination, and implementation of innovations. The health informatics field is increasingly recognizing the importance of implementation science. Implementation frameworks refer to generalized, large-scale frameworks that are focused on performance improvement and institution-wide change.

Cognitive theoretical perspectives focus on human cognitive or psychological processes, which include cognition, motivation, and behavior. Cognitive frameworks attempt to measure how people make decisions, why they made specific choices, and what factors motivate their interest and their behavior.

Technical theoretical perspectives describe the technology itself, the functionality, and the models that guide software development. Such theoretical perspectives often originate from the software engineering domain and describe software development life cycle, (Ruparelia, 2010) software architecture, (Wright & Sittig, 2008) functionality, (McCoy et al., 2014) security, (Fox & Thomson, 2002) and interoperability (Kukhareva et al., 2019).

Evaluation theoretical perspectives are focused on the process of evaluation rather than on socio-technical levels of HIS interventions. Evaluation theoretical perspectives are developed with the aim of improving or standardizing evaluations (Neame et al., 2020). Many comprehensive evaluation frameworks for HISs have been described in literature reviews (Neame et al., 2020; Currie, 2005; Godinho et al., 2021; Vis et al., 2020; Eslami Andargoli et al., 2017; Yusof et al., 2008). For example, a recent systematic review identified 23 evaluation frameworks published from 2000 to 2019 (Neame et al., 2020). Evaluation frameworks are a loose collection of frameworks and models from domains of clinical trials, heath technology assessment, comparative effectiveness research, health services research, health economics and outcome research (Luce et al., 2010). In the next section we describe an evidence-based framework for Grading and Assessment of Predictive tools (the GRASP framework). This framework was recently developed and validated by Khalifa and colleagues at the Australian Institute of Health Innovation (Khalifa et al., 2019, 2020).

Theoretical Perspectives in Health Information System Life Cycle Phases

A short description of several theories, frameworks and models is provided in this section for the purpose of context. We have loosely organized the relevant theories, frameworks, and models within the four phases of the HIS life cycle: planning, development, implementation, and operation. The theories, frameworks and models mentioned below could be useful at other life cycle phases as well.

Planning Phase

Clinical decision support taxonomy. The Clinical Decision Support Taxonomy developed by Adam Wright and colleagues is an example of a technical model (Wright et al., 2011). This taxonomical model describes 53 types of clinical decision support systems, combined into several groups: medication dosing support, order facilitators, point of care alerts/reminders, relevant information displays, expert systems, and workflow support. If the system being evaluated is a clinical decision support system, the evaluator needs to understand what type of system it is to begin to develop an evaluation plan.

Program logic models. Program logical models are types of social models. When planning the development and implementation of a new HIS program, it is useful to think through the components of the program in consultation with project interested parties. A model describing the logic of a specific program is called a program logic model. A specific logic model is a representation of components and mechanisms of a specific program. The logic model usually describes four components of the program: inputs, activities, outcomes, and outputs (Fig. 5.3) (Logic Model Development Guide, 2004).

All evaluations for HISs should develop a program logic model to guide the evaluation process itself. A detailed program model identifies stakeholders, resources, variables, the timing of measures and observations, and the key expectations that reflect their understandings. Most importantly, a model serves as a shared vision between the evaluator team and the other interested parties, creating a unified vision that guides all evaluation activities.

The goal of the logic model is to make sure that the components of the program are easy to see and that the mechanisms are made explicit. The specific methods used to apply a model are not prescribed, although creating a logic model is recommended as the process brings together the various groups who need to work together to ensure success. Use of a wide range of methods and tools is encouraged. Engaging the interested parties is the first step, and that process could involve requirements gathering, technical requirements gathering, cognitive task analyses, contextual inquiry, and ethnographic observation, to name a few approaches. In all cases, the result is a deep description of the program, the expected mechanisms, and the desired outcomes. Once there is agreement on the characteristics of the program at both the superficial level and the deeper structure, designing the evaluation is straightforward.

Fig. 5.4 presents a logic model for the Neonatal Bilirubin Management Application implemented in the University of Utah Health Well Baby nursery and outpatient clinics (Kawamoto et al., 2019). The program logic model was developed through focus groups with public health epidemiologists, data stewards, healthcare administrators, and clinicians.

Naturalistic decision-making framework. Once the idea of a new program becomes clearer, it is important to access workflows, user needs, and user's mental models related to the clinical task which the program intends to change. The cognitive engineering perspective is widely used in health informatics and Human Factors research. One well-respected and well-known framework is the Naturalistic Decision Making Framework (Klein, 1997; Kushniruk & Patel, 2004). The Naturalistic Decision Making Framework emerged from the applied engineering sciences with the goal of understanding human behavior in context—in real-world settings. It is a broad and inclusive framework that covers the cognitive functions such as decision making, sensemaking, situational awareness, and planning focusing on the interaction between the natural settings and the individual, specifically stating that it is essential to watch individuals as they act in the real world. Naturalistic Decision-Making Framework could be used to inform requirement gathering studies.

Situation awareness framework. Situational awareness (SA) is also a cognitive framework derived from engineering psychology. The SA framework is narrower than the Naturalistic Decision-Making Framework and is particularly useful in supporting user requirements gathering and the user-centered design of the HISs. SA combines the cognitive processes of orientation, attention, categorization or sense making, and planning into three levels of performance (Endsley & Garland, 2000). These activities are thought to be critical to human performance in complex environments. Endsley refers to a three-level system of awareness: (1) perception (can I see the stimulus?), (2) comprehension (does it have meaning?), and (3) projection (what is likely to happen given the stimulus, and what can I do?). She defines shared Situation Awareness as the group understanding

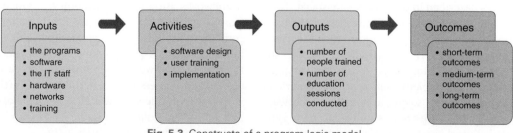

Fig. 5.3 Constructs of a program logic model.

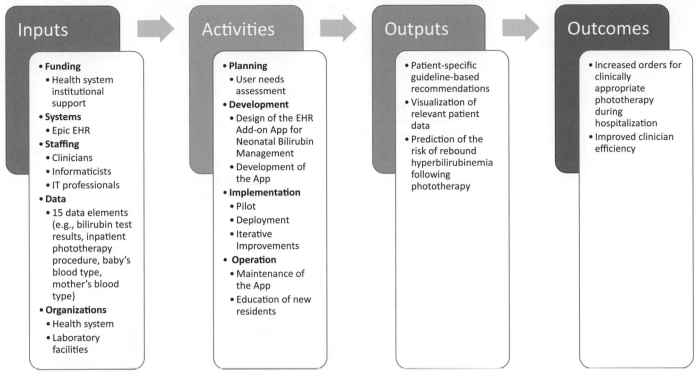

Fig. 5.4 An example of a program logic model for the Neonatal Bilirubin Management App.

TABLE 5.2   **Levels of Situational Awareness**

Level	Description
Perception of the elements in the environment	What is present, active, salient, and important in the environment? Attention will be driven by task needs.
Comprehension of the current situation	Classification of the event is a function of activation of long-term memory. The cognitive processes of classification and task identification drive meaning.
Projection of future status	Expectations of outcomes in the future, are driven by implicit theories and knowledge about the causal mechanisms underlying events.

of the situation (Endsley & Garland, 2000). For example, in one study of health IT, higher Situation Awareness was significantly associated with integrated displays for intensive care unit nursing staff (Koch et al., 2012, 2013). Table 5.2 presents the core components of Situation Awareness and associated definitions.

Development Phase

Plan-Do-Check-Act model. The Plan-Do-Check-Act (PDCA) model is an older evaluation model that emerged from Deming's work on quality improvement in the early 1950s (Deming, 1982). The PDCA model is ubiquitous because of widespread use in quality improvement interventions, as well as for the software prototyping and development. PDCA highlights the iterative nature of quality improvement and software development.

Each cycle of improvement could be as short as 1 hour and could involve as little as one healthcare provider. The PDCA approach combines quick rounds of evaluation and software improvement as illustrated in Fig. 5.5. Evaluation studies are concerned with the "Check" phase of the PDCA cycle. Effective use of evaluation during the HIS life cycle development phase will lead to transforming a high-functioning prototype to an initial functioning system.

Unified theory of acceptance and use of technology. Unified Theory of Acceptance and Use of Technology (UTAUT) is a cognitive theory. Once an initial version of the software is ready, it might be useful to predict whether users will choose to use it before approving the clinical implementation. User intentions to use the software and other factors relative to the planned implementation could be explored using the UTAUT model. UTAUT is an adaptation of the socio-cognitive theories in psychology to the field of information technology (Venkatesh et al., 2003). UTAUT is depicted in Fig. 5.6. The theory predicts users' intentions to use an information system as a function of performance expectancy or self-efficacy beliefs, effort expectancies, social influence, and facilitating conditions. Each of these constructs have been well studied and their relationship validated through hundreds of experimental studies. Significant moderators of these variables of intentions are gender, age, and the degree to which usage is mandated. This model integrates social cognitive theory (Bandura, 1989), theory of reasoned action (Fishbein & Ajzen, 1975), and diffusion of innovations theory (Rogers, 1983).

Venkatesh and Davis have conducted a systematic measurement meta-analysis that tested eight major models of adoption to clarify and integrate the adoption literature. The evaluated

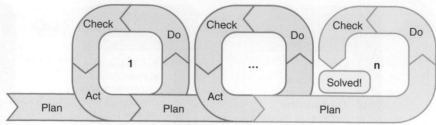

Fig 5.5 A model of Plan-Do-Check-Act (PDCA) cycle.

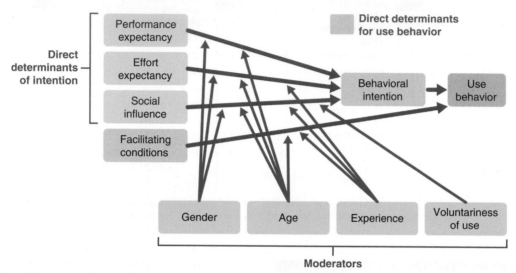

Fig. 5.6 An example of unified theory of acceptance and use of technology. (From Venkatesh, V., Morris, M., Davis, G., & Davis, F. [2003]. User acceptance of information technology: Toward a unified view. *MIS Quarterly, 27*[3], 425–478.)

models were based to some degree on the social cognitive models described above but adapted to the question of IT adoption and use. These empirical studies showed that UTAUT explained around 70% of the variance in *intention to use*, significantly greater than any of the initial models alone. Three key findings of this work are important. First, Venkatesh et al. found that the variables associated with initial *intentions to use* are different from the variables associated with later intentions (Venkatesh et al., 2003; Agarwal & Prasad, 1998; Karahanna et al., 1999). Specifically, the perceived work effectiveness constructs (perceived usefulness, extrinsic motivation, job fit, relative advantage, and outcome expectations) were found to be highly predictive of intentions over time. In contrast, variables such as attitudes, perceived behavioral control, ease of use, self-efficacy, and anxiety were predictors only of early intentions to use (or choice). Second, the authors found that the variables predictive of intentions to use are not the same as the variables predictive of usage behavior itself (Venkatesh et al., 2003). They found that the "effort factor scale" (resources, knowledge, compatible systems, and support) was the only construct other than intention to significantly predict usage behavior. Finally, these authors found that the model differed significantly depending on whether usage was mandated or by choice. In settings where usage was mandated, social norms had a stronger relationship to intentions to use than the other variables. Given these

findings, UTAUT measures can be used to plan implementation studies and to identify contextual factors important for success (Liu et al., 2021).

Implementation Phase

Consolidated framework for implementation research. Consolidated Framework for Implementation Research (CFIR) is a social and organizational framework, created from a combination of many theories. Because the CFIR model is so broad it is useful for giving an overview of the various models in existence (Damschroder et al., 2009). The consequent model is an overarching consolidated framework, consisting of five major domains: intervention characteristics, outer setting, inner setting, individual characteristics, and implementation processes. About 38 constructs were identified across the five major domains, and they include many of the constructs identified in the preceding theories. Although the model is thought to apply to health services implementations broadly, it is particularly applicable to informatics interventions. Readers may be interested in a step-by-step guide for use of this model, sample studies, and more details about the model available at https://cfirguide.org.

Diffusion of innovations theory. Diffusion of innovations is also a social theory focusing on group or cultural change. Diffusion of innovations is an empirically based theory that has driven research in the field of social change for several decades. It was developed by Rogers (a sociologist) after conducting a systematic analysis of over 100 social change interventions (Rogers, 1983; Cooper & Zmud, 1990). In this theory, characteristics of the innovation, the type of communication channels, the duration, and the social system are predictors of the rate of diffusion. The central premise is that diffusion is a process of decreasing uncertainty across a social system. Individuals pass through five stages: knowledge, persuasion, decision, implementation, and confirmation. Social norms, roles, and the type of communication channels all affect the rate of adoption of an innovation. Characteristics of an innovation that affect the rate of adoption include relative advantage as compared with other options; trialability, or the ease with which it can be tested; compatibility with other work areas; complexity of the innovation; and observability, or the ease with which the innovation is visible (Table 5.3). The famous "S" curve of change was derived from the work of Rogers, who demonstrated that change starts out very slowly and then will have a steep upcurve before it flattens out at a higher rate. Other constructs derived from diffusion of innovation include "Early Adopters" (people who adopt change readily).

Normalization process theory. Normalization process theory (NPT) is a social theory that focuses on the organizational level. To further monitor the implementation process and characterize changes that occur in the health system as the new innovation becomes routine, the NPT could be useful. The NPT was formalized by Carl May and Tracy Finch in 2009 (May & Finch, 2009). This theory is centered on the work required to embed and integrate innovations into their social contexts. According to NPT, the key phases leading to successful implementation are coherence, cognitive participation, collective action, and reflexive monitoring. *Coherence* describes whether the interested parties find the practice/program meaningful. *Cognitive participation* describes engagement of individuals and groups. *Collective action* describes interaction between the new practice and preexisting practices. Finally, *reflexive monitoring* describes how the practice is assessed by the interested parties. NPT is often used in the evaluation of implementation

success or failure (Godinho et al., 2021). More information is available at http://www.normalizationprocess.org/

Reach effectiveness adoption implementation maintenance framework. Reach Effectiveness Adoption Implementation Maintenance Framework (RE-AIM) is an evaluation framework. As implementation progresses, it becomes important to measure the implementation process itself. The RE-AIM implementation framework was designed to address the significant barriers associated with implementation of any new intervention, and it is particularly useful for informatics. The five concepts listed in Table 5.4 are important to measure. Most interventions meet with significant resistance, and any useful evaluation should measure the barriers associated with these constructs (Reach, Effectiveness, Adoption, Implementation, and Maintenance). These constructs frame the process of adoption and change of the implementation itself (Glasgow et al., 1999). First, did the intervention actually *reach* the intended target population? In other words, how many providers had the opportunity to use the system? Alternatively, how many patients had access to a new website? Second, for *effectiveness*, did the intervention do what it was intended to do? For instance, did the wound-care decision support work as intended every time? Did it identify the patients it was supposed to identify? Or, did the algorithms miss some key variables in real life? Third, for *adoption*, what proportion of the targeted staff, settings, or institutions used the program? What was the breadth and depth of usage? Did they use it for all relevant patients or only for some? Fourth, for *implementation*, was the intervention the same across settings and time? With most health IT products there is constant change to the software, the skill level of users, and the settings in which they are used. These should be documented and addressed in the evaluation. Finally, for *maintenance*, what were long-term individual or institutional effects? Longer time interval between 6 months and two years should be used to assess maintenance, as well as whether usage continues, and by whom and in what form. For health IT interventions it is especially useful to look

TABLE 5.3   Perceived Attributes of Innovations According to the Diffusion of Innovation Theory

Attribute	Description
Relative advantage	The degree to which an innovation is perceived as being better than the idea it supersedes
Compatibility	The degree to which an innovation is perceived as consistent with the existing values, past experiences, and needs of potential adopters.
Complexity	The degree to which an innovation is perceived as relatively difficult to understand and use.
Trialability	The degree to which the innovation may be experimented with on a limited basis.
Observability	The degree to which the results of an innovation are visible to others.

TABLE 5.4   Reach Effectiveness Adoption Implementation Maintenance Framework: Measures of Implementation Success

Measure	Description
Reach	The absolute number, proportion, and representativeness of individuals who are willing to participate in each program
Effectiveness	The impact of an intervention on important individual outcomes and broader impact including quality of life and economic outcomes
Adoption	The absolute number, proportion, and representativeness of settings and intervention agents
Implementation	The intervention agents' fidelity to the various elements of an intervention's key functions or components
Maintenance	The extent to which a program or policy becomes institutionalized or part of the routine organizational practices and policies

for unintended consequences, as well as workarounds during implementation and maintenance. Readers may be interested in a step-by-step guide for use of this model. Sample studies and more details about the model are available at https://www.re-aim.org.

Operation Phase

Structure-process-outcome model. Structure-process-outcome model is an evaluation model with similar historical origins of the PDCA cycle. The operation phase is a good time to start demonstrating the impact of HISs on process and health outcomes. Donabedian's classic structure-process-outcome model for assessing healthcare quality describes three areas of measurement: structural, process, and outcome measures (Donabedian, 1988). Donabedian defines *structural measures* as the professional and organizational resources associated with the provision of care, such as IT staff credentials, computerized physician order entry systems, or staffing ratios. *Process measures* include the tasks and decisions embedded in care, such as the time it takes to give antibiotics or the proportion of patients on deep vein thrombosis prevention protocols. Finally, *outcome measures* are defined as the final or semifinal measurable outcomes of care, such as the number of amputations due to diabetes, the number of patients with deep vein thrombosis, or the number of patients with drug-resistant pneumonia. These three categories of variables are thought to be mutually interdependent and reinforcing.

DeLone and McLean information systems success theory. DeLone and McLean's information success theory is an evaluation theory that helps to understand the construct of "success" when it comes to information systems (DeLone & McLean, 2003, 2016). Their theory was originally developed in 1992 and revised in 2003 based on significant empirical support. DeLone and McLean used three areas of information: (1) technical (accuracy and efficiency of the communication system), (2) semantic (communicating meaning), and (3) effectiveness (effect on the receiver). These three levels correspond to DeLone and McLean's constructs of (1) "system quality," (2) "information quality," and (3) "impacts" such as use, user satisfaction, and outcomes. DeLone and McLean revised the model in 2003 to include recent literature and added a fourth level, "service quality," referring to the degree to which users are supported by IT staff. Fig. 5.7 depicts an adaptation of the updated 2003

model that adds user satisfaction, user characteristics, and task effectiveness to the original model. This model effectively outlines the various factors that can be used for a full evaluation that can identify possible causes of success and failure.

Socio-technical model for informatics interventions. The socio-technical model proposed by Sittig and Singh describes eight areas to be addressed in a socio-technical implementation and evaluation (Sittig & Singh, 2010). These include: (1) hardware and software, (2) people, (3) clinical content, (4) human-computer interface, (5) workflow and communication, (6) internal organizations features, (7) external rules and regulations, and (8) measurement and monitoring. These categories can serve as a general taxonomy to organize an evaluation study.

Grading and assessment of predictive tools framework. GRASP is an evaluation framework. To compare evidence supporting validity, usefulness, potential impact, and post-implementation effectiveness of the system of interest to other systems, evaluator could use the GRASP framework (Khalifa et al., 2019, 2020). GRASP framework was developed to help healthcare professionals navigate the ever changing landscape of predictive tools in clinical practice (Khalifa et al., 2019, 2020). The framework allows converting existing evidence about a particular clinical decision support or predictive tool into a "grade" ranging from C3 (lowest quality of evidence) to A1 (highest quality of evidence). Table 5.5 shows which grade could be "earned" with which kind of evaluation studies. Clinical predictive tools that could be "graded" using this framework range from the simplest manually applied clinical prediction rules to the most sophisticated machine learning algorithms (Khalifa et al., 2019, 2020).

EVALUATION METHODS

The need for variety in methods is driven by the diversity in population, types of projects, and purposes that are characteristic of research and evaluation studies in informatics. Many evaluation methods are classified as either qualitative methods (stories; direct observation) or quantitative methods (statistical assessments). This division may be artificial and limited but using the terms *qualitative* and *quantitative* to organize

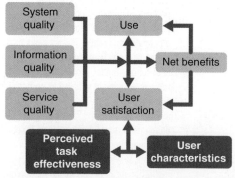

Fig 5.7 A model of information system success. (Adapted from Sharpe, M. E., [1993]. *Journal of Management Information Systems, 19*[4], 9–30.)

TABLE 5.5 Grading and Assessment of Predictive Tools (GRASP) Framework: Evaluation Studies Needed to "Earn" a Grade

Grade	Study Type
C3	Internal Validation of Predictive Performance before Implementation
C2	External Validation of Predictive Performance before Implementation Only Once
C1	External Validation of Predictive Performance before Implementation Multiple Times
B2	Potential Effect Study during Implementation
B1	Usability Study during Implementation
A3	Subjective Studies on Impact after Implementation
A2	Observational Studies on Impact after Implementation
A1	Experimental Studies on Impact after Implementation

methods helps to make them relatively easy to understand. The two main ideas of this section are that (1) the choice of method should fit the question and (2) multiple methods are commonly used in evaluations.

Conclusions of both research and evaluation should be logically and factually sound (validity) and produce similar results if repeated (reliability). Fig. 5.8 illustrates concepts of validity and reliability. While some researchers have denied the need for high validity and reliability in qualitative research, the qualitative methods community has converged on believing that both qualitative and quantitative methods should lead to valid and reliable conclusions (Morse et al., 2002). Morse argues that for qualitative research, these strategies include "investigator responsiveness, methodological coherence, theoretical sampling, and sampling adequacy, an active analytic stance, and saturation" (Morse et al., 2002).

Collecting evaluation information requires the use of systematic procedures that are useful, understandable, and minimize bias. There are several very good guides to conducting qualitative research for health IT evaluation studies (Patton, 2014). The BioMed Central editors now require authors in most informatics journals to self-evaluate their qualitative articles based on the Relevance, Appropriateness, Transparency, and Soundness (RATS) criteria, which also provides good advice for reporting (Clark, 2003). RATS guidelines are: (1) relevance of the study question, (2) appropriateness of qualitative method, (3) transparency of procedures, and (4) soundness of interpretive approach (Clark, 2003).

Study Designs

Both quantitative and qualitative designs require a specific plan for sample size, number of repetitive assessments for each case (cross sectional vs. longitudinal), and sampling methodology (e.g., systematics sampling, representative sampling) (Patton, 2014). Both qualitative and quantitative studies could be observational or experimental, depending on whether the researchers are manipulating the subject's conditions.

Quantitative designs range from observational studies to randomized controlled experimental trials. The study designs presented in this chapter may be particularly useful for health IT and clinical settings. Each of these designs takes advantage of the conditions that are commonly found in health IT projects, including automatically collected data, the ubiquitous use of pre-post design, and outcome-based targets for interventions. Readers may find other quasi-experimental research designs useful for health IT research in the comprehensive textbook by Shadish and colleagues (Shadish et al., 2002).

Qualitative study design is a plan for performing a naturalistic inquiry. In contrast with quantitative study designs, qualitative study designs are often emergent and flexible (Patton, 2014). Evaluation studies using qualitative methods tend to be more applied as the findings are useful and interpretable. Interested parties are usually targeted for enrollment in the study, with small sample sizes of about 12 to 15 participants (Guest, 2006).

Pre-Post Study Design

This study design is very popular because it could be accomplished during the process of implementation. Quality improvements studies are often introduced system-wide to simplify implementation efforts and minimize confusion among providers. These studies gain validity because they repeat themselves in cycles of improvement. However, this study design is the most vulnerable to known and unknown biases.

Interrupted Time Series Analysis

This design is an extension of the simple pre-post format but requires multiple measures prior to and after the introduction of the HIS. Multiple measures help control for trends serve to improve the reliability of the measured effect. Evidence of the impact is found in the differences in mathematical slopes between measures during the pretest and posttest periods. This design has significantly more validity than a simple pre-post one-time measure design and can be very feasible in clinical settings where data collection is automatic. For example, top-level administrators might institute a computerized decision support program to improve patient care for pain management. A straightforward design is to measure the rate of compliance to pain management recommendations during several periods about 12 months before and several periods up to 12 months after implementation, controlling for hospital occupancy, patient acuity, and staffing ratios. This design is highly recommended for health IT implementations where data can be captured electronically and reliably over long periods (Harris et al., 2006; Ramsay et al., 2003).

Randomized Clinical Trials

Randomized controlled trials are considered a gold standard for other health technologies such as pharmaceuticals and medical devices. However, when it comes to health IT, randomized controlled trials are often difficult to administer, as many factors and procedures require strict controls. Adaptive designs can be used as variation an RCT which allows for some factors to change more naturally during an implementation (Mahajan & Gupta, 2010).

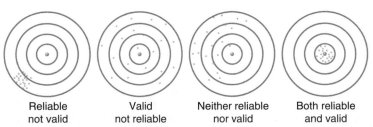

Reliable   Valid   Neither reliable   Both reliable
not valid   not reliable   nor valid   and valid

Fig. 5.8 Possible combinations of validity and reliability of measurement instruments.

Multiple Baseline with Single Subject Design

This design adds significant value to the standard pre-post comparison by staggering implementation systematically (e.g., at 3-month intervals) over many settings while the measurement for *all* settings starts at the same time. In other words, measurement begins at the same time across five clinics, but implementation is staggered every 3 months. Fig. 5.9 illustrates the pattern of responses that might be observed. The strength of the evidence is high if outcomes improve after implementation in each setting and they follow the same pattern (Shadish et al., 2002).

Data Acquisition
Quantitative Data

Quantitative data are commonly gathered by using surveys, direct measurements, and retrieval of EHR data for secondary analysis.

Survey instruments. Constructs of interest could be measured using surveys specifically designed for the project or survey scales which have been developed to work across many projects and previously validated. The advantage of using validated scales is that the results could be compared across multiple studies.

Often, validated scales are aggregated within theoretical perspectives described earlier. For example, the six scales described within UTAUT could be used to measure *perceived usefulness,*

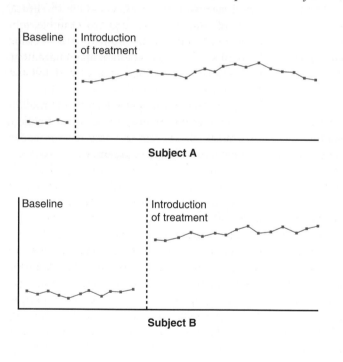

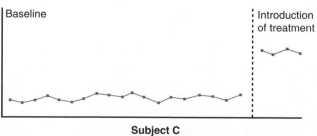

Fig. 5.9 An example of a multiple baseline study design.

social norms and expectations, perceived effort, self-efficacy, ease of use, and *intentions to use* (Venkatesh & Davis, 2000). Reliability for these six scales ranges from 0.92 to 0.95.

A *service quality* (SERVQUAL) survey could be used to measure service quality using five scales that have been thoroughly validated: reliability, assurance, tangibles, empathy, and responsiveness (Pitt et al., 1995). These five scales have been found to have reliability of 0.81 to 0.94.

System usability could be measured using System Usability Scale (SUS), which is widely used outside health IT (Brooke, 1996). It is a 10-item questionnaire applicable to any health IT product. The survey results in a single score ranging from 0 to 100. Bangor et al. endorsed the SUS above other available instruments because it is technologically agnostic (applicable to a variety of products) and easy to administer, and the resulting score is easily interpreted (Bangor et al., 2008). The authors provide a case study of product iterations and corresponding SUS ratings that demonstrate the sensitivity of the SUS to improvements in usability.

Cognitive load could be measured using the NASA Task Load Index (NASA-TLX) scale. The NASA-TLX was developed by Human Performance Group at NASA to measure perceived work load (Hart & Staveland, 1988).

Finally, the Patient Activation Measure (PAM) could be used to measure the degree to which patients take pro-active role in managing their health. The survey results in a single score ranging from 0 to 100. It was developed by Judith Hibbard and colleagues at the University of Oregon (Hibbard et al., 2004).

Direct measurement. Some quantitative data could be directly collected from participants. For example, to access effectiveness of an EHR-based weight maintenance, study evaluators might need to measure participant activity levels using accelerometers, participant weight using scales, and waist circumference using measuring tape.

Software log data. HISs often record in their logs information that could be used in evaluation. Evaluators should check whether important data elements are recorded in the logs before the beginning of the evaluation period. Log data are notoriously difficult to interpret and usually require years of specialized training to process appropriately. However, log data could be successfully used to answer research and evaluation questions about user behavior at scale (Amroze et al., 2019).

Secondary data collection from EHR. The digitization of healthcare leads to aggregation of patient data in the EHRs. This data could be used for analysis of HIS programs. Data analysts could help evaluators to create appropriate data sets from the data warehouse.

Qualitative Data

Qualitative data could be collected through interviews, observations, open-ended surveys, and documents. Qualitative data are usually not intended for transformation into numbers and refer to information in the form of stories, themes, meanings, and metaphors.

Semi-structured interviews. In-person interviews can be some of the best sources of information about an individual's unique perspectives, issues, and values. Interviews vary from a very structured set of questions conducted under controlled conditions to a very informal set of questions asked in an open-ended manner. Typically, evaluators audio-record the interviews and conduct thematic or content coding on the results. For example, user interviews that focus on how health IT affects workflow are especially useful. Some interviews have a specific focus, such as in the critical incident method (Flanagan, 1954). In this method, an individual recalls a critical incident and describes it in detail for the interviewer. In other cases, the interview may focus on the individual's personal perceptions and motivations, such as in motivational interviewing (Miller & Rollnick, 2002). Finally, cognitive task analysis (CTA) is a group of specialized interviews and observations where the goal is to deconstruct a task or work situation into component parts and functions (Hoffman & Militello, 2008; Crandall et al., 2006; Schraagen et al., 2000). A CTA usually consists of targeting a task or work process and having the participant walk through or simulate the actions, identifying the goals, strategies, and information needs.

Observations. An interview may not provide enough information, and, therefore, observing users in action at work is necessary to understand fully the interactions of context, users, and health IT. Observation can take many forms, from using a video camera to using a combination of observation and interview where individuals "think aloud" while they work. The think-aloud procedures need to be analyzed both qualitatively for themes and quantitatively for content, timing, and frequency (Ericsson & Simon, 1993). A related method that is particularly useful for evaluating clinicians is the retrospective think-aloud where the user is videotaped doing their work on the computer without the interruption of having to talk, but then a section is played back to the user and they can then describe their goals and intentions as they watch their own behavior on the screen. This method is integral to user experience evaluations outlined in Chapter 22.

Ethnography and participant observation are derived from the field of anthropology, where the goal is to understand the larger cultural system through observer immersion. The degree of immersion can vary, as can some of the data collection methods, but the overall strategy includes interacting with all aspects of the context. Usually ethnography requires considerable time, multiple observations, interviews, and living and working in the situation if possible. It also includes reading historical documents, exploring artifacts in current use (e.g., memos and minutes), and generally striving to understand a community. These methods are particularly useful in a clinical setting, where understanding the culture is essential (Patton, 2002; Kaplan & Maxwell, 1994).

Less intensive ethnographic methods are also possible and reasonable for health IT evaluations. Focused ethnography is a method of observing actions in a particular context. For example, nurses were observed during patient care handoffs and their interactions with electronic health records were recorded. From these observations, design implications for handoff forms were derived (Staggers et al., 2011, 2012). Another less intensive ethnographic method is Rapid Assessment Method (McMullen et al., 2011). Rapid Assessment Method describes how to plan and conduct intense site visits to inform the design and implementations of HISs (McMullen et al., 2011).

Data Analysis

Quantitative Data Analysis

Two data types often found in evaluation of HISs are *categorical* variables (binary or nominal), such as whether the software was used or not used for a particular case, and *numeric* variables, such as how many times the software was used or the body weight of patients for whom the software was used (interval or ratio data).

Data analysis usually starts with *exploratory analysis*. Evaluators first conduct descriptive analysis by summarizing the participant characteristics and outcomes. Binary data are often summarized using the number of cases and percentages from the whole. For example, in a study of a clinical decision support system for managing neonatal bilirubin levels, 1875 (50%) of newborns in the pre-intervention condition were female (Kawamoto et al., 2019). Continuous data are often summarized using means and 95% confidence intervals (CI). In the same study, mean length of stay for newborns in the pre-intervention period was 3.12 (95% CI: 3.00 to 3.25) (Kawamoto et al., 2019). After the researchers become familiar with the data, they conduct an initial test of association. Association between two binary variables could be explored using a chi-squared test and Fisher exact test. For instance, in the study of the Bilirubin App, there was no statistically significant difference found between mean values of length of stay before and after intervention using chi-squared test ($P = 0.43$). The association between a numeric variable and binary variable could be explored using a t-test and Wilcoxon ranked sum test.

Usually, this simple exploration is followed by a more sophisticated multivariate analysis. For example, in the Bilirubin App study, there was a significant increase in the rate of ordering phototherapy for patients with hyperbilirubinemia based on multivariate regression ($P < .001$) (Kawamoto et al., 2019). We recommend consulting with a statistician before finalizing an analysis. Generalized linear models, such as logistic regression for binary variables and linear regression for continuous variables, are often used to adjust for covariates.

Often the variables which need to be analyzed do not fall into binary or numeric categories. In that case, the evaluator needs to find an appropriate method of analysis. For example, if the evaluator needs to explore connections between people, the Social Network Analysis could be used. As another example, when trying to determine how much utility patients and society receive from a specific program per unit of cost, it might be helpful to conduct a cost-effectiveness analysis. Generalized linear models, social network analysis, and cost-effectiveness analysis are briefly described below.

Generalized linear models. Different forms of generalized linear models, e.g., logistic regression, linear regression, Poisson regression, and gamma regression, are often used to explore associations between variables related to the HISs. Generalized linear models use different distributional assumptions for different types of data. For instance, gamma distribution is especially useful for analyzing length of stay and cost data. Generalized linear models could be implemented using R, SAS, and Stata statistical software.

Social network analysis. Methods that assess the linkages between people, activities, and locations are likely to be very useful for understanding a community and its structure. A social network analysis (SNA) is a general set of tools that calculates the connections between people based on ratings of similarity, frequency of interaction, or some other metric. The resultant pattern of connection is displayed as a visual network of interacting individuals. Each node is an individual, and the lines between nodes reflect the interactions. Although SNA uses numbers to calculate the form of the networked display, it is a qualitative technique because the researcher must interpret the patterns of connections and describe them in narrative form. Conducting an SNA is useful if the goal is to understand how an information system affected communication between individuals. It is also useful for visualizing other connections, such as the relationship between search terms or geographical distances (Durland & Fredericks, 2005). For example, researchers used SNA to examine patient care handoffs from the emergency department to inpatient areas, finding that each handoff entailed 11 to 20 healthcare providers (Benham-Hutchins & Effken, 2010).

Economic evaluation. Economic evaluation includes several types of analysis involving financial outcomes. Economic evaluations attempt to quantify the relative costs and utility of two or more HISs or other conditions such as usual care. Simply measuring additional resources, start-up costs, and labor would be a rudimentary cost analysis. Cost-effectiveness analysis (CEA) is the most common type of economic evaluation. A simple CEA shows a ratio of the cost divided by the change in health outcomes or behavior. For example, a CEA might compare the costs and utility of paying a librarian to answer clinicians' questions versus installing Infobuttons (i.e., an automatic knowledge retrieval tool). Most CEA program evaluations will assess resource use, training, increased staff hiring, and other cost-related information. A full economic analysis requiring a consultation with an economist is not necessarily needed. The specific resources used could be delineated in the logic model, unless it was part of hypothesis testing in a more formal survey. The reader is directed to a helpful textbook if further information is needed (Drummond et al., 2015).

Artificial intelligence-based systems. Evaluation studies shown in Fig. 5.2 could be applied to all types of HISs, from simple clinical reminders to complex systems powered by artificial intelligence (AI). However, each specialized type of HIS would require some modifications to this general approach.

AI-enabled systems are on the more complex end of the spectrum of HISs. AI refers to the ability of information systems to perform intelligent tasks such as reasoning, discovering meaning, generalizing, and learning from experience. In evaluating clinical decision support systems enabled by AI, evaluators should pay attention to the AI design, development, selection, use, and ongoing surveillance (Magrabi et al., 2019). For AI systems, step 4 "technical validation" is more complex compared to simple clinical reminders, incorporating rigorous performance evaluation in a laboratory environment. AI algorithms could be affected by biases in data used for training. Step 10 "technical sustainability assessment" and step 12 "process, clinical, equity, and economic outcomes assessment" are also important for AI to examine effects on the structure, process, and outcome of care delivery. Without rigorous evaluation, AI-driven clinical decision support may fail to deliver on its promise, thus making evaluation a critical step in implementation of AI (Wong et al., 2021). Thus, AI-enabled information systems require continuous evaluation and monitoring to make sure that they are still valid and usable years after development.

Qualitative Data Analysis

Qualitative data consists of audio files, video files, pictures, and notes. Interview audio files could be transcribed using commercial services and imported into qualitative analysis software such as NVivo. There are two approaches to analyzing qualitative data that are really two ends of a continuum: inductive coding and deductive coding. Inductive coding could involve a grounded theory approach (if you are trying to generate a new theory) or an open-ended iterative approach to identify emergent constructs for development of themes (Patton, 2014; Gale et al., 2013). This type of analysis is best done with multiple reviewers of diverse background who have an opportunity to discuss and consensually develop constructs. The process is lengthy, and the product may be a set of themes, metaphors, or stories.

Questions such as "What is the experience of patients with a new symptom tracker?" are best answered using the more inductive approach. In contrast, deductive coding can be used when the constructs are known, such as when using a well-developed theory. Sample questions using this approach could include "What is the nature of social norms or pressure during the implementation process?" Reliability in coding is then more important and is achieved through several iterations of 2 to 3 coders extracting data, assessing agreement, adjusting definitions, and re-coding independently until sufficient agreement is achieved to justify reproducibility. Both can be used with the NVivo software. There are other software tools, such as ATLAS and DEDUCE. CFIR has interview NVivo coding schema available on their website.

Mixed Methods

Quantitative and qualitative methods have their limitations and designs which employ both might be strengthened by combining them in **mixed methods** designs. Such combinations could allow understanding what is happening with the interested parties as well as why it is happening. Evaluation studies increasingly combine qualitative and quantitative methods. Examples of mixed-method designs include Qualitative Comparative Analysis (QCA) (Mattke et al., 2021) and coincidence analysis. In these methods, the content coding derived from the purely qualitative analysis can then be used to "count" constructs across settings or participants. The framework analytic approach proposed by Gale et. al is particularly useful as a first step in these approaches (Gale et al., 2013).

During our work for the University of Utah ReImagine EHR initiative, we often use mixed methods to inform development of interoperable innovations and demonstrate their impact (Kawamoto et al., 2021). For example, we obtained user feedback on a prototype of an app designed to support ambulatory providers managing chronic obstructive pulmonary disease (Curran et al., 2020). Both quantitative and qualitative data were collected during the study. The study found that compared to the EHR alone, the app was associated with improved completion of recommended care (81% vs. 48%, $P < 0.001$), reduced time spent per task, and reduced user frustration (Curran et al., 2020). Analysis of the interviews allowed us to gain a better understanding of the reasons for improved cognitive load, as well as to find areas for improvement of the app (Curran et al., 2020).

CONCLUSION AND FUTURE DIRECTIONS

Evaluation of HISs and programs can range from simple user satisfaction with a new menu to a full-scale analysis of usage, cost, compliance, and patient outcomes. The first step in evaluation is starting with a general theoretical perspective and distilling it to a specific program logic model. Once overall goals and general constructs have been identified, then decisions about measurement and design can be made. In this chapter, evaluation approaches have been framed, focusing on health IT program evaluation, to orient the reader to the resources and opportunities in the evaluation domain. HIS evaluations are typically multidimensional, longitudinal, and complex. HIS interventions and programs present a unique challenge, as they are rarely independent of other factors. Rather, they are usually embedded in a larger program. The challenge is to integrate the goals of the entire program while clarifying the effect and importance of the health IT component. In the future, HIS evaluations should become more theory driven, and the complex nature of evaluations should be acknowledged more readily.

As an HIS becomes integrated at all levels of the information context of an institution, evaluation strategies will necessarily broaden in scope. Outcomes will not only include those related to system effectiveness but also span the whole implementation process. The result will be richer analyses and a deeper understanding of the mechanisms by which HIS has its impact. The incorporation of theory into evaluation will also result in knowledge that is more generalizable and the development of HIS evaluation science. Health practitioners and informaticians will be at the heart of these program evaluations because of their central place in healthcare, IT, and informatics departments.

DISCUSSION QUESTIONS

1. Of the levels of theory discussed in this chapter, what level would be most appropriate for evaluation of electronic health records? Would the level of theory be different if the intervention was for an application targeting a new referral system in a clinic? Why?
2. Assume that you are conducting an evaluation of a new preventative alert targeting primary care providers. What kind of designs would you use in this evaluation study?
3. Using the life cycle as a framework, explain when and why you would use a formative or summative evaluation approach.
4. Review the following article: Harris, A. D., McGregor, J. C., Perencevich, E. N., Furuno, J. P., Zhu, J., Peterson, D. E., et al. (2006). The use and interpretation of quasi-experimental studies in medical informatics. *Journal of the American Medical Informatics Association, 13*(1), 16–23. Explain how you might apply these research designs in structuring a program evaluation.

CASE STUDY

A 410-bed hospital has used a homegrown provider order-entry system for 5 years. Leaders recently decided to put in bar code administration software to scan medications at the time of delivery to decrease medical error. The administration is concerned about medication errors; top-level administration is concerned about meeting the Joint Commission accreditation standards; and the IT department is worried that the scanners may not be reliable and may break, increasing their costs. The plan is to have a scanner in each patient's room; nurses will scan the medication when they get to the room and scan their own badges and the patient's armband. The application makes it possible to print out a list of the patients with their scan patterns, and the nurses sometimes carry this printout because patients' armbands can be difficult to locate or because nurses do not want to disturb patients while they are sleeping. The bar code software was purchased from a vendor, and the facility has spent about a year refining it. The IT department is responsible for implementation and has decided that it will implement each of the four inpatient settings one at a time at 6-month intervals.

The hospital administration wants to conduct an evaluation study. You are assigned to be the lead on the evaluation.

Discussion Questions
1. What is the key evaluation question for this project?
2. Who are the interested parties (stakeholders)?
3. What level of theory is most appropriate at each phase?
4. What are specific elements to measure?

REFERENCES

Agarwal, R., & Prasad, J. (1998). A conceptual and operational definition of personal innovativeness in the domain of information technology. *Information Systems Research, 9*(2), 204–215. https://doi.org/10.1287/isre.9.2.204.

Ainsworth, L., & Viegut, D. (2006). *Common formative assessments.* Thousand Oaks, CA: Corwin Press.

Ammenwerth, E., Brender, J., Nykänen, P., Prokosch, H. U., Rigby, M., & Talmon, J. (2004). Visions and strategies to improve evaluation of health information systems: Reflections and lessons based on the HIS-EVAL workshop in Innsbruck. *International Journal of Medical Informatics, 73*(6), 479–491. https://doi.org/10.1016/J.IJMEDINF.2004.04.004.

Ammenwerth, E. (2015). Evidence-based health informatics: How do we know what we know. *Methods of Information in Medicine, 54*(4), 298–307. https://doi.org/10.3414/ME14-01-0119.

Amroze, A., Field, T. S., Fouayzi, H., et al. (2019). Use of electronic health record access and audit logs to identify physician actions following noninterruptive alert opening: Descriptive study. *JMIR Medical Informatics, 7*(1). https://doi.org/10.2196/12650.

Bandura, A. (1989). Human agency in social cognitive theory. *American Psychologist Journal, 44*(9), 1175–1184. https://doi.org/10.1037/0003-066X. 44.9.1175.

Bangor, A., Kortum, P. T., & Miller, J. T. (2008). An empirical evaluation of the system usability scale. *International Journal of Human-Computer Interaction, 24*(6), 574–594. https://doi.org/10.1080/10447310802205776.

Benham-Hutchins, M. M., & Effken, J. A. (2010). Multi-professional patterns and methods of communication during patient handoffs. *International Journal of Medical Informatics, 79*(4), 252–267. https://doi.org/10.1016/j.ijmedinf.2009.12.005.

Brender, J. (2006). *Handbook of evaluation methods for health informatics.* Elsevier.

Brooke, J. A. (1996). "Quick and dirty" usability scale. In P. W. Jordan, B. Thomas, B. A. Weerdmeester, & I. L. McClelland (Eds.), *Usability Evaluation in Industry* (1st ed., pp. 189–195). London: Taylor & Francis. https://cui.unige.ch/isi/icle-wiki/_media/ipm:test-suschapt.pdf.

Clark, J. (2003). How to peer review a qualitative manuscript. In T. Jefferson & F. Godlee (Eds.), *Peer Review in Health Sciences* (2nd ed., pp. 219–235). London: BMJ Books.

Cooper, R. B., & Zmud, R. W. (1990). Information technology implementation research: A technological diffusion approach. *Management Science, 36*(2), 123–139. https://doi.org/10.1287/mnsc.36.2.123.

Crandall, B., Klein, G. A., & Hoffman, R. R. (2006). *Working minds. A practitioner's guide to cognitive task analysis* (1st ed.). MIT Press: MIT Press.

Cresswell, K., Williams, R., & Sheikh, A. (2020). Developing and applying a formative evaluation framework for health information technology implementations: Qualitative investigation. *Journal of Medical Internet Research, 22*(6), e15068. https://doi.org/10.2196/15068.

Curran, R. L., Kukhareva, P. V., Taft, T., et al. (2020). Integrated displays to improve chronic disease management in ambulatory care: A SMART on FHIR application informed by mixed-methods user testing. *Journal of the American Medical Informatics Association, 27*(8), 1225–1234. https://doi.org/10.1093/jamia/ocaa099.

Currie, L. M. (2005). Evaluation frameworks for nursing informatics. *International Journal of Medical Informatics, 74*(11-12), 908–916. https://doi.org/10.1016/j.ijmedinf.2005.07.007.

Damschroder, L. J., Aron, D. C., Keith, R. E., Kirsh, S. R., Alexander, J. A., & Lowery, J. C. (2009). Fostering implementation of health services research findings into practice: a consolidated framework for advancing implementation science. *Implementation Science, 4*(1), 50. https://doi.org/10.1186/1748-5908-4-50.

DeLone, W. H., & McLean, E. R. (2016). *Information Systems Success Measurement.* Now Publishers Inc. http://doi.org/10.1561/2900000005.

DeLone, W. H., & McLean, E. R. (2003). The DeLone and McLean model of information systems success: A ten-year update. *Journal of Management Information Systems, Vol 19,* 9–30. https://doi.org/10.1080/07421222.2003.11045748. M.E. Sharpe Inc.

Deming, W. E. (1982). *Out of the crisis.* Massachusetts Institute of Technology.

Donabedian, A. (1988). The quality of care. How can it be assessed? *JAMA The Journal of the American Medical Association, 260*(12), 1743–1748. https://doi.org/10.1001/ jama.260.12.1743.

Drummond, M. F., Sculpher, M. J., Claxton, K., Stoddart, G. L., & Torrance, G. W. (2015). *Methods for the economic evaluation of health care programmes* (4th ed.). Oxford: Oxford University Press.

Durland, M., Fredericks, K. (Eds.). (2005). New directions in evaluation: Social network analysis. Hoboken, NJ: Jossey-Bass/AEA.

Endsley, M. R., & Garland, D. J. (Eds.). (2000). *Situation awareness analysis and measurement.* Mahwah, NJ: Lawrence Erlbaum Associates, Inc.

Ericsson, K., & Simon, H. (1993). *Protocol analysis: Verbal reports as data* (Rev. ed.). Cambridge, MA: MIT Press.

Eslami Andargoli, A., Scheepers, H., Rajendran, D., & Sohal, A. (2017). Health information systems evaluation frameworks: A systematic review. *International Journal of Medical Informatics, 97,* 195–209. https://doi.org/10.1016/j.ijmedinf.2016.10.008.

Fetterman, D. (2001). *Foundations of empowerment evaluation.* Thousand Oaks, CA: SAGE.

Fishbein, M., & Ajzen, I. (1975). *Belief, attitude, intention, and behavior: An introduction to theory and research.* Reading, MA: Addison-Wesley.

Flanagan, J. C. (1954). The critical incident technique. *Psychological Bulletin Journal, 51*(4), 327–358. https://doi.org/10.1037/h0061470.

Fox, J., & Thomson, R. (2002). Clinical decision support systems: A discussion of quality, safety and legal liability issues. *Proceedings of the AMIA Symposium,* 265–269. https://pubmed.ncbi.nlm.nih.gov/12463828/. Accessed October 8, 2020.

Gale, N., Heath, G., Cameron, E., Rashid, S., & Redwood, S. (2013). Using the framework method for the analysis of qualitative data in multi-disciplinary health research. *BMC Medical Research Methodology, 13*(1). https://doi.org/10.1186/1471-2288-13-117.

Glasgow, R. E., Vogt, T. M., & Boles, S. M. (1999). Evaluating the public health impact of health promotion interventions: the RE-AIM framework. *American Journal of Public Health, 89*(9), 1322–1327. https://doi.org/10.2105/ajph.89.9.1322.

Godinho, M. A., Ansari, S., Guo, G. N., & Liaw, S.-T. (February 2021). Toolkits for implementing and evaluating digital health: A systematic review of rigor and reporting. *Journal of the American Medical Informatics Association,* https://doi.org/10.1093/jamia/ocab010.

Guest, G. (2006). How many interviews are enough?: An experiment with data saturation and variability. *Field Methods, 18*(1), 59–82. https://doi.org/10.1177/1525822X05279903.

Harris, A. D., McGregor, J. C., Perencevich, E. N., et al. (2006). The use and interpretation of quasi-experimental studies in medical informatics. *Journal of the American Medical Informatics Association, 13*(1), 16–23. https://doi.org/10.1197/jamia.M1749.

Hart, S. G., & Staveland, L. E. (1988). Development of NASA-TLX (Task Load Index): Results of empirical and theoretical research. *Advances in Psychology, 52*(C), 139–183. https://doi.org/10.1016/S0166-4115(08)62386-9.

Hibbard, J. H., Stockard, J., Mahoney, E. R., & Tusler, M. (2004). Development of the patient activation measure (PAM): Conceptualizing and measuring activation in patients and consumers. *Health Services Research, 39*(4 Pt 1), 1005. https://doi.org/10.1111/J.1475-6773.2004.00269.X.

Hoffman, R., & Militello, L. (2008). *Perspectives on cognitive task analysis.* New York, NY: Psychology Press/Taylor and Francis Group.

Kaplan, B., & Maxwell, J. (1994). Qualitative research methods for evaluating computer information systems. In J. Anderson, C. Aydin, & S. Jay (Eds.), *Evaluating Health Care Information Systems: Approaches and Applications* (pp. 45–68). Thousand Oaks, CA: SAGE.

Karahanna, E., Straub, D. W., & Chervany, N. L. (1999). Information technology adoption across time: A cross-sectional comparison of pre-adoption and post-adoption beliefs. *Management Information Systems Quarterly, 23*(2), 183–213. https://doi.org/10.2307/249751.

Kawamoto, K., Kukhareva, P. V., Shakib, J. H., et al. (2019). Association of an electronic health record add-on app for neonatal bilirubin management with physician efficiency and care quality. *JAMA Network Open, 2*(11), e1915343. https://doi.org/10.1001/jamanetworkopen.2019.15343.

Kawamoto, K., Kukhareva, P. V., Weir, C. R., et al. (2021). Establishing a multidisciplinary initiative for interoperable electronic health record innovations at an academic medical center. *JAMIA Open, 4*(3), 1–15. https://doi.org/10.1093/JAMIAOPEN/OOAB041.

Kerlinger, F. N., & Lee, H. B. (1999). *Foundations of behavioral research* (4th ed.). Wadsworth Publishing.

Khalifa, M., Magrabi, F., & Gallego, B. (2019). Developing a framework for evidence-based grading and assessment of predictive tools for clinical decision support. *BMC Medical Informatics and Decision Making, 19*(1). https://doi.org/10.1186/s12911-019-0940-7.

Khalifa, M., Magrabi, F., & Luxan, B. G. (2020). Evaluating the impact of the grading and assessment of predictive tools framework on clinicians and health care professionals' decisions in selecting clinical predictive tools: Randomized controlled trial. *Journal of Medical Internet Research, 22*(7). https://doi.org/10.2196/15770.

Klein, G. (1997). An overview of natural decision making applications. In C. E. Zsambok & G. Klein (Eds.), *Naturalistic Decision Making.* Mahwah, NJ: Lawrence Erlbaum Associates, Inc.

Koch, S. H., Weir, C., Haar, M., et al. (2012). Intensive care unit nurses' information needs and recommendations for integrated displays to improve nurses' situation awareness. *Journal of the American Medical Informatics Association, 19*(4), 583–590. https://doi.org/10.1136/amiajnl-2011-000678.

Koch, S. H., Weir, C., Westenskow, D., et al. (2013). Evaluation of the effect of information integration in displays for ICU nurses on situation awareness and task completion time: A prospective randomized controlled study. *International Journal of Medical Informatics, 82*(8), 665–675. https://doi.org/10.1016/j.ijmedinf.2012.10.002.

Kukhareva, P. V., Warner, P., Rodriguez, S., et al. (January 2019). Balancing functionality versus portability for SMART on FHIR applications: Case study for a neonatal bilirubin management application. *AMIA Annual Symposium Proceedings*, 562–571.

Kukhareva, P., Weir, C., Del Fiol, G., et al. (2022). Evaluation in Life Cycle of Information Technology (ELICIT) Framework: Supporting the innovation life cycle from business case assessment to summative evaluation. *Journal of Biomedical Informatics, 127*(1532-0480), 104014. https://doi.org/10.1016/J.JBI.2022.104014.

Kushniruk A. W., & Patel, V. L. (2004). Cognitive and usability engineering methods for the evaluation of clinical information systems. *Journal of Biomedical Informatics, 37,* 56. https://doi.org/10.1016/j.jbi.2004.01.003

Liu, S., Reese, T. J., Kawamoto, K., Del Fiol, G., & Weir, C. (2021). A systematic review of theoretical constructs in CDS literature. *BMC Medical Informatics and Decision Making, 211, 21*(1), 1–9. https://doi.org/10.1186/S12911-021-01465-2.

Logic Model Development Guide. (2004). *Using logic models to bring together planning, evaluation, and action.* Battle Creek, Michigan: W.K. Kellogg Foundation.

Luce, B. R., Drummond, M., Jönsson, B., et al. (2010). EBM, HTA, and CER: Clearing the confusion. *The Milbank Quarterly, 88*(2), 256–276. https://doi.org/10.1111/j.1468-0009.2010.00598.x.

Magrabi, F., Ammenwerth, E., McNair, J. B., et al. (2019). Artificial intelligence in clinical decision support: Challenges for evaluating AI and practical implications. *Yearbook of Medical Informatics, 28*(1), 128–134. https://doi.org/10.1055/s-0039-1677903.

Mahajan, R., & Gupta, K. (2010). Adaptive design clinical trials: Methodology, challenges and prospect. *Indian Journal of Pharmacology, 42*(4), 201–207. https://doi.org/10.4103/0253-7613.68417.

Mattke, J., Maier, C., Weitzel, T., & Thatcher, J. B. (2021). Qualitative comparative analysis in the information systems discipline: A literature review and methodological recommendations. *Internet Research* https://doi.org/10.1108/intr-09-2020-0529. ahead-of-print(ahead-of-print).

May, C., & Finch, T. (2009). Implementing, embedding, and integrating practices: An outline of normalization process theory. *Sociology, 43*(3), 535–554. https://doi.org/10.1177/0038038509103208.

McCoy, A. B., Thomas, E. J., Krousel-Wood, M., & Sittig, D. F. (2014). Clinical decision support alert appropriateness: a review and proposal for improvement. *Ochsner Journal, 14*(2), 195–202.

McMullen, C. K., Ash, J. S., Sittig, D. F., et al. (2011). Rapid assessment of clinical information systems in the healthcare setting. *Methods of Information Medicine, 50*(4), 299–307. https://doi.org/10.3414/ME10-01-0042.

Miller, W., & Rollnick, S. (2002). *Motivational interviewing: Preparing people to change* (2nd ed.). New York, NY: Guilford Press.

Morse, J. M., Barrett, M., Mayan, M., Olson, K., & Spiers, J. (2002). Verification Strategies for Establishing Reliability and Validity in Qualitative Research. *International Journal of Qualitative Methods, 1*(2), 13–22. https://doi.org/10.1177/160940690200100202.

Neame, M. T., Sefton, G., Roberts, M., Harkness, D., Sinha, I. P., & Hawcutt, D. B. (2020). Evaluating health information technologies: A systematic review of framework recommendations. *International Journal of Medical Informatics, 142,* 104247.

Patton, M. Q. (2002). *Qualitative research & evaluation methods* (3rd ed.). Thousand Oaks, California: SAGE Publications.

Patton, M. Q. (2014). *Qualitative research & evaluation methods* (4th ed.). SAGE Publications, Inc.

Pitt, L. F., Watson, R. T., & Kavan, C. B. (1995). Service quality: A measure of information systems effectiveness. *MIS Quarterly: Management Information Systems, 19*(2), 173–185. https://doi.org/10.2307/249687.

Ramsay, C. R., Matowe, L., Grilli, R., Grimshaw, J. M., & Thomas, R. E. (2003). Interrupted time series designs in health technology assessment: Lessons from two systematic reviews of behavior change strategies. *International Journal of Technology Assessment in Health Care, 19*(4), 613–623. https://doi.org/10.1017/S0266462303000576.

Rogers, E. (1983). *Diffusion of innovations*. New York, NY: Free Press.

Ruparelia, N. B. (2010). Software development lifecycle models. *ACM SIGSOFT Software Engineering Notes, 35*(3), 8–13. https://doi.org/10.1145/1764810.1764814.

Schraagen, J., Chipman, S., & Shalin, V. (2000). *Cognitive task analysis*. Mahway, NJ: Lawrence Erlbaum Associates.

Shadish, W., Cook, T., & Campbell, D. (2002). *Experimental and quasi-experimental designs for generalized causal inference*. Boston, MA: Houghton Mifflin.

Sittig, D. F., & Singh, H. (2010). A new sociotechnical model for studying health information technology in complex adaptive healthcare systems. *Quality & Safety in Health Care, 19*(Suppl 3), i68. https://doi.org/10.1136/qshc.2010.042085. Suppl 3.

Staggers, N., Clark, L., Blaz, J. W., & Kapsandoy, S. (2012). Nurses' information management and use of electronic tools during acute care handoffs. *Western Journal of Nursing Research, 34*(2), 153–173. https://doi.org/10.1177/0193945911407089.

Staggers, N., Clark, L., Blaz, J. W., & Kapsandoy, S. (2011). Why patient summaries in electronic health records do not provide the cognitive support necessary for nurses' handoffs on medical and surgical units: Insights from interviews and observations. *Health Informatics Journal, 17*(3), 209–223. https://doi.org/10.1177/1460458211405809.

Venkatesh, V., & Davis, F. D. (2000). Theoretical extension of the Technology Acceptance Model: Four longitudinal field studies. *Management Science, 46*(2), 186–204. https://doi.org/10.1287/mnsc.46.2.186.11926.

Venkatesh, V., Morris, M. G., Davis, G. B., & Davis, F. D. (2003). User acceptance of information technology: Toward a unified view. *MIS Quarterly, 27*(3), 425–478. https://www.jstor.org/stable/30036540.

Vis, C., Bührmann, L., Riper, H., & Ossebaard, H. C. (2020). Health technology assessment frameworks for eHealth: A systematic review. *International Journal of Technology Assessment in Health Care, 36*(3), 204–216. https://doi.org/10.1017/S026646232000015X.

Wong, A., Otles, E., Donnelly, J. P., et al. (2021, June). External validation of a widely implemented proprietary sepsis prediction model in hospitalized patients. *JAMA Internal Medicine, 181*(8), 1065–1070. https://doi.org/10.1001/JAMAINTERNMED.2021.2626.

Wright, A., Sittig, D. F., Ash, J. S., et al. (2011). Development and evaluation of a comprehensive clinical decision support taxonomy: Comparison of front-end tools in commercial and internally developed electronic health record systems. *Journal of the American Medical Informatics Association, 18*(3), 232–242. https://doi.org/10.1136/amiajnl-2011-000113.

Wright, A., & Sittig, D. F. (2008). A framework and model for evaluating clinical decision support architectures. *Journal of Biomedical Informatics, 41*(6), 982–990. https://doi.org/10.1016/j.jbi.2008.03.009.

Yusof, M. M., Kuljis, J., Papazafeiropoulou, A., & Stergioulas, L. K. (2008). An evaluation framework for Health Information Systems: human, organization and technology-fit factors (HOT-fit). *International Journal of Medical Informatics, 77*(6), 386–398. https://doi.org/10.1016/j.ijmedinf.2007.08.011.

Yusof, M. M., Papazafeiropoulou, A., Paul, R. J., & Stergioulas, L. K. (2008). Investigating evaluation frameworks for health information systems. *International Journal of Medical Informatics, 77*(6), 377–385. https://doi.org/10.1016/J.IJMEDINF.2007.08.004.

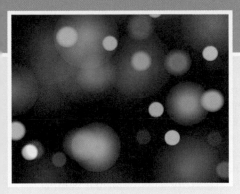

6

Technical Infrastructure

Lisa M. Blair

A sound understanding of the technical attributes of healthcare IT infrastructure, including networking and data security principles, is essential for readers seeking to understand healthcare informatics.

OBJECTIVES

At the completion of this chapter, the reader will be prepared to:
1. Describe how the primary components of healthcare IT infrastructure interrelate.
2. Discuss key components of EHR functionality.
3. Summarize how IT infrastructure enhances quality improvement and patient safety in healthcare.
4. Summarize emerging threats and challenges to healthcare infrastructure.

KEY TERMS

21st Century Cures Act, 87
architecture, 86
central storage, 89
clinical data repository (CDR), 87
clinical decision support tools, 91
cloud, 86
Cures 2.0 Act, 87
cyber security, 91
data life cycle, 87
data sharing networks, 90
data standardization, 89
distributed storage, 89
ehealth exchange, 91

electronic health record (EHR), 87
electronic medical record (EMR), 87
encryption, 92
Genetic Information Discrimination Act (GINA), 86
hardware, 86
Health Information Exchange (HIE), 91
Health Information Organization (HIO), 91
health information portability and accountability act (HIPAA), 86
HITECH Act, 87

infrastructure, 86
interoperability, 89
intranet, 90
master person index (MPI), 90
mobile devices, 86
network, 86
phishing, 92
ransomware, 92
Regional Health Information Organization (RHIO), 91
software 86
thin client, 86
workstation, 86

ABSTRACT ❖

This chapter introduces the concepts of information technology (IT) infrastructure, also called IT architecture, and the life cycle of clinical and administrative healthcare data. Electronic health records (EHRs) and electronic medical records (EMRs) will be discussed in addition to historical and recent developments in infrastructure to support clinical decision-making, research and data access, data processing, data security, and other critical components of quality improvement and enhanced patient safety. Legal and regulatory requirements of healthcare IT and emerging threats and challenges are discussed.

INTRODUCTION

Legal and regulatory requirements and decision-making within healthcare organizations about information technology (IT) infrastructure have important downstream consequences for the care that is delivered to patients at the bedside, clinic, or other points of access. An understanding of the basic components of IT infrastructure is critical to enable informaticists to advocate for and successfully implement systemic adaptations and improvements to empower clinicians, researchers, and patients. In this chapter, you will learn about IT infrastructure and systems that support healthcare informatics, as well as emerging threats to healthcare IT security.

INTRODUCTION TO HEALTHCARE INFORMATION TECHNOLOGY INFRASTRUCTURE

Healthcare IT infrastructure, sometimes called architecture, refers to all components required to operate and manage IT services and environments within a healthcare setting. Traditionally, these components were managed on-site and/or in combination with local data warehouses. Recent trends in IT have increasingly relied on remote components, such as servers and data storage systems that process and store data at great distances or even dispersed over wide networks of computers housed in many different locations. These remote systems are often collectively referred to as "the cloud."

Key Components Defined

Modern healthcare IT is made possible by the meteoric advancement in complexity and functional capacity of computing systems since the development of the first computers in the 1940s. A common lexicon of terms is required to form an understanding of how healthcare IT infrastructure powers much of what we do today. Yet IT is a new field and terminology, components, and ideas continue to rapidly evolve. Here, we identify common and useful terms that will provide a basic language through which infrastructure can be discussed.

Hardware—the collective physical components of computing systems—has changed dramatically, growing smaller in scale and orders of magnitude more powerful. Hardware components may include processors, controller cards, cabling, cooling systems (e.g., fans or heat sinks), power supplies, cases, and display screens. Other specialized components may be integrated depending on the purpose of the individual computing system (e.g., biometric scanners). Required hardware differs between servers or computers that act as central hubs to process and/or store information and computers that users interact with directly. In addition, the term hardware can be used to describe whole physical units within a larger computing network; these individual units may include such things as workstations (computers that connect to a central hub where data is stored and processed), laptops, tablets, servers, data storage devices, networking equipment, and more.

In clinical settings, there are two primary types of hardware that users directly interact with: workstations and thin clients. Workstations—thick clients—are computers that receive input from users, process and store data, and can function independently of a network. Examples in everyday life include desktop or laptop computers. Thin clients, alternatively, may or may not have traditional workstation capabilities; what sets them apart is that their primary work is not done internally. Rather, thin clients connect to servers that store and process data via a network

to request access or make changes to databases. Thin clients are useful in healthcare IT because they enable greater connectivity and real-time access to patient data while providing enhanced data protection. Because no patient information is stored on the local device, physical theft or destruction of a thin client will not result in loss of confidentiality to patients or data loss. Mobile devices other than laptops (e.g., tablets, smartphones, insulin pumps) may use internal or external processing capabilities. These devices often feature stripped-down operating systems and/or applications, and may serve limited functions.

Servers are powerful centralized computing systems. Users must interact with a connected workstation or thin client to access data, and run processes on servers. Servers often require more resources than workstations or thin clients, including orders of magnitude more electricity, environmental cooling capacity, and physical space. Thus, servers are typically housed in secured locations that are remote from the places where users interact with the data and processing capacity. Servers literally "serve up" webpages to browsers or data to applications. In healthcare IT, servers are used for data storage and processing.

Computers may be connected via networks to access remote systems. Networks are collections of computing systems (workstations, thin clients, and servers) that share resources such as data storage or processing power. When a computer connects to the network, it is connecting to a shared space comprised of two or more computing systems (workstations, thin clients, or servers). Networked applications send and request data from servers or other clients.

While hardware forms the physical foundations for computing systems, software is required for computing systems to be functional, and perform the job of storing, processing, retrieving, and displaying information. Software refers to the encoded programs that direct and control how computers function. The major classifications of software include operating systems and applications. Operating systems, such as MacOS, Windows, LINUX, and Android, provide the base for a wide range of computer functions, and act as oversight for applications. All computing systems must have an operating system for baseline functionality, although this may vary widely between workstations. Applications are typically smaller programs that serve individual or integrated functions. One example is a word-processing program that allows text entry, formatting, and printing. In healthcare, one of the primary applications of interest is the software that maintains, stores, processes, and displays patient data.

Legal and Regulatory Considerations

Unlike much of the computing environment for personal use, healthcare IT is strictly regulated by laws in many countries. In the United States, patient data is considered private and confidential. Healthcare entities (including most healthcare providers, health insurance plans, and healthcare clearinghouses) are legally required to safeguard confidentiality and accuracy of data, regardless of how that data is stored. This poses specific challenges to the implementation and administration of healthcare IT.

Furthermore, federal laws such as the Health Information Portability and Accountability Act (HIPAA) and Genetic

Information Discrimination Act (GINA) are two of the many regulations that place specific legal burdens on providers regarding what they may and may not do with data, including the establishment of legal rights of patients to access data themselves, and permit or deny access to others. Under HIPAA, healthcare entities that transmit data are known as "covered entities" and as such are required to meet stringent criteria for data accuracy and security. Similarly, GINA places restrictions on who can access and act on genetic information, a measure put in place to prevent employers and health insurers from discriminating against individuals who have identified genetic risk factors for disease but have not yet manifested symptoms.

Additionally, the 2009 legislation known as the HITECH Act established a requirement that data be shared as electronic health records (EHRs). Reimbursement for services provided to the major US governmental health insurance payer, the Centers for Medicare & Medicaid Services, is tied to healthcare providers and other organizations having, and making meaningful use of electronic systems for recording, storing, processing, utilizing, protecting, and sharing patient data (Centers for Medicare and Medicaid Services, 2010). Such incentives and restrictions necessitate that healthcare IT infrastructure is designed to purpose and strictly controlled.

More recently, the 21st Century Cures Act was passed in 2016 with the goals of accelerating medical product development and enhancing innovations in healthcare. This act goes further than product development and innovation, however. The Office of the National Coordinator (ONC) for Health Information Technology has developed a Cures Act Final Rule to support "seamless and secure access, exchange, and use of electronic health information." (HealthIT.gov, 2021a)

Federal legislative efforts continue to reshape and guide the direction of healthcare services and healthcare IT infrastructure. In 2021, bipartisan legislators in the House of Representatives unveiled a discussion draft of a bill known as the Cures 2.0 Act (Wagner, 2021). If passed in its current form, this act would improve and continue to modernize healthcare delivery and access, authorize the establishment of an agency within the National Institutes of Health, integrate caregivers (typically family members of an ill person) as members of the patient care team, and increase telehealth and genetic testing access.

Introduction to the Data Life Cycle

One of the primary purposes of HIPAA and GINA, among other regulatory efforts, is the protection of confidential patient data and individually identifiable health information. Thus, another concept that must be explored to understand the effect of these protections is the data life cycle. To be useful to healthcare providers and patients (e.g., individuals, families, and communities who need health services), data must not just exist but be usable. Attention to the data life cycle ensures that data can be retrieved and turned into knowledge that prompts action. The data life cycle refers to the eight steps commonly taken in all data-based projects to turn data into actionable knowledge. The eight steps of the data life cycle for general use are: (1) generation, (2) collection, (3) processing, (4) storage, (5) management,

(6) analysis, (7) visualization, and (8) interpretation (Stobrierski, 2021). Additionally, data stored in EHRs requires consideration of a ninth step—sharing (Fig. 6.1).

ELECTRONIC HEALTH RECORDS

Electronic Medical Records and Electronic Health Records

In modern healthcare IT settings, patient data is collected, stored, used, and protected within two basic types of applications: the electronic health record (EHR) and the electronic medical record (EMR). While these terms are often used interchangeably, there are important differences between the two (HealthIT.gov, 2011).

EMRs consist of all the documentation for a single patient at a single location; they are roughly equivalent to what would have once appeared in a paper "chart" for a patient, and include extensive individually identifiable health records. In addition to the function of paper charts, however, EMRs can be used to automatically track follow-up needs and preventive services delivery windows and trend data, such as blood pressure or weight, across visits, and support clinician decision-making using integrated clinical support tools.

EHRs can accomplish all functions of EMRs and much more. Rather than focusing only on patient data generated by clinicians at one location, EHRs are designed to extend the data through sharing with other providers and even across institutions. Furthermore, EHRs incorporate the entire care team, including the patients themselves and (with appropriate caution regarding privacy and regulatory compliance) their families or caregivers.

The widespread adoption of EMRs and, later, EHRs throughout the healthcare system in the United States has been heavily influenced by legislation creating financial incentives to providers to have "meaningful use" of EHRs within their organizations (Centers for Medicare and Medicaid Services, 2010). Meaningful use is a multi-stage plan for improving quality and safety in healthcare by leveraging IT.

Data Collection, Processing, and Storage

The clinical data repository (CDR) is the storage component for patient clinical records. Data stored in a repository may include lab results, medication orders, vital signs, and clinical documentation as well as demographic data, financial information, patient survey or reported outcomes data, historical data on individual health or family medical events, and more. The data may be stored as free text (i.e., unstructured documents) or coded and structured elements that can be analyzed and visualized using additional application components or software. Data within the repository are considered the most essential aspect of the EHR: Without these data, the other components of the EHR are meaningless. Therefore, important aspects of the repository include accessibility, reliability, and security.

Accessibility means the ability to efficiently retrieve data stored within the repository. The repository must provide access methods that allow users of the repository to find information using criteria that are meaningful to the users. For example, the

1. Generation

- Data are generated by the patient and may include demographics, physiological or psychological parameters, family and personal health history, and any other information relevant to human health or the healthcare process (e.g., insurance information)

2. Collection

- Data are collected by patients, clinicians, or equipment and entered into the electronic medical record (EMR) in the form of documentation, assessments, surveys, images or photographs, lab and test results, and more. Some devices, such as insulin pumps, may automatically upload data to the EMR when networked
- Data may also be collected via transfer from outside organizations, providers or institutions in the case of linked electronic health records (EHR)

3. Processing

- Data are processed by the software into a format that can be stored electronically and transfered into a database for storage and further processing
- This may include converting fields in an EMR/EHR record into a format recognizable by the database into which it will be inserted, or even digitizing paper documents via scanning
- Once entered, data may be compressed for more efficient storage and retrieval or encrypted

4. Storage

- Healthcare data are typically stored in databases
- Databases, in turn, are stored either in the workstation or on remote servers (best practice) that enable users to upload and download information through the EMR/EHR application and/or using database query tools
- Legal requirements ensure that data are stored securely to protect patient confidentiality

5. Management

- Data management is a complex, ongoing process requiring balancing between ease of access to enable use of the data and strict control over data integrity
- EMR and EHR data is considered legal documentation
- Managers of healthcare data are legally required to protect data integrity and to enable records to be audited for legal purposes. This often includes time stamping entry, making data read-only to prevent tampering or alteration, and logging who has entered or interacted with the data, when, and in what ways

6. Analysis

- A single patient's data may be accessed to enable care provision and analyzed individually
- Data from many patients may be aggregated and analyzed to enable tracking of trend data across the healthcare system, inlcuding safety and quality assessmments, quality improvement initiatives, or (with ethical approval) anonymized research projects

7. Visualization

- Patient data can be used to create visuals such as graphs to enable quick identification of trends
- Aggregated data may also be visualized to enable identification of trends in outcomes over time or across patient populations, clincians, or clinical units

8. Interpretation

- Interpretation of data may lead to action at individual, organizational, or even national levels though development of patient care plans, facilitation of safety and quality improvement, and development of policies to guide practice or regulation

9. Sharing

- Data are shared between providers and healthcare entities to enable EHRs to contain a comprehensive record of patient data
- Patients have a legal right to review, correct, share, or restrict access to individually identifiable health information/data and safeguards must be in place to prevent unauthorized sharing or access

Fig. 6.1 Healthcare data life cycle.

repository should be able to distinguish data belonging to one patient from that belonging to another based on patient characteristics, such as a patient identifier or an encounter number. Data should also be classified by type, such as lab results, medications, and allergies, to permit easy and quick retrieval of a specific category of data. Data must also be retrievable by the time period in which it was generated, so a picture of current health may be distinguished from historical data. Other important data attributes that help with accessibility include data owners and entry personnel (e.g., ordering physician, charting nurse, and case manager) and location of service or data entry. The access methods for the repository should be robust enough to support current and future users' access needs.

Data Standardization

Data standards must be upheld so that data are able to be processed in a meaningful way. For example, storing blood pressure data in a free-text field eliminates the ability of the application to process and display visualizations, such as trendlines over time. Use of standardized terminology and formatting ensures that data are meaningful and able to be read and processed by machines. The ability to exchange and make meaningful use of data across systems is called *interoperability*; interoperability is a key requirement of healthcare IT systems. *Data standardization* serves numerous functions in healthcare IT, including easing the exchange of information across systems and networks. If all data are coded the same way, no conversion processes need to be applied to integrate them. Standardization is accomplished using libraries or languages that set the standards for terminology and encoding schemes for data that are commonly collected within a setting. In healthcare, the common languages for standardization include **Logical Observation Identifiers Names and Codes (LOINC)** (Werley et al., 1991) and **Systematized Nomenclature of Medicine-CT—Clinical Terms (SNOMED-CT)** (SNOMED International, 2021) (Table 6.1). These are living languages under continual development and expansion. For example, LOINC has been expanded to include nursing terminology. Furthermore, LOINC features a Nursing Subcommittee whose purpose is the development and maintenance of clinical LOINC codes for standardization of nursing terminology, assessments, and interventions (Matney & Anderson, 2021). In addition, data standardization supports public health surveillance, research, quality improvement and safety initiatives, staff scheduling, patient care, trend analysis, and more (Blair & Hardy, 2019).

Repository reliability refers to the dependability and consistency of access to the repository. In a critical healthcare setting, there is little tolerance for downtime when data and data entry are unavailable. Inconsistent repository performance—for instance, longer wait times for data retrieval during high-usage times of the day—also affects the reliability of the repository. Various architectural and procedural models, including redundancy of storage hardware and access routes, system backup policies, bandwidth availability, and regular performance reviews and maintenance, may be employed to increase the reliability of the repository.

Security is essential to the repository because of both the sensitive nature of the data within and the critical role data play in the healthcare environment. Regulations, such as HIPAA, and sound ethical practices demand that organizations provide a high level of privacy and security for the health information they handle. The repository must incorporate security measures, such as data encryption, secure access paths, user authentication, user- and role-based authorization, and physical security of the repository itself to prevent unauthorized access to data, whether inadvertent or malicious. Some security methods may conflict with accessibility and reliability goals, such as when a measure interferes with needed access to a patient's data. User behavior must be considered in developing security tools and protocols; emerging threats to healthcare IT systems often leverage user behavior and inconsistencies in application of user policies (see below). EHR implementers must weigh the benefits and costs of each security practice against its impacts on reliability and accessibility. Good system design can mitigate conflicts while supporting the needs of the healthcare setting.

One characteristic that can be used to distinguish repository models is *central storage* versus *distributed storage*. In the central storage model, a single repository is used to store all (or most) clinical data, and it is used as the primary source for reviewing data. There may still be departmental or function-specific clinical information systems, as well as automated data collection devices, that are used to gather data. Some of these systems may even store copies of their information in their own repositories, but these data are also forwarded to the central repository and stored there. In the case of a healthcare enterprise with multiple facilities, the central model could store information from each of these facilities in one repository. This model improves the ability of a single application to display data from multiple original sources and locations, and it provides the capability to perform clinical decision support (CDS) more efficiently across multiple data types (e.g., combining lab results with medication administration and nutrition data to provide input for medication ordering). Central storage usually requires that data collected from secondary systems be transformed (mapped) to a common storage model

TABLE 6.1	**Examples of Healthcare Data Standardization Languages and Additional Resources**	
Language	**Type of Data Standardized**	**Additional Learning Resources & Examples**
Logical Observation Identifiers Names and Codes (LOINC)	Originally limited to medical laboratory observations, but now includes the Nursing Minimum Data Set (NMDS) to standardize the collection of nursing data	https://loinc.org/downloads/loinc-table/#users-guidehttps://loinc.org/kb/
Systematized Nomenclature of Medicine-Clinical Terms (SNOMED)	Multilingual terminology of clinical health information	https://snomed.org/#
RxNorm	Generic and brand names, meanings, attributes (e.g., strength, dose), and relationships for drugs used in patient care	https://www.nlm.nih.gov/research/umls/rxnorm/index.html

and terminology before being stored in the repository. Data may be replicated to other locations for safety and disaster recovery purposes.

The distributed storage model suggests that each data collection application stores its information in its own repository, and data are federated (joined) through a real-time data access methodology. In this case, a results review application may require access to separate repositories for the lab, microbiology, or radiology, for example, to provide a composite view of information. In the previous example of an enterprise with multiple facilities, each facility might store its own data in a facility-based repository. The distributed model provides some reliability to the EHR because, for example, if one repository goes down, the user may still be able to access information from the other repositories. It also allows the most efficient storage and access for data types and lessens the complexity of having to map data from one system to another. However, the distributed model produces many single points of failure for each repository, limits performance because of the multiple data access paths that may be required, and makes integrated tasks such as CDS much more difficult.

Regardless of storage model, one of the key components of any data repository is the ability to determine to whom the records belong. The **master person index (MPI)**, also known as the master patient index or master member index, is the set of information used to identify each person, patient, or customer of a healthcare enterprise. One or more registration systems may be used at each visit to collect identifying information about the patient that is then sent to the MPI to match against existing person records and resolve any conflicting information. The MPI stores demographic information about the patient, such as names, addresses, phone numbers, date of birth, and sex. Other organizational identifiers, such as social security number, driver's license number, and insurance identification also may be stored. Identifiers from within the healthcare enterprise, such as individual facility medical record numbers, are stored as well. (This is often a vestige of paper medical record systems that used facility-specific identifiers for each patient.)

The MPI record is updated as any information is added. The MPI then serves as both the master of all information collected, forming what is often referred to as the "golden record" for a person and is the source for distinguishing a patient from all other patients in the system. The latter point is important because it helps to ensure that clinical and administrative data are attributed to the correct patient during healthcare encounters. Each MPI record will have a unique patient identifier or number that is used in the repository to associate a clinical record with the appropriate patient and is used by applications to properly retrieve and store information for the right patient. The MPI will typically support standard access methods for storing and retrieving data (e.g., admit/discharge/transfer messages) so that systems that need to use the MPI can rely on a common interface mechanism. A user-facing patient selection application connected to the MPI is typically provided in the EHR so that EHR users can search for and find the record of a particular patient for use in clinical documentation, review, and patient management applications.

Networking and Data Sharing

As described above, networking refers to the interconnectivity of computing systems. The internet is the most widely known and used computing network in the world. It relies on servers and peer-to-peer (workstation to workstation) communication to transmit and receive everything from personal banking records and email to high-definition streaming movies. While this open platform provides a cornucopia of opportunities for sharing, learning, and expanding our understanding of our fellow humans around the globe, it also offers malicious actors widespread opportunities to take advantage of security gaps.

In healthcare, providers and users may rely on the internet to locate research and practice guidelines, download or create patient education materials, and access resources that are available through public or private partners. However, most of the work of healthcare happens on **intranets**. Intranets are smaller, more restricted networks that enable secured transactions between computers within an organization or group; these networks are often administered by local IT resources and professionals. They often have enhanced security protocols, such as two-factor authentication, to ensure that computers and/or individuals connecting to the network are authorized to do so. Traffic on intranets is typically logged to enable IT professionals to conduct optimization of workflows and security protocols.

The protection and preservation of the integrity of data that is transmitted from one healthcare provider or other organization to another must also be considered in healthcare IT infrastructure design and management in accordance with government mandates to share information to enable EHRs. **Data sharing networks** are networks that exchange health information across regions, organizations, or systems. To facilitate data sharing, information exchange networks are designed using either centralized or distributed data architecture (although hybrids of the two are also sometimes deployed). In the centralized model, network participants aggregate, and push their data to a central storage repository (see central storage above). Organizations then retrieve data from the repository as needed. In a distributed model, the network participants keep their data, and provide a mechanism to answer requests for specific data. In either model, the network must provide the ability to match patients between organizations correctly. Without this matching functionality, the network participants are unable to share information accurately. The network may use a global MPI that can map patient identifiers between organizations. In addition, to provide interoperability of the data, the network participants must agree on standards for information exchange. These standards will be discussed in the section titled interoperability standards. Lastly, the exchange network must provide appropriate security mechanisms to authenticate and authorize appropriate use, prevent unwanted access, and accommodate necessary auditing and logging policies.

To connect to the information exchange network, participants may simply treat the network as another interface on their local networks. This allows participants to use existing methods for sharing data, particularly if a centralized model is used, and data are pushed to the central repository.

Another model for linking to the exchange network is to provide a service layer that accepts requests for data. The data request services are accessible by network participants, often in the same way that web pages are made available as URLs on the internet. This method is becoming more popular and is particularly advantageous in the distributed exchange model because it better supports pulling data from an organization as it is needed.

Several models of data sharing networks have evolved in recent decades. A regional health information organization (RHIO) is typically characterized as a quasi-public, nonprofit organization whose goal is to share data within a region. RHIOs were quite often started with a grant or public funding. Meanwhile, health information exchanges (HIEs) have an anchor provider organization and are often started because of financial incentives. The anchor organization frequently provides a data-sharing mechanism to affiliated providers. In practice, the operating characteristics of RHIOs and HIEs may be quite similar, and the distinctions are only in the terminology used. Health information organizations (HIOs) are the latest models, and they support the 2009 HITECH Act mandate for health information sharing between EHRs. The role of an HIO is to facilitate data exchange according to nationally recognized standards. This may mean that an HIO only provides guidance to the organizations in an information exchange network or that an HIO assumes the technical responsibility for providing the exchange mechanism.

ONC facilitated the development of a national "network of networks" whose purpose was to enable healthcare provider organizations and consumers to share information across local information exchange networks. The eHealth Exchange (formerly known as the Nationwide Health Information Network [NwHIN]) created a set of policies and national standards that allows trusted exchange of health information over secured channels via the internet (The Sequoia Project, 2021a). The effort is now managed by a nonprofit industry coalition called The Sequoia Project. The eHealth Exchange includes organizations from all 50 states and four federal agencies (the Social Security Administration and the Departments of Defense, Veterans Affairs, and Health and Human Services) and allows sending and requesting health information from participating organizations. It was instrumental in coordinating data exchange to the Centers for Disease Control and Prevention and state and local health department data during the COVID-19 pandemic (The Sequoia Project 2021b).

INFRASTRUCTURE TOOLS FOR RESEARCH, QUALITY IMPROVEMENT, AND ENHANCED PATIENT SAFETY

One of the primary purposes behind the legislative push toward integrated EHRs and the sharing of patient data involves leveraging the advancement of IT technology to support a mission to improve patient safety, enhance outcomes, and reduce barriers to care. As stated earlier in this chapter, for data to be useful or meaningful, it must be accessible to clinicians, patients, and healthcare administrators when and where they need it to make decisions. Many facets of modern EHR systems directly support this mission.

Key Components to Electronic Health Records Adoption

Clinical decision support tools are a promising method to enhance patient outcomes and clinical decision making. Such tools are often integrated into EHRs and designed to (1) enhance provider attention to important but sometimes overlooked data, such as follow-up screening dates or out of range values, (2) reduce or eliminate certain types of medical error, such as double prescribing, (3) provide early recognition of trends associated with poor outcomes, and (4) enhance efficiency, cost-benefit, and patient and provider satisfaction. Examples of clinical decision-support tools include documentation templates; clinical guidelines; alerts and notifications; order-sets; focused, often disease-specific assessment tools; and more (HealthIT.gov, 2018).

Interoperability is defined in US federal law in the 21st Century Cares Act as technology that (1) enhances secure information exchange across technologies without requiring special effort from users and (2) allows "complete access, exchange, and use of all electronically accessible health information for authorized use" under the law while avoiding the blocking of information exchange. Interoperability is a critical component of EHRs because it ensures that data are transferred in a state that users can access and understand. ONC has developed The Roadmap, (HealthIT.gov, 2019) a document that gives further direction for the technical and operational infrastructure that must be developed to advance true system-wide interoperability. This Roadmap addresses not only data syntax and semantic standards but also identity resolution, data security, access authorization, directories, and resource locators. Most recently, ONC released an Interoperability Standards Advisory whose purpose is to "coordinate the identification, assessment, and determination of 'recognized' interoperability standards and implementation specifications … [to fulfill] clinical health IT interoperability needs." (HealthIT.gov, 2021b)

EMERGING AND ESCALATING THREATS TO HEALTHCARE INFRASTRUCTURE

Due in part to the additional complexities of the regulatory environment, the massive size of healthcare enterprises, and the diversity of users, healthcare IT is anything but nimble. There is often notable delay between the development of software and hardware solutions and their roll-out in healthcare settings. This and other inherent factors of healthcare IT create unique vulnerabilities that can be exploited to become emerging and escalating threats.

Cyber Security Gaps

Just as with crumbling roads and bridges that occur when physical infrastructure is allowed to age, outdated IT infrastructure in healthcare can lead to real-world risks and devastating consequences. The reason for this is that such outdated infrastructure creates many cyber security gaps that may be exploited by malicious actors to steal confidential patient data and employee records and/or hold data, systems, and even patient lives hostage.

Yet the picture is more complicated than just outdated infrastructure. During the COVID-19 pandemic, hospitals and other healthcare systems have had to move more quickly, adapting technologies for telehealth and remote work that had not been thoroughly tested in a healthcare environment (Robinson, 2020). The necessary haste with which these technologies were employed created widespread security vulnerabilities that have been exploited to create havoc using several types of attacks.

In addition, securing critical healthcare IT infrastructure is made even more challenging by the recent adoption of a myriad of external, patient-specific applications and devices that must interface or integrate with the EHR/EMR. Such data are frequently then uploaded directly into patient records. Insulin pumps, which are wearable devices that record and store data on blood glucose levels and insulin usage in patients with diabetes, serve as a cautionary tale. In 2019, IBM worked with researchers to identify a security threat to these devices that would enable hackers to reprogram dosing, alter or obscure glucose readings, and more (Slabodkin, 2020). Physicians and individuals might be misled into acting (or failing to act) in ways that harm health if such data changes are made. Most concerningly, these devices can deliver potentially lethal doses of insulin. The US Department of Homeland Security's Cybersecurity and Infrastructure Security Agency (CISA) issued an advisory about these critical vulnerabilities, and they have since been corrected; however, this case illustrates the importance of overall system design to ensure that data are accurate and protected, regardless of how they enter the EHR environment.

In short, healthcare IT personnel and informaticists must be concerned with the security of data (and devices) for ethical, legal, and regulatory reasons. Robust cyber security practices and teams are essential to ensuring that healthcare IT systems can serve their intended function without compromising patients or the healthcare enterprise.

Responding to Emerging and Escalating Threats to Healthcare Infrastructure

While specific security practices are ever-evolving and beyond the scope of this chapter, such practices have been described as constituting the top two concerns for any healthcare enterprise, along with patients themselves. Thus, two emerging and escalating types of attacks that have recently been plaguing healthcare will be discussed below, along with best security practices for users of healthcare IT infrastructure.

Ransomware attacks are cyber attacks that exploit security gaps to covertly encrypt data, up to and including the full data repository. Encryption is a method of securing data using a digital key and is critical to protecting the privacy of data from theft and unauthorized access; however, in the case of ransomware, perpetrators of an attack use encryption to lock data they do not own and restrict access by those who are authorized to use it. Imagine if instead of stealing a car, someone put a locking mechanism on the wheel, and demanded payment to remove

the lock. Hundreds of hospitals and healthcare systems have been targeted by this type of attack in recent years.

One example from 2020 involves the University of Vermont (UVM) Medical Center (Weiner, 2021). UVM was hit with a ransomware attack that encrypted its EHR, payroll systems, and other vital IT infrastructure, along with a demand from the attackers to pay a ransom. The system was locked down for a month, and while UVM never paid the ransom, the financial cost of the attack was estimated at $50 million. Furthermore, loss of access to critical patient data produced delays in care with real-world consequences to patients in a healthcare system already stressed by an unfolding global pandemic.

Another type of attack has also escalated in recent years. Phishing (pronounced "fishing") is a type of social hacking. Rather than exploiting technical vulnerabilities within infrastructure systems, phishing attacks seek to exploit the human users of an IT system. These attacks often take the form of an email or other communication and rely on fraud and misdirection to take advantage of individuals' goodwill to get them to perform an action. Often, this will involve clicking a web link that uploads dangerous software onto devices or networks, or providing confidential information directly, such as phone numbers, personal identifiers, or passwords. Recently, scammers have begun using impersonation of executives, deans, and other organizational leaders to trick people within an organization to perform actions, such as purchase gift cards and send the codes via email. While the schemes themselves may seem unsophisticated, the rate of success (while small) incentivizes unethical scammers to continue.

As is apparent from the phishing attacks, users are one critical component of healthcare IT security. Without adequate training to recognize threats, users may fall victim to schemes and scams designed to gain access to intranets and/or to steal money, resources, or data. Furthermore, users who do not understand the rationale for security processes, such as two-factor authentication (a method of securing data that attempts to prevent access with stolen passwords) or restrictions on software downloads and installation, may attempt to bypass these measures to improve their workflows or enjoyment of the system. Installing a music streaming app, for instance, may seem like a harmless action that will improve work life for individuals working in offices. However, these actions can have dire consequences for IT systems if that music app has ransomware piggybacked to it. Thus, while robust cybersecurity practices and prevention efforts are necessary in any healthcare IT system, it is just as imperative to ensure that individuals who have access to systems and networks are well trained in security practices and policies and accountable for their actions. Basic best security practices are detailed in Fig. 6.2.

CONCLUSION AND FUTURE DIRECTIONS

Modern healthcare settings deal with an increasingly complex array of data and needs from patients and clinicians. The goals of healthcare IT and healthcare informatics are complementary, supporting not just the health of individual patients and workflows of clinicians but the advancement of healthcare practice

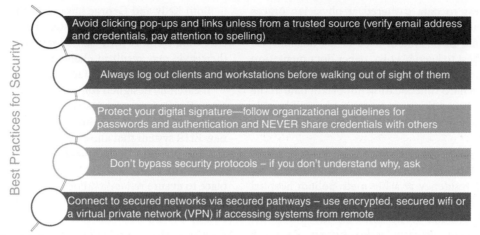

Fig. 6.2 Best security practices for authorized users; for a more comprehensive list, see Norton, 2019.

and the reduction of societal costs associated with healthcare. A clear understanding of the infrastructure used to accomplish these goals is critical for informaticists to promote advances and innovations that will further these goals.

ACKNOWLEDGMENT

The author wishes to acknowledge the contribution of Scott P. Narus to the previous edition of this chapter.

DISCUSSION QUESTIONS

1. What are the advantages and disadvantages of having a local (in-house or on-site) IT infrastructure? What are the advantages and disadvantages of having a distributed or cloud infrastructure? How does the modern healthcare landscape benefit from using a combination approach?
2. In what ways have legislative efforts in the last twenty years shaped the development of healthcare IT?
3. The COVID-19 pandemic has demonstrated that the health of the world and its people is far more interconnected than was previously understood by many people. Discuss the potential consequences in this shift in thinking about health. How might changes in the way the public thinks about health impact the way we gather, store, and use healthcare data?
4. Consider the steps of the data life cycle. Which steps might benefit most from partnerships between IT architects and patients or clinicians? Why?
5. What are the relative strengths of an EHR versus an EMR? Are there any scenarios where an EMR might be preferable?

What potential pitfalls happen when EMRs are combined into an EHR?
6. Data standardization offers many benefits to IT components of the healthcare system. What benefits might it provide to individuals within that system?
7. In what situations might central storage be preferable to distributed?
8. The 2019 cybersecurity vulnerability identified in insulin pumps was a stark reminder of the critical nature of IT security in the healthcare setting. Consider a scenario where data transmitted from a clinical laboratory might be intercepted and altered by bad actors before being integrated into the EHR. What might be the results of such a breach? How might such a breach be prevented?
9. What are some ways to identify a phishing attack? How might a user respond to such an attack in a manner that supports the goal of enhancing security in the organization?

CASE STUDY: CHALLENGES TO HEALTHCARE INFORMATION TECHNOLOGY INFRASTRUCTURE

Meaningful use requires that electronic health record (EHR) data is accessible when, where, and by whom it is needed to make healthcare decisions. Much of the meaningfulness of clinical data, however it is stored, is derived from the way users—clinicians and patients—work and interact with the systems in which data is housed and processed. This is especially true around transitions in healthcare information technology (IT) infrastructure, such as when new software is rolled

out to users. Consider the following scenario: George, a nurse working in a critical care unit at a small, rural hospital, has already seen one major shift in how patient data is collected and recorded at his work site—from paper charts kept at the bedside to a proprietary software electronic medical record (EMR) that relied on a mix of paper and electronic charting that varied by unit. Now, the hospital is moving to a modern EHR system that is supposed to record all patient data in real time and allow access to data gathered at physician offices and other regional hospitals. George's experience with unreliability of the original EMR system used at his hospital has taught him that it is best to keep his own paper documentation and add notes to the digital chart when he gets around to it. Furthermore, he has a hard time locating important data in the EMR when he needs it and does not trust that he will be able to navigate to necessary information quickly enough when the EHR rolls out.

Kelly is excited about the change to complete electronic documentation because that was the system she used during her training and nursing residency at a big metropolitan hospital prior to relocating. She has found the mix of EMR and paper charting to be inefficient and burdensome for her workflows. Kelly plans to adopt a completely paperless system as soon as the EHR is available.

Both Kelly and George have reasonable and understandable reactions to the new EHR system based on their past experiences and comfort with technology. However, the differences in their style may result in challenges to the healthcare IT infrastructure and to patient safety and outcomes.

A carefully designed roll-out of technology will address both cases. For George, administration can set policy regarding when documentation occurs and provide extensive training in the new EHR system that allows users to become familiar and comfortable with how to find the information they need. IT personnel can inform users about the backup systems and processes in place to ensure reliability. For Kelly, IT personnel and administrators can work together to establish downtime protocols and backup systems. Patient care and safety may be enhanced by creating systemic and systematic processes to prepare for outages and other systems issues, especially during IT transitions.

DISCUSSION QUESTIONS

1. What happens if George becomes ill during his shift, and must leave prior to transferring his paper notes to the EHR? How is patient care and the regulatory/legal documentation of care impacted?

2. What happens if there are glitches or unexpected downtime in the initial roll-out phase of the EHR deployment? Will Kelly's patients receive the care they need?

REFERENCES

Blair, L.M., & Hardy, L. (2019). Chapter 8: Data standardization applications—Capturing data. In *Applications of nursing informatics: Competencies, skills, decision-making* (pp. 153–166). Springer Publishing Company.

Centers for Medicare & Medicaid Services. (2010). *CMS finalizes definition of meaningful use of certified electronic health records (EHR) technology.* Centers for Medicare & Medicaid Services. https://www.cms.gov/newsroom/fact-sheets/cms-finalizes-definition-meaningful-use-certified-electronic-health-records-ehr-technology.

HealthIT.gov. (2011, January 4). *EMR vs EHR —What is the difference?* https://www.healthit.gov/buzz-blog/electronic-health-and-medical-records/emr-vs-ehr-difference

HealthIT.gov. (2018). *Clinical decision support.* https://www.healthit.gov/topic/safety/clinical-decision-support

HealthIT.gov. (2019). *Interoperability.* https://www.healthit.gov/topic/interoperability

HealthIT.gov. (n.d.a). *Interoperability Standards Advisory (ISA).* Retrieved September 1, 2021b, from https://www.healthit.gov/isa/

HealthIT.gov. (n.d.b). *ONC's Cures Act Final Rule.* Retrieved September 1, 2021a, from https://www.healthit.gov/curesrule/

Matney, S. A., & Anderson, L. (2021). Logical Observation Identifiers, Names, and Codes Nursing Subcommittee update. *Computers, Informatics, Nursing, 39*(7), 345–346. https://doi.org/10.1097/CIN.0000000000000795.

Robinson, N. (2020). *Emerging threats in healthcare information security: How vulnerable systems lead to hospital cyber attacks.*

Touro College Illinois. http://illinois.touro.edu/news/emerging-threats-in-healthcare-information-security.php

Slabodkin, G. (2020). *Insulin pumps among millions of devices facing risk from newly disclosed cyber vulnerability, IBM says.* MedTech Dive. https://www.medtechdive.com/news/insulin-pumps-among-millions-of-iot-devices-vulnerable-to-hacker-attacks/584043/

SNOMED International. (n.d.). *SNOMED—Home.* Retrieved September 1, 2021, from https://www.snomed.org/

Stobrierski, T. (2021). *8 steps in the data life cycle | Harvard Business School Online.* Business Insights - Blog. https://online.hbs.edu/blog/post/data-life-cycle

The Sequoia Project. (2021b). *EHealth Exchange history.* https://ehealthexchange.org/what-we-do/history/

The Sequoia Project. (n.d.). *EHealth Exchange.* Retrieved August 31, 2021, from https://ehealthexchange.org/

Wagner, C. (2021). *Lawmakers unveil Cures 2.0 Bill to authorize ARPA-H, deliver treatments to patients.* AAMC. https://www.aamc.org/advocacy-policy/washington-highlights/lawmakers-unveil-cures-20-bill-authorize-arpa-h-deliver-treatments-patients.

Weiner, S. (2021). *The growing threat of ransomware attacks on hospitals.* Association of American Medical Colleges (AAMC). https://www.aamc.org/news-insights/growing-threat-ransomware-attacks-hospitals.

Werley, H. H., Devine, E. C., Zorn, C. R., Ryan, P., & Westra, B. L. (1991). The Nursing Minimum Data Set: Abstraction tool for standardized, comparable, essential data. *American Journal of Public Health, 81*(4), 421–426. https://doi.org/10.2105/ajph.81.4.421.

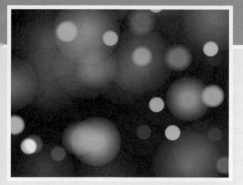

The Electronic Health Record and Precision Care

Charlotte A. Seckman

Today almost all healthcare providers and hospitals are using EHR applications to capture and share patient data across facilities at a local or regional level and, eventually, nationally and internationally.

OBJECTIVES

At the completion of this chapter, the reader will be prepared to:

1. Distinguish between electronic medical record (EMR) and electronic health record (EHR).
2. Discuss factors that have influenced EHR adoption over time.
3. Give examples of various EHR applications used in the clinical environment.
4. Summarize the benefits of EHR use related to cost, access, quality, and safety of care delivery.
5. Discuss challenges associated with EHR use in a technology enabled healthcare environment.
6. Differentiate stakeholder perspectives on EHR use.
7. Summarize how EHRs may contribute to personalized medicine.

KEY TERMS

American Recovery and Reinvestment Act (ARRA), 97
ancillary system, 100
bar code medication administration (BCMA), 101
Coronavirus Aid, Relief, and Economic Security (CARES) Act, 97
clinical decision support (CDS), 103
clinical documentation, 101

computerized provider order entry (CPOE), 101
electronic health record (EHR), 96
electronic medical record (EMR), 96
electronic medication administration record (eMAR), 101

Health Information Technology for Economic and Clinical Health (HITECH) Act, 97
niche applications, 102
patient-generated health data (PGHD), 106
personal health records (PHR), 96
precision medicine, 95

ABSTRACT ❖

The electronic health record (EHR) is one of the most significant innovations introduced in healthcare over the past several decades. Today, almost all healthcare providers and hospitals are using EHR applications to capture and share patient data across facilities at a local or regional level and, eventually, nationally and internationally. Although considerable work is still needed to establish a nationwide interoperable system, EHRs offer many benefits to healthcare organizations, providers, and consumers.

This chapter explores the evolving nature of the EHR to include essential components and functions, how these components are used in the clinical setting, and the benefits related to cost, access, quality, and safety of care. Stakeholder perspectives and key issues associated with EHR use will also be discussed. The chapter concludes with the role of an interoperable EHR in precision medicine as a medium for exploration and translation of evidence into practice along with future directions.

INTRODUCTION

Navigating the complexity of the modern healthcare system has created challenges in managing patient data and information, promoting safety, and providing quality care. Healthcare providers and hospitals endeavor to keep current with billing regulations to receive optimal reimbursement. This requires vigilant monitoring of private insurance contracts and changes in governmental mandates. Provider specialty practices create treatment silos that often hinder continuity of care. Some clinicians find it difficult to maintain competencies and gain access to information related to the latest medical techniques and research. This is compounded by the introduction of personal computers, mobile devices, and the internet of things, which all have boosted consumer demands and a variety of healthcare delivery concerns. The robust nature of the electronic health record (EHR) provides the potential to address many of these issues and transform methods to collect, store, access, process, manage, communicate, and report patient data. However, despite the attention on this technology, alternative views exist regarding what an EHR is, what it does or should do, and how it should be used.

Electronic Medical Record

Terms such as **electronic medical record (EMR)** and **electronic health record (EHR)** are often used interchangeably, but it is important to understand the differences between them. An *EMR* refers to as electronic version of the traditional paper record used and owned by the healthcare provider (Sewell, 2018). In a similar source, Hebda & Czar (Hebda and Czar, 2018) described the EMR as an electronic information resource used in healthcare to capture patient data. The EMR is what most clinicians think of as the automated medical record system used in the clinical setting, and it represents an episodic view of patient encounters. This type of system, seen in hospitals, hospital corporations, and private practices, is predominately controlled by the healthcare organization or provider. Keep in mind the EMR is not just one system but may integrate and/or interface with multiple other systems and applications used by the facility, such as registration, order entry, laboratory, and many other departmental systems. The patient usually does not provide input into the EMR, although portals are now available that provide patient access to test results, problem lists, and other features available during a hospital stay and at home.

Electronic Health Record

So, what are the differences between and EMR and an EHR? In 2008, the National Alliance for Health Information Technology (NAHIT), as a division of the U.S. Department of Health & Human Services (DHHS), convened to clarify and define key health information technology (IT) terms. The EHR was defined as "An electronic record of health-related information on an individual that conforms to nationally recognized interoperability standards and that can be created, managed, and consulted by authorized clinicians and staff across more than one healthcare organization" (The National Alliance for Health Information Technology, 2008). This suggests the availability and use of communication standards, such as nomenclatures, vocabularies, and coding structures, to share patient data across multiple organizations, facilities and providers. In comparison, the EMR is limited to information shared within a single organization or practice, whereas the EHR has the ability to exchange information outside the healthcare delivery system (The Office of the National Coordinator for Health Information Technology [ONCHIT], 2019a). The goal of a nationwide interoperable EHR is that every person will have a birth-to-death (prenatal to postmortem) record of health-related information in electronic form from multiple sources, such as physician office visits, inpatient and ambulatory hospital encounters, medications, allergies, and other medical services that support care, as well as personal input from the consumer perspective. The desired effect of the components of EMRs is to ultimately be part of the larger EHR.

Other definitions stress the importance of the EHR as a way to automate and streamline workflow for healthcare providers, support patient care activities, and provide decision support, quality management, and outcomes reporting (Alexander and Guerra, 2019; McGonigle, 2021; The Office of the National Coordinator for Health Information Technology [ONCHIT], 2019b). In addition, these definitions are often directed toward the needs of the healthcare provider and lack reference to patient and consumer interaction or integration of **personal health records (PHRs)**. Despite the clarification provided by numerous definitions, the acronym EHR has emerged as the preferred term when referring to either an EMR or EHR.

Although an EHR is comprised of many components, it is important to mention the advent of PHR or portals which has added a new dimension to improving patient-provider communications. This type of record is primarily patient or consumer controlled and is discussed in more detail later in this chapter and in Chapter 15. The ultimate goal is that PHR development conform to nationally recognized standards and be integrated into larger systems, allowing the individual to view, manage, and share personal health information with providers. As part of the EHR, this could provide a more comprehensive record of a person's medical history and overall health.

In summary, *EHR* has become the preferred term for the lifetime patient record that would include data from a variety of healthcare specialties and provide interactive access and input by the patient. The term *EHR* is distinct in meaning from the term *EMR*. As with other expressions in the past, the term *EMR* may eventually fade away. Although some disagreement exists on exactly what the terms *EHR* and *EMR* mean, the EHR is clearly an essential tool that has rapidly evolved to better manage patient care in a complex healthcare delivery system.

HISTORICAL AND CURRENT SOCIOTECHNICAL PERSPECTIVES

In two landmark reports, the Institute of Medicine (IOM) (Institute of Medicine, 2000; Institute of Medicine, 2001) identified significant issues related to providing care in the healthcare environment. Both prompted a need to design and implement EHR systems as a method to increase patient safety, reduce medical and medication errors, and improve the quality of care. As a result, numerous federal initiatives to facilitate nationwide adoption and expansion of EHR technologies emerged. The outcome of this expansion has shown that EHRs save time, provide real-time access to patient information at the point of care, facilitate the work of the clinician, provide decision support capabilities, support clinical care and research, and improve quality and safety of care (Rathert, Porter, Mittler, & Fleig-Palmer, 2019; The Office of the National Coordinator for Health Information Technology [ONCHIT], 2017a). This section explores historical and current factors associated with EHR adoption and use to include federal requirements, promoting interoperability and certification, interoperability and standards, and the role of the health practitioner.

Federal Initiatives

Over the years, federal regulations were promulgated to guide adoption and use of EHRs in the U.S. In response to the IOM reports, the Bush administration initiated national mandates and guidelines from collaborative working groups to address safety and quality issues in healthcare but these were not enough to accelerate the development and adoption of health IT. In 2009, public law 111-5—the American Recovery and Reinvestment Act—was passed to stimulate the U.S. economy, which included a critical component, called the Health Information Technology for Economic and Clinical Health (HITECH) Act, to expand the adoption and use of EHR technology. This act authorized programs designed to improve healthcare quality, safety, and efficiency using health IT (U.S. Department of Health and Human Resources DHHS, 2017). More details about the HITECH Act plus other related legislation can be found in Chapter 29. A key for this chapter is the provision that targeted the stimulation and adoption of EHRs and the development of secure health information exchange (HIE) networks. Details of this program are presented in the next section.

In 2020, a new $2 trillion dollar stimulus package was enacted by Congress, the Coronavirus Aid, Relief, and Economic Security (CARES) Act—H.R. 748— in response to the COVID-19 pandemic to aid families and businesses. In addition, 127 billion was allocated to healthcare facilities to cover expenses related to the pandemic such as the purchase of ventilators, protective gear, medications, and other medical devices; coverage for COVID-19 testing and vaccines; support for prevention and treatment in underserved populations; and the implementation and use of telemedicine (Library of Congress, 2020). The Coronavirus Preparedness and Response Supplemental Appropriations Act, 2020—H.R. 6074—allocated 8.3 billion to various agencies for research and the development of a vaccine and/or cure for COVID-19. The wide-spread adoption and use of EHR systems became a critical resource for managing healthcare challenges encountered during the pandemic to include the rapid deployment of telehealth services, enhanced use of PHRs, modules for documenting vaccination administration, mobile devices for communication, the development and implementation of new standards and coding structures for billing and care processes, and tracking the prevalence of COVID-19. Certified EHR systems allowed for greater interoperability and sharing of data across multiple healthcare providers and patients.

Promoting Interoperability Program and Certification

In 2011, the Center for Medicare and Medicaid Services (CMS) established a monetary incentive program for providers and healthcare organizations to encourage the implementation and "meaningful use" of certified EHRs. Meaningful use is now an outdated term and the program was renamed in 2018 to Promoting Interoperability (PI). Historically, this program was designed to leverage technology to improve quality, safety, and efficiency in patient care and deployed in three stages (The Office of the National Coordinator for Health Information Technology [ONCHIT], 2013). Criteria for each stage varied based on whether the EHR system was implemented in ambulatory practices or hospitals. The first stage focused on electronic data capture and tracking of key clinical conditions, communication, data sharing and coordination of care, reporting public health information and quality measures, and engaging patients and families (Centers for Medicare & Medicaid Services [CMS], 2020). Stage 2 encouraged patient engagement and the robust use of health IT through continuous quality improvement efforts, HIE networks, structured data capture, information exchange, population health, and research (Centers for Medicare & Medicaid Services [CMS], 2020). The final Stage 3, released in 2017, expanded on the objectives for the first two stages to support further quality initiatives; improve safety, efficiency, and patient outcomes; address population health requirements; provide enhanced decision support; and promote patient-centered HIE (Centers for Medicare & Medicaid Services, 2021). More recently, the focus of the PI program is to increase interoperability and enhance patient access to personal health information. An important change, the Medicare Access and CHIP Reauthorization Act (MACRA) of 2015 shifted reimbursement criteria from the traditional fee-for-service to a value-based care system (see details in Chapter 29). As a result, several models emerged under the umbrella of the CMS Merit-based Incentive Payment System (MIPS), which includes the PI program and other alternative payment models (APMs) (Centers for Medicare & Medicaid Services, 2019; The Office of the National Coordinator for Health Information Technology [ONCHIT], 2019c).

In order to increase interoperability between systems, standards and certification criteria were created by ONCHIT under several regulations such as the 21st Century Cures Act, the 2015 Edition Health Information Technology Certification Criteria, and the ONCHIT Certification Program (The Office of the National Coordinator for Health Information Technology [ONCHIT], 2020; Azar, 2020). The sole purpose of certification is to promote patient safety, security, and interoperability of EHR systems that are developed by health IT vendors. In order to comply with CMS quality improvement programs, such as Promoting Interoperability, providers and hospitals were encouraged to replace legacy systems and/or implement certified EHR systems. Today when ONCHIT issues new criteria, vendors respond by incorporating required functionality in their products and updates are offered to existing customers. According to a 2019 survey, 94% of U.S. hospitals have adopted certified EHR technology to support patient care processes, and over half utilize state, regional, or local HIE's to share data (Johnson and Pylypchuk, 2021).

Interoperability and Standards

A major component of the HITECH Act was to promote interoperability or the sharing of data across organizations. Critical to achieving this goal is the utilization and harmonization of standards in order to support interoperability. There are a number of organizations that develop and approve standards used in healthcare today. According to the Health Information Management Systems Society (HIMSS), (Health Information Management Systems Society [HIMSS], 2021) standards development centers around five items: (1) vocabularies and terminologies, (2) data or document content, (3) transport of messages, (4) privacy and security, and (5) unique identifiers. See Chapter 4 for more detail about standards and standard setting. In order to expedite a nationwide exchange of data, DHHS has been actively involved in advancing the use of standards to support interoperability through advisory groups and provisions outlined in the 21st Century Cures Act (Azar, 2020; Health Information Management Systems Society [HIMSS], 2021). This includes developing standards for data collected from nontraditional sources such as mobile health devices and social determinants of health. Health information exchange (HIE) networks provide standardized data and information for public health agencies, hospitals, and providers in order support continuity of care.

From an international perspective, the European Commission launched several initiatives to improve the safety and quality of care through information sharing such as the e-Health Digital Service infrastructure that provides guidance on implementing digital services, the Smart Open Services (epSOS) project that supports healthcare providers and patients access to critical medical information, and the deployment of numerous European Reference Networks (European Commission, 2021). Overall, EHR adoption and interoperability has the potential to reach beyond the borders of this nation to meet the needs of a mobile society.

Healthcare Providers Role

Healthcare providers play an important role as the primary users of EHR technology. Interdisciplinary involvement is important throughout the systems life cycle, from participating in strategic planning and selecting a system (see Chapters 17 and 18) to testing, implementing, and maintaining systems (see Chapter 20). Clinicians may serve in various roles such as project leader, champion, committee member, participant in conducting workflow analysis, testing system features and functions, or be a super user or trainer during implementations or upgrades. Once a system change is implemented, clinical users have a responsibility to report any issues with functionality, usability, workflow, and impact on patient care. Healthcare providers can assist in designing clinical decision support (CDS) systems to enhance patient adherence to disease management, develop data set standards to improve outcomes, identify areas to increase patient safety, and evaluate quality of care. Many are engaged in local, regional, and national strategic initiatives to improve care coordination using EHRs and expand utilization of HIE (McBride and Tietz, 2019).

A typical EHR is designed to allow access and input by a variety of healthcare providers as a way to manage care. In the same way, fulfillment of documentation requirements involves contributions from multiple disciplines to produce high-quality data for processing claims, providing continuity of care, and analyzing patient outcomes. With the current nursing shortage, executives are pressured to find ways to increase productivity while they struggle to recruit/retain qualified healthcare personnel. Expanding and maintaining a robust EHR system can enhance access to patient information, provide more accurate and complete documentation, improve data availability, and provide decision support capabilities, often leading to increased staff productivity and satisfaction (Hebda and Czar, 2018; American Association of Colleges of Nursing [AACN], 2020).

ELECTRONIC HEALTH RECORD APPLICATIONS IN THE CLINICAL SETTING

An EHR is not one system but is composed of multiple systems, applications, or components designed to support the functions of various departments or user roles. Depending on the setting, an EHR may differ in terms of integration between the components, data presentation, usability, and clinical workflow. This section discusses the initial driving forces and key attributes for EHR development along with a discussion of various applications currently used in the clinical setting.

Driving Forces and Key Attributes

In 2003, a group called the EHR Collaborative was formed to support rapid adoption and develop standards for EHR design (Institute of Medicine, 2004). This group included sponsors from the American Medical Association, the American Nurses Association (ANA), HIMSS, and a variety of other informatics organizations. The EHR Collaborative held forums and gathered input from stakeholder communities such as healthcare providers, insurance companies, HIT vendors, researchers, pharmacists, public health organizations, and consumers. As a result, the IOM (Institue of Medicine, 2003) released a report outlining eight essential care delivery components for an EHR with an emphasis on functions that promote patient safety, quality, and efficiency. These components are still prominent today in all EHR systems and incorporate unique functions that contribute to the integration of a comprehensive patient record (see Table 7.1). In addition to the various components and functions, there are 12 key attributes prescribed by the IOM (Institue of Medicine, 2003) as the gold standard components of an EHR. These attributes serve as guidelines to organizations and vendors involved in the design and implementation of EHRs and include the information shown in Box 7.1.

Transactional Versus Translational Systems

Early hospital information systems were developed to address the business side of healthcare through a variety of transactions such as billing, scheduling, managing resources, and inventory control. Administration applications; admission, discharge, and transfer (ADT); order entry; and various aspects of ancillary department applications are examples of transactional systems. The advent of evidence-based practice and an increased interest in translational medicine prompted a need for systems that addressed care coordination, patient safety, best practice, and quality of care in the context of improving patient outcomes. Examples of translational systems designed to support these efforts are clinical documentation, clinical decision support, electronic medication administration, barcoding, and other specialty practice applications. Both transactional and translational systems work together to provide data and information that can be utilized to generate knowledge and wisdom for managing care, improving practice, and conducting research (see Fig. 7.1). Each application will be discussed in more detail in the following sections.

TABLE 7.1 Summary of the Electronic Health Record Essential Components and Functions for Care Delivery

Component	Essential Functions	Application Examples
Administrative processes	Ability to conduct all financial and administrative functions associated with institutional operations and patient management	Admissions, Discharge, Transfers (ADT)/Registration Scheduling Claims processing Administrative reporting
Communication and connectivity	Provides a medium for electronic communication between healthcare providers and patients	E-mail Mobile devices Text/web messaging Integrated health records Telemedicine
Decision support	Provides reminders, alerts, and resource links to improve the diagnosis and care of the patient	Medication dosing, allergies Risk screening/prevention Clinical guidelines Resource links
Dentistry and optometry	Ability to incorporate dental records and vision prescriptions	Dental records Vision records
Health information and data	Ability to enter and access key information needed to make clinical decisions	Patient demographics Problem lists Medical/nursing diagnoses Medications/allergies Results reporting
Order-entry management	Ability to enter all types of orders via the computer system	Laboratory Pharmacy Radiology Other orders
Patient support	Provides patient education and self-monitoring tools	Discharge instructions Computer-based learning Telemonitoring
Results management	Provides the ability to manage current and historical information related to all types of diagnostic reports	Laboratory tests Radiology reports Other procedures
Population health management	Provides data collection tools to support public and private reporting requirements	Public health system Disease surveillance Bioterrorism

Adapted from Institute of Medicine, Committee on Data Standards for Patient Safety: Board of Health Care Services. *Key Capabilities of an Electronic Health Record System: Letter Report.* Washington, DC: The National Academies Press; 2003.

BOX 7.1 The Institute of Medicine's Key Attributes of an Electronic Health Record

1. Provides active and inactive problem lists for each encounter that link to orders and results; meets documentation and coding standards.
2. Incorporates accepted measures to support health status and functional levels.
3. Ability to document clinical decision information; automates, tracks, and shares clinical decision process/rationale with other caregivers.
4. Provides longitudinal and timely linkages with other pertinent records.
5. Guarantees confidentiality, privacy, and audit trails.
6. Provides continuous authorized user access.
7. Supports simultaneous user views.
8. Access to local and remote information.
9. Facilitates clinical problem solving.
10. Supports direct entry by physicians.
11. Cost measuring/quality assurance.
12. Supports existing/evolving clinical specialty needs.

Adapted from Institute of Medicine, Committee on Data Standards for Patient Safety: Board of Health Care Services. *Key Capabilities of an Electronic Health Record System: Letter Report.* Washington, DC: The National Academies Press; 2003.

Administrative Applications

Although administrative applications are often discussed as a separate entity, a fully integrated EHR system will include many of these systems in order to facilitate care (see Chapter 8). ADT or registrations systems for example are critical to organizing patient data such as demographics (age, birth data, race, marital status, gender, and social determinates of health); insurance and provider information; diagnosis, procedures, chief complaint and problem lists; allergies; and unique identifiers. ADT systems also track patient status such as inpatient vs outpatient, location, current and past procedures, length of stay, and much more. Patient identifying data is stored in a Master Patient Index for retrieval across other EHR applications and for HIE (U.S. Department of Health and Human Services [DHHS], 2021).

Financial applications are necessary for billing patients, submitting claims, and keeping track of an organization's fiscal health. These systems may connect to payer systems for quicker processing. Standards used may include coding structures such as the International Classification of Diseases (ICD); Current

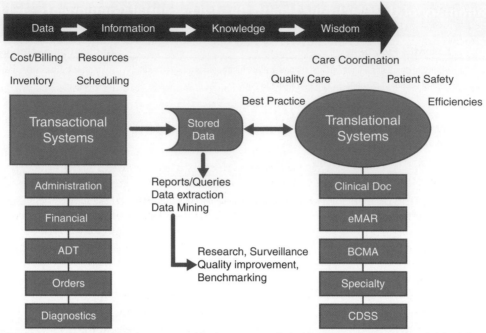

Fig. 7.1 Information transformation: transactional versus translational systems in healthcare. Original diagram ©2012 by Charlotte Seckman, PhD, RN, BC, FAAN, Associate Professor, University of Maryland School of Nursing, Nursing Informatics Program, Baltimore, MD. *ADT*, Admission, discharge, transfers; *BCMA*, barcode medication administration; *CDS*, clinical decision support; *Clinical Doc*, clinical documentation; *eMAR*, electronic medication administration record

Procedural Terminology (CPT), and Diagnosis-Related Group (DRG). Case, quality, and practice management systems may also be used to facilitate reimbursement, improve patient satisfaction, and meet various government and accreditation regulations. Not all administrative systems are patient-focused. Some applications assist the organization with staffing and scheduling, provider credentialing, and human resource tracking. Add to the list business intelligence software for analyzing the massive amounts of data being collected in EHRs today.

Ancillary Applications

An **ancillary system** refers to software applications used by departments such as laboratory, radiology, pharmacy, cardiology, respiratory, physical therapy, and material management. Laboratory information systems (LIS) and radiology information systems (RIS) were available long before the concept of an interoperable EHR system was introduced. Both LIS and RIS are designed to address the specific needs of the department related to collecting, processing, and reporting test results along with managing resources and costs. The LIS consists of several subcomponents including hematology, chemistry, microbiology, immunology, blood bank, and pathology (Farzandipour, Meidni, Sadeqi, & Dehghan, 2019). The LIS interfaces with other devices, such as blood analyzers, for direct input of blood test results. Coding structures are used to track and identify resources and provide cost data for billing. Logical Observation Identifier Names and Codes (LOINC) is a universal coding system used to identify laboratory and other clinical observations, whereas the Systematized Nomenclature of Medicine (SNOMED) coding structure is commonly used in pathology (Bodenreider, Cornet, & Vreeman, 2018; Stram et al., 2020). A LIS interfaced with other clinical applications in the EHR improves workflow, decreases

turnaround times and errors, and provides quicker access to results (Petrides et al., 2017).

The RIS is similar to the LIS in that it incorporates data from multiple services to include X-rays, fluoroscopy, mammography, ultrasound, magnetic resonance imaging scans, computed tomography scans, and other special procedures. It also uses coding structures such as CPT or ICD to identify procedures, resources, and billing (Rubin and Kahn, 2017). However, the global standard for the transmission, storage, and display of medical imaging information is called Digital Imaging and Communications in Medicine (DICOM). The RIS may integrate data from a picture archiving and communication system (PACS), which stores digital versions of diagnostic images for display in the EHR. The PACS provides better contrast and clarity of images along with the ability to enlarge details, which enhances satisfaction with providers and radiology staff (Abbasi et al., 2020; Aldosare, Saddik, & Al Kadi, 2017).

The pharmacy department typically has a system to assist with inventory, prescription management, billing, and dispensing of medications. The FDA requires that all drugs be registered and reported using a National Drug Code (NDC) which serves as a universal identifier for medicines (Anderson, 2018). Besides the NDC, other coding structures include the National Drug File-Reference Terminology (NDF-RT) and RxNorm. The NDF-RT groups drugs according to classes such as anticoagulants, antibiotics, and so on, whereas RxNorm contains specific brand/generic names to include active ingredients, strength, dose, and interactions (National Library of Medicine, 2017; National Library of Medicine, 2021). Clinical screening can be done by monitoring medication usage throughout the hospital and identifying potential adverse drug events. Dispensing and transcription errors decrease when the pharmacy application is integrated with automated dispensing systems, CPOE, eMAR and barcoding devices (Carroll and Richardson, 2020). Prescriptions can be tracked along with printing of labels and medication instructions for patients or staff. The pharmacy system can provide patient drug profiles that include current and past medications, allergies, and contraindications. These features are designed to reduce errors and enhance patient safety.

Computerized Provider Order Entry

Computerized provider order entry (CPOE) is a component of the larger EHR system. The "P" in CPOE may also refer to prescriber or practitioner signifying those who are authorized to write/enter orders such as physicians, nurse practitioners, physician assistants, dentists, osteopathic doctors, and anesthesiologists. CPOE is software designed to allow providers to enter a variety of orders—such as medications, dietary services, consults, ADT, nursing orders, laboratory, and other diagnostic tests—via a computer. In fact, the term *order entry* can be misleading, as CPOE is truly an orders management (transactional) system that allows orders to be entered, processed, tracked, updated, and completed. For most organizations, handwritten orders no longer exist which eliminates transcription errors related to misplaced decimal points and illegible handwriting. Now, prescribers enter orders directly into the computer. During the ordering process, alerts (such as drug allergy warnings), duplicate orders, and other decision support rules are available to assist the healthcare provider to make informed choices. Once an order is entered, the CPOE system interfaces or integrates with other EHR components, such as a laboratory or pharmacy system, to process the order. Results from the LIS, RIS and other ancillary systems are then displayed, not in CPOE, but in a results management component of the EHR. Decision support rules may be applied to flag abnormal results and/or reminders for pending or repeat procedures.

Studies have consistently demonstrated the benefits of CPOE in reducing medication errors. Early studies found the implementation of CPOE decreased the length of hospital stay, lowered costs, improved quality of care and better drug dosing, and decreased the number of allergic reactions (Bates et al., 1998; Gandhi et al., 2005; Mekhjian et al., 2002). More recent studies concur with these findings and suggested that medical and medication errors can be reduced along with improving data integrity, accuracy, workflow, and patient outcomes (Wiegel et al., 2020; Lyons et al., 2017; Prgomet et al., 2017; Sutton et al., 2020).

Electronic Medication Administration and Barcoding

The electronic medication administration record (eMAR) provides a medium to view and document medication use for individual patients. When medication orders are entered into the CPOE system, this information is sent to the pharmacy system for verification and dispensing. New orders appear on the patient's medication list in the eMAR and include the drug name, administration time, dose, and route. Usually, the eMAR contains all types of medications and intravenous fluid orders, with the ability to sort the list in a variety of ways. For example, users can display scheduled, as needed (prn), pending, past due, or completed medications and can query the list for specific entries. Some systems will color code medication order types for quick sorting and identification. The eMAR may be integrated with the clinical documentation system to allow for documentation of a pain response associated with giving pain medications or to enter vital signs before administering certain medications. Efforts to decrease medication administration errors focus on eMAR use in combination with bar coding devices. An example of an eMAR screen is shown in Fig. 7.2.

Bar Code Medication Administration (BCMA) is a method used to address patient safety and reduce errors that occur during the actual administration of medicines. The idea of barcoding patients was first introduced in 1992 by a nurse at a Veterans Health Administration (VHA) hospital after observing a scanner used for car rental (U.S. Department of Veterans Affairs, 2002). This system is most effective when combined with CPOE, a pharmacy dispensing system, and the eMAR. Bar codes can be read by optical scanners or bar code readers. The medication administration process with BCMA in the clinical setting starts with the nurse scanning their badge, the patient's wristband bar code, and the medication bar code. The scanner verifies the five "rights" of medication administration—right patient, right drug, right dose, right time, and right route—and documents the actual administration in the eMAR.

Radio frequency identification (RFID) is also used for medication administration. This technology uses electronic tags embedded in an identification badge or band to track and monitor activities. Passive RFID works in a similar way to regular bar coding with the use of a scanner. Active RFID does not require a scanner; rather, it automatically transmits signals to a computer or wireless device without disturbing the patient. This technology is becoming more common in hospitals to track patient care activities, including medication dispensing and administration. Research supports many advantages related to the use of BCMA and eMARs, which includes a reduction in medication error rates and potential adverse events; accuracy and completeness of medication records; increased staff satisfaction; less cognitive burden; and enhanced patient care (Zheng et al., 2021; Hariyati et al., 2021; Naidu and Alicia, 2019; Strudwick et al., 2018).

Clinical Documentation

Clinical documentation applications provide a medium for recording, managing, and reporting patient care activities by a variety of disciplines. The American Nurses Association (ANA) advocates for the use of various vocabularies and terminologies in order to promote standardization of data, reporting, and information exchange (Sewell, 2018). (See Chapter 4 for more detail about standards.) Structured notes using standardized languages or organizational terms may come in the form of pull-down menus, decision trees, or keywords embedded in a sentence. Some documentation applications contain functionality to store and retrieve predefined notes of normal findings or interventions associated with clinical practice guidelines. Some organizations use "charting by exception," wherein normal values are pre-filled according to established guidelines so clinicians only document abnormal findings. The danger of this method is allowing "normals" to automatically copy over without validation or updates from the clinician on the true status of the patient.

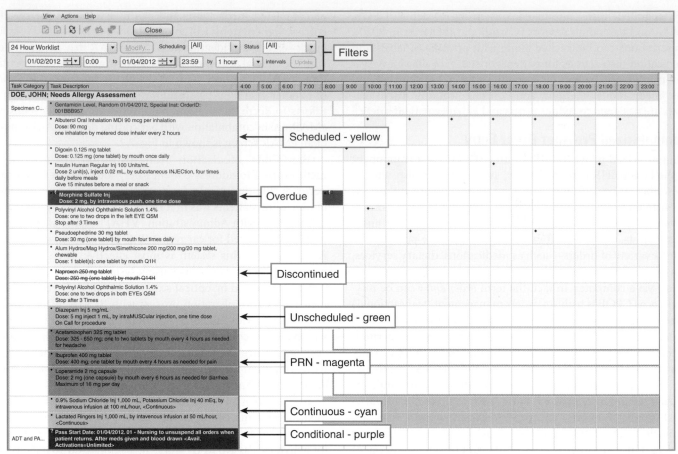

Fig. 7.2 Example of an eMAR. (Copyright 2012 Allscripts. Used with permission.)

Clinical documentation applications contain functionality to support workflow processes associated with conducting physical assessments, creating plans of care, performing interventions and other activities. Often electronic flow sheets or grids are used to record vital signs and other procedures quickly. An effective documentation system includes decision support rules that alert the clinician about abnormal values, missing content, the need for additional assessments, or to verify essential information. Many systems provide the ability to graph numeric data such as vital signs and lab values. Depending on the type of data collected, various clinical, administrative, and research reports can be generated.

Overall, clinical documentation systems are reported to support better communication between healthcare providers, promote professional accountability, streamline workflow, and improve care management (Asmirajanti, Hamid, & Hariyati, 2019). Unfortunately, there are concerns that the increasing complexity of this technology coupled with information overload, outdated practices, and expanding documentation requirements, has become burdensome for clinicians (Baumann, Baker, & Elshaug, 2018; Padden, 2019). Nurses and other healthcare providers are starting to advocate for change in documentation practices and to re-evaluate what is important for data capture and reporting. Efforts related to application re-design, creating new practice models, utilization of data dashboards, and incorporating voice recognition technology may pave the way to addressing documentation burden (Padden, 2019; Blackley et al., 2019; Joseph et al., 2020; Kravet and Bailey, 2018).

Specialty Applications

EHR components, such as CPOE, eMAR, and clinical documentation, are commonly available in organizations to all healthcare providers, but often there is a need for unique functionality beyond what is provided in these applications. Specialty or niche applications are software programs created to address the requirements of specific departments and groups of users. Although many niche applications can function as stand-alone systems, integration with or interface to the hospital-wide EHR is preferred to decrease redundancy, enhance communication, and provide a more comprehensive patient record. Some examples of departments that may use specialty applications include perioperative or surgical services, maternity care, neonatal intensive care, and the emergency department (ED). Applications specific to these four areas will be discussed, but keep in mind there are many other niche systems available for a wide variety of healthcare needs.

A surgical information system (SIS) incorporates functionality to improve clinical, operational, and financial outcomes throughout the entire perioperative experience. Functionality may include operating room scheduling; management of equipment, supplies, and inventory; clinical documentation; patient and specimen tracking; and administrative reporting capabilities. It is not uncommon for the anesthesiology department to have their own system for documentation which, if not interfaced with the main EHR, can create gaps in the clinical record.

Some organizations solve this problem by scanning paper documents or requiring double entry of data.

A maternity care information system (MCIS) is another type of niche system used to address the needs of obstetrics staff and patients. A MCIS is used to support clinical protocols for maternity care, track mother and baby progress, capture fetal-uterine monitoring data, and record results of Doppler blood flow and other diagnostic tests. Key features of this system include electronic forms for documenting and reporting all aspects of antenatal, intrapartum, and postnatal care, as well as normal, healthy, or adverse pregnancy outcomes. In most states, maternity and child care records must be maintained for 25 years, so storage of this data is critical.

Likewise, a neonatal information system (NIS) that interfaces with other EHR components would contain much of the same information found in the primary system. Unique to an NIS would be growth charts, nutritional calculations, monitor parameters, and coding structures specific to the needs of critically ill newborns. Clinical staff in these specialty units can benefit from user-defined logbooks, resource utilization, quality improvement data, and statistical reports designed for their specific needs.

An emergency department information system (EDIS) provides unique functionality related to ED clinical workflow, documentation of triage and patient encounters, tracking of patient location, treatment progress, charge capture and reimbursement management, clinical rules for risk mitigation, and patient education and referral. Once again, not unlike other niche systems, the EDIS is designed to improve clinical, operational, and financial outcomes throughout the entire ED experience. Since the ED is seen as the portal to inpatient care, the EDIS is integrated as part of the overall EHR, so data are readily available to care providers in all areas of the hospital.

Clinical Decision Support

Clinical decision support (CDS) systems assist the healthcare provider with some aspect of decision making and are crucial to the design of an effective EHR. For example, the earliest CDS were alerts developed for CPOE related to duplicate orders, allergies, and medication dosing errors. A CDS system can provide alerts related to changes in a patient's condition, abnormal lab or diagnostic test results, and reminders about important tasks such as follow-up visits, preventive care, immunizations, and updates to critical patient information. Although these types of alerts are easy to program and provide clinicians with information for decision making, too many warnings can lead to alert fatigue. Most simple alerts, warnings and reminders provide a recommended action, but it is always the clinician's decision whether to comply, take an alternate action, or ignore. (See Chapter 12 for details on CDSS.)

For more complex decisions, some EHRs may contain web links to external resources such as medication information, educational materials, or search engines like PubMed or Medline. Many healthcare systems also have intranets that provide links to policies and procedures, clinical guidelines, and evidence-based protocols. In 2006, the National Institutes of Health (NIH), in collaboration with the National Library of Medicine (NLM), developed a personalized decision support application called the EBP InfoBot which is still used by the NIH Clinical Center (Demner-Fushman, Seckman, Fisher, & Thoma, 2013). This system was designed to augment a patient's EHR by automatically searching various literature sources and providing information that could be used to develop plans of care and assist with decision making. Operating behind the scenes are rule sets programmed to extract key data from the patient's medical record, map free text data to standardized terminology, and create a series of EBP-type queries from extracted data. These questions are used to search multiple NLM databases, internal standards of care and guidelines, and other external clinical resources, then provide a summary of the information based on clinical user-group preference directly into the EHR. The application functions in real time and provides flexibility to adapt to the requirements of the decision maker. Overall, the EBP InfoBot decreased provider search time, reduced information overload, and provided current and timely resources to support decision making at the bedside. An example of the EBP InfoBot summary screen is shown in Fig. 7.3. CDS technology is rapidly evolving and the advent of machine learning and artificial intelligence (discussed in a later section) provides powerful tools to predict disease and supplement human decision making skills (Medic et al., 2019; Middleton, Sittig, & Wright, 2016).

ELECTRONIC HEALTH RECORD BENEFITS

Most health policy initiatives are designed to address concerns that focus on cost, access, quality and safety of care. For example, concerns regarding the increasing cost of prescription drugs and how organizations are reimbursed for care became the focus of Medicare reform legislation and a transition to value-based care models. The 21st Century CURES Act addressed information blocking by requiring healthcare organizations to allow patients secure, free access to select personal health information (Azar, 2020). This rule is designed to foster patient/provider communications, provide data to make informed choices, and ultimately improve the quality of care. With this in mind, the benefits of an EHR will focus on cost, access, quality, and safety of care delivery.

Cost Savings

Cost savings is always a big motivator, especially if a healthcare provider or institution wants to stay in business. Since the mandate to adopt EHR technology, many studies have reported and continue to report a positive financial return on investment for healthcare organizations (Atasoy, Greenwood, & McCullough, 2019; Highfill, 2020; Moncho, Marco-Simo, & Cobarsi, 2021; Najmi et al., 2021). Cost benefits include increased productivity, efficiency in billing, improved reimbursement rates, improved verification of coverage, faster turnaround for accounts, lower medical record costs, support for pay-for-performance, and enhanced regulatory requirement compliance.

Access to Patient Care Information

An EHR provides better and faster access to patient care information for providers and consumers. An EHR allows

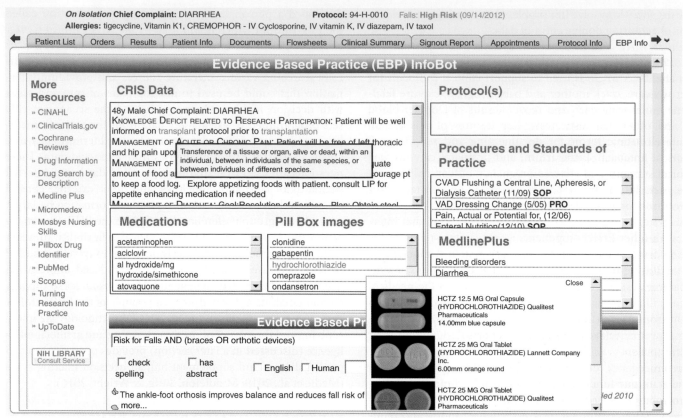

Fig. 7.3 EBP InfoBot. (EBP Infobot developed by the National Library of Medicine [NLM] in collaboration with the National Institutes of Health, Clinical Center [NIHCC] Patient Care Services. Screenshot used with permission from NLM.)

simultaneous access to patient records and restricts users' access to only the information that they are permitted to view. Many systems contain functionality such as graphs, charts and data, dashboards that trend on demand, and tools that facilitate comparison of current and past data. Another benefit is that clinicians have access to drug information, decision support tools, and resources to supplement patient care. Conducting research or quality improvement initiatives often involve reviewing chart data and can be a cumbersome process if done manually. The EHR provides a more effective and efficient method to access and aggregate data through the use of sophisticated reporting tools and machine-learning applications. As EHR functionality continues to expand, this will improve data access across multiple facilities and provide better continuity of care.

Consumer demand for access to personal healthcare information (PHI) is increasing. Portals or PHRs tethered to a provider and/or hospital EHR can enhance communications and facilitate management and control of disease, which leads to better outcomes (Han et al., 2019; Paydar et al., 2021). The expanded use of portals provide consumers with the ability to send electronic messages, schedule appointments, receive reminders, view laboratory and test results, track progress, and access educational resources. (See Chapter 15 for details about Personal Health Records.)

Quality and Safety

Health care quality can be defined as "care that is safe, effective, patient-centered, timely, efficient, and equitable." (Office of Disease Prevention and Health Promotion, 2021). EHR

technology contains functionality designed to foster quality through: (1) timely access to patient information; (2) decision support tools for safe, effective care; (3) patient engagement using portals and mobile devices; and (4) coordination and management of care. All this is predicated on maintaining the integrity of collected data. Safety and efficiency are much easier to quantify. Over the years, reducing medication errors has been a major focus of CPOE and BCMA implementations. Systems that support clinical decision making and provide early warnings of changes in patient status can be used to avert medical errors. Diagnosis and treatment options can be explored using decision support technology. Clinical and operational efficiencies in communication, workflow, documentation, and administrative functions are reported benefits of EHR technology (Hebda and Czar, 2018; McGonigle, 2021).

ELECTRONIC HEALTH RECORD CHALLENGES

The actual and potential benefits of an EHR are evident, but challenges also exist. This section focuses on several issues associated with EHR technology related to cost, data integrity, privacy and confidentiality, standards, documentation burden, patient access, ownership, and patient-generated health data (PGHD).

Cost

The cost to implement, upgrade, and maintain an EHR is a major barrier. There are basically five financial components to consider when purchasing a system: (1) hardware, (2) software, (3) design and implementation assistance, (4) training, and (5) ongoing maintenance (The Office of the National Coordinator for Health Information Technology [ONCHIT], 2014). Physicians in a large private practice can expect first-year costs around $233,297 to purchase and implement a certified EHR, whereas hospitals spend $25 million up to $10 billion on this initial endeavor (American Medical Association, 2019; Pearl, 2017). Annual maintenance is an added expense that can be approximately 18% to 20% of the purchase price. In both scenarios, financial planning for initial and ongoing training, technical support, and software upgrades must be considered. Since each healthcare organization purchases its own EHR applications, they are responsible for internal interfaces and connections to other facilities, which is another cost factor. Incorporating standards are very important for interoperability and the development of local, regional, or national EHRs. The bottom line—implementing, upgrading and maintaining an EHR system is very expensive.

Data Integrity

Data integrity refers to the accuracy, consistency, reliability, and completeness of stored and transmitted data that can be compromised when information is entered incorrectly or is deliberately altered, or when system protections are not working correctly or a system suddenly fails (University of Illinois Chicago, 2021; Zarour et al., 2021). As EHR adoption expands to include data from multiple healthcare entities, more opportunities for human error exist. Poor screen designs that are confusing and cumbersome and lack of system training often lead to data entry errors. How this is monitored and who is responsible for correcting inaccurate information is an issue. Critical patient information, such as allergies, medical history, and medications, should always be validated and updated at each episode of care. Education on how to use the EHR should be provided to all staff before implementing a new system, when changes are made to an existing system, and during orientation for new employees. Stringent security measures that include audit trails, penalties for fraudulent activities, and detailed policies and procedures are other measures that protect data integrity.

Data integrity can also be affected if a system is not working correctly or suddenly fails. Unfortunately, users do not always recognize when an application is not functioning, such as a broken alert or incorrect calculations, and this leads to inaccuracies in data. When an interface from one application to another is not working, this may not be readily noticeable. For example, a physician is able to enter orders using CPOE, but the interface to the pharmacy department system fails and medication orders are not received or dispensed, or orders do not arrive in the laboratory and the blood is not drawn. Subsequently, a healthcare provider may discover the problem only when it is time to administer medications or when test results are not available. These kinds of problems ultimately affect patient care. If the interface resumes functioning, the orders may cross over, but depending on the time the order was placed, some data may be lost or corrupted or a new order may have been placed. Support mechanisms, such as the customer help desk to track issues, rigorous system testing, and safeguards to prevent human error, are extremely important to ensuring data integrity.

Privacy and Confidentiality

Despite advances in technology used to secure EHR data, privacy and confidentiality continue to be major concerns for both the healthcare professional and consumer. With the expansion of the EHRs and HIEs as a driving force to automate and share health information, clinicians may find government and regulatory requirements for controlled access to patient information too restrictive or an invasion of privacy. In this respect, providers may be less inclined to use the EHR or may be more cautious when documenting patient care to avoid litigation. The increase in cybercrimes, especially the use of ransomware, to steal or lock patient data exposes vulnerabilities in our healthcare system and is a breach of trust for the consumer. The fear is that a large-scale EHR system could allow access to personal data without adequate protection against the unauthorized use of information. Some consumers prefer that sensitive health information (such as psychiatric care) never be shared, which creates problems because this can represent critical information missing from a medical record. Before a nationwide interoperable EHR can be fully implemented, major issues related to privacy and security need to be addressed. This topic is discussed in more detail in Chapter 28.

Standard Language for Clinical Care

Healthcare professionals have been discussing the need for standardized vocabularies and terminologies that capture clinical care activities for many decades. Although the use of billing codes (i.e., ICD, DRG, CPT) is commonplace, clinical and nursing languages are constantly evolving and underutilized. Despite the fact that standardization would allow for a mutual understanding of terms, improved communication among healthcare professionals, and provide a common way to a capture, access, and report data, many organizations still resist this change.

Implementation has been hindered by numerous factors such as disagreement on which terminologies to use, lack of harmonization between multiple standardized structures, licensing fees and copyrights, and customization of EHR systems that don't allow for the application of certain terminologies (The Office of the National Coordinator for Health Information Technology [ONCHIT], 2017b). Other factors include cultural and language barriers, threats to autonomy, and user resistance.

Documentation Burden

A significant amount of time is spent by all healthcare providers in processing and documenting patient-related data, but using an EHR system for these activities can be perceived as a frustrating and burdensome experience (Padden, 2019; Yin et al., 2021). Current research on documentation burden identified issues with poorly designed flowsheets (Yin et al., 2021) and the cumbersome charting of assessment data (Swietlik and Sengstack, 2020). Problems of usability are compounded by complex human-computer interfaces, poorly designed decision support tools, and a lack of training that leads to significant medical errors and resistance to accept the technology.

The complexities of EHR technology add concerns that new types of errors are beginning to emerge. Many clinicians complain that information systems increase their workload, which decreases productivity and efficiency. The volume of data needed to comply with government and organizational requirements, documenting routine tasks, and information overload increases the cognitive workload, which leads to errors and issues with data integrity. The burden of documentation is often disruptive to the natural workflow of clinicians with complaints that this impacts time spent at the bedside providing patient care. Padden (2019) suggests documentation should be re-evaluated for value and the impact it has on improving patient outcomes. Addressing this issue is complex and requires user involvement and attention to system design and testing in order to streamline processes and reduce documentation burden.

Consumer Access to Electronic Health Records

Despite advancements in portal technologies, barriers still exist related to providing patient/consumer access to EHR data. The EHR was not originally created for consumer use and required a great deal of redesign and financial investment to allow outside access. Another consideration is that patients are often seen by a variety of healthcare providers so information may be fragmented across several different facilities and practices. The technical infrastructure to integrate (or interface) data from these disparate systems is difficult as well as costly. Recent reports of health insurance and government data violations fuel concerns over privacy, confidentiality, and security of personal health data. The Health Information Portability and Accountability Act (HIPAA) security rules for electronic health data were established to require entities to take appropriate "administrative, physical, and technical safeguards to ensure the confidentiality, integrity, and security of electronic protected health information" (U.S. Department of Health & Human Services [DHHS], 2020). The 21st Century Cures Act also proposed specific policies for patient access to include participation in HIEs (Azar, 2020; Lye et al., 2018). But providers may be at risk for lawsuits if strict precautions are not taken and patient data is compromised, resulting in limited involvement in data sharing.

Consumers have a legal right to request access to PHI, but control of the data is still debatable. Even though access to PHI is available, consumers are restricted from viewing certain entries, such as physician and other clinical provider notes, along with the inability to update or correct information (Azar, 2020). Providers are concerned that patients may not have the knowledge or skills to interpret the information in the health record. Studies have reported that sharing notes and other health information with patients may be confusing or harmful and cause the patient undue anxiety; therefore, some providers may avoid encouraging portal use (Dendere et al., 2019; Roehrs et al., 2017).

Disagreements related to e-mail use and what can be addressed online versus routine office visits can lead to dissatisfaction with care. The fear of increased workload or workflow interruptions may hinder online engagement by clinicians, although the rapid deployment of telemedicine services in response to the COVID-19 pandemic altered some of these perceptions. Some clinicians are concerned that patients may find mistakes in the record, which could prompt legal action. Patients who lack computer skills may have difficulty accessing and using EHR portal systems. A common practice is to provide patients with a link to an EHR portal without any training on how to navigate the site. Chronic illnesses, debilitating diseases, or pain can hinder interest or the ability to access a portal. Once access is achieved, consumers may lack the knowledge to interpret the medical results or information provided. Some providers prefer to delay release of test results until after they discuss findings with the patient verbally. Advocates for immediate and timely access to data contend that bias exists for those with lower socioeconomic status and literacy skills. They propose that alternate methods should be available to address issues associated with data access (Irizarry et al., 2017; Showell, 2017).

Ownership

Traditionally, health records have been the property of the service institution. A comprehensive, interoperable EHR would cross institutional boundaries, making the determination of ownership more complex. Consumer access and ownership to the larger volume of EHR data opens the door to a plethora of legal, ethical, and medical issues requiring serious discussion and research (Chiruvella and Guddati, 2021; Mirchev, Mircheva, & Kerekovska, 2020). As discussed earlier, consumers have access to their PHI through portals, and what they are allowed to access is expanding, but there are still unanswered questions related to ownership. For example, who will be responsible for updating and ensuring data accuracy? Who will store the shared data? Should "ownership" and "access" be completely separate concepts so that those responsible for storing, updating, and ensuring data accuracy are considered data stewards but not owners? (That is, the consumer may own the data but the responsibilities of data stewardship may reside with a healthcare institution.) Would consumers have access to all the data or a subset of the data? What role would the government play in monitoring the access, quality, security, privacy, and confidentiality of patient records?

Consumer access and consent is a critical element of the EHR initiatives and has significant implications for healthcare organizations and the issue of ownership. Some providers may be uncomfortable with the prospect of patients reading their notes and may alter what and how they document to accommodate consumer access (Chiruvella and Guddati, 2021). Health professionals must have consent to retrieve or share patient records between facilities to ensure that personal information is not accessed inappropriately. This rule could affect quality of care if the consumer is concerned about confidentiality and denies permission. Ultimately, ownership may be driven by who has control of the data, or ownership may become irrelevant as access becomes the driving force in answering these many questions.

Patient-Generated Health Data

Patient-generated health data (PGHD) are defined as "health-related data created, recorded, or gathered by or from patients (family members or care givers) to help address a health concern" (The Office of the National Coordinator for Health Information Technology [ONCHIT], 2018). Although most EHR systems provide a patient portal that "push" data for viewing, few offer the flexibility and functionality to capture PGHD to augment care. The internet and mobile technologies are a growing trend for collecting PGHD (Jim et al., 2020; Lai et al., 2017). Sharing on social media sites; the use of mobile devices such as smartphones, laptops, and wearable items (wristbands, clothing, etc.); genetic testing; and other types of biometric sensors generate massive amounts of data that could be captured for clinical care and research (Demiris et al., 2019). PGHD transmitted or entered into an EHR portal provides an opportunity to monitor and track progress and actively engage patients in care management (Lai et al., 2017).

Despite these benefits, use of PGHD is met with some scrutiny by healthcare professionals. There are several major concerns associated with PGHD related to (1) volume and quality of data, (2) how data will be used, (3) privacy and security, and (4) user characteristics (Nittas et al., 2019). The volume of data reported by patients can be overwhelming to providers, leading to information overload and workflow concerns. Discerning which data are pertinent or not could be very time consuming. Detailed data might be useful in gaining insight into a patient problem but could also hinder effective analysis because of challenges associated with screening large amounts of data. This also raises questions about who is responsible for checking the data, when and how often, and what are the liabilities if timely review and response to data do not occur. Patients may provide more detail than needed, as well as deviate from the actual problem to include experiences of others or data unrelated to their condition. Patients may not be aware of which data should be included when reporting an issue or decide not to report a change because they think it is not important. Some patients may try to manipulate data to force a certain outcome, such as obtaining certain prescription medications. Patients may underreport or overreport based on the need to fill in the blanks or comply with the healthcare provider's directions. Incorrect data entry is a concern because treatment options may be unrelated to status and cause harm or ineffective disease management. In addition, personal opinions or inappropriate comments could be problematic and cause discomfort for healthcare providers.

As with patient access to EHR data, privacy and security is a major concern with PGHD (Nittas et al., 2019). Patients and providers need assurance that the data are from an authenticated source and linked to the correct patient through a secure portal.

Patient characters such as literacy level (health, computer and digital), social determinants of health, and attitudes around technology are a concern and may impact collecting reliable and credible PGHD (Nittas et al., 2019). Poorly designed devices and applications may be difficult for some patients to understand or use, not to mention that mobile devices can be very expensive and cost-prohibitive to certain demographics. Some EHR vendors are beginning to integrate data from PGHD sources directly or through questionnaires, but there is still a need for technologies with the ability to transform and filter PGHD into meaningful information to improve decision making and clinical outcomes (Lai et al., 2017; Nittas et al., 2019).

STAKEHOLDER PERSPECTIVES

In most organizations, EHRs are utilized by multiple groups or stakeholders that share an interest in leveraging this tool to support patient care. Stakeholders may have similar concerns about the technology but different needs and approaches for resolution. It is important to consider the perspectives of essential stakeholders, which include consumers, healthcare providers, healthcare administrators, insurance payers, and state and national governments.

Consumers

Healthcare consumers or patients have a unique vantage point for evaluating the effect of EHRs. They see multiple providers in a variety of settings and are the victim when gaps in care coordination occur. They often provide the same information repeatedly and are aware of technology failures that threaten their personal data. In 2019, the Kaiser Family Foundation (KFF) conducted a health survey of 1440 adults to determine patients' expectations and perceptions regarding EHRs and health IT. The majority of respondents (88%) indicated their provider uses an EHR system. Only half (45%) indicated that EHRs improved care and communication with their physician, whereas the other half (44%) maintained there was no difference (Munana, Kirzinger, & Brodie, 2019). Although consumers acknowledge the potential for EHR technology to improve care, there are still concerns about the privacy, security, and accuracy of these systems. In this same survey, older adults were more concerned about unauthorized access to PHI than younger respondents (Munana, Kirzinger, & Brodie, 2019). One in five respondents reported errors in their medical record and nearly half (45%) were concerned this could affect the care they received. With patient volume increasing in hospitals and provider practices along with the massive data collected on a daily basis, the likelihood of human error is great. As consumers demand more access to EHR data and become more involved in care decision-making, these concerns must be addressed (Wass, Vimarlund, & Ros, 2019).

Healthcare Providers

In the early stages of EHR adoption, there was a lot of resistance from physicians especially related to CPOE. Entering orders was seen as a clerical task better suited for lower-level staff. These attitudes have drastically shifted as EHR systems became more commonplace, a new generation embraced technology, and mandates to enforce provider involvement prevailed. In a recent study, providers' attitudes toward the implementation of a new EHR significantly improved over time (Krousel-Wood et al., 2018). Providers noted numerous benefits that influenced this change related to easy access to current and past medical records; improved communication between provider and patient; availability of various prompts to support preventive care, ordering medications and other care related activities; improved care coordination; and sharing of medical information through HIE networks. Other studies supported these benefits and noted improvements in workflow, safety, and quality of care (Wani and Malhotra, 2018; Denton et al., 2019).

But not all providers agree the current state of EHR systems is the best solution and is a major cause of physician burnout. Liebman, Chiang, and Chodosh (Liebman, Chiang, & Chodosh, 2019) noted that EHRs offer little in terms of "meaningful clinical assistance, knowledge synthesis or targeted learning" (p. 331). Lack of integration with other systems, higher costs, overuse of alerts and warnings, and the time-consuming nature of data input is disruptive to the normal workflow associated with providing care (Liebman et al., 2019; Lim et al., 2018). Another study indicated that the increasing documentation requirements related to numerous government initiatives produced a stressful environment and led to less time with the patient (Hanauer et al., 2017). Although perceptions about EHR vary among providers, the potential for expanding functionality by incorporating virtual technologies, the use of machine learning and artificial intelligence, and radical interoperability are exciting prospects for the next generation of providers (Abrams et al., 2020).

Nurses constitute one of the largest groups of EHR users and their perspective is critical to the successful integration of current and future technology. Nurses' attitudes toward EHRs are positive, reporting the system increased productivity, improved performance, enhanced effectiveness, decreased medication administration errors, and supported evidence-based practice and clinical care activities (McGonigle, 2021; Graham, Nussdorfer, & Beal, 2018; Michaels, 2020). Knowledge-based systems may include functionality that integrates clinical guidelines, protocols and other decision support tools to assist nurses in the development of plans of care and monitor outcomes.

As mentioned in an earlier section, documentation burden has surfaced as a serious issue for the nursing community. As technology becomes more robust and patient care more complex, nurses struggle to meet documentation demands imposed by the employing facility, practice organizations, and government mandates. In a systematic review, Baumann, Baker, & Elshaug (Baumann et al., 2018) reported nurses spent significantly more time documenting care post-EHR implementation (23%) then pre-EHR (9%). Nurses also observed a duplication of efforts among care providers, fragmented or incomplete documents, and a decrease in physician–nurse communication. These inefficiencies in workflow were compounded by multiple interruptions, competing tasks, and dissatisfaction with the lack of time to spend with patients.

Health Care Organizations and Organizational Culture

An important question for healthcare organizations is how to stay financially viable in an environment determined to control escalating healthcare costs. Added to this burden is the mandate to implement comprehensive EHR systems to meet value-based criteria for reimbursement and expanding interoperability to a national-wide level. Depending on the size and complexity of each organization, costs for implementing and upgrading EHR technology are a significant investment. Beyond the initial expenses are fees associated with consultants, IT staff, programmers, internal staff resources, training, licensing, and ongoing maintenance. For the healthcare executive, EHR systems improve operational efficiency, strengthen communication throughout the organization, increase patient safety, support compliance with regulatory requirements, improve medical record security and storage, improve care coordination, enhance the quality of care, and provide faster turnaround for procedure authorization, billing, and claims submission (The Office of the National Coordinator for Health Information Technology [ONCHIT], 2019d). Healthcare executives and leaders must look at leveraging this technology not only to control costs but also to increase safety, improve patient outcomes and quality of care, and provide tools for better decision making (Pearson and Frakt, 2018). Healthcare executives must also reflect beyond single-facility implementation to the possible benefits of system integration that will foster collaboration at local, national, and international levels.

The healthcare environment is filled with many cultures, subcultures, and traditions, and the implementation or upgrade of EHR components is always disruptive to the sociocultural system. Cell phones, e-mail, and social media have significantly changed our interpersonal, professional, and business communications. In this respect, the use of EHR technology challenges social and cultural norms and has altered how we communicate with patients and other providers. Nurses are often unaware of new orders or alerts until they sign on to the EHR. This can create delays in care and disruptions in workflow, especially when monitoring a critically ill patient.

The healthcare organization itself is a culture where a common purpose, rules, processes, and mindset are shared by all employees (Ballaro and Washington, 2016). Healthcare organizations are challenged with issues surrounding the evolving nature of EHR technology. Whether in a hospital setting or private practice, nurses, physicians, and other caregivers are required to use an EHR as part of their daily routine, but some find it difficult to comply. Reasons for this vary and may include poor computer skills, complexity of the application, poorly designed systems, lack of available hardware, or difficulty adjusting to change. Organizations that recognize cultural standards and support employee needs foster positive perceptions of EHR technology use.

Insurance Payers

The EHR provides several benefits for insurance companies through better disease management and reporting of services. Pay-for-performance requirements are supported and can be submitted in a timely manner. Claims that are incorrectly coded or lack coding standards can confuse payers when they attempt to reimburse organizations for services. Systems that integrate patient data with coding and billing structures can provide data to control costs and manage expensive procedures. Medicare and Medicaid claims require significant documentation and review by CMS staff to determine if reimbursement criteria are met. Nursing and physician documentation are critical to capturing quality measures to meet payer requirements along with evidence for the provision of a variety of electronic services such as information exchange, security measures, and patient access to data.

State and National Government

In 2018, the cost of healthcare in the U.S. was over $3.6 trillion, and it is expected to grow faster than the national income (National Center for Health Statistics, 2021). In 2020, the coronavirus (COVID-19) pandemic added substantially to medical costs through massive hospitalizations, vaccination programs, and long-term care. One proposed measure for cost containment focuses on improving coordination and quality of care. The implementation of a nationwide interoperable EHR was recommended as a solution that would significantly reduce medical errors, improve care quality, and save the U.S. healthcare system major expense (The Office of the National Coordinator for Health Information Technology [ONCHIT], 2021). A major challenge is how to support the sharing of patient data across multiple organizations which requires a nationwide technology infrastructure and communication standards, such as standardized nomenclatures, vocabularies, and coding structures. Although the initial expenditures for EHR adoption was high, the benefits to our nation is the ability to identify and address safety issues in a timely fashion, notify patients and populations at risk for disease or environmental exposure, detect epidemics (such as COVID-19), and prepare for bioterrorism attacks (The Office of the National Coordinator for Health Information Technology [ONCHIT], 2019e). A clinical dataset of essential information is available as a result of the increased use of EHRs, which would allow researchers to explore preventive and curative solutions that address the nation's health and healthcare issues. Ultimately, a nationwide, interoperable EHR system would assist government agencies to improve the overall healthcare for all U.S. citizens.

ELECTRONIC HEALTH RECORD AND PRECISION CARE

Precision medicine or personalized care is an emerging science predicated on the use of big data, genomics, and machine learning techniques to foster the translation of evidence into clinical practice (Abdul-Husn and Kenny, 2019; Naithani, Sinha, Misra, Vasudevan, & Sahu, 2021). The underlying premise is that people are different in terms of genetics, how they live, and sociocultural factors, therefore treatment and preventive measures should be "personalized" and directed toward these variances. The EHR is a major source of "big data" that can be analyzed to identify specific biomarkers, clinical characteristics, disease progression, and treatment response by various phenotypes or clinical diseases.

Biobanks

Biobanks, which are repositories of medical, biological and/or genetic material, could be linked to EHR systems to create a more comprehensive set of data for research (Glicksberg, Johnson, & Dudley, 2018). But since EHRs were primarily created to support clinical care they may harbor missing data, redundancies, and documentation errors, which are not ideal for conducting research. On the other hand, data harvested from an actual clinical setting on a continuous basis would be more realistic than data from a controlled trial (Glicksberg

et al., 2018). Researchers are currently using biobanks linked to EHRs to confirm prior variable/phenotype relationships and to uncover new relationships, (Haggerty et al., 2017) create innovative drugs and enhance drug effectiveness and tolerance, (Shameer et al., 2017) and identify gene mutations associated with specific diseases like BRCA1/2 for breast cancer (Buchanan et al., 2019). Genomics and phenotyping hold the key to disease detection and treatment with the promise of designer medications that target the unique characteristics of each individual.

Customized medications will likely eliminate prescribing drugs or doses that do not work, help minimize side effects, and decrease costs. Other treatments, such as diet and exercise, can be personalized to avoid guesswork and trial and error. For example, if a patient's genetic code and phenotype reveal a risk for colon cancer, then preventive measures can start earlier. More frequent exams, colonoscopies, and diets that promote colon health can be the focus of care. In the future, an individual's genome sequence may be part of a comprehensive medical record, not unlike recording medications and allergies.

Machine Learning

Machine learning is a powerful evaluation tool that can be used to facilitate healthcare providers and consumers in the decision-making process, as well as advance research in personalized medicine. Massive amounts of data are being collected daily in EHRs and it would be impossible for the average clinician to analyze without assistance. Machine learning is basically a set of statistical and computational algorithms that can map complex relationships between biologic, genotype, and disease data. The clinical utility of these mathematical models is the ability to predict response to treatment or potential for disease (Ho et al., 2019). But EHRs are limited to data collected in clinical settings related to episodic care and contain gaps in understanding the big picture. Non-traditional sources such as PGHD from mobile devices, dental repositories, and smart home technologies have the potential to enhance existing methods and advance the field of precision medicine (Glicksberg et al., 2018; Thyvalikakath et al., 2020).

CONCLUSION AND FUTURE DIRECTIONS

EHR is the preferred acronym for the lifetime patient record that includes healthcare data from the consumer and a variety of provider sources. Common EHR applications used in the clinical setting include CPOE, eMAR, BCMA, clinical documentation, specialty applications, and CDS. The EHR has many benefits related to cost savings, access, quality, and safety of care delivery. Although there are many advances in the technology, issues associated with ownership, data integrity, privacy and confidentiality, organizational culture, patient access, documentation burden, PGHD, and the development of an infrastructure to support a nationwide EHR still need to be addressed. Despite similar concerns, stakeholders maintain a positive overall attitude about the benefits of EHR technologies related to easy access to records, improved communications, support for decision making, and increased safety and quality of care. As EHRs become more sophisticated and documentation needs increase, this places new demands on the user. Documentation burden is a common complaint among providers due to organizational, professional, and regulatory charting requirements; coupled with high patient acuity, which has resulted in less time to provide direct care.

The EHR plays a pivotal role in personalized medicine as a medium for data, information, knowledge exchange, and exploration. The EHR contains a wealth of information related to disease, interventions, and treatment responses that can be used for research. Access to an interoperable EHR with links to biobanks can be used to diagnose, prevent, and treat preexisting and potential health issues based on unique biological responses, resulting in highly individualized care. Analysis of these huge databases, utilizing machine learning algorithms, can reveal patterns and predictions on how to reverse or prevent disease. Future directions are promising for the EHR in supporting research efforts, mobilizing care coordination across national and international boundaries, and advancing precision care.

DISCUSSION QUESTIONS

1. It is anticipated that EHR functionality will expand to allow consumers to enter data into the system along with direct input of other types of PGHD. What are some benefits and challenges associated with this change from the perspective of consumers, providers, and healthcare organizations?
2. Patients expect full access to their personal health data. What limitations, if any, would be in the best interest of patients? Should patients be permitted to correct entries? Why or why not?
3. Documentation burden is a recognized issue among nurses. What factors contribute to this phenomenon and what strategies could be used to decrease documentation requirements?
4. Discuss the advantages and disadvantages associated with implementing and using a national EHR.
5. Discuss legal, ethical, and social issues associated with the introduction of precision medicine.

CASE STUDY

Although your facility has a state-of-the art electronic health record (EHR), it lacks specific functionality to address the needs of emergency care. In the interest of patient safety and to integrate activities into the EHR your team has been tasked to explore the following three options: (1) implement and integrate a triage system; (2) incorporate clinical vocabularies in the EHR to support nursing and physician documentation requirements; and (3) implement RFID technology for patient tracking.

DISCUSSION QUESTIONS

1. What are the advantages and disadvantages of each option? Which option would you recommend implementing first and why?
2. Your team and the Vice President of Patient Care Services are working together to address the needs of the Emergency Department. Who would you identify as stakeholders in the implementation of each solution and why? What steps would you take to minimize user resistance?
3. The EHR is not fail-proof, and human error is an issue. Discuss potential decision support tools and functionality that could be implemented to increase patient safety.

REFERENCES

Abbasi, R., Jabali, M. S., Khajouei, R., & Tadayon, H. (2020). Investigating the satisfaction level of physicians in regards to implementing medical picture archiving and communication system (PACS). *BMC Medical Informatics and Decision Making, 20*(180), 1–8. https://doi.org/10.1186/s12911-020-01203-0.

Abdul-Husn, N., & Kenny, E. (2019). Personalized medicine and the power of electronic health records. *Cell, 177*(March 21, 2019), 56–68. https://doi.org/10.1016/j.cell.2019.03.0392.

Abrams, K., Shah, U., Korba, C., & Elsner, N. (2020, July 9). How the virtual health landscape is shifting in a rapidly changing world: Findings from the Deloitte 2020 Survey of U.S. Physicians. *Deloitte*. Retrieved August 30, 2021, from https://www2.deloitte.com/us/en/insights/industry/health-care/physician-survey.html

Aldosare, H., Saddik, B., & Al Kadi, K. (2017). Impact of picture archiving and communication system (PACS) on radiology staff. *Informatics in Medicine Unocked, 10*(2018), 1–16. https://doi.org/10.1016/j.imu.2017.11.001.

Alexander, S., & Guerra, D. (2019). The electronic health record. In S. Alexander, K. H. Frith, & H. Hoy (Eds.), *Applied clinical informatics for nurses* (2nd ed., pp. 163–180). Burlington, MA: Jones & Bartlett.

American Association of Colleges of Nursing (AACN). (2020, September). Nursing shortage. *American Association of Colleges of Nursing*. Retrieved August 25, 2021, from https://www.aacnnursing.org/News-Information/Fact-Sheets/Nursing-Shortage

American Medical Association. (2019). *Impact of high capital costs of hospital EHRs on the medical staff. Board of Trustees*. Chicago: American Medical Assocation. Retrieved August 20, 2021, from. https://www.ama-assn.org/system/files/2019-04/a19-bot32.pdf.

Anderson, L. (2018, February 8). National drug codes explained and the ONC Health IT Certificati. *Drugs.com*. Retrieved August 23, 2021, from https://www.drugs.com/ndc.html

Asmirajanti, M., Hamid, A., & Hariyati, R. (2019). Nursing care activities based on documentation. *BMC Nursing, 18*(32), 1–5. https://doi.org/10.1186/s12912-019-0352-0.

Atasoy, H., Greenwood, B., & McCullough, J. S. (2019). The digitization of patient care: A review of the effects of electronic health records on health care quality and utilization. *Annual Review of Public Health, 40*(2019), 487–500. https://doi.org/10.1146/annurev-publhealth-040218-044206.

Azar, I. I. (2020). 21st Century Cures Act: Interoperability, information blocking, and the ONC Health IT Certification Program. *Federal Register: The Daily Journal of the United States Government* 2020-05.

Ballaro, J., & Washington, E. (2016). The impact of organizational culture and percerived organizational support on successful use of electronic healthcare record (EHR). *Organization Development Journal, 34*(2), 11–29. Retrieved from https://eds-b-ebscohost-com.proxy-hs.researchport.umd.edu/eds/pdfviewer/pdfviewer?vid=2&sid=8bcf1a63-56d7-408e-8187-e6cf75bf8718%40sessionmgr4006.

Bates, D. W., Leape, L. L., Cullen, D. J., Laird, N., Petersen, L., Teich, J., et al. (1998). Effect of computerized physician order entry and a team intervention on prevention of serious medication errors. *JAMA, 280*(15), 1311–1316. https://doi.org/10.1001/jama.280.15.1311.

Baumann, L., Baker, J., & Elshaug, A. (2018). The impact of electronic health record systems on clinical documentation times: A systematic review. *Health Policy, 122*(2018), 827–836. https://doi.org/10.1016/j.healthpol.2018.05.014.

Blackley, S., Huynh, J., Wang, L., Korach, Z., & Zhou, L. (2019). Speech recognition for clinical documentation from 1990 to 2018: A systemati review. *JAMIA, 26*(4), 324–338. https://doi.org/10.1093/jamia/ocy179.

Bodenreider, D., Cornet, R., & Vreeman, D. J. (2018). Recent developments in clinical terminologies: SNOWMED CT, LOINC, and RxNorm. *Yearbook of Medical Informatics, 27*(01), 129–139.

Buchanan, A., Kandamurugu, M., Meyer, M. N., Wagner, J., Hallquist, M., Williams, J. L., et al. (2019). Early cancer diagnoses through BRCA1/2 screening of unselected adult biobank participants. *Genetics in Medicine, 20*(5), 554–558.

Carroll, N., & Richardson, I. (2020). Enablers and barriers for hospital pharmacy information systems. *Health Informatics Journal, 26*(1), 406–419. https://doi.org/10.1177/1460458219832056.

Centers for Medicare & Medicaid Services (CMS). (2020, July 20). Requirements for previous years. *CMS.gov*. Retrieved August 24, 2021, from https://www.cms.gov/Regulations-and-Guidance/Legislation/EHRIncentivePrograms/RequirementsforPreviousYears

Centers for Medicare & Medicaid Services. (2019, November 18). MACRA. *CMS.gov*. Retrieved August 25, 2021, from https://www.cms.gov/Medicare/Quality-Initiatives-Patient-Assessment-Instruments/Value-Based-Programs/MACRA-MIPS-and-APMs/MACRA-MIPS-and-APMs

Centers for Medicare & Medicaid Services. (2021, August 17). Promoting interoperability programs. *CMS.gov*. Retrieved August 24, 2021, from https://www.cms.gov/regulations-and-guidance/legislation/ehrincentiveprograms?redirect=/ehrincentiveprograms/#BOOKMARK1

Chiruvella, V., & Guddati, A.K. (2021). Ethical issues in patient data ownership. *Interactive Journal of Medical Research*, 10(2), e22269 1-9. Retrieved from https://www.i-jmr.org/2021/2/e22269

Demiris, G., Iribarren, S. J., Sward, K., Lee, S., & Yang, R. (2019). Oatient generated health data use in clinical practice: A systematic review. *Nursing Outlook, 67*(4), 311–330. https://doi.org/10.1016/j.outlook.2019.04.005.

Demner-Fushman, D., Seckman, C., Fisher, C., & Thoma, G. (2013). Continual development of a personalized decision support system. *MEDINFO, 2013*, 175–179.

Dendere, R., Slade, C., Burton-Jones, A., Sullivan, C., Staib, A., & Janda, M. (2019). Patient portals facilitating engagement with inpatient electronic medical records: A systematic review. *Journal of Medical Internet Research, 21*(4), e12779. https://doi.org/10.2196/12779.

Denton, C., Soni, H., Kannampallil, T., Serrichio, A., Traub, S., & Patel, V. (2019). Emergency physicians' perceived influence of EHR use on clinical workflow and performance metrics. *Applied Clinical Informatics, 9*(3), 725–733. https://doi.org/10.1055/s-0038-1668553.

European Commission. (2021, June 21). *Exchange of electronic health records across the EU. Shaping Europe's digital future*. Retrieved August 25, 2021, from https://digital-strategy.ec.europa.eu/en/policies/electronic-health-records

Farzandipour, M., Meidni, Z., Sadeqi, J. M., & Dehghan, V. E. (2019). Designing and evaluating functional laboratory information system requirements integrated to hospital information systems. *Journal of Evaluation in Clinical Practice, 25*(5), 788–799. https://doi.org/10.1111/jep.13074.

Gandhi, T., Weingart, S., Seger, A., Borus, J., Burdick, E., Poon, E., et al. (2005). Outpatient prescribing errors and the impact of computerized prescribing. *Journal of General INternal Medicine, 20*, 837–841. https://doi.org/10.1111/j.1525-1497.2005.0194.x.

Glicksberg, S., Johnson, K., & Dudley, J. (2018). The next generation of precision medicine: Observational studies, electronic health records, biobanks and continuous monitoring. *Human Molecular Genetics, 27*(R1), R56–R62. https://doi.org/10.1093/hmg/ddy114.

Graham, H., Nussdorfer, D., & Beal, R. (2018). Nurses attitudes related to accepting electronic health records and bedside documentation. *CIN Plus, 36*(11), 515–520.

Haggerty, C., James, C., Calkins, H., Tichnell, C., Leader, J., Hartzel, D., et al. (2017). Electronic health record phenotype in subjects with genetic variants associated with arrhythmogenic right ventricular cardiomyopathy: A study of 30,716 subjects with exome sequencing K. *Genetic Medicine, 19*(11), 1245–1252. https://doi.org/10.1038/gim.2017.40.

Han, H., Gleason, K. T., Sun, C., Miller, H., Kang, S. J., Chow, S., et al. (2019). Using patient portals to improve patient outcomes: Systematic review. *JMIR Human Factors, 6*(4), 1–11. https://doi.org/10.2196/15038.

Hanauer, D. S., Brandford, G., Greenberg, G., Kileny, S., Couper, M., Zheng, K., & Choe, S. (2017). Two-year longitudinal assessment of physicians' perceptions after replacement of a longstanding homegrown electronic health record: Does a J-curve of satisfactio really exist? *JAMIA, 24*(e1), e157–e165. https://doi.org/10.1093/jamia/ocw077.

Hariyati, S., Tutik, R., Mediawati, A., & Eryando, T. (2021). The effectiveness of electronic medication administration record: A systematic review. *International Journal of Nursing Education, 13*(3), 97–103.

Health Information Management Systems Society (HIMSS). (2021). *Interoperability in healthcare. HIMSS*. Retrieved August 25, 2021, from https://www.himss.org/resources/interoperability-healthcare#Part6

Hebda, T., & Czar, P. (2018). *Handbook of informatics for nurses and healthcare professionals* (6th ed.). Boston: Pearson.

Highfill, T. (2020). Do hospitals with electronic health records have lower costs? A systematic review and meta-analysis. *International Journal of Healthcare Management, 13*(1), 65–71. https://doi.org/10.1080/20479700.2019.1616895.

Ho, D., Schierding, W., Wake, M., Saffery, R., & O'Sullivan, J. (2019). Machine learning SNP based prediction for precision medicine. *Frontiers in Genetics, 10*(267), 1–10. https://doi.org/10.3389/fgene.2019.00267.

Institiue of Medicine. (2003). *Key capailities of an electronic health record system: Letter report.* Washington, DC: National Academies Press. doi: https://doi.org/10.17226/10781.

Institute of Medicine. (2000). *To err is human: Building a safer health system.* In L. T. Kohn, J. M. Corrigan, & M. S. Donaldson (Eds.), Washington, DC: The National Academies Press. https://doi.org/10.17226/9728.

Institute of Medicine. (2001). *Crossing the quality chasm: A new health system for the 21st century.* Washington, DC: The National Academies Press. https://doi.org/10.17226/10027.

Institute of Medicine. (2004). *Patient safety: Achieving a new standard for care.* In P. Aspden, J. M. Corrigan, J. Wolcott, & S. M. Erickson (Eds.), Washington, DC: National Academies Press.

Irizarry, T., Shoemake, J., Nilsen, M., Czaja, S., Beach, S., & Dabbs, A. (2017). Patient portals as a tool for health care engagement: A mixed-method study of older adults with varying levels of health literacy and prior patient portal use. *Journal of Medical Internet Research, 19*(3), e99. https://doi.org/10.2196/jmir.7099.

Jim, H., Hoogland, A., Brownstein, N., Barata, A., Dicker, A., Knoop, H., et al. (2020). Innovations in research and clinical care using patient-generated health data. *CA: A Cancer Journal for Clinicians, 70*(3), 182–199. https://doi.org/10.3322/caac.21608.

Johnson, C., & Pylypchuk, Y. (2021, February). *Use of certified health IT and methods to enable interoperability by U.S. non-federal acute care jospitals, 2019.* Washington DC: Office of the National Coordinator for Health Information Technology. ONC Data Brief, no. 54.

Joseph, J., Moore, Z., Patton, D., O'Connor, T., & Nugent, L. (2020). The impact of implementing speech recognition technology on the accuracy and efficiency (time to complete) clinical documentation by nurses: A systematic review. *Journal of Clinical Nursing, 29*(13-14), 2125–2137. https://doi.org/10.1111/jocn.15261.

Kravet, S., & Bailey, J. (2018). Deriving value from data and data dashboards. *The Journal of Medical Practice Management, 336,* 341–343.

Krousel-Wood, M., McCoy, A., Ahia, C., Holt, E. W., Trapani, D. N., Luo, Q., et al. (2018). Implementing electronic health records (EHRs): health care provider perceptions before and after transition from a local basic EHR to a commercial comprehensive EHR. *JAMIA, 25*(6), 618–626. https://doi.org/10.1093/jamia/ocx094.

Lai, A. M., Hsueh, P., Choi, Y. K., & Austin, R. (2017). Present and future trends in consumer health informatics and patient-generated-health data. *Yearbook of Medical Informatics, 26*(01), 152–159. https://doi.org/10.15265/IY-2017-016.

Library of Congress. (2020). H.R. 748-Cares Act: 116th Congress (2019-2020). Retrived September 29, 2021 from Congress.gov: https://www.congress.gov/bill/116th-congress/house-bill/748

Liebman, D. L., Chiang, M. F., & Chodosh, J. (2019). Realizing the promise of electronic health records: Moving beyond "paper on a screen." *American Academy of Ophthalmology, 126*(3), 331–334. https://doi.org/10.1016/j.ophtha.2018.09.023.

Lim, M., Boland, M., McCannel, C., Saini, A., Chiang, M., Epley, D., & Lum, F. (2018). Adoption of electronic health records and perceptions of financial and clinical outcomes among ophthalmologists in the United States. *JAMA Ophthalmology, 136*(2), 164–170. https://doi.org/10.1001/jamaophthalmol.2017.5978.

Lye, C., Forman, H., Daniel, J., & Krumholz, H. (2018). The 21st Century Cures Act and electronic health records one year later: Will patients see the benefits? *JAMIA, 25*(9), 1218–1220. https://doi.org/10.1093/jamia/ocy065.

Lyons, A., Sward, A., Deshmukh, V., Pett, M., Donaldson, G., & Turnbull, J. (2017). Impact of computerized provider order entry (CPOE) on length of stay and mortality. *JAMIA, 24*(2), 303–309. https://doi.org/10.1093/jamia/ocw091.

McBride, S., & Tietz, M. (2019). *Nursing Informatics for the advanced practice nurse.* New York: Springer Publishing Company, LLC.

McGonigle, D. M. (2021). *Nursing informatics and the foundation of knowledge* (5th ed.). Burlington, MA: Jones & Bartlett.

Medic, G., Klieb, M., Atallah, L., Weichert, J., Panda, S., Postma, M., & El-Kerdi, A. (2019). Evidence-based clinical decision support systems for the prediction and detection of three disease states in critical care: A systematic literature review. *F1000Research, 8*(2019). https://doi.org/10.12688/f1000research.20498.2.

Mekhjian, H. S., Kumar, R. R., Kuehn, L., Bentley, T., Teater, P., Thomas, A., et al. (2002). Immediate benefits realized following implementation of physician order entry at an academic medical center. *JAMIA, 9*(5), 529–539. https://doi.org/10.1197/jamia.M1038.

Michaels, D. (2020, March 26). Nursing Documentation: Historical review Florence Nightingale to Computer EHR. *American Nursing History.* Retrieved 18 1, 2021, from https://www.americannursinghistory.org/documentation

Middleton, B., Sittig, D., & Wright, A. (2016). Clinical Decision Support: A 25 year retrospective and a 25 year vision. *IMIA Yearbook of Medical Informatics, 25*(S01), S103–S116. https://doi.org/10.15265/IYS-2016-s034.

Mirchev, M., Mircheva, I., & Kerekovska, A. (2020). The academic viewpoint on patient data ownership in the context of big data: Scoping review. *Journal of Medical Internet Research, 22*(8), e22214. https://doi.org/10.2196/22214.

Moncho, V., Marco-Simo, J.M., & Cobarsi, J. (2021). EHR implementation: A literature review. In A. Rocha, C. Ferras, D. Lopez-Lopez, & T. Cuarda (Ed.), *ICITS: International Conference on Information Technology & Systems. 2,* pp. 3–12. Libertad City, Ecuador: Springer, Cham. doi: https://doi.org/10.1007/978-3-030-68418-1-1

Munana, C., Kirzinger, A., & Brodie, M. (2019, March 18). Data Note: Public's Experiences with Electronic Health Records. *KKF.* Retrieved August 28, 2021 from https://www.kff.org/other/poll-finding/data-note-publics-experiences-with-electronic-health-records/

Naidu, M., & Alicia, Y. (2019). Impact of bar-code medication administration and electronic medication administration record system in clinical practice for an effective medication administration process. *Health, 11*(05), 511–526. https://doi.org/10.4236/health.2019.115044.

Naithani, N., Sinha, S., Misra, P., Vasudevan, B., & Sahu, R. (2021). Precision medicine: Concept and tools. *Medical Journal Armed Forces India, 77*(2021), 249–257. https://doi.org/10.1016/j.mjafi.2021.06.021.

Najmi, U., Haque, W., Ansari, U., Yemane, E., Alexander, L., Lee, C., et al. (2021). Inpatient insulin pen implementation, waste, and potential cost savings: a community hospital experience. *Journal of Diabetes Science and Technology, 15*(4), 741–747. https://doi.org/10.1177/19322968211002514.

National Center for Health Statistics. (2021, May 8). *Health expenditures.* Centers for Disease Control and Prevention (CDC).

Retrieved August 29, 2021, from https://www.cdc.gov/nchs/fastats/health-expenditures.htm

National Library of Medicine. (2017, May 8). National Drug File—Reference terminology source. *National Library of Medicine.* Retrieved August 20, 2021, from https://www.nlm.nih.gov/research/umls/sourcereleasedocs/current/NDFRT/index.html

National Library of Medicine. (2021, July 9). RxNorm. *National Library of Medicine.* Retrieved August 20, 2021, from https://www.nlm.nih.gov/research/umls/rxnorm/index.html

Nittas, V., Lun, P., Ehrler, F., Puhan, M. A., & Mutsch, M. (2019). Electronic patient-generated health data to facilitate disease prevention and health promotion: Scoping review. *J Med Internet Res, 21*(10), e13320. https://doi.org/10.2196/13320.

Office of Disease Prevention and Health Promotion. (2021, August 24). *About health care quality. Health.gov.* Retrieved September 29, 2021, from https://health.gov/our-work/national-health-initiatives/health-care-quality/about-health-care-quality#:~:text=Health%20care%20quality%20is%20a%20broad%20term%20that,care%20quality%20and%20a%20key%20priority%20for%20ODPHP.

Padden, J. (2019). Documentation burden and cognitive burden: How much is too much information? *CIN: Computers Informatics Nursing, 37*(2), 60–61.

Paydar, S., Emami, H., Asadi, F., Moghaddasi, H., & Hosseini, A. (2021). Functions and outcomes of personal health records for patients with chronic diseases: A systematic review. *Perspectives in Health Information Management, 18*(Spring), 1–15. Retrieved from. https://www.ncbi.nlm.nih.gov/pmc/articles/PMC8314040/.

Pearl, R. (2017, June 15). What health systems, hospitals and physicians need to know about implementing electronic health records. *Harvard Business Review.* Retrieved August 27, 2021, from https://hbr.org/2017/06/what-health-systems-hospitals-and-physicians-need-to-know-about-implementing-electronic-health-records

Pearson, E., & Frakt, A. (2018). Administrative costs and health information technology. *JAMA Forum, 320*(6), 537–538. Retrieved from https://jamanetwork.com/.

Petrides, A. K., Bixho, I., Goonane, E. M., Bates, D. W., Shaykevich, S., Lipsitz, S. R., et al. (2017). The benefits and challenges of an interfaced electronic health record and laboratory information system. *Archives of Pathology & LaboratoryMedicine, 141*(3), 410–417.

Prgomet, M., Li, L., Niazkhani, Z., Georgiou, A., & Westbrook, J. (2017). Impact of commercial computerized provider order entry (CPOE) and clinical decision support systems (CDSS) on medication errors, length of stay, and mortality in intensive care units: A systematic review and meta-analysis. *JAMIA, 21*(2), 413–422. https://doi.org/10.1093/jamia/ocw145.

Rathert, C., Porter, T. H., Mittler, J. N., & Fleig-Palmer, M. (2019). Seven years after Meaningful Use: Physicians' and nurses' experiences with electronic health records. *Health Care Management Review, 44*(1), 30–40.

Roehrs, A., Da Costa, C., da Rosa Right, R., & De Oliveira, K. (2017). Personal health records: a systematic literature review. *Journal of Medical Internet Research, 19*(1), e13. https://doi.org/10.2196/jmir.5876.

Rubin, D. L., & Kahn, C. E., Jr. (2017). Common data elements in radiology. *Radiology, 283*(3), 837–844.

Sewell, J. (2018). *Informatics and nursing: Opportunities and challenges* (6th ed.). Philadelphia: Williams & Wilkins.

Shameer, K., Blicksberg, B., Hodos, R., Johnson, K., Badgeley, M., Readhead, R., … Dudley, J. (2017). Systematic analyses of drugs and disease indications in RepurposeDB reveal pharmacological, biological and epidemiological factors influencing drug repositioning. *Briefings in Bioinformatics, 19*(4), 656–678. https://doi.org/10.1093/bib/bbw136.

Showell, C. (2017). Barriers to the use of personal health records by patients: A structured review. *PeerJ,* 1–24. https://doi.org/10.7717/peerj.3268.

Stram, M., Gigliotti, G., Hartman, D., Pitkus, A., Huff, S. M., Riben, M., et al. (2020). Logical observation identifiers names and codes for laboratorians. *Archives of Pathology & Laboratory Medicine, 144*(2), 229–239.

Strudwick, G., Warnock, C., Kalia, K., Clark, C., & Booth, R. (2018). Factors associated with barcode medication administration technology that contribute to patient safety. *Journal of Nursing Care Quality, 33*(1), 79–85. https://doi.org/10.1097/NCQ.0000000000000270.

Sutton, R., Pincock, D., Baumgart, D., Sadowski, D., Fedorak, R., & Kroeker, K. (2020). An overview of clinical decision support systems: Benefits, risks and strategies for success. *Digital Medicine, 3*(17), 1–10. https://doi.org/10.1038/s41746-020-0221-y.

Swietlik, M., & Sengstack, P. (2020). An evaluation of nursing admission assessment documentation to identify opportunities for burden reduction. *Journal of Informatics Nursing, 5*(3), 6–11.

The National Alliance for Health Information Technology. (2008). *Defining key health information technology terms. Office of the National Coordinator for Health Information Technology.* Washington, DC: Department of Health & Human Resources. Retrieved August 24, 2021, from. https://www.citizenshealthinitiative.org/sites/citizenshealthinitiative.org/files/media/common/HITTermsFinalReport_051508.pdf.

The Office of the National Coordinator for Health Information Technology (ONCHIT). (2019a, May 2). What are the differences between electronic medical records, electronic health records, and personal health records? *HealthIT.gov.* Retrieved from https://www.healthit.gov/faq/what-are-differences-between-electronic-medical-records-electronic-health-records-and-personal

The Office of the National Coordinator for Health Information Technology (ONCHIT). (2019b, September 10). What is an electronic health record (EHR)? *HealthIT.gov.* Retrieved August 24, 2021, from https://www.healthit.gov/faq/what-electronic-health-record-ehr

The Office of the National Coordinator for Health Information Technology (ONCHIT). (2017a, October 5). Impact of EHRs on care. *HealthIT.gov.* Retrieved Augutst 24, 2021, from https://www.healthit.gov/topic/health-it-and-health-information-exchange-basics/benefits-ehrs

The Office of the National Coordinator for Health Information Technology (ONCHIT). (2013, June 1). What is meaningful use? *HealthIT.gov.* Retrieved August 24, 2021, from https://www.healthit.gov/faq/what-meaningful-use

The Office of the National Coordinator for Health Information Technology (ONCHIT). (2019c, October 22). Meaningful use. *HealthIT.gov.* Retrieved August 25, 2021, from https://www.healthit.gov/topic/meaningful-use-and-macra/meaningful-use

The Office of the National Coordinator for Health Information Technology (ONCHIT). (2020, November 2). Certification criteria. *HealthIT.gov.* Retrieved August 24, 2021, from https://www.healthit.gov/topic/certification-ehrs/certification-criteria

The Office of the National Coordinator for Health Information Technology (ONCHIT). (2014, November 12). *How much is this going to cost? HeathIT.gov.* Retrieved August 19, 2021, from https://www.healthit.gov/faq/how-much-going-cost-me

The Office of the National Coordinator for Health Information Technology (ONCHIT). (2017b). *Standard Nursing Terminologies: A Landscape Analysis.* Washington, DC: ONHIT. Retrieved August

28, 2021, from. https://www.healthit.gov/sites/default/files/snt_final_05302017.pdf.

The Office of the National Coordinator for Health Information Technology (ONCHIT). (2018, January 19). What are patient-generated health data? *HealthIT.gov.* Retrieved fromhttps://www.healthit.gov/policy-researchers-implementers/patient-generated-health-data/

The Office of the National Coordinator for Health Information Technology (ONCHIT). (2019d, May 16). What are the advantages of electronic health records? *HealthIT.gov.* Retrieved August 30, 2021, from https://www.healthit.gov/faq/what-are-advantages-electronic-health-records

The Office of the National Coordinator for Health Information Technology (ONCHIT). (2021). *Interoperbility roadmap.* HealthIT.gov. Retrieved August 30, 2021, from https://www.healthit.gov/topic/interoperability/interoperability-roadmap

The Office of the National Coordinator for Health Information Technology (ONCHIT). (2019e, May 21). How can electronic health records improve public and population health outcomes? *HealthIT.gov.* Retrieved August 30, 2021, from https://www.healthit.gov/faq/how-can-electronic-health-records-improve-public-and-population-health-outcomes

Thyvalikakath, K., Duncan, W., Siddiqui, Z., LaPradd, M., Eckert, G., Schleyer, T., et al. (2020). Leveraging electronic dental record data for clinical research in the National Dental PBRN Practices. *Applied Clinical Informatics, 11*(2), 305–314. https://doi.org/10.1055/s-0040-1709506.

U.S. Department of Health & Human Services (DHHS). (2020, September 23). The Security Rule. *HHS.gov Health Informatoin Privacy.* Retrieved August 28, 2021, from https://www.hhs.gov/hipaa/for-professionals/security/index.html

U.S. Department of Health and Human Resources (DHHS). (2017, June 17). HITECH Act Enforement Interim Final Rule. *HHS.gov.* Retrieved August 24, 2021, from https://www.hhs.gov/hipaa/for-professionals/special-topics/hitech-act-enforcement-interim-final-rule/index.html

U.S. Department of Health and Human Services (DHHS). (n.d.). Mater Patient Index (MPI). *Indian Health Services.* Retrieved August 20, 2021, from https://www.ihs.gov/hie/masterpatientindex/

U.S. Department of Veterans Affairs. (2002, June 18). VA nurse's idea: Bar code scanning to support patient care. *VAntage Point.* Retrieved August 26, 2021, from https://blogs.va.gov/VAntage/75902/va-nurses-idea-bar-code-scanning-support-patient-care/

University of Illinois Chicago. (2021, July 22). *What is data integrity and why is it important in healthcare?* Retrieved August 17, 2021, from https://healthinformatics.uic.edu/blog/data-integrity/

Wani, D., & Malhotra, M. (2018). Does the meaningful use of electronic health records improve patient outcomes? *Journal of Operations Management, 60*(2018), 1–18. https://doi.org/10.1016/j.jom.2018.06.003.

Wass, S., Vimarlund, V., & Ros, A. (2019). Exploring patients' perceptions of accessing electronic health records: Innovation in healthcare. *Health Informatics Journal, 25*(1), 203–215. https://doi.org/10.1177/1460458217704258.

Wiegel, V., King, A., Mozaffar, H., Cresswell, K., Williams, R., & Sheik, A. (2020). A systematic analysis of the optimization of computerized physician order entry and clinical decision support systems: A qualitative study in English Hospitals. *Health Informatics Journal, 26*(2), 1117–1132. https://doi.org/10.1177/1460458219868650.

Yin, Z., Liu, Y., McCoy, A., Malin, B., & Sengstack, P. (2021). Contribution of free-text comments to the burden of documentation: Assessment and analysis of vital sign comments in flowsheets. *Journal of Medical Internet Research, 23*(3), e22806. https://doi.org/10.2196/22806.

Zarour, M., Alenezi, M., Ansari, M., Pandey, A., Ahmad, M., Agrawal, A., et al. (2021). Ensuring data integrity of healthcare information in the era of digital health. *Healthcare Technology Letters, 8*(3), 66–77. https://doi.org/10.1049/htl2.12008.

Zheng, W., Lichtner, V., Van Dort, B., & Baysari, M. (2021). The impact of introducing automated dispensing cabinets, barcode medication administration, and closed loop electronic medication management systems on work processes and safety of controlled medications in hospitals: A systematic review. *Research in Social and Administrative Pharmacy, 17*(2021), 832–841. https://doi.org/10.1016/j.sapharm.2020.08.001.

8

Administrative Applications in Healthcare

*Michael H. Kennedy, Kathy H. Wood, Gerald R. Ledlow,
Michele Bosworth, and Michael Morris*

*If a health care system cannot effectively track the total cost of all materials
used to treat an individual patient and aggregate data to determine the cost of
treating groups of patients, managing the cost of health care is not possible.*

OBJECTIVES

At the completion of this chapter, the reader will be prepared to:

1. Describe how vendors inform healthcare organizations of potentially useful administrative software applications.
2. Discuss the basic Financial Information Systems (FISs) and their application in healthcare organizations.
3. Give examples of different practice management systems and integrated healthcare systems.
4. Explain how health information technology applications can be leveraged to improve delivery of care to diverse populations.
5. Describe the attributes of an efficient supply chain (materials management) system in a healthcare organization.
6. Describe the role of human resources information systems in supporting and streamlining human resource management actions.
7. Give examples of applications that manage and use healthcare business data.

KEY TERMS

accountable care organization (ACO), 120

accounts payable, 117

accounts receivable, 117

assets, 117

business intelligence (BI), 131

charge description master file, 127

claims denial management, 118

claims processing and management, 118

financial information system (FIS), 116

fixed asset management, 118

general ledger, 116

materials management, 127

patient accounting, 117

pay for performance (P4P), 120

payroll, 117

population health management, 124

practice management systems (PMSs), 122

supply chain management (SCM), 118

supply-item master file, 127

transaction history file, 127

value based care, 124

vendor master file, 127

ABSTRACT ❖

This chapter addresses the administrative applications within health information systems that are designed to facilitate the delivery of healthcare, such as financial, practice management, value-based care, supply chain and materials management, human resources, and business intelligence systems.

INTRODUCTION

Health information systems are "complexes or systems of processing data, information and knowledge in healthcare environments" (Haux, 2006, p.270). These environments comprise a variety of settings, including hospitals, ambulatory settings, long-term care facilities, and managed care organizations.

Typically, the applications within health information systems are categorized as clinical or administrative. This chapter focuses on the administrative applications within health information systems designed to facilitate the management of healthcare delivery. The chapter considers in turn financial, practice management, value-based care, supply chain management, human resources, and healthcare business intelligence systems.

VENDOR RESOURCE GUIDES

Vendors

The applications required to process information in healthcare settings are primarily provided by vendors. The vendor market for hospital information systems alone in 2013 had total revenues of almost $14 billion, with the top five vendors in terms of revenue being McKesson ($3.4 billion), Cerner ($2.9 billion), Siemens ($1.8 billion), Epic Systems Corporation ($1.7 billion), and Allscripts (almost $1.4 billion). These revenue statistics were based upon published earnings reports, direct contact with vendors, research of websites, and estimates for privately held companies or to exclude non-health revenues (Ciotti & Alcaro, 2014). A recent market forecast estimates the valuation of products and services from healthcare software vendors will reach $25 billion by 2024 (Pang et al., 2021).

Types of Vendors

Vendors that deploy a comprehensive suite of applications are referred to as enterprise vendors. Specialized applications are also provided by niche vendors. When specialty vendors and vendors targeting nonhospital markets are included, the health information system marketplace becomes a confusing morass of products whose capabilities are difficult to assess. Fortunately, professional organizations such as the Healthcare Information and Management Systems Society (HIMSS—https://www.himss.org/), hard copy and online content publishers such as Health Data Management (https://www.healthdatamanagement.com/), and trade and technology research companies such as Gartner (https://www.gartner.com/) and KLAS (https://klas-research.com/) help stakeholders assess their options and make informed decisions.

Gartner and KLAS provide fee-based ratings services. Gartner states, "We deliver the technology-related insight necessary for our clients to make the right decisions, every day" (Gartner, Inc, 2016). KLAS declares, "Healthcare technology is rapidly changing, and KLAS is dedicated to being the source that holds vendors accountable and amplifies the voice of your peers" (KLAS, 2016). This is done by monitoring vendor performance based on feedback from healthcare providers and by conducting independent analyses of products and services. KLAS publishes a *Best in KLAS Awards* report annually for software, professional services, and medical equipment. KLAS's reports should be used with some caution, as the vendors cited by KLAS represent the rankings of just one ratings service, but they do serve as a resource.

FINANCIAL INFORMATION SYSTEMS (FISS) APPLICATIONS

A financial information system (FIS) is a system that stores and records fiscal (financial) operations within an organization that are then used for reporting and decision making. Healthcare organizations (HCOs), like any other business, must perform various "financial" types of functions to remain viable. These involve the following components:

- A customer (patient) purchasing the product (receiving the service).
- Salespeople (healthcare personnel) providing the service or product.
- A facility to receive the service or product (healthcare facility).
- Supplies needed for a procedure (materials management).
- Payment received by the HCO for the product (service) received (receivables).
- Monies received to be deposited in accounts (accounting).
- Payment made to healthcare personnel and support staff for services performed (payroll).
- Expenses paid (payables) to external constituents that made it possible to perform a procedure (e.g., mortgage and utilities).

The architecture of a typical FIS is illustrated in Fig. 8.1. As Siwicki noted, finance systems in healthcare should never be underestimated in keeping HCOs up and running (Siwicki, 2019). Although it is true that financial functions are usually not a matter of life or death for the patient, an ill-fitted FIS can be life or death for the fiscal viability of the organization. Therefore one must choose wisely and update the FIS often to keep up with the ever-changing regulations and variations that affect the revenue and profitability of the organization.

Evolution of Healthcare Financial Information Systems

Automated FISs were the first type of systems used in many healthcare facilities. The main purpose of these initial FISs was basic bookkeeping and payroll. Basic accounting systems were then put into place to help with the billing function. Rosario emphasizes the importance of managing revenue flow and meeting goals (Rosario, 2021). The original revenue flow was getting cash flow by capturing charges and collecting from the patient or the patient's third-party payment system. Entering charges and creating claims to send to insurance companies and patients were some of the first, and easiest, functions for an FIS. Payroll was also a very simple function for an FIS to perform. Initially, there was no need for analytics or importing to spreadsheets, and reporting functions were limited, but that has changed with the new demands for information from the patient and public (Rosario, 2021). HCOs embraced the basic financial functions to remain financially viable. Fig. 8.1 shows how financial transactions fit within the FISs.

Some of the basic financial systems required by HCOs and other businesses are general ledger, payroll, patient accounting, claims processing, claims denial management, contracts management, and fixed asset management.

General Ledger

The general ledger consists of *all* financial transactions made by the HCO. This is similar to a personal checking ledger where any checks written or deposits made are recorded in the account. Numerous financial areas need to be tracked. Therefore, an HCO will maintain various subsidiary ledgers. Each of these ledgers tracks customer and vendor names, dates of transactions, types of transactions, and balances remaining. The FIS managing the general ledger must be able to track and

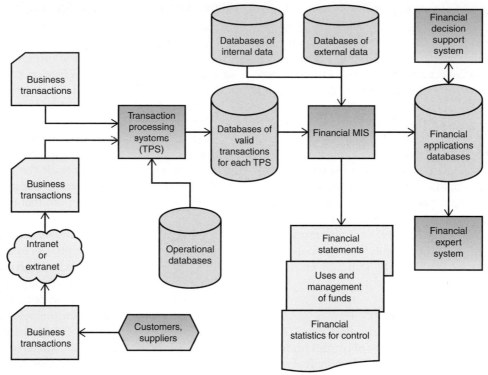

Fig. 8.1 Financial information system architecture. (Healthcare Financial Management Association Certification Professional Practicum PowerPoint.)

report information in a variety of ways to meet the needs of the decision makers. Types of financial data that need to be tracked include:

- *Assets:* Assets are property items that can be converted easily into cash. Assets are classified as tangible and intangible. Tangible assets include current and fixed assets such as inventory or buildings and equipment. Intangible assets include nonphysical resources such as copyrights or computer systems.
- *Accounts payable:* Accounts payable are the monies that are owed to vendors and suppliers for items purchased on credit (very similar to using a personal credit card and then paying back the amount on a monthly basis). These usually occur in the form of invoices or statements. This would fall under the category of disbursements in many systems. Because many vendors offer discounts when paid by a certain date, the FIS needs to be able to track the dates that payments need to be made in order to receive the discount or avoid the penalties that may be applied for late payments.
- *Accounts receivable:* The opposite of accounts payable, accounts receivable are monies that are owed to the institution. The vast majority of the dollars owed to the HCO come in the form of patient-generated revenues. Once claims have been submitted to insurance companies (if the patient is covered by insurance), the remaining balance is sent to the patient for payment. The FIS has to be able to track the amount owed by the insurance, minus any negotiated rate such as managed care contracting, and the remaining balance owed by the patient. Ideally, the system estimates the amounts owed up front so the collection process can begin at the time of the visit.

Payroll Application

The application that handles compensation payments to employees is the payroll system. This is also referred to as a disbursement system. The FIS application must be able to deduct taxes, benefits, possibly savings amounts, and other deductions. At the onset of FISs for payroll, the minimal functions could be performed. In advanced systems, automatic payroll deposits and much more can be performed. In addition, overtime pay, pay rates, and payroll histories must be tracked and reported. At the end of the calendar year, the system must be able to generate W2 forms for the employee to use in income tax preparation.

Patient Accounting Application

A patient accounting (or patient finance) application tracks the accounting transactions related to patient services. All charges incurred because of the patient visit need to be tracked and added to the patient's financial record. This can include inpatient fees if the patient is hospitalized, healthcare provider (e.g., physicians and nurse practitioners) and medication fees associated with the treatment, and procedure costs, including surgeries, radiology, and whatever else is necessary for the care of the patient. The procedural and diagnostic codes also become part of the patient billing record to complete the information necessary for the insurance payer to submit payment for the claim. Without critical information, such as charges and coding, the claim process is delayed, resulting in reduced cash flow for the HCO.

The collection process can begin at the time of the visit. This statement implies that the patient can receive services without paying anything up front. This is the reality in emergencies.

Because of the Emergency Medical Treatment and Active Labor Act (EMTALA), patients must be treated in the case of emergency regardless of their ability to pay. This can lead to hundreds of thousands of dollars outstanding that the healthcare facility will try to collect after the service has been performed. The collection process in healthcare is much different from the process in a traditional business that requires payment before the product or service is provided. The FIS also needs to be able to track outstanding balances and assist in tracking these for the patient accounts personnel who will be attempting to collect the balances. The older the balances are, the more difficult they are to collect. The FIS needs to be able to differentiate the balances based on several factors, including, but not limited to, amount, payer, age of the account, and so forth. The features needed in FISs are now much more complex than in the past. For example, managers now may need to track the revenue generated by staff as a measure of productivity.

Claims Processing and Management System

As patients present for registration and admission, a single healthcare facility must be prepared to bill numerous insurance companies (third-party payers) representing hundreds of coverage and payment plans across government and private insurance. Some patients have primary coverage and supplemental coverage (e.g., Medicare as primary insurer and another insurer for supplemental coverage). Other patients receiving charity care or those with no insurance are categorized as private pay patients.

Claims processing and management is the submission of the insurance claim or bill to the third-party payer, either manually or electronically, and the follow-up on the payment from the payer. The application must be able to keep each of the payer types separate and know the requirements of how to bill the claims, who to bill for the balances, or if the balances need to be written off and not billed to anyone. Collections can be very challenging for the healthcare facility. Many new standards have been adopted for claims processing, but numerous different standards and requirements must be followed for the various insurance companies and plans. Insurance marketplaces and the shift towards more patient financial responsibility have caused claims processing to be even more complex than in previous years (Reiner, 2021).

Sending "clean" claims is the key to getting payment quickly. Clean claims are those claims that contain all critical information such as patient demographics, charges, procedures performed, procedural and diagnostic coding, and other information required by the insurance company to remit prompt payment. Timely claims processing and collection are key to the fiscal health of institutions so they can meet the financial obligations in their disbursements and accounts payable functions. The claims-processing application must review the claim before it is submitted to ensure that all necessary data fields are complete and accurate. If the claim is not clean, it will be denied, creating a delay and generating increased labor costs to correct errors before payment can be received for the service provided.

Claims Denial Management Application

Denials from insurance companies are tracked, and they require follow-up. The claims denial management application can prevent denials imposed by the insurance carrier in a variety of ways. For example, the application can issue an alert on a request by clinical personnel for a patient to stay an additional day in his or her current patient status (i.e., observation, inpatient) if that request is likely to be denied by the insurer. The submitted insurance claim for a patient's stay may also be denied for improper coding or missing information. When the denial occurs, the application must track the update and the progress on having the denial reversed. Because a claim or request was denied initially does not mean that the decision cannot be reversed. Persistence and proper documentation can be the deciding factors leading to reversal. Be proactive and handle the denied claims early in the process by using the right mix of education, technology, services, and advisory support (Reiner, 2021). In addition, the communications that took place between each area of patient care must be documented, collected, and stored in an orderly manner for the proof to be shown. This is just one example of why the FIS must be carefully integrated with the clinical systems. Although 31% of providers are still using manual claims denial processes, most recognize the benefits of these systems, including automatic updates in diagnostic codes and insurance requirements (Reiner, 2021).

Contract Management Application

HCOs have a variety of contracts they must track, including those for supply chain management (SCM) and managed care. These types of contracts affect the bottom line of the organization, so the contracts must be tracked and managed for the organization to obtain maximum financial gain. SCM contracts include group purchasing, where healthcare systems negotiate a price for using a standard vendor. Vendor price comparisons and usage need to be tracked, and the system must ensure that employees are adhering to the purchasing policies. Additional SCM functions can include providing incentives for healthcare providers to reduce the cost of their preferred supplies. For example, some surgeons may have particular instruments or supplies they prefer for surgical procedures. These supplies may be much more expensive than an alternative brand. The FIS could help the organization track the supply costs and the costs for procedures and provide reports for physicians to accompany requests for their assistance in reducing those costs.

Managed care contracting can be very challenging and complex. The contracts can be numerous, and each contract can have different terms. The FIS needs to be able to track these contracts and manage the terms and results of each contract individually. For example, when a patient is covered by a nongovernmental insurance plan, the insurance company may have negotiated an agreed-upon amount for reimbursement per service or per patient. The insurance and patients need to be billed according to that contract's terms, and any negotiated discount should not be billed.

Fixed Asset Management Application

Fixed asset management applications manage the fixed assets in a healthcare facility that cannot be converted to cash easily, sold, or used for the care of a patient, such as land, buildings, equipment, fixtures, fittings, motor vehicles, office equipment, computers, software, and so forth. Each fixed asset must be tracked by location, person, age, and other factors. In an HCO, the assets can be issued to a person, a procedure room, a department, and others. The FIS must handle the vast number of assets and the various areas in which the assets can be located. This system tracks depreciation, maintenance agreements, warranties related to the assets, and when assets will need to be replaced.

Healthcare Financial Information Systems—In Perspective

Healthcare FISs during the first decade of the twenty-first century supported a number of improvements in the business processes, including patient scheduling, laboratory and ancillary reporting, medical record keeping and reporting, and billing and accounting. In addition to the previous FISs, there are many applications to improve efficiency, productivity, and quality. These include fiscal decision support through clinical and financial analytics, (HealthLeaders, 2018) automated patient outreach via text messaging for appointment reminders, pre-visit instructions, and missed appointment notifications (Providertech, 2018). In addition, there are three key areas in future FIS planning tools: visualization, artificial intelligence, and Blockchain, all delivered via cloud services (Siwicki, 2018).

Financial Reporting

One of the primary functions of an FIS is providing the reports that demonstrate the financial condition of the organization. The most common reports for HCOs are summarized in Table 8.1. Note that the titles may vary depending on whether the organization is for profit or not for profit.

The income statement or statement of operations is a good representation of the bottom line, or money left over (net income or loss), of the organization (Table 8.2). This report lists all revenues (monies coming in) and expenses (monies going out), and these are often compared with those of prior years and with the budget plan.

The balance sheet or statement of financial position shows a glimpse of the organization's financial condition at any given point in time (Table 8.3). The FIS needs to pull the financial data from assets, liabilities, and equity to present the report, so the organization can determine whether the numbers in the categories are balanced. Balance sheet data are based on a fundamental accounting equation (Assets = Liabilities + Owner's equity), so each side must "balance" to show the financial condition of the organization.

The cash flow statements show whether the organization will be successful in paying its bills (have more money than it owes). Table 8.4 provides an example of a cash flow statement.

TABLE 8.3 Balance Sheet

Assets		Claims on Assets	
Current Assets		**Current Liabilities**	
Cash	$123,000	Accounts payable	$100,000
Marketable securities	$200,000	Notes payable	$150,000
Accounts receivable	$345,000		
Inventories	$100,000	Total Current Liabilities	$250,000
		Long-term note	$300,000
Total Current Assets	$768,000		
		Total Liabilities	$550,000
Long-Term Assets		Owner's equity	$843,000
Building (gross)	$350,000		
Accumulated depreciation	($50,000)	Total Claims	$1,393,000
Net building	$300,000		
Land	$325,000		
Total Long-Term Assets	$625,000		
Total Assets	$1,393,000		

From Healthcare Financial Management Association Certification Professional Practicum PowerPoint.

TABLE 8.4 Statement of Cash Flows

Cash Flow from Operations	$1800.00
Net income	$259.00
Adjustments	$1541.00
Depreciation expense	($100.00)
Accounts payable	$130.00
Credit card account	$50.00
Patient credits	$0.00
Sales tax payable	$1.23
Accounts receivable	$986.77
Inventory asset	$473.00
Cash Flow from Investing	($1000.00)
Equipment	($1000.00)
Cash Flow from Financing	$1500.00
Opening balance equity	$2000.00
Owner's equity	($500.00)
Draw	($500.00)
Investment	$0.00
Net Change in Cash	$2300.00

From Healthcare Financial Management Association Certification Professional PracticumPowerPoint.

TABLE 8.1 Financial Statements

For Profit	Not for Profit
Balance sheet	Statement of financial position
Income statement	Statement of operations
Statement of cash flows	Statement of cash flows

TABLE 8.2 Income Statement

Revenue	$1,195,450.25	100.00%
Cost of goods sold	870,175.83	72.79%
Gross margin	$325,274.42	27.21%
Overhead	29,879.65	2.50%
Net ordinary income (loss)	$295,394.77	24.71%
Interest expense	1,269.08	0.11%
Interest income	5,387.08	0.45%
Net income (loss)	$299,512.77	25.05%

From Healthcare Financial Management Association Certification Professional Practicum

An HCO keeps track of certain financial ratios to help it evaluate its financial condition; these can be important when borrowing for future capital investments. The FIS must be able to calculate and report ratios on demand so that at any given time the organization can assess its financial condition. Ratios are classified into several categories, such as solvency, debt, management or turnover, profitability, and market value. Several ratios are unique to the healthcare industry, such as Length of Stay and Bed Occupancy. Average Length of Stay in the United States for most procedures is 4.8 days. Decision makers can analyze the length of stay for their hospitals to determine whether they are on track for most procedures. Keep in mind, however, that a shorter length of stay does not necessarily mean lower costs. Bed occupancy provides a quick glance at how many inpatient beds are being used. The occupancy is typically higher during flu season and other epidemics. The ratio, Accounts Receivable Days in an HCO, is generally higher than in other organizations because the services are provided before payment is made by the patient or insurance company.

Challenges With Financial Information Systems

One of the challenges that large HCOs face with the implementation of FISs is ensuring that the various systems in place at numerous locations are integrated. Larger HCOs can include 20 or more facilities, and within each of these facilities can be numerous sub-facilities. The different financial systems, applications, and SCM systems can become very complicated when they are merged and the information systems do not interface well (Siwicki, 2019).

The purpose of HCOs is to provide quality patient care. While generating maximum revenue is not its defining purpose, an organization must generate income to stay in business and advance new programs and services. What this means is that patient care systems can be seen by some as a higher priority compared with FISs. Decision makers may have a more challenging time realizing the return on investment or understanding the importance of the investment in FISs because IT software applications such as patient accounting or revenue are considered an intangible asset. The key is to ensure the integration of the various applications (Siwicki, 2019). If an information system meets the requirements needed for patient care and includes integrated applications such as patient accounting, the organization will have the best of both worlds. True integration supports the effective transfer of captured data across all applications. This leads to improved efficiency and enhanced cash flow, and the total cost of ownership is lower (Siwicki, 2019).

Historical Approaches to Financing Healthcare

Historically healthcare was financed using a "fee-for-service" approach. With this approach, each time a service (e.g., an office visit, an injection, delivery of a baby, or surgery) is completed, payment is provided. There are two key problems with this approach. First, such an approach encourages the provider to increase the amount of services performed. For example, a healthcare system that does more procedures is able to make more money compared with a healthcare system that is more conservative. Second, such an approach does not consider the quality of the service provided. With a fee-for-service approach, a postoperative infection provides the healthcare institution with additional income because they can now charge to treat that infection. "The predominant fee-for-service system under which providers are paid leads to increased costs by rewarding providers for the volume and complexity of services they provide. Higher intensity of care does not necessarily result in higher quality care, and can even be harmful" (James, 2012, p. 1). As healthcare costs have increased and problems with healthcare safety have become more obvious, there have been increasing efforts to use a different approach to funding healthcare.

During the 1990s, a managed care approach was introduced to reduce excessive and unnecessary care. By paying providers a lump sum per patient to cover a given set of services, there was no advantage for increasing the amount of service provided. In addition, poor quality could increase the institution's cost with no financial gain. However, this approach presented new concerns because a managed care approach motivated payers to control costs by restricting services. Concerns about compromised quality and constraints on patients having access to providers of their choice led to a backlash (James, 2012).

Analyzing Accountable Care Organizations and Pay for Performance

The most recent regulation affecting healthcare finance to date is the Affordable Care Act (ACA). Officially called the Patient Protection and Affordable Care Act (PPACA), and sometimes called ObamaCare, the ACA is a U.S. law aimed at reforming both the healthcare delivery system and the health insurance industry. The ACA includes a number of provisions designed to encourage improvements in patient outcomes as a basis for payment. For example, Medicare's Hospital Readmissions Reduction Program reduces payments by 1% to hospitals that have excessively high rates of avoidable readmissions for patients experiencing heart attacks, heart failure, or pneumonia (James, 2012).

Another key aspect of the ACA is the concept of pay for performance. The concept of pay for performance ties payment to the quality of the care provided or to patient outcomes as opposed to the service delivered. The most familiar program that **pay for performance (P4P)** is the voluntary **accountable care organization (ACO)**. An ACO is a network of doctors and hospitals that share responsibility for providing care to a specific group of patients and in return receives bonuses when these providers keep costs down and meet specific quality benchmarks (James, 2012).

Three other P4P programs include value-based purchasing, physician quality reporting, and Medicare Advantage plan bonuses (James, 2012). These programs are intended to provide financial incentives for physicians and HCOs to have accountability over controlling costs while gaining more efficiency and higher quality in their operations. HCOs are also going beyond the clinical aspect of healthcare by looking at social determinants (e.g., age, gender, geographical location, socioeconomic position, nutritional habits, drug uses or abuses, and work environment) that may cause health issues in certain populations.

Since the inception of the ACA in 2010, over 440 Medicare ACOs have been created nationwide. Of the Medicare ACOs initiated, 54% lowered expenditures and generated $383 million in net savings for Medicare, resulting in significant shared savings payments for the ACOs. The Medicare Shared Savings Program (MSSP) is voluntary and encourages teams of healthcare providers to collaborate as an ACO (Shared Savings Program, 2021); public reporting is one of the requirements for the MSSP (Schulz et al., 2015). As ACOs continue to grow in numbers, their overall financial viability will be determined.

There are challenges to the participants in these P4P programs. One of the key challenges is determining the quality "perceived" by patients, because this can vary tremendously because of opinions and expectations. In addition, complying with the structural suggestions such as adding health information technology can be costly, so the participants would need to know how much they are receiving in incentives to determine if the costs of the structural changes result in an overall positive gain financially.

As regulations and financial incentives continue to be put into place, HCOs need a means to track the effect of such regulations. Tracking demographics and social determinants will allow any trends to be discovered. The FIS will provide tools to help the HCOs and the ACOs analyze the feasibility and results of the shared savings in the P4P incentive, as well as to track information for the prevention of health issues.

Financial Information Systems Integration

- Financial systems matured much faster than clinical systems (CSs) did (Williams, 2002); therefore, the degree of integration of the FIS with CSs was somewhat limited. However, there are several advantages to integration within the FIS and across CSs. For example, this approach eliminates duplication of effort, which also reduces the number of potential errors. Benefits of integration include
- A transition is provided between front-end and back-end operations.
- Information required for billing such as demographics and insurance can be gathered and verified at the point of service or admission so that the information is immediately available for patient care and financial personnel.
- Eligibility checking for insurance can be done online; automated charging is supported, eliminating the need for charge entry.
- Availability of clinical records with detailed charges that have been secured through proper access allows staff to respond to questions from patients, payers, or others without having to access paper charts (Williams, 2002).

All these features of integration improve the bottom line, which is the aim in healthcare finance. In addition to the basic accounting systems, such as general ledger, accounts payable, and accounts receivable (AR), FISs handle functions that are more complex such as activity or project management. Advanced revenue cycle IT, or new generation, is often referred to as integrated "bolt-ons" (Hammer & Franklin, 2008). TechTarget describes a bolt-on as a product or system similar to an add-on but one that can be attached *securely* to

an existing system (Bolt-ons, n.d.). Besides integrated bolt-ons, there are workflow rules engines, advanced executive scorecards, and single-database clinical and revenue cycle systems (Hammer & Franklin, 2008). Workflow rules engines help to manage workflow. For example, documents can be stored in a document management system and e-mail or event reminders can be automatically sent to the people involved with the tasks. Advanced executive scorecards are strategic management tools that aggregate data from electronic health records (EHRs) in concert with an FIS, thereby providing a snapshot of how the healthcare institution is performing in certain areas. For example, the snapshot may show a quarterly increase in the hospital's cost to deliver a baby. Investigating these data may demonstrate an increase in cesarean-sections or a decrease in babies delivered by midwifes. These "scores" can then be compared with the data of other hospitals offering obstetrical services. A single-database clinical and revenue cycle system is a system used to ensure accuracy, availability, and data integrity for patient care and billing for the HCO. When changes are made to information contained within the database, those changes are managed throughout the system. In other words, the user does not need to make the change in multiple locations; the database management system will do that for the user to ensure that all necessary changes have been made. This is particularly important when dealing with procedures, documentation for those procedures, and the charges that accompany those procedures. In line with the original accounting systems, these advanced systems are designed to improve billing by reducing billing errors, improving the timeliness of billing to cash collected, decreasing the cost of collections, providing real-time eligibility for services, and providing improvements to current operational efficiencies via other functions (Hammer & Franklin, 2008).

Improvement in cash flow has remained a constant goal since the onset of FIS. Adaptability and flexibility in healthcare is the key to successful patient care and quality, and the same applies to FIS choices. An example of the revenue cycle is provided in Fig. 8.2.

One of the more recent IT tools used to positively affect the revenue cycle is a communication management system. The variety of communications (e.g., patient care, insurance coverage, and patient admission), the method of communication (e.g., face to face, phone, fax, and internet via patient portal, email, or social media), and the number of people engaged in communications make organizing and tracking communications a complex process. As Reiner points out, communications surrounding care of the patient and payment can be very difficult to track and retrieve (Reiner, 2021). A centralized management tracking system could assist in this area. An audit trail needs to be very detailed and include all communications that capture and travel with the patient, as well as the authorizations associated with each step. In other words, these communications need to be captured, indexed, and archived for future retrieval (Reiner, 2021).

Efficiency Tools

Decision makers need tools to capture productivity for various activities within the financial services area of the organization.

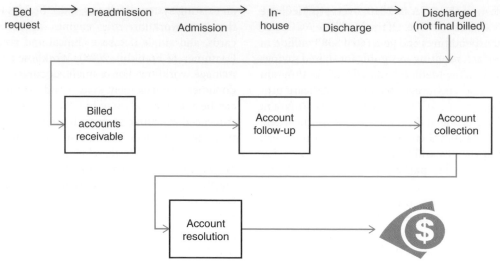

Fig. 8.2 Revenue cycle function. (Healthcare Financial Management Association Certification Professional Practicum PowerPoint.)

For example, collecting balances from the patient may fall within the responsibilities of a handful of employees. At the front end (before services are received), patients who have been preregistered can be asked for payment on the estimated amount owed. At the back end (after services have been received), patients who have a remaining balance after insurance has paid will need to pay that balance. How does an organization know which employees are having success at collecting payments? The reporting tools must provide a snapshot of the data so the decision makers can immediately analyze financial events within a particular area.

In addition to reporting tools, the application needs to be able to assist end users with the questions that need to be asked, and when. For example, if a patient has an outstanding balance from a previous visit, the patient access personnel may need to know whether they should request payment. Information needed should be readily available and easy to access. When adaptable and flexible designs between clinical and financial systems are combined, powerful analytics are deployed via the web to every desktop; many activities are self-service, freeing up valuable time and resources for the HCO (Hammer & Franklin, 2008).

Managing services has become more complex, resulting in a need for improved AR management. For example, capturing charges has increased in complexity just as medical care has (Hammer & Franklin, 2008). As a result, FISs are an integral part of the technology within a healthcare environment and CIOs and CFOs work together to maximize these IT systems so organizations can achieve their goals (Siwicki, 2020). A dashboard provides users with a visual analysis of specific data points so an organization can gauge how it is performing in certain areas (it is called a *dashboard* because it resembles the visual data points provided on an automobile dashboard). Efficiency may be improved by applications that allow for coding edits or overriding default values as needed, that are easy to use, and that include executive dashboard capabilities (Siwicki, 2020).

PRACTICE MANAGEMENT SYSTEMS

Practice management systems (PMSs), or Physician Office Management and Medical Information systems (POMIS), are very similar to the information systems supporting integrated healthcare systems, only on a smaller scale. These applications focus on the services provided in a healthcare provider's office compared with the services provided in a large healthcare system or hospital. Similar to the hospital revenue cycle management system, the PMS is designed to collect patient demographic and insurance information, manage appointment scheduling, document the reason for the visit and patient care procedures performed for the patient, post charging information for the billing process, and manage collection and follow-up. As with inpatient or acute care systems, PMSs require integration. The primary differences between PMSs and information systems supporting hospitals are specific provider scheduling templates and types of visits, transaction or line-item provider billing compared with account-driven hospital billing, and provider-based medical record content (orders, referrals, provider documentation, and problem lists) that differs from the typical comprehensive hospital medical record (Sorrentino & Sanderson, 2001). The charges from a medical practice office are connected to codes used for practice management billing and include Healthcare Common Procedure Coding System (HCPCS) and Current Procedural Terminology (CPT), with Relative Value Units (RVUs) and work RVUs (wRVUs). Each CPT code has an RVU attached (defined by Medicare). Since physicians may be reimbursed through this "work" component of the RVU, the information system being used needs to be able to calculate the productivity of the physician. The information system must also be able to generate claims using this type of coding, usually through an electronic submission. Electronic medical records (EMRs) have become more common if not essential modules within a PMS after the U.S. government incentives supporting EHRs. An explanation of the difference between an EMR and an EHR can be found at https://www.healthit.gov/buzz-blog/

electronic-health-and-medical-records/emr-vs-ehr-difference (also discussed in Chapter 7). Information on the episodes of care maintained in the EMR can be shared with the hospital or health center should the patient need to be admitted. Sharing this information helps ensure that the information in the EMR becomes part of the EHR. However, this is often not a "plug and play" environment. Creating a successful interface to share data between the EMR of a practice and a hospital or health center information system is a complex process. Chapter 6 includes additional information on health information exchanges (HIEs) and health information organizations (HIOs) and the issues involved with these.

In outpatient settings, healthcare providers can spend much of their time documenting the details of the patient visit. There are a variety of ways to accomplish this, including documenting and recording what is being said and done while the patient is in the examination room, dictating and transcribing based on written notes, or using voice recognition software during or after the visit. Traditionally, visit notes were often transcribed by a third party, leaving room for error through misreading of handwriting or mishearing of dictation. There is also a time delay until the documentation becomes part of the patient record because of the multiple processes required. The healthcare provider is required to review and sign off on the final documentation, but time constraints can encourage the provider to rush and perhaps overlook some details.

A method using more enhanced technology and providing quicker turnaround is voice recognition. Voice recognition software capabilities have greatly improved over the last few years. Voice recognition eliminates the need for a third party and allows healthcare providers to input information themselves, saving steps, time, and money. The application allows text to be viewed in real time, and providers can edit and approve it immediately. The time savings can result in much more timely billing and improved cash flow versus waiting for dictated notes to be approved after being transcribed.

Patient Outreach System

Some practices specialize in providing preventive care to manage patients with chronic illnesses. In these practices, an electronic registry of the clinic's entire patient population can be used in a patient outreach system. The registry includes the demographic and medical record information needed to notify patients, and an automated reminder capability (Curtis & Schelhammer, 2011). Patient outreach systems should incorporate evidence-based, specialty-specific protocols—or recommended care guidelines—for chronic and preventive care. Then, once the outreach system identifies patients due for preventive screenings and follow-up care for chronic diseases, the patients are contacted via an automated phone messaging system or another computerized method.

Online Billing and Payment Tool

Collections in a practice can be just as challenging as collections in a hospital, except that few emergency cases occur in a provider practice setting, allowing office staff to determine the acceptability of denying services to a patient until a payment plan has been established. In addition to routine collection practices, implementing an online billing and payment tool (e.g., using a credit card to pay online) can help improve the management and collection of fees owed by patients. Conley states that the healthcare facility can realize increased patient satisfaction and improved staff efficiencies by implementing an online payment tool (Conley, 2009). Benefits for the patient and the provider's office are outlined in Box 8.1.

Free and Charitable Clinics

There are approximately 1400 Free and Charitable Clinics throughout the nation who provide affordable, quality healthcare services to the uninsured and the underinsured (About us, n.d.). Some of the services provided include medical, dental, pharmaceutical, behavioral health, vision, and health education (Public policy, n.d.). Although many of the staff are paid, the majority of healthcare services are provided through volunteers. These may be retired physicians, nurses, nurse practitioners, physician assistants, dentists, ophthalmologists, and others. Some of the clinics partner with local college programs who offer degrees in the health sciences areas.

There are various applications used for the care and case management in the free and charitable clinics. One of the ways these clinics reduce costs while having the financial resources to provide these services is through grants. For example, there are product-based grants through the Point of Care, Enhancing Clinical Effectiveness (PcCECE). These point-of-care diagnostic testing tools allow clinicians to evaluate patients on site and get the test results before the patient leaves the clinic (Free and charitable clinics receive grant for point-of-care diagnostics, n.d.). The clinics must also document in an EMR like other clinics, manage their cases, collect minor fees when applicable, and communicate with the financial systems used throughout the larger organization when other services are provided. To learn more about possible information system solutions, reach out to

BOX 8.1 Benefits of Implementing an Online Payment Tool for Patients and Provider Offices

- Self-management of their open accounts
- Ability to pay outstanding balances
- Secure communication on a 24/7 basis with the business office (the practice will determine the turnaround time of communications to the patient)
- Ability to update address or demographic changes
- Ability to update changes to insurance coverage (which often occur annually)
- Preregister for services or appointments
- Enhanced customer service capabilities
- Ability for staff to accept payments in person or over the phone
- Ability for staff to view the patient statement exactly as submitted to the patient, which helps to improve communications and efficiencies for payment collection

Data from Conley, C. (2009). Improve patient satisfaction and collections with efficient payment processes. Emdeon Express Winter Edition. http://emdeonexpress.blogspot.com/2009/02/its-no-secret-that-health-care-is.html;.

the National Association of Free and Charitable Clinics (https://www.nafcclinics.org/).

Hospital–Healthcare Provider Connection

PMSs integrated with the hospital information system can be more efficient for healthcare providers in a clinic or private practice. According to Cash, physicians, nurse practitioners, physician assistants, and others with staff privileges who participate in the hospital network have certain expectations about the IT, including that it should:

- Provide a single sign-on to an integrated information system from all key system entry points.
- Automate the provider's day as much as possible using mobile access (automation means that access is available wherever the clinician is and that the information is in a useful format).
- Have 24/7 support for any device, anywhere.
- Provide a dashboard to view critical clinical and financial information with the ability to act on it immediately (Cash, 2008).

Healthcare provider dissatisfaction can occur if the information system:

- Slows performance of the task
- Reduces the ability to bill insurance or the patient
- Adds more administrative duties to clinical responsibilities

All healthcare providers have patient care as a top priority. The provider's focus may be on care of the patient, whereas office personnel must focus on receiving maximum payment for the care of that patient. The records stored at the practitioner level must be accessible and transferable to the hospital in the case of an admission or referral. HIEs are making this possible for referrals, consultations, admissions, discharges, and transfers. IT solutions such as EMRs, digital storage of patient data, voice recognition software, and e-mailing of correspondence can offer efficiency, cost savings, and improved patient care, which should be the priorities of practice management (Gates and Urquhart, 2007).

VALUE-BASED CARE APPLICATIONS

Since the early 2000s, healthcare leaders have focused on addressing the high cost and comparatively poor outcomes produced by the U.S. health system. Central to their efforts is the concept of generating and rewarding healthcare value. Value is defined as delivering the best outcome for the dollars invested (Porter & Teisberg, 2006; Porter, 2009). This transition from a volume focused payment system to value-based care requires that managers take the integration of clinical and financial data to new levels to create actionable information where the outcomes and costs of patient care at the population level are monitored and managed in unison (Scherpbier, 2014). This demand for actionable data is driving healthcare organizations (HCO) to undertake substantial capital investments in information systems in order to be competitive in the market.

Population health management (PHM) is the cornerstone of the ongoing value-driven transformation of the U.S. health system. In this context, population health management is the focus on improving health outcomes for a specified population, such as the panel of patients treated by a physician or all diabetic individuals cared for by a HCO (Berwick et al., 2008). In order to deliver effective and efficient PHM, data from multiple traditional health information systems must be integrated with and augmented by newly evolving information packages that provide additional data on the social and economic determinants of health as well as the community level resources that support individual level health.

Health information systems for PHM vary widely in their design and manufacture. Some are proprietary systems that integrate data from existing clinical and business applications, while others are additional modules that expand the capabilities of existing infrastructure such as EHR systems. In the early era of PHM, independent systems were common but more recently, applications from legacy providers, particularly EHRs, have grown in market share. Regardless of the design or manufacturer, PHM systems must be able to integrate data from multiple sources, perform analyses on the data for population risk stratification and performance management, and facilitate the management and coordination of patient care through functionalities such as the generation of care lists and reminders for providers and patients (Scherpbier, 2014).

Because of the tremendous diversity of PHM systems, it would be impossible to discuss all possible arrangements for such infrastructure. In the interest of providing a more concise discussion, we will focus on PHM applications that are supplemental modules developed by EHR manufacturers. While this restricts our coverage, all PHM applications, regardless of their design, depend on data from the EHR as the backbone of their operation

Population Health Applications in the Electronic Health Record

When medical facilities had paper charts, information was written onto paper, papers were collected into charts, and charts were filed on shelves in storage rooms. The information on those papers sat idle and did not inform further decisions about the patient, the populations, or the organization unless it was pulled from the shelf and manually reviewed. Imagine the millions of data points segregated in time and space due to the paper format. Enter the EHR. The EHR allows for real-time capture, organization, connection, analysis, and use of data to support clinical decisions to improve the health of populations. EHRs can slice data into thousands of iterations such as all diabetics within a health system, practice, or physician panel. Multiple specifications can be applied to delve further into that diabetic population such age, gender, vaccination status, cardiovascular risk, readmission risk, and risk of diabetic complications. The slicing of data allows HCOs to prioritize care delivery efforts to improve health outcomes for the population of interest.

To provide these capabilities, the right constructs must be in place with strategically designed data architecture, tools, and analytics. Many EHRs provide built-in reports for the end user to run. However, less sophisticated EHRs lack these functionalities, forcing HCOs to rely on consultants and customization fees to access population health data. HCOs exist to provide the right care to the right patient at the right time for the right indication at the right price without harm; all received and perceived by the patient to have occurred in the right way. Managing populations in this "right" way requires the use of meaningful data that is acquired from the EHR. Exploring many popular EHR platforms' websites, it is evident that population health is a core menu item in their solutions and services offerings.

Though varying by vendor, dashboards are derived from patient data, arranged, and benchmarked. The ability to manage a population relies on data quality; thus defined data entry standards are key. The reason to manage populations is to make populations healthier, improve outcomes, and hopefully decrease healthcare costs. As such, there are many factors that contribute to poor health outcomes such as social determinants of health, chronic disease burden, access to care, health literacy, and receipt of recommended preventive services such as vaccines and cancer screenings. The goal would be to follow

the Population Health Sieve and Support Model as shown in Fig. 8.3. Once patient data are filtered to identify patients at highest risk for poor health outcomes or needing preventive services, the HCO care team should determine the appropriate layers of care to envelop the patient with. Imagine a fragile piece of glassware receiving multiple layers of bubble wrap to protect it. This is the approach to the layers of care in this model, represented by assessment and provision of needed social resources, preventive services, lifestyle change programs, chronic disease indicator management to name a few. These layers of support expand the care team led by physicians to enhance patient touchpoints and care services through non-clinical and clinically licensed personnel. The predicted results would be improved health outcomes, less complications, earlier diagnosis and treatment of severe disease, prevention, and decreased healthcare costs. Healthier patients equate to healthier and more productive communities. However, this places immense

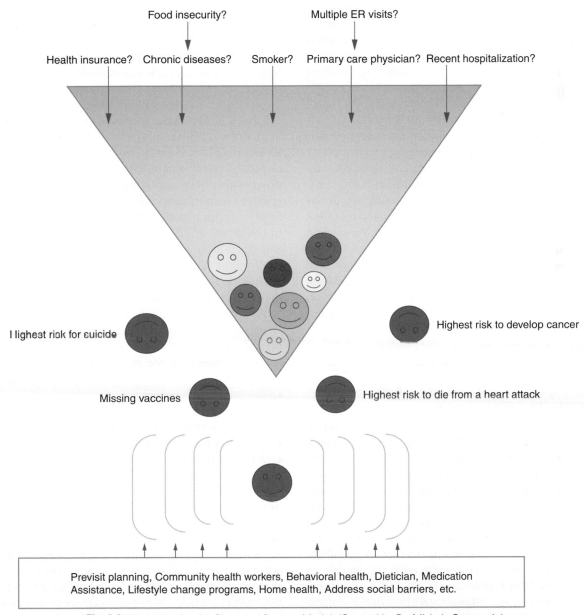

Fig. 8.3 Population Health Sieve and Support Model. (Created by Dr. Michele Bosworth.)

importance on the data captured, stored, and utilized within the EHR that feeds into this model. The adage holds true, garbage in equals garbage out.

Integrating Social Determinants of Health With the EHR

As mentioned, the clinical care that an individual receives is only one of many factors that determine the overall health outcome from care (Evans et al., 1994). Social determinants, including the economic and physical environment that an individual lives within influences not only the underlying health of the individual but also the effectiveness of the healthcare system's actions. Because of this, the introduction of community level socioeconomic, infrastructure and geospatial factors into the clinical needs assessments of the patient population(s) served by an HCO can add a layer of richness to the organization's predictive and prescriptive analytics. Additionally, such contextual data are also instrumental for the population health and case management teams. For example, consider a patient who is being discharged from the hospital and will need to follow up with her primary care physician within 7 days. If the patient does not have access to transportation, the best discharge planning will be of little value. The patient will never get to the appointment unless a connection is made for transportation. In the past discharge planners had to keep lists of contact numbers for services that their patients might need, now many PHM systems allow for the integration of secondary data sources that can provide instant access to up to date resources available in the patient's community.

There are a substantial number of different social determinants focused platforms available. The platform findhelp (previously known as Aunt Bertha) (https://www.findhelp.org) is one example of an application that can be directly linked into EHR systems such as EPIC. findhelp provides access to information on social and community services nationwide at the county level. If we return to our example of a patient being discharged from the hospital, a discharge planner retrieve data on relevant transportation services using findhelp or a similar application without exiting the EHR system. Additionally, these data services provide up-to-date contact information, hours of operation, eligibility for service use, and other material needed to provide a smooth transition for the patient.

Assessing Organizational Capabilities for Population Health Management

As HCOs attempt to navigate developing the infrastructure and skills needed to support a PHM care model, the vast array of decisions can be overwhelming for leaders. This is particularly true because of financial capital limitations that force most organizations to stage their investments in PHM. To assist industry with these strategic decisions, the HIMSS tasked their Clinical and Business Intelligence Committee to examine what organizational and information system capabilities are essential to operate a PHM model of care and to assess how these essential capabilities vary based on the payment models an HCO faces. The HIMSS Population Health and Management Model is available at https://www.himss.org/resources/himss-population-health-management-and-capabilities-model.

SUPPLY CHAIN MANAGEMENT

SCM includes the acquisition of materials of care and the logistics or movement of those materials to caregiving facilities and organizations. Routinely, health systems deploy information system solutions to support the functions of SCM.

Healthcare Supply Chain and Informatics

What is a supply chain? The Council of Supply Chain Management Professionals defines *supply chain* in two ways: (1) starting with unprocessed raw materials and ending with the final customer using the finished goods, the supply chain links many companies together, or (2) the material and informational interchanges in the logistical process stretching from acquisition of raw materials to delivery of finished products to the end user. All vendors, service providers, and customers are links in the supply chain (Glossary, 2013).

Integrated information systems that share data, embedded with analytics (formulas that produce user decision support information) are growing more and more commonplace in healthcare and the healthcare supply chain. With over 30 billion transactions (business of healthcare hand-offs to include purchasing supplies) in healthcare each year, innovative information systems are required to reduce costs (half of those transactions are still fax based or manual) and improve efficiency. Block chain innovations are a testament to this needed evolution in information systems. According to the Blockbox, "Blockchain in healthcare improves overall security of patients' electronic medical records, resolves the issues of drugs authenticity and drugs supply chain traceability, and enables secure interoperability between healthcare organizations" (https://theblockbox.io/blog/blockchain-technology-in-healthcare-in-2021/). The ability to verify the traceability and trackability of healthcare supplies, consider counterfeit medications for example; block chain is a new and exciting addition to the information system and data infrastructure in the healthcare supply chain.

A supply chain is much more than procurement of materials. Many times, the potential advantages of SCM are missed because the term is thought to relate only to the supply side of an organization or to the purchasing of materials. In addition, SCM is not:

- Inventory management
- Logistics management
- Forming partnerships with suppliers
- A strategy for shipping
- A logistics pipeline
- A computer system

The healthcare supply chain is complex, with requirements that go across, for example, the equipment for operating suites, pharmaceuticals, and medical and surgical supplies for all settings. In any health system with hospitals, clinics, and employees ordering from the supply chain, thousands of transactions occur daily across hundreds of vendors. Medical and surgical supplies, pharmaceuticals, and equipment are the "technology" that enables the delivery of healthcare services. These technologies couple with clinician knowledge and expertise within an appropriate healthcare facility function to provide efficacious services to patients.

Materials management in healthcare is the storage, inventory control, quality control, and operational management of supplies, pharmaceuticals, equipment, and other items used in the delivery of patient care or the management of the patient care system. As such, materials management is a subset of the larger function of SCM. It should be noted that the term *materials management* is also sometimes used as a synonym for the healthcare supply chain.

Typically, an organization named Materials Management or Central Supply in the hospital bears the burden of having the right item at the right place at the right time. The leading professional association, the Association for Healthcare Resource and Materials Management or AHRMM, lists common functions of the supply chain in healthcare. Several of these functions occur in the Purchasing Department, which is a key department within Materials Management.

As a department within Materials Management, Purchasing traditionally controls or participates in several functions (Blount et al., 2012):

- Budgeting
- Replenishing inventory
- Evaluating and selecting capital
- Negotiating
- Maintaining the Materials Management Information System (MMIS)
- Reviewing product use and analyzing value
- Maintaining vendor relationships
- Monitoring the product selection process to ensure selection is competitive
- Coordinating with Finance to ensure reimbursement of products
- Providing information to end users regarding product use, costs, and alternatives

All these items can be a part of the SCM strategy, but the misconceptions behind what is considered SCM have slowed implementation. As healthcare institutions increasingly need to understand and control actual costs, SCM and in turn materials management is now an area of growth because of the potential for cost savings (Lummus & Vokurka, 1999). Because the acquisition, logistics, and management of materials in healthcare are complex, a sophisticated information system is required to provide effective, efficient, and efficacious materials as needed.

The sophistication in automating this process has increased tremendously since the late 1990s. Applications now include electronic catalogs; information systems such as enterprise resource planning (ERP) systems from vendors such as Infor (https://www.infor.com/) or McKesson (https://www.mckesson.com/); warehousing and inventory control systems from vendors such as TECSYS (https://www.tecsys.com/) and Manhattan (https://www.manh.com); exchanges from vendors such as Global Health Exchange (GHX) (https://www.ghx.com/); and integration with other systems such as clinical, revenue management, and finance. An innovative technology in this area is radio frequency identification (RFID); more information can be found at https://advantech-inc.com/.

With increased automation, these systems have improved supply chain performance and management in healthcare, with more innovations expected in the future. The healthcare supply chain is an untapped resource of financial savings and revenue enhancement opportunities (Roark, 2005). Recognizing these opportunities, HIMSS advocated for more improvements in a white paper titled *Healthcare ERP and SCM Information Systems: Strategies and Solutions*. HIMSS indicated that ERP systems will be tools for quality and safety because they integrate capabilities such as procure-to-pay, order-to-cash, and financial reporting cycles. These functions should help institutions match needed materials with care in a more timely and cost-effective manner (HIMSS, 2007).

Integrated Applications in Supply Chain Management

The importance of these ERP and SCM systems should be apparent, including the technology associated with them, such as bar code scanners and electronic medication cabinets (e.g., Pyxis [www.carefusion.com/our-products/medication-and-supply-management/medication-and-supply-management-technologies/pyxis-medication-technologies/pyxis-medstation-system] and Omnicell [https://www.omnicell.com/]). The basic components of an integrated healthcare supply chain system include the following:

- Supply item master file: A list of all items used in the delivery of care for an HCO that can be requested by healthcare service providers and managers. This file typically contains between 30,000 and 100,000 items.
- Charge description master file: A list of all prices for services (e.g., Diagnosis-Related Groups [DRGs], HCPCS, and CPT) or goods provided to patients that serves as the basis for billing.
- Vendor master file: A list of all manufacturers or distributors (vendors) that provide the materials needed for the HCO along with the associated contract terms and prices for specific items. This file typically contains 200 to 500 different vendors or suppliers.
- Transaction history file: A running log of all material transactions of the HCO. In a computerized system, it is a running list of all supplies and materials being used to deliver care or manage the operations of the institution.

These four files must be integrated to support the operations and management of the supply chain. The integration necessary in the modern HCO is illustrated in Fig. 8.4 as a diagram of interfaces across supply chain, clinical, and financial systems (Corry et al., 2005).

Supply Cost Capture

As a survey of supply chain progress (Poirer & Quinn, 2004) demonstrates, "In all industries, not just healthcare, three out of four chief executive officers consider their supply chains to be essential to gaining competitive advantage within their markets" (Ledlow et al., 2007, p. 2). According to Moore, if the trend in the cost of the healthcare supply chain continues to grow at the current rate, supply chain could equal labor cost in annual operating expenses for hospitals

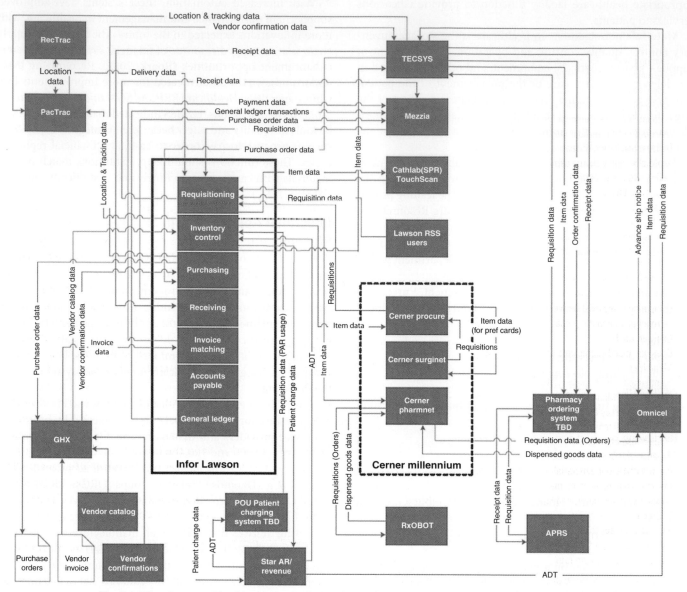

Fig. 8.4 Wire diagram of healthcare supply chain information systems. (Dr. Jerry Ledlow, personal files.)

and health systems between 2020 and 2025 (Moore, 2008). Clearly, maximizing efficiency of the healthcare supply chain is an increasing concern.

Consider supply charge capture events in which patient-specific supplies are ordered for the care of that patient and the items are then billed separately to the patient. "Every year, hospitals lose millions of dollars when items used in the course of a patient's care somehow slip through the system without ever being charged or reimbursed" (Bacon & Pexton, 2010, p. 1). Point-of-use technology, or capturing charges when supplies or materials are used, allows healthcare institutions to increase productivity, increase accountability, and reduce downtime through improvements in their internal supply chain. Automated dispensing machines for medications or supplies can be used to decentralize store operations, capture charges, and bring supplies and materials to employees without compromising security and accountability (Evahan Technology, 2005). These systems, if integrated with a

solid business process, can enhance efficiency and effectiveness of the healthcare supply chain.

Strategic factors associated with supply success and enhancement are important as well. These include the following (Ledlow et al., 2007):

- Information system usefulness, electronic purchasing, and integration
- Leadership supply chain expertise
- Supply chain expenditures
- Provider level of collaboration
- Nurse and clinical staff level of collaboration
- Leadership team's political and social capital
- Capital funds availability

This section has provided a high-level overview of technology in materials management. Box 8.2 details specific considerations for automating SCM and materials management (Ledlow et al., 2011).

BOX 8.2 Process Standardization

Process Standardization in Conjunction with Utilization of an Information System

- Develop standard (or *more standardized*) processes for:
- Item master and charge description master maintenance and synchronization
- Supply stock selection, reduction, compression, and management
- Supply charge item capture (accurate and timely)
- Accountability measures for Central Supply and clinical units
- Standardize clinical/floor stocked supplies replenishment processes
- Daily reconciliation of pharmaceuticals and medical/surgical supply items, especially supply charge capture items
- Taking into consideration:
- Clinical unit needs
- Physical layout variations may require modification to an accepted standard
- The business process must be efficient before a technological solution can be integrated into the process
- "One-size" solution will not fit all

Process Standardization in Process Improvement: Balancing Trade-Offs

- Competing goals exist between various stakeholder groups; trade-offs will be required to find the proper balance that best meets all needs
- Clinician Goals
- Does not impede caregivers or patient care delivery
- Minimize rework
- Right supplies, right place, right time
- Supply Chain Managers/Central Supply Goals
- Improve accuracy for supplies consumed
- Improve timeliness for supply consumption
- Efficient use of labor
- Revenue and Cost Avoidance Goals
- Procure and acquire material wisely with contracted compliance goals
- Efficient management of materials considering utilization rates, preferences, expiration dates, and Food and Drug Administration requirements
- Reduce number of supply charge capture items
- Improve accuracy for charge capture
- Improve timeliness for charge capture
- Improve charge capture rate

From Ledlow JR, Stephens JH, Fowler HH. Sticker shock: an exploration of supply charge capture outcomes. *Hosp Topics.* 2011;89(1):9. Reprinted by permission of the publisher (Taylor & Francis Ltd, http://www.tandf.co.uk/journals).

HUMAN RESOURCES INFORMATION SYSTEMS

Human resources information systems (HRISs) leverage the power of IT to manage human resources. They integrate "software, hardware, support functions and system policies and procedures into an automated process designed to support the strategic and operational activities of the human resources department and managers throughout the organization" (Chauhan et al., 2011, p. 58). The authors distinguish between operational, tactical, and strategic HRISs. Operational HRISs collect and report data about employees and the personnel infrastructure to support routine and repetitive decision making while meeting the requirements of government regulations. Tactical HRISs support the design of the personnel infrastructure and decisions about the recruitment, training, and compensation of persons filling jobs in the organization. Strategic HRISs support activities with a longer horizon such as workforce planning and labor negotiations. In contrast, Targowski and Deshpande state that generic HRISs typically include the following subsystems defined by function: recruitment and selection from among candidates; administration of personnel processes; time, labor, and knowledge management; training and career development; administration of compensation and benefits for active workers and pensions for retirees; payroll interface; performance evaluation; transitioning and outplacement; labor relations; organization management; and health and safety (Targowski & Deshpande, 2001).

Human Resources Information Systems as a Competitive Advantage

Khatri argues that the management of human resources in HCOs is a central function because the healthcare and administrative services delivered are based on the knowledge of staff delivering these services (Khatri, 2006). Human resources management should focus on employee training, as well as developing and refining the work systems to improve the work climate and the quality of service to customers. Although HCOs should include the effective management of human resources as part of strategic planning, most fail to do so. Khatri offers three reasons why many HCOs do not employ optimal human resource practices. First, he argues that the responsibilities and activities of human resources personnel are institutionalized and undervalued in many HCOs. Second, the provider culture of healthcare focuses on the clinical delivery of care with less attention paid to the effective management of resources. Finally, lack of expertise and low skills in the human resource function have limited the ability of human resource managers to engage effectively in strategic and operational planning. Khatri's premise is that improving human resource capabilities should help human resource managers engage more effectively in managing human resources (Khatri, 2006).

Khatri further proposed five dimensions of human resources capability. The first four are a competent human resources executive in the C-suite, a skilled human resources staff, an organizational culture that elevates human resources to a central function, and commitment to continuous learning. An integrated, computerized HRIS is the final capability (Khatri, 2006).

Vendors may offer comprehensive or component human resource information system applications to HCOs. Three examples of vendors offering comprehensive human resource information system solutions within a larger suite of ERP products are Infor Human Capital Management for Healthcare (https://www.infor.com/industries/healthcare), Oracle PeopleSoft (https://www.oracle.com/industries/healthcare/products.html), and UKG (https://www.ukg.com). Simplr (https://www.symplr.com/) is an example of a company with a narrower focus on workforce management.

Human Resources Subsystems

The human resources subsystems described below reflect a modification of the subsystems described by Targowski and Deshpande, and they represent a taxonomy of functions typically described by the vendor websites for HRISs (Targowski & Deshpande, 2001).

Personnel Administration

The centralized and integrated management of employee data is a key feature of HRISs. Personnel records are maintained and updated with information such as employee identification and demographics, dates of service, position and job code, location code, and employment status (permanent or temporary, full time, or part time). Systems also maintain records of licensure, credentials, certifications, and skill proficiency levels. Increasingly, self-service capabilities allow employees to maintain a personal profile with the ability to access and modify personal information such as name, address, contact information, marital status, and information about dependent family members.

Managing Human Resources Strategically and Operationally

HRISs can be used to address, in whole or in part, the challenge of managing human resources from a strategic and operational perspective. First, strategic management of human resources can be accomplished by accurately reflecting the organizational structure of the healthcare institution. This can be accomplished by using a wiring diagram to illustrate the hierarchy of positions in the organization, the job descriptions associated with each position, and whether the positions are filled or vacant. This analysis is then used to support the recruiting process for vacant positions. Functions that support this process include posting job announcements and application forms; providing status reports for submitted applications; maintaining interview schedules; and providing selection tools such as dynamic interview guides, multistage testing, computer adaptive testing, and mini simulations. Once a decision is made, the formal job offer letter and new employee benefits can be viewed online. HRISs should also have the capability to assist employees in transitioning out of the organization when discharged, displaced by reductions in the workforce, or retiring (Targowski & Deshpande, 2001).

Staffing and Scheduling

Staffing and scheduling replaces the subsystem "time, labor, and knowledge management" as a more accurate representation of the activities supported by this HRIS subsystem. Staffing and scheduling are two different activities. Staffing involves the assignment of personnel to job positions while ensuring that they are qualified by virtue of degree, licensure, certification, training, and experience. Scheduling involves the assignment of qualified personnel to a scheduling template within a work area in the organization to fulfill the mission of that organization. Scheduling of personnel such as nursing staff is extremely challenging, so much so that nurse scheduling can be considered a definitive representative of the archetypal multishift scheduling problem found in operations research and management sciences literature. Kronos (https://www.kronos.com/industry-solutions/health-systems), now a part of UKG, is among a number of vendors providing nurse scheduling solutions for health systems. Vendors typically offer both staffing and scheduling modules. Other modules manage scheduling for staff development and facilitate self-scheduling in conjunction with temporary staff management

to fill openings in the schedule. Key requirements for staffing and scheduling include cost-effective staffing while meeting constraints imposed by required qualifications, scheduling visibility, and matching the level and number of caregivers to patient classification and acuity levels as mandated by law or regulation.

Once scheduled, employees' time and attendance are tracked. Key elements include accurate time collection, implementation of user-defined pay rules, compliance with a variety of labor laws, and expeditious identification of productivity or overtime issues.

Just as schedules must be explicitly developed, time-off policies must be proactively managed because of their effect on the schedule. These time-off policies are designed to meet the requirements of federal labor laws such as the Family and Medical Leave Act (FMLA) and state and local laws. In addition to meeting legal and regulatory constraints, time-off policies must enforce organizational policy for vacation, maternity leave, and sick leave. The software used to do this is referred to as "leave management" or "absence management" and is typically a rules-based application designed to manage absence requests while interfacing with workload scheduling.

Because of the difficulty of scheduling in healthcare, flexible scheduling solutions are becoming increasingly common. Solutions representative of representative of many scheduling systems are found with Simplr (https://www.symplr.com/workforce-management/workforce-management) to include self-scheduling, shift trading and open-shift management using mobile technology.

CareSystems (https://caresystemsinc.com/healthcare/) also provides solutions in the healthcare staffing and scheduling arena, with a suite of products that manage time and attendance, assess patient acuity and estimated nurse workload, and employ intelligent scheduling algorithms to create optimal nursing schedules.

Training and Development

IT solutions should be able to be used as the infrastructure to plan and manage employee training, to serve as the delivery mechanism synchronously and online, and to link training with the developmental plan for each employee by identifying shortfalls in skills and competencies and then recording when those shortfalls have been remediated (Targowski & Deshpande, 2001).

Compensation, Benefits, and Pension Administration-Payroll Interface

"Compensation and benefit plans can vary from company to company. They include various plans such as flexible and nonflexible healthcare plans, short- and long-term disability plans, saving plans, retirement plans, pension plans, and flexible spending accounts." (Targowski & Deshpande, 2001, p. 46).

When coupled with personnel administration and staffing and scheduling systems and supported by timekeeping and absence management software, the management of compensation, benefits, and pension administration becomes more accurate and less time consuming.

Performance Evaluation

Talent management and *performance management* are terms used by several vendors. From the healthcare provider's perspective, the focus is on recruiting and training employees and developing competencies required to fulfill institutional goals and objectives. The individual career goals of employees are also considered. Information capabilities in this area include:

- Profiling employee competencies and any gaps.
- Identifying when employee and organizational goals are met.
- Identifying top performers.
- Managing dashboards to display unit performance.

BUSINESS INTELLIGENCE SYSTEMS

Since the late 1990s, healthcare institutions have been building data warehouses and integrating data. Along with the technical aspects, data warehousing includes improving data quality, developing protocols for governance, and facilitating the employment of appropriate analytic measures. This is difficult because of practice variation and changes to the standards of practice over time. As quoted in an article by Erickson, 2009, Dick Gibson, the CIO of Legacy Health, notes,

"We generate and use data like any other industry, but healthcare does not lend itself to the use of discrete data because the outcomes are necessarily fuzzy and ongoing. Airlines have seats, schedules, and know if you landed on time. In healthcare, we know if you are alive, but the big money goes to broad sets of descriptive terms around patient care that are very qualitative." (Erickson, 2009, p. 29).

These descriptive terms can be captured more succinctly by the use of diagnostic and procedural codes, but data quality and integration is a problem because of the number of procedures and number of providers engaged in the delivery of care (Erickson, 2009).

Business Intelligence Systems Applications

Many organizations are turning to business intelligence (BI) software to provide tools to effectively manage and use their massive amounts of data. BI software is purported to lead to an improvement in financial (particularly revenue cycle) and operational performance, as well as patient care (Glaser & Stone, 2008). Implementing BI in healthcare that successfully integrates financial and clinical data is regarded as one of the four pillars of the Value Project undertaken by the Healthcare Financial Management Association (Clarke, 2012). Business intelligence (BI) is defined as the "acquisition, correlation, and transformation of data into insightful and actionable information through analytics, enabling an organization and its business partners to make better, timelier decisions." (Giniat, 2011, p. 142). However, Glaser and Stone warn that for the BI to be most effective, the BI tools must be placed in the hands of the people who actually do the work, training must be done initially and throughout the project so that users will have time to use the basic functions and expand their knowledge, questions that arise throughout the analysis must be reviewed and

answered, and the BI should be used for long-term planning (Glaser & Stone, 2008). Glaser and Stone describe the BI platform as "a stack—one technology on top of another." (Glaser & Stone, 2008, p. 69). Their description was used to construct Fig. 8.5. Effective management of this stackable technology involves making the business case for BI, establishing implementation targets, enlisting BI champions, governing effectively, and establishing BI roles to include data stewards, data owners, business users, and data managers (Glaser & Stone, 2008).

As with the other information systems discussed in this chapter, BI systems may be part of an enterprise system, provided as component software, or employed at application level. Most of the major healthcare information system vendors have BI software imbedded in their products.

Dimensional Insight (https://www.healthcare.dimins.com) was ranked #1 in annual best in KLAS Report for healthcare business intelligence/analytics for 2021 followed by Health Catalyst Analytics Platform (https://www.healthcatalyst.com/) and Epic Cognito.

Given the cost, time, and complexity of the large-scale implementation of enterprise BI, application-level BI should be employed strategically to address "key processes, functions, or service lines." (Hennen, 2009, p. 95). Application-level BI software provides some of the data integration and visualization of enterprise packages, analyzes existing data that may be overlooked in traditional reporting, and creates actionable knowledge. However, some caution is necessary. Glaser and Stone note that ad hoc, smaller-scale analysis may lead to the creation of data

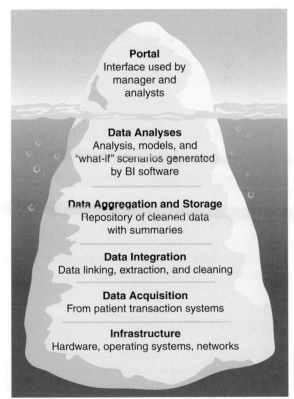

Portal
Interface used by manager and analysts

Data Analyses
Analysis, models, and "what-if" scenarios generated by BI software

Data Aggregation and Storage
Repository of cleaned data with summaries

Data Integration
Data linking, extraction, and cleaning

Data Acquisition
From patient transaction systems

Infrastructure
Hardware, operating systems, networks

Fig 8.5 Business intelligence platform. (Data from Glaser, J., & Stone, J. [2008]. Effective use of business intelligence. *Healthcare Financial Management*, 62[2], 68–72.)

silos, inefficient or repetitive management of data, and unnecessary duplication (Glaser & Stone, 2008). These are appropriate cautions, but application-level BI can complement the development of enterprise BI by producing results in the interim as the enterprise capabilities are developed (Hennen, 2009).

Employment of Artificial Intelligence

The scope, scale, and format of data collected in healthcare environments present a challenge to decision makers. Artificial Intelligence (AI) is a set of technologies that can be used to transform data to knowledge to support decision-making in both clinical and administrative environments. Davenport and Kalakota note that AI technologies currently employed in healthcare include machine learning where algorithms (often structured as neural networks) are employed to autonomously improve predictions based upon the accuracy of past predictions, natural language processing used to address the challenge of a primarily text-based medical record, rule-based expert systems to capture the if-then logic employed by human experts, and process automation (Davenport & Kalakota, 2019). Chen and Decary add AI voice technology and assistants to the mix and note that consumer acceptance of AI assistants with limited capacity such as Alexa, SIRI and Google Assistant foreshadow the development of more sophisticated applications in healthcare AI. They note that continued development of health-related AI technologies will come from technology companies currently dominating the marketplace, EHR vendors, and niche specialists in healthcare AI (Chen & Decary, 2020).

CONCLUSION AND FUTURE DIRECTIONS

Given the magnitude of the investment in health information systems, and that administrative applications are more mature than clinical applications, a salient question is whether these administrative applications have made healthcare delivery more productive. In "Unraveling the IT Productivity Paradox—Lessons for Healthcare," Jones, Heaton, Rudin, and Schneider explore the paradoxical relationship between "the rapid increase in IT use and the simultaneous slowdown in productivity." (Jones et al., 2012, p. 2244). Several lessons emerge from the authors' analysis:

- Mismeasurement partially contributed to the paradox. The authors suggest, "assessment of the value of healthcare outputs could be improved through the more sophisticated use of clinical data to understand access, convenience, and health outcomes" (Jones et al., 2012).
- New information technology often requires redesign of the processes that were previously tailored to the technology or manual system just replaced.
- New information technology compromises productivity when it fails to be user centered.
- Finally, HCOs can no longer afford to have an abundance of untapped data that fails to improve decision making. Improvements in healthcare information systems, BI, and analytics must continue to improve the quality of decision making (Jones et al., 2012).

Administrative systems in this chapter were listed as separate applications because they evolved independently of CSs. Many of the future benefits will accrue from integrating data from all systems. For example, if a healthcare system cannot effectively track the total cost of all materials used to treat an individual patient and aggregate data to determine the cost of treating groups of patients, managing the cost of healthcare is not possible. AI will have an increasing important role in effectively managing big data in healthcare and transforming data to actionable information for administering the environment in which care is delivered and the health of populations (Stanfill & Marc, 2019). As new information becomes available for decision making, healthcare professionals on both the administrative and the clinical sides of the organization will need to learn new interprofessional approaches to using these data in making decisions.

DISCUSSION QUESTIONS

1. Explain why healthcare facilities are critical to the effective operation of health systems.
2. Describe how a decision maker would use the financial information system reporting function to make decisions, and provide a summary of what the various reports tell the decision maker.
3. Explain the benefits of incorporating an online billing and payment in a provider practice setting.
4. Explain how point-of-use technology facilitates supply charge capture.
5. Discuss how self-service applications are typically deployed in human resources information systems.
6. Discuss the advantages and disadvantages of using business intelligence at the application level as opposed to the enterprise level.

CASE STUDY

Michael H. Kennedy, Kim Crickmore, and Lynne Miles[1]

Managing the flow of patients and bed capacity is challenging for any hospital, especially for unscheduled admissions. For Zed

---

[1]Kim Crickmore and Lynne Miles are past Advisory Board members for the East Carolina University Health Services Management Program.

Medical Center, a large regional referral center in the South and a member of the University Health System Consortium, the challenge is even greater. As the flagship hospital for a multihospital system with more than 750 licensed beds and a Level 1 trauma center with 50-plus trauma beds, approximately 70% of annual admissions are unscheduled.

The vice-president for Operations has a PhD in Nursing, is a fellow of the Advisory Board Company, and has more than 20 years' tenure at Zed Medical Center. Three of the ten departments under her purview (Patient Care Coordinator, Bed Control, and Patient Transfers) are directly engaged in managing patient flow and bed capacity. The division is also responsible for system-wide care coordination for patients discharged to skilled nursing facilities, to home health, and to home without planned service delivery. Current operational goals include (1) decreasing the current length of stay by 0.3 days from 5.7 to 5.4 days and (2) "ED to 3"—a slogan incorporating the intention to place patients from the emergency department into a bed within 3 hours of the decision to admit. With the Centers for Medicare & Medicaid Services clarifying penalties for readmissions within 30 days, Zed Medical Center has been preparing to effectively manage readmissions based on CMS guidelines.

The eight staff members assigned to Patient Transfers coordinate with hospitals within the region wanting to transfer patients to Zed Medical Center. They take calls, connect outside transfers with accepting physicians, and arrange transport. The accepting physician determines the patient's needed level of care, special care needs (e.g., diabetic), and the time frame for transfer. The

Patient Transfer Department uses the TransferCenter module of TeleTracking (www.teletracking.com) to manage the transfer and admission of patients. After a patient has been accepted for admission by the admitting physician, Bed Control makes the bed assignment. The staff members of Bed Control assign incoming patients to specific beds once the Patient Placement Facilitators from the Patient Care Coordinator Department identify the nursing unit to which patients should be assigned. This determination is made based on the level of care required, physician preferences in choice of nursing unit, and the scope of care supported by the nursing units. The Bed Control Department uses the Capacity Management Suite of the TeleTracking software. The PreAdmitTracking module keeps track of bed status with an "electronic bedboard," which provides a graphical user interface through which planned admissions, transfers, and discharges can be annotated. The status of a bed freed by patient discharge for which a cleaning request has been made is also noted (dirty, in progress, or cleaned). The Bed Tracking module uses the medical center's paging network to notify the environmental services staff of a cleaning request and the unit director of the unit that a patient is incoming. The TransportTracking module automatically dispatches patient transport requests via phone or pager.

DISCUSSION QUESTIONS

1. How are patients prioritized for bed assignment?
2. Describe some of the advantages and disadvantages of this new software. Include the stated organizational goals in your answer.
3. Discuss how this software might share data with other institutional applications to provide a dashboard view of census-type activity.

REFERENCES

About us. (n.d.). Welcome to National Association of Free and Charitable Clinics. National Association of Free and Charitable Clinics. https://www.nafcclinics.org/content/about-us

Bacon, S., & Pexton, C. (2010). Improving patient charge capture at Yale-New Haven. iSixSigma. http://www.isixsigma.com/index.php?option=com_k2&view=item&id=997:&Itemid=49../../200353/AppData/Local/Temp/2/XmlTemp/0007.html-sLink29ir0205.

Berwick, D. M., Nolan, T. W., & Whittington, J. (2008). The triple aim: Care, health, and cost. *Health Affairs*, 27(3), 759–769.

Blount, D., Chaney, V., Fohey, L., Goodhue, R., Greiner, T., & Hinkle, D. (2012). *Materials management review guide* (4th ed.). Chicago, Illinois: Association for Healthcare Resource & Materials Management of the American Hospital Association.

Bolt-ons. (n.d.). Computer glossary, computer terms—Technology definitions and cheat sheets from WhatIs.com—The tech dictionary and IT encyclopedia. https://whatis.techtarget.com/search/query?q=bolt-ons

Cash, J. (2008). Technology can make or break the hospital-physician relationship. *Healthcare Financial Management*, 62(12), 104–109.

Chauhan, A., Sharma, S., & Tyagi, T. (2011). Role of HRIS in improving modern HR operations. *Review of Management*, 1(2), 58–70.

Chen, M., & Decary, M. (2020). Artificial intelligence in healthcare: An essential guide for health leaders. *Healthcare Management Forum*, 33(1), 10–18. https://doi.org/10.1177/0840470419873123.

Ciotti, V., & Alcaro, B. (2014). Top 2013 HIS vendors by revenue. *Health Data Management*, 22(6), 16.

Clarke, R. (2012). Rethinking business intelligence. *Healthcare Financial Management*, 66(2), 120.

Conley, C. (2009). *Improve patient satisfaction and collections with efficient payment processes*. Emdeon Express Winter Edition. http://emdeonexpress.blogspot.com/2009/02/its-no-secret-that-health-care-is.html../../200353/AppData/Local/Temp/2/XmlTemp/0007.html - sLink17ir0195.

Corry, A. P., Ledlow, G. R., & Shockley, S. (2005). Designing the standard for a healthy supply chain. *Montgomery Research*

Curtis, E., & Schelhammer, S. (2011). *Patient outreach system helps clinic boost care visits, revenues*. Healthcare Financial Management Association. http://www.hfma.org/Leadership/E-Bulletins/2011/August/Patient_Outreach_System_Helps_Clinic_Boost_Care_Visits,_Revenues/../../200353/AppData/Local/Temp/2/XmlTemp/0007.html - sLink16ir0190.

Davenport, T., & Kalakota, R. (2019). The potential for artificial intelligence in healthcare. *Future Healthcare Journal*, 6(2), 94–98. https://doi.org/10.7861/futurehosp.6-2-94.

Erickson, J. (2009). BI's march to health care. *Information Management*, 19(7), 29–34.

Evahan Technology. (2005). Point of use technology in the supply chain. Ferret. http://www.ferret.com.au/c/Evahan/Point-of-use-technology-in-the-supply-chain-n698823../../200353/AppData/Local/Temp/2/XmlTemp/0007.html - sLink30ir0210.

Evans, R., Barer, M., & Marmor, T. (1994). *Why are some people healthy and other not? The determinants of health of populations.* New York, NY: Aldine de Gruyter.

Free and charitable clinics receive grant for point-of-care diagnostics. (n.d.). Welcome to National Association of Free and Charitable Clinics. National Association of Free and Charitable Clinics. https://www.nafcclinics.org/content/free-and-charitable-clinics-receive-grant-point-care-diagnostics

Gartner, Inc. Why Gartner? http://www.gartner.com/technology/why_gartner.jsp. Accessed June 13, 2016.

Gates, P., & Urquhart, J. (2007). The electronic, "paperless" medical office: has it arrived? *Internal Medicine Journal, 37,* 108–111.

Giniat, E. J. (2011). Using business intelligence for competitive advantage. *Healthcare Financial Management, 65*(9), 142–146.

Glaser, J., & Stone, J. (2008). Effective use of business intelligence. *Healthcare Financial Management, 62*(2), 68–72.

Glossary 2013 01 080513. Council of Supply Chain; 2013. http://cscmp.org/sites/default/files/user_uploads/resources/downloads/glossary-2013.pdf../../200353/AppData/Local/Temp/2/XmlTemp/0007.html-sLink20ir0200.

Hammer, D., & Franklin, D. (2008, February). Beyond bolt-ons: Breakthroughs in revenue cycle information systems. *Healthcare Financial Management, 62*(2), 52–60.

Haux, R. (2006). Health information systems—past, present, and future. *International Journal of Medical Informatics, 75,* 268–281.

HealthLeaders. (2018, March 8). *Clinical and financial analytics lead healthcare IT investment and ROI.* HealthLeaders Media. https://www.healthleadersmedia.com/innovation/clinical-and-financial-analytics-lead-healthcare-it-investment-and-roi.

Hennen, J. (2009). Targeted business intelligence pays off. *Healthcare Financial Management, 63*(3), 92–98.

HIMSS. Healthcare ERP and SCM Information Systems: Strategies and Solutions. In: A White Paper by the HIMSS Enterprise Information Systems Steering Committee; 2007.

James, J. (2012). Health policy brief. http://healthaffairs.org/healthpolicybriefs/brief_pdfs/healthpolicybrief_78.pdf. Accessed June 13, 2016.

Jones, S. S., Heaton, P. S., Rudin, R. S., & Schneider, E. C. (2012). Unraveling the IT productivity paradox—lessons for healthcare. *New England Journal of Medicine, 366*(24), 2243–2245.

Khatri, N. (2006). Building HR capability in health care organizations. *Health Care Management Review, 31*(1), 45–54.

KLAS. Our story. http://www.klasresearch.com/about-us/our-story. Accessed June 13, 2016.

Ledlow, G., Corry, A., & Cwiek, M. (2007). *Optimize Your Healthcare Supply Chain Performance: A Strategic Approach.* Chicago, Illinois: Health Administration Press.

Ledlow, J. R., Stephens, J. H., & Fowler, H. H. (2011). Sticker shock: an exploration of supply charge capture outcomes. *Hospital Topics, 89*(1), 9.

Lummus, R. R., & Vokurka, R. J. (1999). Defining supply chain management: a historical perspective and practical guidelines. *Industrial Management & Data Systems, 99*(1), 11–17.

Moore, V. (2008). *Clinical supply chain.* Chicago, Illinois: Paper presented at American College of Healthcare Executives National Congress;.

Pang, A., Markovski, M., & Ristik, M. (2020, November 20). Top 10 healthcare software vendors and market forecast 2019-2024. APPS RUN THE WORLD. Retrieved September 13, 2021, from https://www.appsruntheworld.com/top-10-healthcare-software-vendors-and-market-forecast/#.

Poirer, C., & Quinn, F. (2004). A survey of supply chain progress. *Supply Chain Management Review, 8*(8), 24–31.

Porter, M. E., & Teisberg, E. O. (2006). *Redefining health care: creating value-based competition on results.* Boston: Harvard Business School Press.

Porter, M. E. (2009). A strategy for health care reform-toward a value based system. *The New England Journal of Medicine, 361*(2), 109–112.

Providertech. (2018, September 4). *Text messaging in healthcare: Automated patient outreach.* Providertech. https://www.providertech.com/automated-patient-outreach/

Public policy. (n.d.). Welcome to National Association of Free and Charitable Clinics. National Association of Free and Charitable Clinics. https://www.nafcclinics.org/public-policy

Reiner, G. (2021, May 18). Success in proactive denials management and prevention. HFMA. https://www.hfma.org/topics/hfm/2018/september/61778.html

Roark, D. C. (2005). Managing the healthcare supply chain. *Nursing Management, 36*(2), 36–40.

Rosario, C. (2021, February 19). How important is financial & clinical reporting for healthcare? EHR, RIS, Practice Management & Medical Billing Software | ADS. https://www.adsc.com/blog/how-important-is-financial-and-clinical-reporting-for-healthcare

Scherpbier, H. (2014). Data analytics in population health. *Population Health Matters, 27*(2).

Schulz, J., DeCamp, M., & Berkowitz, S. A. (2015). Medicare shared savings program: public reporting and shared savings distributions. *The American Journal of Managed Care, 21*(8), 546–553.

Shared Savings Program. (2021, June 22). Centers for Medicare & Medicaid Services | CMS. https://www.cms.gov/Medicare/Medicare-Fee-for-Service-Payment/sharedsavingsprogram/about

Siwicki, B. (2018, July 12). *What to expect in the next generation of healthcare finance technologies.* Healthcare Finance News. https://www.healthcarefinancenews.com/news/what-expect-next-generation-healthcare-finance-technologies.

Siwicki, B. (2019, May 16). Implementation best practices: Ringing up success with finance IT. Healthcare IT News. https://www.healthcareitnews.com/news/implementation-best-practices-ringing-success-finance-it.

Siwicki, B. (2020, January 30). *Tech optimization: Keeping financial IT humming.* Healthcare IT News. https://www.healthcareitnews.com/news/tech-optimization-keeping-financial-it-humming.

Sorrentino, P. A., & Sanderson, B. B. (2001). Managing the physician revenue cycle. *Healthcare Financial Management, 65*(12), 88. 90, 92, 94.

Stanfill, M. H., & Marc, D. T. (2019). Health Information Management: Implications of artificial intelligence on healthcare data and information management. *Yearbook of Medical Informatics, 28*(1), 56–64. https://doi.org/10.1055/s-0039-1677913.

Targowski, A. S., & Deshpande, S. P. (2001). The utility and selection of an HRIS. *Advances in Competitiveness Research, 9*(1), 42–56.

Williams, B. (2002). "Gaining with integration: three healthcare organizations use integrated financial-clinical systems to achieve ROI, process improvement, and patient care objectives." *Health Management Technology, 23*(6), 10–13, 15.

9

Community Health Systems

Karen S. Martin and Jeanette M. Olsen

No matter how dreary and gray our homes are, we people of flesh and blood would rather live there than in any other country, be it ever so beautiful. There is no place like home.

Baum, L. F. (1900). *The wonderful wizard of Oz*. Chicago, IL: George M. Hill Co.

OBJECTIVES

At the completion of this chapter, the reader will be prepared to:

1. Summarize the origins of community health services and information systems in the United States.
2. Differentiate between at least three community health practice models.
3. Describe two standardized datasets commonly used in community-based settings.
4. Explain the value of using standardized terminologies in community-based settings.
5. Demonstrate the utility and applications of the Omaha System in community-based care settings.
6. Summarize the value of clinical data and information technology in community health practice.

KEY TERMS

community-based public health, 137
electronic health records, 135
home health, 137
hospice care, 138
Hospice Item Set (HIS), 140
Intervention Scheme, 143

nurse-managed health centers, 138
Omaha System, 140
Outcome and Assessment Information Set (OASIS), 139
palliative care, 138
Problem Classification Scheme, 141

Problem Rating Scale for Outcomes, 143
standardized datasets, 139
standardized terminologies, 140

ABSTRACT ❖

Community health systems located in the United States are changing rapidly. Information technology is accelerating those changes. This chapter will address (1) community-based public health, home health, hospice and palliative care, nurse-managed health centers, and other practice models; (2) the electronic health records (EHRs) and information systems used at community-based practice sites; and (3) the value and power of clinical data and information generated by these information systems. Core values of community health clinicians include patient-centered care and services that are of high quality, efficient, and cost effective. Information systems began with billing systems and evolved to point-of-care solutions in the 1990s. The Outcome and Assessment Information Set (OASIS) and Hospice Item Set (HIS) are examples of standardized datasets. Using standardized terminologies is an important strategy that complements community-based core values. The Omaha System, one of the standardized terminologies developed in a community health setting and recognized by the American Nurses Association, is described and clinical examples illustrate how practice, documentation, and information management can enhance the quality of care.

INTRODUCTION

Community health systems located in the United States are changing rapidly and becoming increasingly linked to other providers in the healthcare community. Information technology (IT) related technological advances, the emphasis on big data, national initiatives—including the transition to value-based care—and the recent pandemic are accelerating these changes. Numerous references describe community-related research, economics, and patient personal preference, suggesting that home is the optimal location for diverse health and nursing services (American Nurses Association [ANA], 2014; National Hospice and Palliative Care Organization

[NHPCO], 2020, 2021; Ankota, 2021; Omaha System Website, 2021; Riekert, 2021; Avalere Health, 2020). Patient residences include houses, apartments, dormitories, trailers, boarding and care homes, hospice houses, assisted-living facilities, shelters, and cars. Although residences are the primary location where community-based care is provided, many organizations offer services at workplaces, schools, churches, community buildings, and other sites.

This chapter addresses community-based public health, home health, palliative care and hospice, nurse-managed health centers, and other community-based practice models; the supporting electronic health records (EHRs) and other information systems used at the practice sites; and the value of clinical data and information generated by these information systems. The assessment, planning, intervention, and evaluation services that are part of these models range from promoting wellness and preventing disease to caring of the sick and dying. Ideally, these services are captured in EHRs so they may be quantified, analyzed, and used to measure the outcomes of care. Formal community-based caregivers include nurses, social workers, physical and occupational therapists, speech-language pathologists, registered dietitians, home health aides, chaplains, physicians, and others. Team approach and interprofessional collaboration are required to address the intensity of the patient's and family's needs. Although the term *patient* is used consistently in this chapter, *client*, *customer*, *consumer*, and *member* are alternative terms often used in community health systems.

EVOLUTION AND MILESTONES

Community health systems have a long and distinguished history in this country. In the early years, care for those who were ill or dying was typically informal and provided by women living in the household or neighborhood. Home health provided by formal caregivers originated in the 1800s and was based on the district nursing model developed by William Rathbone in England. In many communities, the initial programs evolved into visiting nurse associations (VNAs) and the movement expanded rapidly in the United States, resulting in the formation of 71 agencies before 1900 and 600 by 1909 (Dieckmann, 2017; Buhler-Wilkerson, 2002).

In 1893, Lillian Wald and Mary Brewster established the Henry Street Settlement House in New York City and developed a comprehensive program staffed by nurses and social workers. One of Wald's most impressive innovations was to convince the Metropolitan Life Insurance Company to include home visits as a benefit and to examine the cost effectiveness of care, a partnership that continued until 1952 (Dieckmann, 2017; Buhler-Wilkerson, 2002).

Public health departments were established and expanded during the early years of the 20th century. Health department staff members were primarily nurses who focused on care of immigrants, milk banks for mothers and babies, communicable disease, and environmental issues. They were concerned about consistent practice standards, patient record, and the collection of statistics (Stanhope & Lancaster, 2020).

Home health services were included as a major benefit when Medicare legislation was enacted in 1965 and resulted in significant changes nationally. The benefit was designed to provide intermittent, shorter visits with temporary lengths of stay to persons aged 65 and older; health promotion and long-term care services were not reimbursed. Nurses continued to represent the largest group of agency staff members; however, involvement of other professions was required. When a patient was admitted to service, the home health agency was required to develop a plan of care, obtain the signature of a physician, and follow additional regulations (Dieckmann, 2017; Centers for Medicare and Medicaid Services [CMS], 2017).

Hospice care was introduced in the 1970s. Florence Wald is acknowledged as the founder of the hospice movement in the United States, establishing Connecticut Hospice with interprofessional staff in 1974. The concept of hospice grew from a commitment to provide compassionate and dignified care to people who were at the end stage of life, offering care in the comfort of home with an emphasis on quality of life. Medicaid reimbursement for hospice care began in 1980 and Medicare reimbursement began in 1983; reimbursement determines many aspects of the hospice programs (NHPCO, 2020, 2021; Stanhope & Lancaster, 2020; Wright & Stanley, 2022).

Nurses employed in community health settings were concerned about documentation, standardization, and accountability in addition to practice. Their concerns were similar to those of other healthcare professionals. For example, physicians advanced systems for nomenclature and classification beginning with the International Classification of Diseases (ICD) in 1893. The modern-day emphasis on standardization began in the 1960s. In 1966, Avedis Donabedian, a physician, described the well-known structure, process, and outcome framework for evaluating the quality of medical care (Donabedian, 1966). Another physician, Lawrence Weed, developed a problem-oriented medical record in 1968 that was adaptable to computerization (Weed, 1968). In 1986, Mary Elizabeth Tinetti developed and published a tool to measure mobility problems in elderly patients (Tinetti, 1986). In 1990, Pamela Duncan developed a balance measure referred to as "functional reach" that is especially useful for her physical therapist colleagues who work in community settings. Functional reach can serve as a measure of frailty in elders to predict fall risk and help identify appropriate interventions (Duncan, Weiner, Chandler, & Studenski, 1990). Numerous studies have been conducted to confirm the value of Tinetti's and Duncan's tools and original research. Over the last 25 years, many other respected and validated tools have been adopted into practice, including the use of required standardized data sets for home health and hospice. These tools ensure that objective data are captured as care is being delivered.

Information systems were first adopted by home health agencies in the early 1980s. The development and use of these systems in home health, hospice, and other community-based settings have generally evolved in the following historical sequence to (1) support billing, (2) collect data at the point of patient care to support the financial needs of the business,

(3) manage and support collection of standard clinical datasets, and (4) provide clinical decision support (CDS). This evolution is analogous to the progression described in the data, information, knowledge, and wisdom continuum.

Billing Solutions

Initially, data within systems moved in one direction from the community health agency to the third-party payer as an electronic claim. The payer, upon receiving the claim, reviewed and paid the claim. As financial systems and electronic capabilities advanced, bidirectional exchange of claims information management became commonplace. This allowed the payer to receive the electronic claim and return an acknowledgment of payment to the healthcare provider electronically.

Clinical Decision Support Systems

CDS systems are part of the next frontier for some community-based practice settings including home health. These systems are applications that analyze data and help healthcare providers make clinical decisions (Office of the National Coordinator for Health Information Technology [ONC], 2018). CDS systems generally use one of two approaches: (1) presenting the best practices and evidence-based practice options to the clinician by finding and displaying what is known about the patient to a knowledge base using rule sets and an interface engine, or (2) using a process of machine learning that presents or displays best practices and evidence-based practice options to the clinician after analyzing the data and comparing them to similar patterns or scenarios that exist in the system. These systems have been challenging to implement because they are dependent on understanding a clinicians' workflow, which usually varies among patients and lacks structured clinical concepts, characteristics that are required to develop a knowledge base or machine learning (ONC, 2018). In addition, standardized terminologies are required to develop effective CDS systems. The next goal for CDS systems is to achieve rapid learning systems that can support quick and widespread adoption of evidence-based practices. When these learning systems are used, the time needed to implement best practices and evidence-based practice will be significantly reduced. Reaching this goal will require health information networks which can collect and support analysis of large amounts of data in simple, clear terms and return the findings to clinicians though CDS systems at the point of care (Office of the National Coordinator for Health Information Technology [ONC], 2020). See Chapter 12, for a more detailed discussion of CDS systems.

PRACTICE MODELS

Community-Based Public Health

The basis of community-based public health practice is the individual, family, and community. Public health nurses and other clinicians provide services that address and include health education and wellness campaigns, immunization clinics, screening events, parent-child health and safety, communicable disease, family planning, environmental health, substance use, and sexually transmitted disease. The recent pandemic increased the importance, visibility, and challenges of health departments, and required altered practices (Public Health Informatics Institute, 2021). Approximately 2800 city, county, metropolitan, district, and tribal health departments exist in the United States. Since 2008, local health departments have lost 31,000 of approximately 184,000 positions because of decreasing budgets, layoffs, and attrition. Many public health nursing positions have been lost because of lack of funds (National Association of County and City Health Officials [NACCHO], 2019). In this chapter the emphasis is on computerization to support these types of public health services that are provided to individuals and families across the community.

Increasingly, public health services are directed toward the community with a focus on the entire population and primary prevention. Principles of public health and epidemiology or causality, as well as community assessment and public policy, are usually components of these types of public health programs. Chapter 10 focuses on public health informatics with an emphasis on population health of communities, countries, and global health.

Home Health

Home health is the delivery of intermittent health-related services in patients' places of residence with the goal of promoting self-care and independence rather than institutionalization. The intensity of services has increased dramatically as hospital stays have become shorter and patients have been discharged with serious illnesses or soon after surgery and with complex treatment needs. The care delivered often focuses on supporting a safe transition back to the home following an episode of illness or exacerbation that required an inpatient or extended care facility stay (ANA, 2014; Riekert, 2021; Avalere Health, 2020; Stanhope & Lancaster, 2020).

Home health interventions include medication reconciliation; teaching and coaching to improve the ability of patients, families, and caregivers to manage independently; coordination of care with other healthcare providers and community resources; and early detection of decline or exacerbation. Common treatments and procedures now include ventilators, renal hemodialysis, and intravenous therapy for antibiotics, chemotherapy, and analgesia, as well as delivery of total parenteral nutrition and blood products.

An estimated 35,000 agencies provide home health services across the country (Ankota, 2021). Of those, 11,356 are Medicare-certified agencies. As the largest payers for Medicare-certified agencies, Medicare accounts for 23% and Medicaid accounts for 17% of total home health reimbursement. State and local governments, private pay, and private insurance are the other sources (Medicare Payment Advisory Commission [MedPAC], 2012). All types of home health agencies provide services to approximately 12 to 15 million patients with more than 600 million visits annually to those who range in age from infants to elders. More than 85% of all home health patients are over the age of 65 and more are women than men. Recipients of home health services have diverse needs. Diagnoses of type 2 diabetes, history of falls and aftercare for orthopedic and other procedures, chronic obstructive pulmonary disease, and hypertensive heart disease are listed most often for all home health patients. Septicemia or severe sepsis and major hip and knee joint replacements top the list for patients discharged from hospitals to home health (Ankota, 2021; Avalere Health, 2020; Dieckmann, 2017; MedPAC, 2021; Harris-Kojetin, et al., 2019).

Hospice and Palliative Care

Hospice care involves the delivery of services by teams of interprofessional clinicians for those who have exhausted curative treatment measures. Palliative care focuses on quality of life for patients and their families facing the problems associated with life-threatening illness. Whereas palliative care often begins once a cure is no longer possible and may be long term, hospice care is limited to patients with life expectancies of 6 months or less. Both hospice and palliative care involve holistic care, an emphasis on dignity, and being surrounded by the comforts of home and family; however, the programs have differences. Typically, palliative care services focus on comfort, quality of life, and end-of-life or advanced care planning. Hospice involves symptom management with the goal of providing as much comfort and dignity as possible at the end of life, including bereavement follow-up for families after a patient's death. In this country, a stigma may be associated with end-of-life care. It is associated with giving up and the refusal to accept death as a natural process, although this is changing as evidenced by the growth in hospice programs (NHPCO, 2020, 2021; Wright & Stanley, 2022; Harris-Kojetin, et al., 2019; ANA & Hospice and Palliative Nurses Association [HPNA], 2014).

There were approximately 5800 hospice programs in 2018; about 4639 were Medicare-certified. Approximately 1.55 million Medicare beneficiaries received hospice services in 2018, with an average stay of 89.6 days (NHPCO, 2020). The average length of stay is increasing as hospice becomes more widely accepted. Medicare is the largest payer of hospice services with approximately 51% of beneficiaries using services at the end of life (MedPAC, 2021). Medicaid, Veterans Benefits, and private insurance also cover hospice care.

Nurse-Managed Health Centers

Community health nurses, as well as advanced practice registered nurses—including clinical nurse specialists, nurse practitioners, and certified nurse midwives—provide care at urban and rural centers called nurse-managed health centers. These centers may have collaborative agreements with physicians and other interprofessional colleagues and are a part of or associated with educational institutions. They provide clinical experiences for students and are in underserved areas. Target populations include pregnant teens, fragile elders, low-income mothers and children, and others who may be underinsured or uninsured. Nurse-managed health centers offer primary care services, preventive care, chronic illness care, and care for specific conditions such as obesity. More than 250 centers exist in the United

States, and Philadelphia has more than any other city (National Nursing-led Care Consortium [NNCC], 2020).

Other Practice Sites

School, faith community, and occupational health nurses, as well as other clinicians, provide healthcare in noninstitutionalized settings. School nurses typically participate in classroom instruction, screen the school setting for safety hazards, provide medications in collaboration with parents and healthcare providers, work with children who have special needs, monitor immunization status, and provide and follow-up on screening procedures. Faith community nurses may function as case managers when they help their parishioners obtain needed healthcare services, food, shelter, and supplies. Some provide educational and surveillance interventions for those who have chronic illnesses such as diabetes and cardiovascular disease. Occupational health nurses are often employed by businesses with a high risk of injury or with an emphasis on health promotion and wellness such as smoking cessation, weight loss, and regular exercise.

Similarities Among Community Practice Settings

Because community-based clinicians have the opportunity to work with patients and their families over time, they embrace core values that influence their practice. Interprofessional collaboration and a seamless healthcare environment are essential. Practice is based on the consumer movement: people have rights and responsibilities, must be knowledgeable about their own healthcare, and must participate as partners in healthcare decisions. These values are linked to themes of access, cost, quality, and IT.

The power of the patient and family is an important core value. When a nurse or other healthcare professional enters a patient's home, the patient and family are in charge, not the clinician. Clinicians immediately observe indicators and collect data about patients' lifestyles, resources, and motivation. While providing care, clinicians identify patients' strengths and incorporate those strengths in the care process. The goal of community practice settings is to provide patient-centered care and include patients, their families, and their caregivers in care planning and delivery. In the hospital or long-term care facility, the nurse gives medications, changes dressings, and controls many aspects of care. In the community, nurses assist patients to provide their own care or assist family members or informal caregivers to provide that care (Riekert, 2021; Stanhope & Lancaster, 2020; Martin, 2005; National Academies of Sciences, Engineering, & Medicine [NASEM], 2021).

Clinicians who work in community settings need skills that demonstrate dedication, flexibility, and independence. Although they develop plans for their day and for each visit or encounter, those plans often need to be adapted and modified. It may not be possible to accomplish Plan A, so Plan B, C, or D may be substituted at a moment's notice. Colleagues, equipment, and references are not readily available to the extent that they are in hospitals and long-term care facilities. Selected help and supplies may be available in the trunk of a

BOX 9.1 The Quadruple Aim for Healthcare

The Triple Aim for Healthcare (2008)
- Better care for individuals, described by the six dimensions of healthcare performance: safety, effectiveness, patient-centeredness, timeliness, efficiency, and equity.
- Better health for populations, through attacking "the upstream causes of so much of our ill health," such as poor nutrition, physical inactivity, and substance abuse.
- Reducing per-capita costs.
- The Quadruple Aim for Healthcare (added 2014)
- Improved clinical experience/care team well-being.

Adapted from Berwick, D. M., Nolan, T. W., & Whittington, J. (2008). The triple aim: Care, health, and cost. *Health Affairs, 27*(3), 759–769; Bodenheimer, T., & Sinsky, C. (2014). From triple to quadruple aim: Care of the patient requires care of the provider. *Annals of Family Medicine, 12*(6), 573–576.

car or via cellphone, in the EHR, from the internet, or from a pager request. Clinicians always need to consider their safety. Environments may be difficult, dysfunctional, or even dangerous. Many patients and families welcome clinicians, although that does not always happen. Clinicians need to develop and rely on their basic education, ongoing education, life experiences, and common sense to function self-sufficiently and to enjoy their work responsibilities.

The Triple Aim model for healthcare was published in 2008; the fourth concept was added in 2014 (Box 9.1) (Berwick, Nolan, & Whittington, 2008; Bodenheimer & Sinsky, 2014). However, the primary concepts of the model have been the foundation and core values of home health and related community-based services from their inception: services that are patient-centered, high in quality, efficient, cost effective, and focus on positive partnerships between patients and providers. Although the size, staffing, organization, board structure, and financial arrangements of the practice models summarized in this chapter vary markedly, all deal with clinical data and limited financial resources. Clinicians who work in community settings must leave a reasonable data trail about their patients and the services they provide for themselves, their colleagues, and their managers/administrators. In addition, they must be knowledgeable about costs and funding; frequently, they help patients and families understand and manage health-related financial issues. In many situations, Medicare and Medicaid funding regulations are the primary determinant of the type and length of home health and hospice services. Private insurance companies determine their own guidelines but typically follow Medicare's policies. Ever-changing regulations and reimbursement patterns, interest in private pay services, and the aging population contribute to altered services. Although the momentum is moving slowly, the Centers for Medicare and Medicaid Services (CMS) is beginning to implement value-based payment rather than volume-based payment (Centers for Medicare and Medicaid Services [CMS], 2020b; Remington, 2021). Agencies that provide Medicare- and Medicaid-certified services must meet strict national regulations. Most states have additional licensing rules (Centers for Medicare and Medicaid Services [CMS], 2017).

STANDARDIZED DATASETS

Standardized datasets are required in Medicare-certified and hospice settings and are found in other community-based settings. The concept of a standardized dataset in the community began more than 25 years ago with the Resident Assessment Instrument (RAI). This approach was adopted in response to a public outcry regarding the inadequate quality of care occurring in long-term or extended nursing facilities and to the government's effort to bring visibility and transparency to care provided in these institutions. Over time, the use of standardized datasets has expanded from long-term care to home health, renal dialysis units, and other care settings. This approach provides a means to collect patient characteristics and measurements in a standardized manner that allows data aggregation for analysis. The aggregated data offers the opportunity for data-driven decision making related to care delivery and correlating payment systems to a predicted level of care needed by the patient (Centers for Medicare and Medicaid Services [CMS], 2021c; Rand, Smith, Jones, Dargan, & Hogan, 2021).

Standardized datasets have largely evolved without the adoption of standardized point-of-care and reference terminologies in practice settings. Although standardized terminologies in medicine have existed for centuries, the adoption of standardized terminologies in nursing and the other health professions began about 45 years ago. However, adoption in practice has been limited and even more limited among the information systems commonly purchased by home health, hospice, and other community-based care settings. Although standardized datasets have served an important purpose, healthcare providers need additional strategies to achieve the care communication and coordination necessary to transform healthcare and achieve the Quadruple Aim for healthcare (see Box 9.1). Strategies need to include a focus on patient-centered care, best practices and evidence-based care, interprofessional care teams, and a value-based approach that can be quantified, analyzed, and used to measure the outcomes of care (ANA, 2014; Ankota, 2021; ONC, 2020; Remington, 2021; Demiris, et al., 2019). Two examples of standardized datasets commonly used in community-based settings are described below.

Outcome and Assessment Information Set

The Outcome and Assessment Information Set (OASIS) is the standardized dataset that home health agency clinicians complete with their patients (Centers for Medicare and Medicaid Services [CMS], 2021d). It is designed to determine payment and measure the quality and outcomes of practice. OASIS consists of questions and response sets; collection requirements vary according to specific times during the process of care (i.e., admission, transfer, resumption of care, follow-up, or discharge). Public reporting, another benefit of the data and outcomes collected using the OASIS dataset, began in

2003. It allows the public to compare outcomes of home health agencies in a local community to the state and national outcome averages (Centers for Medicare and Medicaid Services [CMS], 2021a).

The OASIS dataset has undergone four major revisions. OASIS-D was implemented January 1, 2019, and use of OASIS-D1 began January 1, 2020. The proposed starting date for OASIS-E is January 1, 2023; it has 31 pages arranged in A-Q sections (Centers for Medicare and Medicaid Services [CMS], 2021d). Each major revision has involved modifications to the data collected including exclusions, modifications, and additions. OASIS will continue to evolve in effort to harmonize quality measures across care settings to improve data collection and analysis.

Hospice Item Set

The Affordable Care Act of 2010 required that the Secretary of Health and Human Services publish selected quality measures that must be reported by hospice programs. Those measures are referred to as the Hospice Item Set (HIS); the current version became effective February 16, 2021 (Centers for Medicare and Medicaid Services [CMS], 2021b). The approach to develop a standardized dataset for hospice agencies has been industry-driven rather than mandated by the CMS. The Conditions of Participation for Hospice, effective in 2008, describe the expectation that the hospice industry determines the appropriate measures to collect and report nationally (Centers for Medicare and Medicaid Services [CMS], 2020a). This approach reflects the fact that hospices had been collecting and reporting key quality measures through their associations and other data analysis partners for almost 20 years. The CMS mandated that hospices begin their reporting processes with two measures: one that is patient related and one that is structural. It is expected that the number of measures will increase as the industry continues to identify, propose, and refine a dataset (NHPCO, 2020, 2021; ANA & HPNA, 2014).

STANDARDIZED TERMINOLOGIES

The American Nurses Association (ANA) recognizes 12 reference and point-of-care or interface terminologies. These terminologies are described in detail in Chapter 4 and the references that accompany that chapter. Use of standardized terminologies is increasing in response to diverse factors. The national initiative to link reimbursement to value instead of volume serves as an important factor because providers will need quantitative data to confirm improved patient outcomes (Fennelly, et al., 2021; Graves & Corcoran, 1989; Healthcare Information and Management Systems Society [HIMSS], 2021; Matney & Settergren, 2018; American Nurses Association [ANA], 2018; Minnesota Department of Health, 2014; Nelson & Joos, 1989; Sewell, 2019). As noted by the Alliance for Nursing Informatics, the use of standardized nursing and other health terminologies:

...is necessary and a prerequisite for decision support, discovery of disparities, outcomes reporting, improving performance, maintaining accurate lists of problems and

medications, and the general use of and reuse of information needed for quality, safety, and efficiency (Sensmeier, 2010, p. 66).

Point-of-Care and Reference Terminologies

It is critical that point-of-care terminologies are mapped to reference terminologies to enable current and future interoperability and data sharing described in this chapter. The point-of-care terminologies recognized by the ANA have been or are being mapped.

Ideally, students are introduced to and become somewhat familiar with the 12 terminologies in their entry programs and clinical sites during their basic education. In addition, students should understand the difference between reference terminologies including Systematized Nomenclature of Medicine—Clinical Terms (SNOMED CT) and Logical Observation Identifier Names and Codes (LOINC), and point-of-care terminologies as discussed in Chapter 4.

Use of Terminologies in Care Settings

Similarities and differences are evident when the terminologies are compared and contrasted (Fennelly, et al. 2021; ANA, 2018; Sewell, 2019). A terminology that is especially pertinent to this chapter, the Omaha System, is summarized in the next section. Many authors note that whereas point-of-care terminologies were initially intended for use in specific settings (i.e., community, acute, or long-term care), healthcare delivery has changed dramatically and boundaries have blurred. It is possible to implement most of the terminologies across the continuum of care. Developing a structure that is computer compatible was not the initial goal in the development of point-of-care terminologies. With the IT explosion and proliferation of software vendors, relationships are evolving between the terminologies and software developers of clinical information systems. When discussing point-of-care terminologies, it is important to remember the distinction between terminologies and the individual software applications that may incorporate a terminology. Any one terminology can be used in the development of systems by multiple developers and vendors.

OMAHA SYSTEM

The Omaha System is an example of a point-of-care terminology recognized by the ANA that is mapped to SNOMED CT and LOINC, the two reference terminologies. It was initially developed to (1) be used by public health, home health, and community-based agencies, (2) operationalize the problem-solving process, (3) provide a practical, easily understood, computer-compatible guide for daily use in community settings by interprofessional clinicians, and (4) provide a tool to quantify, analyze, and improve the quality of care. From the early public health, home health, hospice, and school health focus, adoption began to expand in the 1990s, with both automated applications and paper-and-pen forms. Current use represents the continuum of care and has extended far beyond the early community-based settings. In 2014, more than 22,000 interprofessional clinicians, educators, and researchers were using the Omaha System in the United States and a number of other countries with various types of software based on the Omaha System. Since then, the number of users has increased significantly, and the number of users can no longer be estimated. Details about the application, users, clinical examples (case studies), inclusion in reference terminologies, research, best practices and evidence-based practice, and listserv are described in publications and on the website (https://www.omahasystem.org) (Omaha System Website, 2021; Martin, 2005).

Description of the Omaha System

The Omaha System consists of the Problem Classification Scheme, the Intervention Scheme, and the Problem Rating Scale for Outcomes. Reliability, validity, and usability were established when the fourth federally funded research project was completed in 1993 (Box 9.2). The three components, designed to be used together, are comprehensive, relatively simple, hierarchical, multidimensional, and computer compatible. Since the first developmental research project in 1975, the Omaha System has existed in the public domain; thus, the terms, definitions, and codes are not held under copyright. They are available for use without permission from the publisher or developers and without a licensing fee; however, the terms and structure must be used as published (Omaha System Website, 2021; Martin, 2005).

The conceptual model is based on the dynamic, interactive nature of the problem-solving process, the clinician-client relationship, and concepts of diagnostic reasoning, clinical judgment, and quality improvement (Fig. 9.1). The patient as an individual, a family, or a community appears at the center of the model, reflecting a patient-centered approach. The central location suggests the many ways in which the system can be used, the importance of the patient, and the essential partnership between patients and clinicians.

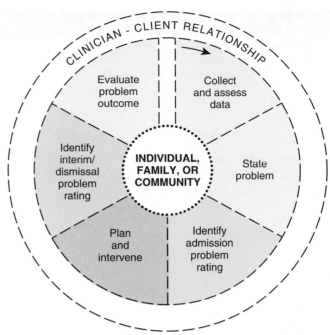

Fig. 9.1 Omaha System model of the problem-solving process. (From Martin, K. S. [2005]. *The Omaha System: A key to practice, documentation, and information management.* Reprinted 2nd ed. Omaha, NE: Health Connections Press.)

The system was intended for use by nurses and all members of healthcare delivery teams. The goals of the research were to (1) develop a structured and comprehensive system that could be both understood and used by members of various disciplines, (2) foster collaborative practice, and (3) generate accurate and consistent aggregate data. Therefore, the system was designed to guide practice decisions, sort and document pertinent patient data uniformly, and provide a framework for an agency-wide, interprofessional clinical information management system capable of meeting the daily needs of clinicians, managers, and administrators (Omaha System Website, 2021; Martin, 2005; Monsen, et al. 2021a; Monsen, Kelechi, McRae, Mathiason, & Martin, 2018; Monsen, Martin, & Bowles, 2012).

Problem Classification Scheme

The **Problem Classification Scheme** is a comprehensive, orderly, non-exhaustive, mutually exclusive taxonomy designed to identify diverse patients' health-related concerns. It has simple and concrete terms that are used to organize a comprehensive assessment—an important standard of interprofessional practice. The Problem Classification Scheme consists of four levels. Four domains appear at the first level and represent priority areas. Forty-two terms, referred to as client problems or areas of patient needs and strengths, appear at the second level. The third level consists of two sets of problem modifiers: health promotion, potential and actual, as well as individual, family, and community. Clusters of signs and symptoms describe actual problems at the fourth level. The content and relationship of the domain and problem levels are outlined in Box 9.3 and are further illustrated by the clinical example in Box 9.4. Understanding the meaning of and relationships among the terms is a prerequisite to using the scheme accurately and

---

BOX 9.2 Development of the Omaha System

As early as 1970, the clinicians and administrators of the Visiting Nurse Association (VNA) of Omaha, Nebraska, began addressing practice, documentation, and information-management concerns. Their goal was to identify a strategy that would translate theory into practice and share pertinent qualitative and quantitative data with healthcare professionals and the public. At that time, clinicians were not using computers, and there was no systematic nomenclature or classification of patient problems and concerns, interventions, or patient outcomes to quantify clinical data and integrate with a problem-oriented record system. These realities provided the incentive for initiating research and involving community test sites throughout the country. Between 1975 and 1993, the staff of VNA of Omaha conducted four extensive, federally funded development and refinement research studies that established reliability, validity, and usability. The work of Larry Weed was recognized. Avedis Donabedian, who developed the structure, process, and outcome approach to evaluation, was a valuable consultant.

Data from Donabedian, A. (1966). Evaluating the quality of medical care. *The Milbank Memorial Fund Quarterly, 44*(3), 166–206; Martin, K. S. (2005). *The Omaha System: A key to practice, documentation, and information management.* Reprinted 2nd ed. Omaha, NE: Health Connections Press.

BOX 9.3   Domains and Problems of the Omaha System Problem Classification Scheme

Environmental Domain
Material resources and physical surroundings both inside and outside the living area, neighborhood, and broader community:
- Income
- Sanitation
- Residence
- Neighborhood/workplace safety

Psychosocial Domain
Patterns of behavior, emotion, communication, relationships, and development:
- Communication with community resources
- Social contact
- Role change
- Interpersonal relationship
- Spirituality
- Grief
- Mental health
- Sexuality
- Caretaking/parenting
- Neglect
- Abuse
- Growth and development

Physiological Domain
Functions and processes that maintain life:
- Hearing
- Vision
- Speech and language

- Oral health
- Cognition
- Pain
- Consciousness
- Skin
- Neuro-musculo-skeletal function
- Respiration
- Circulation
- Digestion-hydration
- Bowel function
- Urinary function
- Reproductive function
- Pregnancy
- Postpartum
- Communicable/infectious condition

Health-related Behaviors Domain
Patterns of activity that maintain or promote wellness, promote recovery, and decrease the risk of disease:
- Nutrition
- Sleep and rest patterns
- Physical activity
- Personal care
- Substance use
- Family planning
- Health care supervision
- Medication regimen

From Martin, K. S. (2005). *The Omaha System: A key to practice, documentation, and information management.* Reprinted 2nd ed. Omaha, NE: Health Connections Press.

BOX 9.4   Ernest Morales: A Man Who Received Home Health Services

Kelly S. Nelson, PT, DPT, PCS, CWS
*Assistant Professor, Department of Physical Therapy,
School of Pharmacy and Health Professions, Creighton University
Omaha, Nebraska*

Information Obtained during the First Visit/Encounter
Ernest Morales, age 79 years, had a fracture of his left femur surgically repaired two- and one- half weeks ago. Ernest spent three days in the acute care hospital followed by 14 days at the subacute rehabilitation facility. He was discharged to his home yesterday.

During the home health nurse's first visit, Ernest's wife seemed relatively well informed. In Ernest's presence she stated, "I am going to need help caring for him. It's a difficult time for us." The nurse summarized the agency's services including interprofessional providers, and the goals of care for both Mr. and Mrs. Morales. The couple agreed when the nurse suggested that a home health aide visit to provide personal care.

Ernest was resting in his hospital bed with added side rails. He shifted in bed with difficulty and required assistance to roll or sit up. Mrs. Morales could not find the bed mobility and transfer technique instructions they reviewed yesterday prior to discharge from the subacute facility. Ernest and his wife reported being unsure of the assistance and guarding techniques needed for him to safely use his wheeled walker when moving from the bed to a sturdy chair in the kitchen. However, his wife demonstrated the ability to independently don and doff the gait belt used for safety during assisted transfers and gait. Ernest, his wife, and the nurse discussed plans and goals for the physical therapist's visit later today and the occupational therapist's visit tomorrow.

The nurse indicated that the surgical site and Ernest's skin were in excellent condition and offered evidence-based suggestions about bed mobility and prevention of skin shearing and breakdown. Mrs. Morales reported that she could manage Ernest's diet, fluid intake, and elimination. She said she would appreciate the use of a raised toilet seat and a shower chair.

Although Ernest was reluctant to admit he had pain, he rated it as a 4 out of 10 on the Visual Analog Scale pain scale. Mrs. Morales administered pain medication at least three times a day and as needed, indicating that she "would not wait for Ernest to look miserable." She described how she evaluated Ernest's pain and used the pain scale as the nurse instructed. The nurse showed Mrs. Morales a website describing evidence-based pain management and gave her some printed instructional materials. Mrs. Morales agreed to keep the nurse informed as Ernest's need for pain medications changed and if other symptoms such as constipation occurred. The nurse mentioned several methods for achieving nonpharmacological pain relief and asked the couple to discuss their preferences before the nurse's next visit. They said they would do so.

Application of the Omaha System
Domain: Physiological
Problem: Pain (High Priority Problem)
Problem Classification Scheme
Modifiers: Individual and Actual
Signs/Symptoms of Actual:
- expresses discomfort/pain
- compensated movement/guarding

BOX 9.4   Ernest Morales: A Man Who Received Home Health Services—cont'd

Intervention Scheme
Category: Teaching, Guidance, and Counseling
Targets and client-specific information:
- anatomy/physiology (diagnosis and surgery in relation to pain, joint, and pain management)
- relaxation/breathing techniques (consider options and decide)

Category: Surveillance
Targets and client-specific information:
- signs/symptoms—mental/emotional (attitude, emotions)
- signs/symptoms—physical (ability/willingness to move)

Problem Rating Scale for Outcomes
Knowledge: 3—basic knowledge (knows pain causes, need for medication, but not other options)
Behavior: 3—inconsistent knowledge (not tried additional options for pain relief, but willing)
Status: 3—moderate signs/symptoms (caused by injury and surgery)

Problem: Neuro-musculo-skeletal function (High Priority Problem)
Problem Classification Scheme
Modifiers: Individual and Actual
Signs/Symptoms of Actual:
- limited range of motion
- gait/ambulation disturbance
- difficulty transferring
- fractures

Intervention Scheme
Category: Teaching, Guidance, and Counseling
Targets and Client-Specific Information:
- occupational therapy care (plan of care)
- physical therapy care (plan of care)

Category: Surveillance
Targets and client-specific information:
- durable medical equipment (bed set-up adequate, needs raised toilet seat and shower chair)
- mobility/transfers (bed mobility)
- signs/symptoms—physical (surgical site, skin condition)

Problem Rating Scale for Outcomes
Knowledge: 3—basic knowledge (recalls some instructions, can't find handout)
Behavior: 2—rarely appropriate behavior (limited mobility/activity)
Status: 2—severe signs/symptoms (minimal activity)

Domain: Health-related Behaviors
Problem: Personal Care (High Priority Problem)
Problem Classification Scheme
Modifiers: Individual and Actual
Signs/Symptoms of Actual:
- difficulty with bathing
- difficulty with toileting activities
- difficulty dressing lower body
- difficulty dressing upper body
- difficulty shampooing/combing hair

Intervention Scheme
Category: Case Management
Targets and client-specific information:
- paraprofessional/aide care (schedule 3 times/week)

Problem Rating Scale for Outcomes
Knowledge: 4—adequate knowledge (knows help needed)
Behavior: 4—usually appropriate behavior (requested assistance)
Status: 2—severe signs/symptoms (care is difficult because of John's physical condition)

Problem: Medication regimen
Problem Classification Scheme
Modifiers: Individual and Actual
Signs/Symptoms of Actual:
- unable to take medications without help

Intervention Scheme
Category: Teaching, Guidance, and Counseling
Targets and Client-Specific Information:
- medication action/side effects (reports of pain, movement, non-verbal cues)
- medication administration (scheduling doses appropriately)

Category: Surveillance
Targets and Client-Specific Information
- signs/symptoms—physical (discussed effectiveness, constipation, other symptoms; will use pain scale)

Problem Rating Scale for Outcomes
Knowledge: 4—adequate knowledge (informed about pain medication, watch for changing needs)
Behavior: 4—usually appropriate behavior (good administration schedule)
Status: 3—moderate signs/symptoms (pain scale = 4)

---

consistently to collect, sort, document, analyze, quantify, and communicate patient needs and strengths.

Intervention Scheme

The Intervention Scheme is a comprehensive, orderly, non-exhaustive, mutually exclusive taxonomy designed for use with specific problems. It consists of three levels of actions or activities that are the basis for care planning and services, providing the structure and terms to organize care plans and actual care. An important standard of interprofessional practice is providing interventions and leaving a data trail regarding the care that was provided. Four broad categories of interventions appear at the first level of the Intervention Scheme. An alphabetical list of 75 targets or objects of action and 1 "other" appear at the

second level. Client-specific information generated by clinicians is at the third level. The contents of the category and target levels are outlined in Boxes 9.5 and 9.6, respectively, and are further illustrated by the clinical example in Box 9.4. The Intervention Scheme enables clinicians to describe, quantify, and communicate their practice, including improving or restoring health, describing deterioration, or preventing illness.

Problem Rating Scale for Outcomes

The Problem Rating Scale for Outcomes consists of three five-point, Likert-type scales used to measure the entire range of severity for the concepts of Knowledge, Behavior, and Status. Each of the subscales is a continuum that provides a framework for measuring and comparing problem-specific patient outcomes at

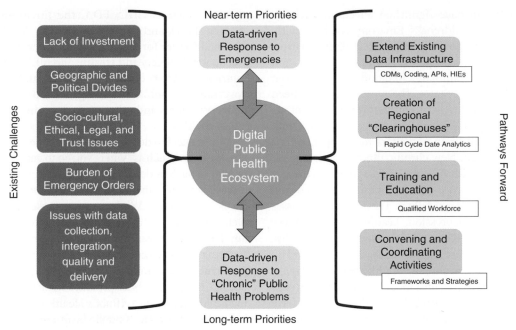

Fig. 10.2 Conceptual Model for the digital public health ecosystem. *HIEs*, Health information exchanges. (Adapted from Madhavan, S., Bastarache, L., Brown, J. S., Butte, A. J., Dorr, D. A., Embi, P. J. et al. [2021]. Use of electronic health records to support a public health response to the COVID-19 pandemic in the United States: a perspective from 15 academic medical centers. *Journal of the American Medical Informatics Association, 28*[2], 393–401.)

Applying a Systems Approach to Public Health

A systems approach is parallel to the definition of public health, notably where a *system* and *public health* are reflective of their environments and the interactions and relationships among the components. Aristotle said that "the whole is greater than the sum of its parts" suggesting that public health (as a system) is greater than each of its parts. The public health "system," for the purposes of this book, includes the sociological context, behavioral context, and sociopolitical challenges.

Systems model indicates that, for functionality, required input leads to a process, which results in an output (Fig. 10.3). This system is affected by behaviors, the environment, and other sociological issues. Adapting this model to public health "Input" can be notation of an illness (e.g., COVID-19) that results in a "process" (e.g., tracking, illness identification, leading to an output [e.g., recovery, hospitalization, mortality]). This system is impacted by "behaviors"—presence of a vaccine and protective behaviors, such as social distancing and use of masks. The environmental exposure impact could be determining if the individual were in an enclosed area or outside; what was the area occupancy. Sociological exposure could be the determination of social determinants of health or the social and political environment existing within the system. These all impact the output results. Sociological input, political challenges, and behaviors are all necessary components to the system to affect an appropriate public health informatics output.

Public Health Practices

There is a continuous need for the prevention and control of infectious and non-infections chronic illnesses, injuries, and

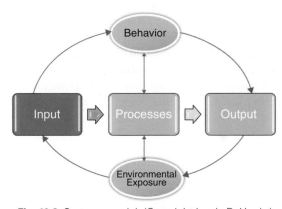

Fig. 10.3 Systems model. (Copyright Lynda R. Hardy.)

behaviors (such as smoking) that cause high rates of morbidity and mortality (Boyles et al., 2021). An example are the environmental factors involved in maternal morbidity and mortality (Boyles et al., 2021). The stress of pregnancy increases the vulnerability of the female body during the stress of pregnancy, where certain organs are more susceptible to damage. Emerging data have identified prenatal stress exposure increases the risk of autism spectrum disorder and autistic traits (Varcin et al., 2017). Environmental factors, such as water, soil, food, and other contaminants, also impact maternal health. These contaminants include heavy metals, air pollutants, and pesticides (Boyles et al., 2021).

Children are at a greater risk of environmental effects of contaminants because their bodies are still growing. The exposure children have to environmental contaminants, meaning anything they touch, can have significant effects on a child's development (CDC, Children's' Environmental Health: https://ephtracking.cdc.gov/showChildEHMain.action). Recently, aging drinking water pipes, gasoline additives, and paint showed spikes of contaminants in blood levels have been noted in areas of the United States. These increases have been noted in toxic blood lead levels of children (Swaringen et al., 2022). Elevated blood lead levels in children cause issues with bone marrow, kidney, and brain and affect their appetite, irritability, and ability to learn. New chronic illness trends suggest they present earlier in life. Chronic disease diagnosis on the rise in children and adolescents are asthma, obesity, hypertension, stroke, type 2 diabetes, and renal failure. These chronic illnesses are increasing the rate of depression. Leading causes of these chronic illnesses are poor dietary habits, sedentary lifestyles, and poor access to health care (Sentell et al., 2020). The WHO identifies new environmental threats for children citing greenhouse gas emissions, addictive substances, and road injury suggesting that "climate change and ecological degradation" have become threats to the lives of children (https://www.who.int/news-room/fact-sheets/detail/children-new-threats-to-health).

Addressing these public health challenges involves a diverse set of professionals and agencies, as illustrated in Fig. 10.4, that all have one common goal: to improve people's health and protect them from health risks. The interdisciplinary professionals specialize in public health nursing, behavioral sciences, health education, epidemiology, environmental health, injury control, biostatistics, emergency medical services, health services, international health, maternal and child health, nutrition, public health laboratory practice, public health policy, and public health clinical practice. The agencies involved are the local (city and county), state, and tribal health departments and federal

agencies, such as CDC, FDA, the Environmental Protection Agency (EPA), and the Census Bureau. The CDC includes the National Center for Health Statistics, the National Institute for Occupational Safety and Health, and other centers that focus on injuries, infectious diseases, genomics, and global health. These governmental public health agencies partner with healthcare delivery systems and others to ensure the conditions for population health.

When asked to define public health, people often mention service functions, such as "where you go to get your child immunized or to get a birth or death record," or job duties, such as "employing disease detectives that respond to outbreaks and inspectors who check restaurants." While correct, these responses are incomplete. Public health agencies provide direct clinical services like any healthcare organization but also provide services, such as outbreak management and surveillance, which are not otherwise performed in a community. The Public Health Development and Social Cognition website provides the latest information regarding health and wellness (Public Health Development, n.d.). Some less visible examples of public health activities include monitoring of air and water, prevention and control of injuries, building of safe roadways, protection of the food supply, proper disposal of solid and liquid waste and medications, rat control and mosquito abatement, surveillance of infectious and chronic diseases, and prevention and preparedness research. This diverse set of activities can be summarized in the core functions and essential services for effective public health systems that were defined by the Institute of Medicine (IOM) Committee for the Study of the Future of Public Health. There are many opportunities to use informatics strategies with these services.

The National Academies of Sciences, Engineering, and Medicine's (previously the IOM) framework developed in 1988 is still valid today. Public health agencies are mandated to perform three core functions: (1) assessment—"to regularly and systematically collect, assemble, analyze, and make available information on the health of the community, including statistics on health status, community health needs, and epidemiologic and other studies of health problems" (Institute of Medicine US, 1988); (2) policy development—"to exercise its responsibility to serve the public interest in the development of comprehensive public health policies by promoting use of the scientific knowledge base in decision-making" (Institute of Medicine US, 1988); and (3) assurance—"to assure their constituents that the services necessary to achieve agreed upon goals are provided, either by encouraging actions by other entities (private or public sector), by requiring such action through regulation, or by providing services directly" (Institute of Medicine US, 1988). The essential services related to these functions are described in Box 10.2.

APPLYING INFORMATICS TO PUBLIC HEALTH

History of Public Health Informatics

Chapter 6 provides an understanding of information technology infrastructure, including the networking of data principles

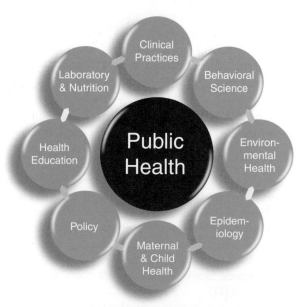

Fig. 10.4 Public health practices.

for health informatics. This section identifies the inception and rationale for public health informatics and its relationship to the health of the public. The development of computers or counting machines provided a path for the collection, analyses, prediction, and prevention of health-related illnesses. Health informatics can be traced to the 1950's literature noting the association of computers in the provision of healthcare and information processing (Fenton & Biedermann, 2014). The maximization of technology, or the systematic application of computers to science, in public health provided an environment and a vision of population and public health (Panth & Acharya, 2015).

We can trace public health informatics back to Florence Nightingale's impact on the digital age through her systematic collection of health information during the Crimean War. A born statistician, Nightingale systematically collected data related to soldier mortality to modify healthcare provision and reduce infection rates. Her work, while not performed in silico, enabled an informatics approach to informed decision-making in the field and applied a predictive approach to reducing mortality by modifying procedures improving population health. Nightingale used data visualization (the Nightingale Rose Diagram) to show how data and informatics could modify patient-related outcomes (Hardy & Bourne, 2017). Retrospectively, informaticians scoured the data related to the 1918 influenza pandemic and attempted to model it for the COVID-19 pandemic.

The discipline of public health informatics was separated from medical and nursing informatics by clarifying that public health informatics principles applied to populations, whereas medical and nursing informatics applied to individuals (Lumpkin & Magnuson, 2020).

BOX 10.2 Core Functions and the Ten Essential Services for Effective Public Health Systems

Core Function: Assessment
Essential Services

- Monitor health status to identify community health problems.
- Diagnose and investigate health problems and health hazards in the community.

Core Function: Policy Development
Essential Services

- Inform, educate, and empower people about health issues.
- Mobilize community partnerships to identify and solve health problems.
- Develop policies to support individual and community health efforts.

Core Function: Assurance
Essential Services

- Enforce laws and regulations that protect health and ensure safety.
- Link people to health services and assure the provision of healthcare when otherwise unavailable.
- Assure a competent public health and personal healthcare workforce.
- Evaluate effectiveness, accessibility, and quality of personal and population-based health services.
- Research for new insights and innovative solutions to health problems.

Adapted from Committee for the Study of the Future of Public Health. (1988). *The future of public health.* Washington, DC: The National Academies Press.

Influence of Modern Public Health Informatics Infrastructure

The public health informatics infrastructure incorporates three interconnecting components (Fig. 10.5), a qualified workforce, up-to-date information systems, and the interoperability to connect with essential systems and agencies to ensure the protection of the public's health. A qualified workforce is one that is educated and proficient at managing health informatics. The American Medical Informatics Association has two certifications for informaticians, one in clinical informatics and the other in health informatics. These certification programs ensure that trained individuals can obtain, track, and manage health-related data.

HIS are moving targets and rapidly updated to ensure efficiency and effectiveness. A broad definition of HIS is any system that houses and manages health data. Examples of HIS are electronic health records (EHRs), health-related registries, patient portals, and decision support systems. Public health requires a variety of HIS to monitor, predict, and prevent illnesses and injuries. Public health personnel interface with HIS at local, state, and federal levels with a focus on understanding health-related trends that help in forecasting or predicting. Early examples of health information use are Florence Nightingale's Rose Diagram, previously discussed, which indicated her use of statistics to evaluate soldier mortality (Brixey et al., 2020), and John Snow's use of health information (e.g., an HIS) with the formation of maps to determine the cause of cholera in 1854 in London. Today, we use multiple types of HISs such as **surveillance** databases, health information exchanges (HIEs), registries (often illness specific), public health records, death certificates, and occasionally the Internet of things. These HISs allow public health officials a high-level view of population health with the potential to narrow the focus to specific populations. The crux of these systems is interoperability—the ability to share and integrate all data. The health interoperability layer provides an example of how health interoperability is essential to health informaticians from a systems perspective (Fig. 10.6). This image can be extrapolated to the public health domain where business domain services are local, state, and federal services, terminology services becomes the focal point for data standardization, while health, facility, healthcare, and product (drugs and devices) registries become additional points of information for understanding and predicting health and wellness.

Systems Approach to Public Health Informatics

Fig. 10.7 illustrates a systems approach for informatics for health technology, informatics, and digital health in a global

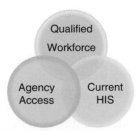

Fig. 10.5 Public Health Informatics infrastructure requirements.

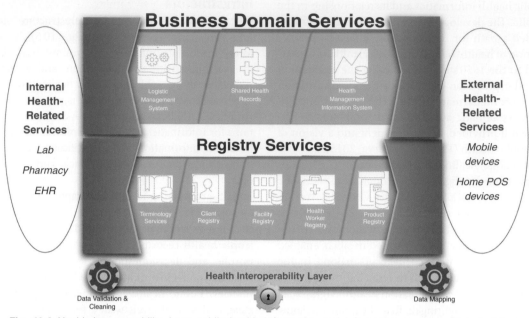

Fig. 10.6 Health interoperability layer public health informatics and information systems. (Adapted from OpenHIE. This work is licensed under a Creative Commons Attribution 4.0 International License.)

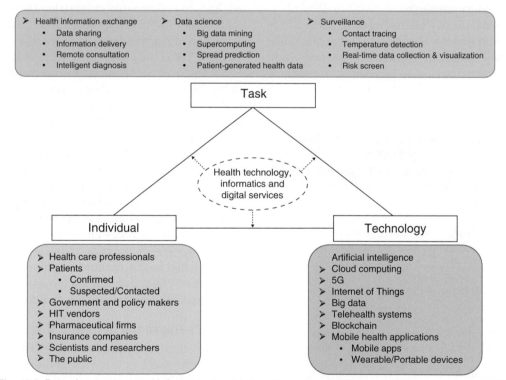

Fig. 10.7 Role of technology and informatics in global public health emergency. (Adapted from Ye, J. [2020]. The role of health technology and informatics in a global public health emergency: practices and implications from the COVID-19 pandemic. *JMIR Medical Informatics, 8*[7], e19866.)

public health crisis, as experienced with COVID-19. This illustration is divided into three sections for health technology, informatics, and digital services: the individual, the technology, and the task. The individual refers to all the healthcare professionals, patients and the public, governmental and policy makers, and companies and vendors with inputs for technology, treatments, and reimbursement. The technology refers to the current and evolving technologies used by the individuals described to process for information. The tasks are further divided into HIE, data science, and surveillance. These are discussed in the following section. An example of informatics in global public health emergencies is the healthcare provider conducting a rapid COVID-19 point of care testing with a patient testing positive. This step reflects involvement with the government with reporting and insurance company for diagnosis and reimbursement. The positive test is documented and reported to the NDDSS. At this point, contact tracing is conducted and spread prediction is analyzed. This has also been conducted with recent cases of measles outbreaks in the United States.

INFORMATICS IN THE PUBLIC DOMAIN

Health Information Exchange

To succeed in its mission and conduct core functions, public health entities rely on data and partnerships with healthcare and other settings in a community. Health Information Exchange (HIE) initiatives and organizations provide an infrastructure to improve the required communication between public health and community partners. In the past, the primary aim of an HIE was to bring unavailable clinical data from patients' disparate health records to the point of care where clinicians and patients need it the most. The motivation for exchanging health data has been to create a complete health records to address safety and quality concerns, gain efficiencies, reduce duplication of effort and control costs, notify participants about problems and potential drug seekers, and perform research. Box 10.3 includes HIE applications for achieving these public health benefits. When public health agencies participate in an HIE, they can both provide and receive value from their participation. Public health benefits from participating in an HIE include the following additional benefits:

- More timely and complete receipt of disease reports.
- Faster transmission of better information to public health case managers (for communicable disease control or newborn screening follow-up).
- Easier identification and analysis of gaps in preventive health services (immunizations and Papanicolaou smears) and of patterns that could improve performance.

BOX 10.3 Potential Health Information Exchange Applications for Use in Public Health

- Mandatory reporting of laboratory findings
- Non-mandatory reporting of laboratory data
- Mandatory reporting of physician diagnoses
- Non-mandatory reporting of clinical data
- Public health investigation
- Clinical care in public health clinics
- Population-level quality monitoring
- Mass casualty events
- Disaster medical response
- Public health alerting: patient level
- Public health alerting: population level

Adapted from Shapiro, J. S., Mostashari, F., Hripcsak, G., Soulakis, N., & Kuperman, G. (2011). Using health information exchange to improve public health. *American Journal of Public Health, 101*, 616–623.

- Easier identification and analysis of follow-up failures (treatment of sexually transmitted diseases or environmental evaluation of lead poisoning) and of patterns that could improve performance.
- Analysis and display of geographic distribution of illness or injury to focus public health interventions or services.
- Analysis and display of the temporal and geographic epidemic spread.
- Improved ability to communicate with selected healthcare providers and patients (Foldy & Ross, 2005).

Public health also provides value to the HIE partners (Foldy & Ross, 2005; Shapiro et al., 2011). Public health can provide patient information (e.g., immunization records, newborn screening results, tuberculosis clinical findings, and child health clinic records) and epidemiologic information to improve diagnosis (e.g., distribution and incidence of Lyme disease to improve a clinician's estimation of pretest probability). A public health agency may serve as a trusted neutral party for confidential health information or may maintain a community master person index that can support the HIE using identifiers generated by healthcare organizations, birth records, and other sources (Duncan et al., 2015). Public health involvement in an HIE can reduce the cost and labor of reporting. Finally, public health can provide personalized patient care information available in the community and alert healthcare providers to urgent community health issues.

Fig. 10.8 illustrates an approach for informatics for health technology, informatics, and digital health in a global public health crisis, as experienced during the COVID-19 pandemic. This illustration is divided into three sections for health technology, informatics, and digital services: the individual, the technology, and the task. The individual refers to all the healthcare professionals, patients and the public, governmental and policy makers, and companies and vendors with input for technology, treatments, and reimbursement. The technology refers to the current and evolving technology used by all the individuals described to process for information. The tasks are further divided into health information exchange (HIE), data science, and surveillance. An example for using informatics in global public health emergencies is the healthcare provider conducting a rapid Covid point of care testing with a patient testing positive. This step reflects involvement with the government with reporting and insurance company for diagnosis and reimbursement. The positive test is documented and reported to the NDDSS. At this point, contact tracing is conducted and spread prediction is analyzed. This has also been conducted with recent cases of measles outbreaks in the United States.

Public Health Surveillance and Information Systems

Public health surveillance is the ongoing collection, analysis, interpretation, and dissemination of data for a stated public health purpose. The primary goal of surveillance is to provide actionable health information to public health staff, government leaders, and the public to guide public health policy and programs (Smith et al., 2013). Hence, surveillance activities and the information generated guide decisions and monitor progress. These are critical for meeting all three functions

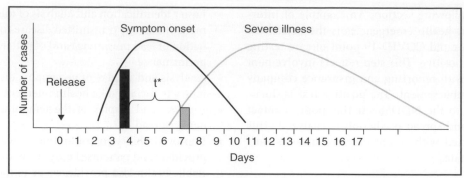

Fig. 10.8 Traditional and syndromic surveillance reporting—rationale for early detection. *t**, Time between detection by syndromic (prediagnostic) surveillance and detection by traditional (diagnosis-based) surveillance. (Adapted from Centers for Disease Control and Prevention [CDC]. Henning, K. J. [2004, September 24]. Overview of syndromic surveillance: What is syndromic surveillance? *MMWR*. Available at: https://www.cdc.gov/mmwr/preview/mmwrhtml/su5301a3.htm.)

TABLE 10.1 Examples of Matching Surveillance Purposes With Methods

Purpose	Method
Provide case management; notify exposed partners; provide prophylaxis to contacts; detect outbreaks; quarantine exposed contacts; isolate cases; take regulatory actions to prevent exposure; target interventions to remediate hazards to exposed persons	Case reporting to local and state health departments by clinicians, healthcare facilities, and laboratories
Monitor common diseases for which routine detection is not needed (e.g., influenza, Lyme disease)	Sentinel surveillance (collection of detailed information about a subset of cases) or sampling of suspected cases for full investigation
Monitor population vital statistics	Birth and death certificate reporting to states
Monitor population cancer incidence	Case reporting to state health department cancer registries by clinicians, healthcare facilities, and pathology laboratories
Monitor prevalence of childhood vaccination rates	Reporting of all childhood vaccinations by clinicians to state immunization information systems
Monitor population prevalence of risk factors and health-related conditions	Public health telephone, school-based, community, or other self-reported surveys; public health examination surveys; analysis of de-identified electronic health records, hospital data, claims data, and other clinical encounters
Measure population levels of environmental and occupational risk factors	Public health or community and worker surveys; environmental monitoring and modeling; biomonitoring
Monitor antibiotic resistance in communities	Electronic laboratory reporting
Monitor characteristics and quality of care for health events and conditions (e.g., myocardial infarction, stroke, cardiac arrest, and diabetes)	Quality improvement registries (e.g., Paul Coverdell National Acute Stroke Registry)
Detect evidence for unreported changes in community health or track situational awareness during public health emergencies	Analysis of de-identified clinical data by public health to detect changes in population health (syndromic surveillance)
Evaluate effectiveness of public health programs and interventions; monitor health trends in a population	Trend analysis of vital statistics reports, case reports, vaccination prevalence, clinical and billing data, population survey data, worksite injury and death reports, law enforcement records, and special surveys
Characterize the epidemiology of specific diseases or injuries and develop hypotheses about and target interventions toward their risk factors	Analysis of population data or case-based data to describe disease or injury characteristics and risk factors

Adapted from Smith, P. F., Hadler, J. L., Stanbury, M., Rolfs, R. T., & Hopkins, R. S. (2013). Blueprint version 2.0: Updating public health surveillance for the 21st century. *Journal of Public Health Management and Practice, 19*(3), 231–239 https://doi.org/10.1097/PHH.0b013e318262906e.

required of a public health system: assessment, policy development, and assurance. It is important to note that surveillance is an activity that often requires partnerships with private and public entities in the community and legislation to enforce it. Surveillance is difficult to delegate to others in the community,

so it has been a public health department activity. The surveillance purpose should match the methods used to achieve the best data (Table 10.1).

Syndromic surveillance is the process used by public health officials to detect, understand, and monitor health events. This allows tracking even prior to a diagnosis for public health to identify unusual levels of illness and determine if and what a response should be. Fig. 10.8 depicts the time between traditional and syndromic surveillance reporting and potential data sources for syndromic reporting. Syndromic surveillance is an early warning system. An example of this, was following the COVID-19 outbreak in China and then worldwide. The goals of the COVID-19 surveillance are (Center for Disease Control and Prevention [CDC], 2021a, 2021b):

- Visualize data related to volume and proportion positive in geographic areas.
- Incorporate COVID-19 data from six commercial laboratories for the health department to monitor orders, test results and more.
- Provide timely updates to plan and execute the national response.
- Support the state and local health departments' use of data to analyze, visualize, and share the findings.
- Collaborate to use data better from the state and local health departments, CDC, academic, and industry to share insightful analysis strategies.

Public Health Reporting Considerations

In the United States, public health reporting to perform surveillance and implement control measures has been going on since the eighteenth century, when tavern owners were asked to report persons with illnesses to a local board of health. Today, public health reporting to recognize and control communicable diseases in a community is a quintessential public health activity. The rules concerning the diseases that should be reported and the actions to take if reporting is necessary vary among the fifty states, may vary among cities or counties within a state, may vary by disease, and sometimes vary by reporting entity (i.e., whether the reporter is a laboratory or a clinician) and other factors. As shown in Fig. 10.6, a local health department is often the agency responsible for (1) receiving reports from laboratories, clinicians, hospitals, and other reporters (e.g., schools and daycare centers); (2) investigating

the situation; and (3) implementing control measures (Fig. 10.6). Information gathered during the investigation informs the public health response and helps establish whether to count the event for surveillance purposes.

Local and state agencies may share a single web-based system, or the two levels of governmental public health may have separate systems. Either way, more data are collected during an investigation than are needed for "notification" from the local to state health department. The information shared is often summary information ascertained after completing the investigation. Depending on the information available from the completed investigation, a disease report may be classified as a "confirmed" or a "probable" case, for example. This classification is used when summarizing surveillance data to consistently report similar events over time while still quantifying the unconfirmed but relevant events.

The information used by the state health department for surveillance is a subset of the information gathered during an investigation. When information is sent to the CDC as a "notifiable report," the record is de-identified and filtered again to include only the data needed for national surveillance. Finally, the set of conditions included in the NNDSS is not reported in every local and state authority and does not include all conditions reported everywhere.

There are many complexities associated with the detailed processes of public health reporting, but the high-level process shown in Fig. 10.9 illustrates a set of activities that is commonly conducted across the United States. Informatics solutions may be applied to each step in the process. For example, the first step in public health reporting concerns the publishing of reporting criteria (e.g., specifications). Currently, the guidance and regulations that laboratories and other reporters need to follow are described on websites and posters and can often be found by using search terms such as "communicable disease reporting regulations for [state A or city B]." The information cannot be processed by electronic systems; it changes periodically, especially during an outbreak; and it differs among states and between states and the CDC. Case reporters must interpret the

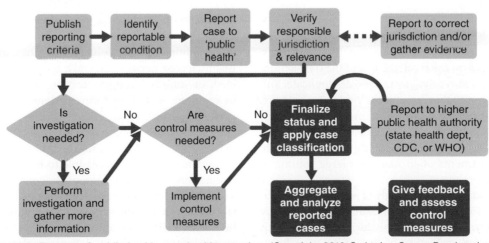

Fig. 10.9 Process of public health case health reporting. (Copyright 2010 Catherine Staes. Reprinted with permission.)

criteria expected and maintain the reporting criteria in their systems. This situation could be improved using knowledge management strategies that allow public health authorities to author structured content and disseminate the laboratory and clinical reporting specifications in both a human-readable format and a structured format for use by automated laboratory and clinical systems. This strategy is being employed using the Reportable Condition Knowledge Management System, which is under development by the Council of State and Territorial Epidemiologists (Council of State and Territorial Epidemiologists [CSTE], 2015).

Several factors make it difficult for clinicians, laboratories, and others to identify reportable conditions. Underreporting is common when manual processes are involved and reporting relies on clinicians to remember to report (Angulo et al., 2021; Overhage et al., 2008). Studies have shown a lack of knowledge among clinicians about reporting requirements (Cusimano et al., 2017; Staes et al., 2009). In addition, even as the use of detection logic is becoming more common in laboratory and clinical systems, the sensitivity and specificity of logic can vary by the reportable condition. For example, a single lab test result is sufficient for detecting chlamydia, a clinical diagnosis is required for identifying culture-negative tuberculosis or suspected measles, and a combination of laboratory and clinical findings is required to identify chronic hepatitis B infections (Klompas et al., 2008). There are informatics opportunities for defining and publishing detection logic (including codes such as International Classification of Diseases-10 [ICD-10], Logical Observation Identifiers Names and Codes [LOINC], and Systematized Nomenclature of Medicine-Clinical Terms [SNOMED-CT]) and using surrogate markers for reportable events, such as administration of hepatitis B immunoglobulin to newborns as an indicator of an infected mother.

Challenges in the process of reporting a case or lab result to public health agencies result in delayed reporting, inefficient data gathering with incomplete reports, variable data collection, and nonstandard formats used to transfer the information (e.g., fax, phone, email, mail, web forms, electronic laboratory reports). Some challenges are being addressed by increased the use of EHRs, Meaningful Use incentives, and Health Level Seven (HL7) standards.

Challenges of Data Collection

While these factors improve the capabilities for the sender, there are also challenges on the receiving end of the transaction. Health departments must receive, sort, filter, de-duplicate, and consolidate information that arrives "at their doorstep" via fax, phone, online web forms, and electronic messaging systems, and from records routed from their state or other local health departments using statewide electronic disease surveillance systems. Health departments often manage a large volume of reports using manual processes.

For example, in an observational study of workflow in a local health department, 3454 reportable conditions were manually entered into an electronic data system during an 18-month period. In a prospective evaluation of the information being received, 18% of the reports were for other counties, 3% were not reportable, 16% were duplicates, and 18% were updates on previously reported cases (Rajeev et al., 2011). Personnel resources are used to manage all the paper arriving to find the new, relevant information among all incoming paper.

In an ideal world, a health department would receive complete information in a timely manner only once, and updates and duplicates would be managed automatically. There are numerous informatics opportunities to do the following: Enable the use of specifications (computable logic) to define where and how the reports should be sent, the urgency of reporting, and the information to include in a report:

- Automate information extraction of additional information in the EHR.
- Improve standardization of message structure and content.
- Enable secure information exchange.
- Create public health information systems to receive case reports and allow access by local and state public health entities.

Systems are being built to receive laboratory reports, but this is only part of the information required to manage persons with communicable diseases in municipalities, counties, and states.

- The processes associated with performing an investigation and implementing control measures (such as excluding a person with salmonella from food service or daycare or vaccinating contacts of a person with meningitis) can be complex. Decisions must be made on incomplete and evolving information, and guidelines are often ambiguous. The situation could be improved by automated linkage between clinical and electronic lab reports with information concerning updated or redundant reports.
  - Improved quality of the information in a report (e.g., include additional associated lab findings needed for investigation).
  - Improved tools to explore the existing information (Livnat et al., 2010).
  - Decision support tools that improve the management of current information and apply guidelines.

The processes associated with aggregating information across jurisdictions and sharing subsets of information with a higher authority could be addressed using new strategies. Currently, aggregation occurs by copying information and sending it up the chain. However, "central" aggregation is defined differently among different stakeholders and does not support sudden unanticipated needs. Currently, ad hoc queries must be initiated, or informal communication and data aggregation may be required. A goal for future systems should be the ability to perform dynamic aggregation across jurisdictions and to access complete data in their native environments, with appropriate permissions. In addition, future systems should allow surveillance data to be more accessible to healthcare systems and the community for decision support in near real time.

In summary, case reporting and management will benefit from computable knowledge managed and served by public health authorities about what, how, where, and when to report; automated event detection; electronic, standardized information exchange; improved systems for receiving and integrating case reports; and the ability to access disparate systems with appropriate permissions to dynamically aggregate data across jurisdictions and respond to new situations, data, and priorities.

MAINTAINING PUBLIC HEALTH AND PUBLIC HEALTH STANDARDS

Standards can be found in nearly every aspect of life, but why are they important? Standards, defined by a compilation of ideals and principles, are an agreed-upon method for measurement that are repeatable, harmonized, and outcome related for a way of doing something. They provide an estimation of goal completion and determine if the goal has been reached or if additional work is required. Standards can be found in every discipline. This section focuses on public health standards and the use of informatics to meet that need.

Maintaining Privacy in an Open Ecosystem

Historically, healthcare data has maintained an elevated level of protection and privacy. Regulations, like HIPAA, were instituted to protect the safety and privacy of an individual's personal healthcare data. We have evolved into a digital world or ecosystem where maintaining privacy is difficult. The institution of an open ecosystem, including social media, suggests that personal health information is no longer private. The advancement of sites, like Facebook's Preventive Health tool, opened the flood gates of health information and decreased the ability to maintain privacy and provided a treasure trove of data for that platform to manipulate. Other sites capturing health-related data, like genomic evaluation sites and EHR vendors, have made health care data more available for sharing (Bari & O'Neill, 2019). Some academic institutions have added language to their research informed consent, suggesting that data collected within a research project can be sold.

Individuals share their health-related data with third-party app developers not covered by HIPAA regulations. Recently, US federal regulations required that healthcare providers be directed to submit medical information through third party apps if the individual requests them. For the public, this means that many apps can sell or share data. Grundy et al. (2019) noted that 79% of healthcare apps do, indeed, sell or share the data they collect. The expectation of privacy (for health-related data) should be carefully reviewed by all individuals prior to sharing their data.

Public Health in Pandemics

To improve the timeliness with which outbreaks are detected (COVID-19 and influenza outbreaks in particular), informatics researchers have been testing new signals for event detection, evaluating statistical models for finding noteworthy events among normal variation, and devising new strategies for visualizing information and engaging a broader community. Table 10.2 illustrates the relationship between illness-related events and the variety of surveillance systems that may capture these events. The quest to identify early events must balance the potentially less predictive quality of the information with improved opportunities to identify infections and outbreaks, and then implement control measures to prevent further spread. Events that occur earlier in the chain of illness-related events may be less specific and lead to false-positive signals. The quality of the detected signals must be evaluated prior to routine use in public health practice. Finally, there are new opportunities to use personal health records (PHRs) and social media to monitor indicators of health status and attitudes and beliefs in the community. A scoping review was conducted on what social media told us about COVID-19. This review analyzed 81 studies and five public health themes were identified:

- Surveying public attitudes.
- Identifying infodemics (information with epidemic and refers to rapid, wide-spread information about something that has both accurate and inaccurate data).
- Mental health assessment.
- Analysis of governmental response to the pandemic.
- Evaluating the quality of health prevention educational videos.

During the COVID-19 pandemic, social media has been instrumental and played a critical role in disseminating and tackling infodemic, health information, and misinformation.

Significant Public Health Issues

Healthcare Effectiveness Data and Information Set (HEDIS) measures relate to significant public health issues (cancer, smoking, asthma, heart disease, and diabetes). Health plans collect, monitor, and report data regarding their performance in almost 100 areas. Data are reported to the National Committee for Quality Assurance (NCQA) and provide a rating on the quality of care provided. HEDIS measures compliance with best practices for better patient outcomes. Some important areas monitored are:

- Antibiotic stewardship
- Colorectal screening
- Treatment of COPD
- Hypertension management
- Beta-blockers after a heart attack
- Antidepressant medication management

HEDIS allows the public to measure the quality of healthcare plans to make informed decisions about their care. NCQA impacts the health of the public through implementation of evidence-based healthcare practices, thereby improving patient outcomes and saving healthcare dollars (https://ncqa.org/about-ncqa).

PUBLIC HEALTH INFORMATICS AND FUTURE PANDEMICS

Informatics Weaknesses Identified Using Previous Public Health Responses

Public health crises are known for exposing the weaknesses and potential threats to our healthcare systems and responses. WHO and CDC have experienced crises with previous public health outbreaks and pandemics: H1N1 influenza and Ebola

TABLE 10.2	Relevant Surveillance Systems for Illness-Related Events
Illness-Related Event	**Surveillance Systems That Capture the Event**
Actions in the Home or Community	
Search for information about "flu" in Google	Google flu trends (www.google.org/flutrends/; http://www.healthmap.org/flutrends/)
Stay home from school	School absenteeism surveillance
Buy over-the-counter cough medicine	National Retail Data Monitor (https://www.rods.pitt.edu/site/content/blogsection/4/42/)
Read news article about possible outbreak in the community	HealthMap (www.healthmap.org/en)
Healthcare Surveillance	
Visit an urgent or emergency care setting and report chief complaint	Syndromic surveillance of chief complaints from all or sentinel clinics
Have a medically attended visit for influenza-like illness	U.S. outpatient influenza-like illness surveillance network (ILINet)
Be diagnosed with a reportable disease	National electronic disease surveillance system
Be hospitalized with influenza	Influenza hospitalizations CDC's flu activity & surveillance (www.cdc.gov/flu/weekly/fluactivitysurv.htm)
Get a laboratory test for a viral pathogen	Pathogen surveillance (GermWatch: https://intermountainhealthcare.org/health-information/germwatch/)
Receive positive lab result	Electronic laboratory reporting
Mortality Surveillance	
Succumb to illness and die	Death registration system (i.e., vital records)
Child less than 5 years	Influenza-associated pediatric mortality
Resident of a city included in the 122-city system	122 cities mortality reporting system

CDC, Centers for disease control and prevention.

outbreaks in the United States. These crises have demonstrated the need for improving the infrastructure of public health systems, especially informatics. The weaknesses that have been identified are data collection, processes, responses, policy, and communication (Basit et al., 2021; Carney & Weber, 2015; Lombardo, 2009).

H1N1 Influenza Pandemic

In 2009, the WHO elevated the influenza alert to the level of a pandemic for H1N1 Influenza. Because of the surveillance and preparedness for the avian H5N1 influenza outbreak at the time, WHO and CDC were able to detect H1N1 progression and fast-track its vaccination program for the H1N1 pandemic. This pandemic led to the creation of automated case specific disease monitoring application to collect, analyze, and access to information faster between local, state, and national levels (Lombardo, 2009). Another advancement because of this pandemic is the use of the internet for educational material for the public and healthcare providers (Lombardo, 2009).

The Ebola Outbreak

During the 2015 Ebola virus outbreak in the United States, the importance of global monitoring and disease positive patient contract tracing was illuminated. Americans had felt safe from Ebola contact within its borders. However, with the 2015 outbreak, it became clear change was needed within our public health informatics. There were US healthcare workers that were exposed to and contracted Ebola from international undiagnosed patients during this time (Centers for Disease Control and Prevention, 2021c). The 2015 outbreak resulted in a call to action for improving the electronic monitoring systems to prepare and responds to outbreaks and pandemics. It also exposed the need for improved coordinated care and sharing of trustworthy information to the public, known as public health intelligence (Carney & Weber, 2015).

Carney and Weber (2015) called for the formation of a "national center to guide public health intelligence gathering and synthesis" (Carney & Weber, 2015). This would shift the focus from public health surveillance on people to for people by sharing accurate information about diseases, contagions, and other public health issues. The national center would coordinate and organize the public health intelligence to improve situational awareness within geographic regions or globally. There was a call for a consumer centric model of public health intelligence to meet all groups, organizations, and governmental and personal stakeholders.

The COVID-19 Pandemic

The COVID-19 pandemic in early 2000 highlighted the disjointed and outdated healthcare reporting system, which had been identified in earlier public health crisis and pandemics. The same issues identified from H1N1 and Ebola reared from the neglect to act upon identified gaps to address public health issues with accurate data from health care informatics. Some of the public lost faith and trust in governmental agencies due to conflicting or duplication of data, and the time lag in actual occurrences and real-time delay reporting. This created a chasm that needed to be addressed immediately. Johns Hopkins University efforts in monitoring COVID-19 began on January 22, 2020, with global tracking maps with the number of deaths. On March 3, 2020, this evolved into the Johns Hopkins Coronavirus Resource Center (JHCRC), which provided real-time outbreaks and number of cases and mortality. The JHCRC is an interprofessional collaboration that collects data from 260 sources, including 182 local, state, and federal agencies. The disciplines are public health, medicine, science and engineering, civic impact center, and health security center. The JHCRC provided real-time data for situational awareness and orchestrated responses to the pandemic. Johns Hopkins was able to demonstrate with a concerted and interprofessional effort that real-time, accurate data could be obtained and disseminated (Basit et al., 2021).

Public Health in Future Pandemics

The world was clearly unprepared for the COVID-19 pandemic as was the US's unpreparedness of the 1918 influenza pandemic. The need to harness data, as the two exemplars (Nightingale and Snow) identified, was not appreciated at the local, state, and federal levels (Brixey et al., 2020). The Johns Hopkins University struggled to obtain data but provided maps and tables indicating the spread of COVID-19, but a concerted effort to capture essential public health information (e.g., demographics, testing) may have provided key predictors to mitigate the rapid increase in cases. Basit et al. provide detailed information related to required data to inform pandemics (Basit et al., 2021).

Craven et al. (2020) identified there are five shifts in healthcare systems that need to occur to reduce future pandemics. The largest risk is related to the public health surveillance systems. This continues to be outdated and lacks systems integration which allows systems to communication, share data, and decrease the number of times and type of data has entered to coordinate a response to public health crises. The five-pillar approach to preparedness focuses on the public health system to always ready and able to respond system, disease surveillance, prevention agenda, healthcare capacity, and research and development. With the approach, the recognition and response to potential/actual threats will be improved with a more coordinated response.

The McKinsey report identified the issues and needs during the COVID-19 pandemic with clear recommendations for the future or the *new normal*. Their profound statement, *"Healthcare has found itself tested by the pandemic. The frontlines are delivering heroically, but the next normal for healthcare will look nothing like the normal we leave behind"* (Singhal et al., 2020), provides a warning to healthcare and health informatics personnel about the needs for the next pandemic. Their warning further articulates the need for unprecedented *resolve*, a visceral look at our *resilience*, a plan for *return* to normal after potential shut down. It also emphasizes the need for clear plans for individuals and providers and response preferences and expectations to *reimagine* healthcare (Sneader & Singhal, 2020).

CONCLUSION AND FUTURE DIRECTIONS

The H1N1 Influenza, Ebola Virus, and COVID-19 pandemic have clearly demonstrated a drastic need for infrastructure enhancement in informatics for our public health system. Accurate and timely reporting of data, leveraging the data to better understand the disease spread, evaluation of institutions to treat the public, establishing guidelines and responses nationally and globally, and improvements related to lessons learned from previous public health crisis should be the foundation of our public health system to respond to future potential or actual crisis.

ACKNOWLEDGMENT

The authors wish to acknowledge the contribution of Catherine Janes Staes to the previous edition of this chapter.

▌ DISCUSSION QUESTIONS

1. How might you begin to develop a data and information exchange between acute care, subacute care, and home health settings that would support the work of public health? Do such systems already exist?

2. Monitoring population health status is a central public health activity. A variety of survey systems, such as the CDC's National Health and Nutrition Examination Survey (NHANES) and National Health Interview Survey (NHIS), as well as state and national reporting systems, such as the Behavioral Risk Factor Surveillance System (BRFSS), Pregnancy Risk Assessment Monitoring System (PRAMS), and National Electronic Disease Surveillance System (NEDSS), provide public health practitioners with the ability to assess health trends, identify and respond to emerging health hazards, and guide development of interventions and policies that address serious health conditions, such as obesity, smoking, and diabetes. With the proliferation of EHRs within acute and ambulatory care systems, how much of this survey activity do you think can be folded in under routine data collection and exchange activities?

3. The primary goal of public health is to affect population health and ensure a healthy community. How might you see public health nurses using web-based tools to reach, manage, and educate populations of patients residing in targeted communities?

4. Part of the job of the public health informatician is to develop the tools required to translate between clinical and public health worldviews as they relate to information system development and data sharing across the specialties. As a clinical leader, by what means would you advocate to enable this sharing?

5. Personal health records are technological tools that are being implemented within the acute care setting to enable data exchange with EHRs and to encourage patient activation in healthcare. How might you foresee the use of patient-entered data from a PHR or patient portal as a public health surveillance tool?

CASE STUDY

You have been hired as an informatician at a state health department. The health department is developing systems to receive laboratory and clinical case reports from clinical settings, such as hospitals and doctor's offices. Your state has had an immunization registry in operation for several years and has been successful in getting cooperation from healthcare settings to send data to the system.

DISCUSSION QUESTIONS

1. Why is the system for reporting immunizations and receiving results at the health department so successful, particularly in comparison to the struggles you are observing as the health department sets up its laboratory and case reporting systems?
2. What is the difference between the information required to report the administration of an immunization and the information required to report a person with a communicable disease?
3. What standard vocabulary is used to code a vaccine name and how is this vocabulary different from the LOINC or SNOMED-CT vocabularies required for laboratory and clinical case reporting?
4. What is the value proposition for a healthcare provider to participate in an immunization registry?

REFERENCES

Angulo, F. J., Finelli, L., & Swerdlow, D. L. (2021). Estimation of US SARS-CoV-2 infections, symptomatic infections, hospitalizations, and deaths using seroprevalence surveys. *JAMA Network Open*, *4*(1), e2033706-e2033706.

Arias, E., Tejada-Vera, B., Ahmad, F., & Kochanck, K. D. (July 2021). National Center for Health Statistics (July 21, 2021). Life expectancy in the U.S. declined a year and half in 2020. Available from NVSS at https://www.cdc.gov/nchs/pressroom/nchs_press_releases/2021/202107.htm.

Bari, L., & O'Neill, D. P. (2019). *Rethinking patient data privacy in the era of digital health*. Health Affairs Blog. https://www.healthaffairs.org/do/10.1377/hblog20191210.216658/full/.

Basit, M. A., Lehmann, C. U., & Medford, R. J. (2021). Managing pandemics with health informatics: Successes and challenges. *Yearbook of Medical Informatics*, *30*(1), 17–25. https://doi.org/10.1055/s-0041-1726478.

Boyles, A. L., Beverly, B. E., Fenton, S. E., Jackson, C. L., Jukic, A. M. Z., Sutherland, V. L., Baird, D. D., Collman, D. D., Ferguson, K. K., Hall, J. E., Martin, E. M., Schug, T. T., White, A. J., & Chandler, K. J. (2021). Environmental factors involved in maternal morbidity and mortality. *Journal of Women's Health*, *30*(2), 245–252.

Brixey, J., Salyer, P., & Simmons, D. (2020, July). Nightingale power: The advent of nursing informatics. *Nursing Management (Springhouse)*, *51*(7), 51–53. https://doi.org/10.1097/01.NUMA.0000669104.92938.0a.

Carney, T. J., & Weber, D. J. (2015). Public health intelligence: learning from the Ebola crisis. *American Journal of Public Health*, *105*(9), 1740–1744. https://doi.org/10.2105/AJPH.2015.302771.

Centers for Disease Control and Prevention, (2016). Regulations and Laws that may apply during a pandemic. https://www.cdc.gov/flu/pandemic-resources/planning-preparedness/regulations-laws-during-pandemic.htm.

Center for Disease Control and Prevention (CDC). (2018). Health Insurance Portability and Accountability Act of 1996 (HIPAA). Available at https://www.cdc.gov/phlp/publications/topic/hipaa.html.

Center for Disease Control and Prevention (CDC). (2021a, August 19), National Syndromic Surveillance Program (NSSP). https://www.cdc.gov/nssp/overview.html.

Center for Disease Control and Prevention. (CDC). (2021b, April 15). NSSP supports the Covid-19 response https://www.cdc.gov/nssp/covid-19-response.html.

Centers for Disease Control and Prevention. (2021c). *History of Ebola virus disease (EVD) outbreaks*. https://www.cdc.gov/vhf/ebola/history/chronology.html.

Council of State and Territorial Epidemiologists (CSTE). (2015). Surveillance/informatics: Reportable condition knowledge management system. http://www.cste.org/group/RCKMS.

Craven, M., Sabow, A., Van der Veken, L., & Wilson, M. (2020). Not the last pandemic: Investing now to reimagine public health systems. *McKinsey Report*.

Cusimano, M. D., Zhang, S., Topolovec-Vranic, J., Hutchison, M. G., & Jing, R. (2017). Factors affecting the concussion knowledge of athletes, parents, coaches, and medical professionals. *SAGE Open Medicine*, *5*, 2050312117694794.

Duncan, J., Eilbeck, K., Narus, S. P., Clyde, S., Thornton, S., & Staes, C. (2015). Building an ontology for identity resolution in healthcare and public health. *Online Journal of Public Health Informatics*, *7*(2), e219. https://doi.org/10.5210/ojphi.v7i2.6010.

Fenton, S. H. & Biedermann, S. (2014). *Introduction to healthcare informatics*. American Health Information Management Association (AHIMA).

Foldy, S., & Ross, D. A. (2005). *Public health opportunities in health information exchange*. Atlanta, GA: Public Health Informatics Institute.

Green, L. W. (2006). Public health asks of systems science: to advance our evidence-based practice, can you help us get more practice-based evidence? *American Journal of Public Health*, *206*, 406–409.

Grundy, Q., Chiu, K., Held, F., Continella, A., Bero, L., & Holz, R. (2019). Data sharing practices of medicines related apps and the mobile ecosystem: Traffic, content, and network analysis. *BMJ (Clinical Research ed.)*, *364*, l920. https://doi.org/10.1136/bmj.l920.

Hardy, L. R., & Bourne, P. E. (2017). Data science: Transformation of research and scholarship. In C. Delaney, C. Weaver, J. Warren, T. Clancy, & R. Simpson (Eds.), *Big data-enabled nursing. Health informatics.* Cham: Springer. https://doi.org/10.1007/978-3-319-53300-1_10.

Institute of Medicine (US) Committee for the Study of the Future of Public Health. (1988). *The future of public health.* Washington (DC): National Academies Press (US). Available from: https://www.ncbi.nlm.nih.gov/books/NBK218218/ doi: 10.17226/1091.

Klompas, M., Haney, G., Church, D., Lazarus, R., Hou, X., & Platt, R. (2008). Automated identification of acute hepatitis B using electronic medical record data to facilitate public health surveillance. *PLoS ONE, 3*(7), e2626.

Leischow, S. J., Best, A., Trochim, W. M., Clark, P. I., Gallagher, R. S., Marcus, S. Ess., & Matthews, E. (2008). Systems thinking to improve the public's health. *American Journal of Preventive Medicine, 35*(2 Suppl), S196–S203. https://doi.org/10.1016/j.amepre.2008.05.014.

Livnat, Y., Gesteland, P., Benuzillo, J., Pettey, W., Bolton, D., Drews, F., … Samore, M. (2010). Epinome-a novel workbench for epidemic investigation and analysis of search strategies in public health practice *AMIA Annual Symposium Proceedings* (Vol. 2010, pp. 647). American Medical Informatics Association.

Lombardo, J. (2009, Dec 10). Public health informatics and the H1N1 pandemic. *Online journal of public health informatics, 1*(1), e4. https://doi.org/10.5210/ojphi.v1i1.2778.

Lumpkin, J. R., & Magnuson, J. A. (2020). History of public health information systems and informatics. In J. Magnuson & B. Dixon (Eds.), *Public health informatics and information systems. Health informatics.* Cham: Springer. https://doi.org/10.1007/978-3-030-41215-9_2.

Madhavan, S., Bastarache, L., Brown, J. S., Butte, A. J., Dorr, D. A., Embi, P. J., Friedman, C. P., Johnson, K. B., Moore, J. H., Kohane, I. S., OPayne, P. R., Tennenbaum, J. D., Weiner, M. G., Wilcox, A. B., & Ohno-Machado, L. (2021). Use of electronic health records to support a public health response to the COVID-19 pandemic in the United States: A perspective from 15 academic medical centers. *Journal of the American Medical Informatics Association, 28*(2), 393–401.

National Center for Health Statistics (July 21, 2021). Life expectancy in the U.S. declined a year and half in 2020. Available at https://www.cdc.gov/nchs/pressroom/nchs_press_releases/2021/202107.htm.

National Center for Health Statistics. Health, United States. (2019) Table 04. Hyattsville, MD. 2021. Available from: https://www.cdc.gov/nchs/hus/contents2019.htm.

Overhage, J. M., Grannis, S., & McDonald, C. J. (2008). Comparison of the completeness and timeliness of automated electronic laboratory reporting and spontaneous reporting of notifiable conditions. *American Journal of Public Health, 98*(2), 344–350.

Panth, M., & Acharya, A. S. (2015). The unprecedented role of computers in improvement and transformation of public health: an emerging priority. *Indian Journal of Community Medicine: Official Publication of Indian Association of Preventive & Social Medicine, 40*(1), 8–13. https://doi.org/10.4103/0970-0218.149262.

Public Health Development & Social Cognition (n.d.). Available at https://phdsc.org/.

Rajeev, D., Staes, C., Evans, R. S., Price, A., Hill, M., Mottice, S., … Rolfs, R. (2011). Evaluation of HL7 v2. 5.1 electronic case reports transmitted from a healthcare enterprise to public health. *AMIA Annual Symposium Proceedings* (Vol. 2011, pp. 1144). American Medical Informatics Association.

Sentell, T., Choi, S. Y., Ching, L., Quensell, M., Keliikoa, L. B., Corriveau, É., & Pirkle, C. (2020). Prevalence of selected chronic conditions among children, adolescents, and young adults in acute care settings in Hawai'i. *Preventing Chronic Disease, 17*, 190448. https://doi.org/10.5888/pcd17.190448.

Shapiro, J. S., Mostashari, F., Hripcsak, G., Soulakis, N., & Kuperman, G. (2011). Using health information exchange to improve public health. *American Journal of Public Health, 101*, 616–623.

Singhal, S., Reddy, P., Dash, P., & Weber, K. (2020). *From "wartime" to "peacetime": Five stages for healthcare institutions in the battle against COVID-19.* McKinsey & Company. https://www.mckinsey.com/industries/healthcare-systems-and-services/our-insights/from-wartime-to-peacetime-five-stages-for-healthcare-institutions-in-the-battle-against-covid-19.

Smith, P. F., Hadler, J. L., Stanbury, M., Rolfs, R. T., & Hopkins, R. S. (2013). "Blueprint version 2.0": Updating public health surveillance for the 21st century. *Journal of Public Health Management Practice, 19*(3), 231–239. https://doi.org/10.1097/PHH.0b013e318262906e.

Sneader, K., & Singhal, S. (2020). *Beyond coronavirus: The path to the next normal.* McKinsey & Company. https://www.mckinsey.com/~/media/mckinsey/industries/healthcare%20systems%20and%20services/our%20insights/beyond%20coronavirus%20the%20path%20to%20the%20next%20normal/beyond-coronavirus-the-path-to-the-next-normal.pdf?shouldIndex=false.

Staes, C. J., Gesteland, P., Allison, M., Mottice, S., Rubin, M., Shakib, J., … Byington, C. L. (2009). Urgent care providers' knowledge and attitude about public health reporting and pertussis control measures: implications for informatics. *Journal of Public Health Management and Practice: JPHMP, 15*(6), 471.

Swaringen, B. F., George, E. G., Kamenov, D., McTigue, N. E., Cornwell, D. A., Bonzongo, J-C. J. (2022). Children's exposure to environmental lead: A review of potential sources, blood levels, and methods used to reduce exposure. *Environmental Research, 204*(B), 112025, https://doi.org/10.1016/j.envres.2021.112025.

Varcin, K. J., Alvares, G. A., Uljarević, M., & Whitehouse, A. J. O. (2017). Prenatal maternal stress events and phenotypic outcomes in autism spectrum disorder. *Autism Research, 10*(11), 1866–1877. https://doi.org/10.1002/aur.1830.

Ye, J. (2020). The Role of Health Technology and Informatics in a Global Public Health Emergency: Practices and Implications From the COVID-19 Pandemic. *JMIR Medical Informatics, 8*(7), e19866. https://doi.org/10.2196/19866.

11

Evidence-Based Informatics

Juliana J. Brixey and Zach Burningham

High-quality cost-effective care requires health information systems that present the evidence needed for providers to make best-practice decisions at the point of care and then capture the data by which the effectiveness of those decisions can be measured.

OBJECTIVES

At the completion of this chapter, the reader will be prepared to:
1. Give examples of trends in evidence-based quality improvement.
2. Describe effective models in structuring evidence-based practice (EBP) initiatives.
3. Discuss the role of informatics in EBP.
4. Discuss the relationship between EBP and practice-based evidence (PBE).
5. Summarize key components of the practice-based evidence (PBE) research designs.
6. Discuss the synergistic role of EBP and PBE in developing informatics-based solutions for managing patients' care needs.

KEY TERMS

clinical practice guidelines (CPGs), 172
comparative effectiveness research, 183
evidence-based practice (EBP), 166
knowledge transformation, 170
learning health system (LHS), 166
practice-based evidence (PBE), 166

ABSTRACT ❖

This chapter links evidence-based practice (EBP) and practice-based evidence (PBE) with informatics by exploring the central, shared construct of knowledge. The discussion offers a foundation for understanding EBP and PBE, as well as their interrelationships. The narrative describes how EBP and PBE are supported and integrated through a variety of current informatics applications. The chapter concludes by exploring opportunities for applying informatics solutions to maximize the advantages offered by the synergistic implementation of EBP and PBE in providing cost-effective, safe, quality healthcare for individuals, families, populations, and communities.

INTRODUCTION

Informatics solutions and tools hold promise for enhancing evidence-based clinical decision making and for measuring the effectiveness of those decisions in real-time. The field of informatics and the concepts of evidence-based practice (EBP) and practice-based evidence (PBE) intersect at the crucial junction of knowledge for clinical decisions, with the goal of transforming healthcare to be reliable, safe, and effective.

A foundational paradigm for informatics is the framework of data, information, knowledge, and wisdom (DIKW) discussed in Chapter 2. The DIKW framework indicates that, as data are organized into meaningful groupings, the information within those data can be seen and interpreted. The organization of information and the identification of the relationships between the facts within the information create knowledge. The effective use of knowledge, such as the process of providing personalized care to manage human healthcare needs, is wisdom. The DIKW framework is foundational to developing a learning health system (LHS), emphasizing the importance of real-world data and analytics to continually deliver new knowledge to providers and stakeholders, leading to wiser action and enhanced decision-making.

An LHS is now possible through advancements in computerization and the electronic health record (EHR). These tools provide the technologies to collect, organize, label, and efficiently and effectively deliver evidence-based information and knowledge at the point of decision making where clinicians can apply them. Patient-specific data is captured through documentation in the patient's EHR as care is delivered, thereby providing a feedback loop for evaluating the effectiveness of patient-care decisions, creating cycles of continuous quality improvement (CQI). These data can be aggregated across patients, demonstrating the effectiveness of evidence-based decisions across groups of patients in various settings.

A challenge to achieving this ideal is the complexity of issues surrounding standardized terminology in healthcare and the lack of a common framework across the field of EBP and PBE. Standardized terminology is requisite for naming, classifying, tagging, locating, and then analyzing evidence to use in practice.

EVIDENCE-BASED PRACTICE

Knowledge is the heart of EBP. Knowledge must be transformed to increase its utility at the point of care (POC) within the EBP paradigm (Stevens 2015). EBP's ultimate goal is improving systems and microsystems within healthcare based on science. Using computerized methods and resources to support the implementation of EBP has the potential for improving healthcare. Delivering evidence to the point of patient care can align care processes with best practices.

Evidence-based Practice Evolution

The evolution of EBP underscores its potential impact on quality of care and health outcomes. *To Err Is Human*, a well-known Institute of Medicine report, estimated that approximately 100,000 patients were harmed annually by the healthcare system (Institute of Medicine, 2000). The report emphasized the significance of preventable harm and death. Experts in 2014 considered 100,000 deaths as an underestimation suggesting that more recent data indicate the mortality rate of medical errors ranges from 210,000 to 400,000 annually (McCann, 2014; James, 2013; Makary & Daniel, 2016; Anderson & Abrahamson, 2017). There is a debate that the actual number of deaths attributed to medical errors has been overestimated (Jarry, 2021). Nonetheless, healthcare organizations have not irradicated avoidable medical errors.

Crossing the Quality Chasm (Chasm), a 2001 Institute of Medicine report following *To Err Is Human*, reported that national leaders identified the gap between what is known about best care and what is practiced. Moreover, the *Chasm* report cited more than 100 surveys of quality of care with scores on the "report card" indicating healthcare performance as poor. Box 11.1 presents findings from these surveys, comparing current care to what was deemed the best care or standards of care. These results indicated that improvement was needed if every patient is to receive consistent, high-quality care. The report identified EBP as a solution to achieve the goal of quality healthcare.

BOX 11.1 Institute of Medicine Findings on 2001 Level of Current Care Compared With Standards of Care

- 47% of myocardial infarction patients did not receive beta blockers
- 50% of children with asthma did not receive written instructions
- 48% of the elderly did not receive their annual influenza vaccine
- 63% of smokers were not advised to quit smoking
- 84% of Medicare patients with diabetes were not tested with the A1c blood test

Data from the Institute of Medicine. (2001). *Crossing the quality chasm: A new health system for the 21st century* [Committee on Health Care in America & Institute of Medicine]. Washington, DC: National Academies Press.

Another set of reports demonstrating this challenge is the National Healthcare Quality Report (NHQR) and the National Healthcare Disparities Report (NHDR) produced by the Agency for Healthcare Research and Quality (AHRQ). These reports, published annually since 2003, have provided an annual snapshot of the quality of care across the country (Agency for Healthcare Research and Quality [AHRQ], 2015). Beginning in 2014, findings on healthcare quality and healthcare disparities were integrated into a single document titled the *National Healthcare Quality and Disparities Report* (QDR). This report highlights the importance of examining quality and disparities together to gain a more comprehensive picture of healthcare. "The report demonstrates that the nation has made clear progress in improving the health care delivery system to achieve the three aims of better care, smarter spending, and healthier people, but there is still more work to do, specifically to address disparities in care." (AHRQ, 2015). For example, patient safety improved, as demonstrated by a 17% reduction in rates of hospital-acquired conditions (HACs) between 2010 and 2013. However, across a broad range of measures, recommended care is delivered only 70% of the time. Similarly, the downward trend for the HACs continued for the years between 2014 and 2017, as evidenced by a 13% reduction (AHRQ, 2020). Failure of care delivery, including clinician-related inefficiencies such as variability in care, has not been resolved, resulting in continued waste and cost (Shrank, Rogstad, & Parekh, 2019).

Solutions to the healthcare quality gap are offered in the *Chasm* report (Institute of Medicine [IOM], 2001). The IOM expert panel issued recommendations for urgent action to redesign healthcare so that it is **s**afe, **t**imely, **e**ffective, **e**fficient, **e**quitable, and **p**atient-centered, often referred to as the STEEEP principles (IOM, 2001). Each of the STEEEP redesign principles is described further in Table 11.1.

The *Chasm* report continues to be a major influence, directing national efforts targeted at transforming healthcare. For example, the STEEEP recommendations are now reflected in health profession education programs. The American Association of Colleges of Nursing (AACN) educational competencies include requirements for programs to prepare nurses who contribute to quality improvement (American Association of Colleges of Nursing [AACN], 2021). AACN *Essentials*, updated in 2021, specify that professional nursing practice be grounded in translation of current evidence into practice and further point to the need for knowledge and skills in information management

TABLE 11.1	Descriptions of the STEEEP Principles for Redesigning Healthcare
Principle	**Description**
Safe	Avoid injuries to patients from the care that is intended to help them.
Timely	Reduce wait time and sometimes harmful delays for both those who receive and those who give care.
Effective	Provide services based on scientific knowledge to all who could benefit, and refrain from providing services to those not likely to benefit.
Efficient	Avoid waste, including waste of equipment, supplies, ideas, and energy.
Equitable	Provide care that does not vary in quality because of personal characteristics such as gender, ethnicity, geographic location, and socioeconomic status.
Patient centered	Provide care that is respectful of and responsive to individual patient preferences, needs, and values, and ensure that patient values guide all clinical decisions.

Adapted from Institute of Medicine. (2001). *Crossing the quality chasm: A new health system for the 21st century* (Committee on Health Care in America & Institute of Medicine) (pp. 39–40). Washington, DC: National Academies Press.

as being critical in the delivery of quality patient care (AACN, 2021). Likewise, the Accreditation Council for Graduate Medical Education (ACGME) requires medical education in quality improvement (Accreditation Council for Graduate, 2020). The STEEEP principles are also reflected in clinical practice resources, such as the AHRQ Health Care Innovations Exchange, where the STEEEP elements are the selection criteria for inclusion in this unique clearinghouse (AHRQ, 2021).

Quality of Care

Quality of care and EBP are conceptually linked, and form the hub of healthcare improvement. The descriptions and definitions reflect the overlap of these concepts and offer reference points against which to expand their understanding. In particular, the focal point of both is the use of knowledge in practice.

The definition of *quality of care* includes two essential connections to EBP and knowledge that provide a linkage to informatics. First, quality healthcare services increase the likelihood of reaching the goals of care or expected outcomes. This implies that processes of EBP must assist clinicians in knowing which options in health services are effective. The strongest cause-and-effect knowledge is discovered through formal research. Second, EBP is connected to quality insofar as healthcare is consistent with current knowledge. *Using knowledge* presumes accessibility to it at the POC. The overlap of EBP and knowledge is further underscored by the definition of the STEEEP principle "effective." *Effectiveness* is defined in the STEEEP framework as evidence-based decision making, suggesting, "Patients should receive care based on the best available scientific knowledge" (p. 62) *Knowledge* is the point of convergence across the areas of EBP, informatics, and improvement. Using informatics approaches can make evidence available and accessible at the POC.

POC testing can occur within the LHS framework. Through informatics, a health system can implement an evidence-based approach to learn what is and what is not working in healthcare quality and safety. An LHS is broadly defined as "any entity that routinely and continuously seeks to generate and learn from data, for purposes of improving individual and population health." (Guise et al., 2018). It is important to note that an LHS is not designed to replace more a time-intensive rigorous research design but seeks to compliment such efforts. There are tradeoffs to relying solely on a less controlled approach in determining optimal health care delivery practices.

The LHS recognizes the vital role the patient plays in the continual learning process. Providing a patient-centered approach to health outcomes is achieved by using patient data to formulate, evaluate, and update processes. With the advancements in informatics and IT, organizations now seek to develop "rapid" LHSs by creating well-orchestrated pipelines of near-real time data that flows back to the clinician and allows for iterative and continual refinement of the knowledge base (Abernathy et al., 2010). It must be noted that while beneficial, the LHS is not without implementation difficulties (Smoyer et al., 2016). For example, an LHS requires substantial IT investment, including a well-constructed backend data architecture, and advanced analytic capabilities, all of which can be resource-intensive. Both data storage and analytic capabilities are equally necessary. An LHS can begin to provide the environment to initiate precision medicine. For example, if genetic test results are simply stored as scanned image files without further analytic processing, then the data interpretation is still left for busy clinicians to complete. Data capture coupled with advanced analytics is required in rendering these data suitable for clinical use, such as being able to quickly determine a patient's genetic attributes and appropriate model for treatment (Williams et al., 2018). New infrastructures are recommended for the future, including computable representations, augmented with traditional human-readable representations (e.g., text, graphs, and figures) due to the quantity of evidence and the time to change practice. Computable representations include other types of evidence (e.g., rules and predictive models). Notably, the novel representations can be digitized as knowledge objects (DKOs). The DKOs would be available through digital libraries.

The primary impetus for EBP in healthcare is the selection of the option that improves the patient's health. Evaluation and use of research evidence support this option. In concert with the use of research evidence is the use of an institutional LHS using patient data (evidence) and analytics to assess a personalized, evidence-based approach, to the current medical issue. Clients present multiple actual or potential health problems requiring management or resolution (e.g., living with asthma, learning disabilities, and obesity management). Clinical actions may not be based on the best available scientific knowledge and, therefore, offer less effective client care (IOM, 2001). The essential role of a healthcare provider is to select and provide interventions providing a positive patient outcome and the most effective strategies for changing the microsystem or system of care. Clinicians choose from and interpret various clinical data and information while facing pressure to decrease the uncertainty, risks to patients, and costs. Knowledge underlies these decisions and plays a primary role in the care provided.

Evidence-based clinical decision making can be described as a prescriptive approach to making choices in diagnostic and intervention care, based on the idea that research-based care improves outcomes most effectively. Research-based care provides evidence about which option is most likely to produce the desired outcome. EBP is seen as a key solution in closing the gap between what is known and practiced.

However, essential questions lie between accepting this as true and the clinician's and system's ability to enact it: How do clinicians know which interventions will most likely diminish or resolve the health problem and help the client reach their health goal? What resources are available to apply EBP principles directly in clinical decision making? Answering these questions begins with analyzing the different models of EBP.

EVIDENCE-BASED PRACTICE MODELS

Several EBP models are useful in understanding various aspects of EBP and elucidating connections between informatics and EBP. An overview of models in the field reflects several challenges for developing informatics approaches. The primary challenge is the lack of a common framework that could be used to organize and implement EBP principles.

Effective EBP Models

Prominent EBP models can be grouped into one of three categories of models for designing and implementing systematic approaches to strengthen evidence-based clinical decision making (Mitchell et al., 2010). Table 11.2 describes the critical attributes and provides examples in three categories.

TABLE 11.2 Models for Evidence-Based Practice

Focus	Description	Examples of Models
Evidence-based practice, research use, and knowledge transformation processes	Direct a systematic approach to synthesizing knowledge and transforming research findings to improve patient outcomes and the quality of care. Address both individual practitioners and healthcare organizations. Focus on increasing the meaningfulness and utility of research findings in clinical decision making.	• Stevens Star Model of Knowledge Transformation (Stevens, 2015) • Advancing Research and Clinical Practice Through Close Collaboration (ARCC) Model of Evidence-Based Practice in Nursing and Healthcare (Melnyk et al., 2008) • Johns Hopkins Nursing Evidence-Based Practice Model and Guidelines (Newhouse et al., 2007) • Iowa Model of Evidence-Based Practice (Titler, Kleiber, & Steelman, 2001) • Stetler Model of Research Utilization (Stetler et al., 2007)
Strategic and organizational change theory to promote uptake and adoption of new knowledge	Trace mechanisms by which individual, small group, and organizational contexts affect diffusion, uptake, and adoption of new knowledge and innovation. The premise is that interventions, outcomes evaluations, and feedback are important methods to promote practice change.	• Promoting Action on Research Implementation in Health Services (PARiHS) (Kitson et al., 2008; Rycroft Malone, 2004; Rycroft Malone et al., 2002) • Vratny and Shriver Model for Evidence-Based Practice (Vratny & Shriver, 2007) • Pettigrew and Whipp Model of Strategic Change (Stetler et al., 2007) • Outcomes-Focused Knowledge Translation (Doran & Sidani, 2007) • Determinants of Effective Implementation of Complex Innovations in Organizations (Weiner et al., 2009) • Ottawa Model of Research Use (Graham & Tetroe, 2007; Logan & Graham, 1998)
Knowledge exchange and synthesis for application and inquiry	Structure ongoing interactions among practitioners, researchers, policy-makers, and consumers to facilitate the generation of clinically relevant knowledge and the application of knowledge in practice; all parties are engaged in bidirectional collaboration across the translation continuum.	• Collaborative Model for Knowledge Translation between Research and Practice Settings (Baumbusch et al., 2008) • Framework for Translating Evidence into Action (Swinburn et al., 2005) • Knowledge Transfer and Exchange (Mitton et al., 2007) • Canadian Institutes of Health Research Knowledge Translation within the Research Cycle Model or Knowledge Action Model (Armstrong et al., 2006; Brachaniec et al., 2006; Graham et al., 2006) • Interactive Systems Framework for Dissemination and Implementation (Wandersman et al., 2008)

From Mitchell, S. A., Fisher, C. A., Hastings, C. E., Silverman, L. B., & Wallen, G. R. (2010). A thematic analysis of theoretical models for translational science in nursing: Mapping the field. *Nursing outlook*, *58*(6), 287–300. Used with permission.

TABLE 11.5 Characteristics of Practice-Based Evidence

Characteristic	Practice-Based Evidence
Description	Participatory research approach requiring documentation of predefined processes and outcome data and analysis
Goal	Determine the effectiveness of multiple interventions on multiple outcomes in the actual practice environment
Design classification	Observational (descriptive)
Temporal aspects	Prospective
Typical sample size	800–2000+

- Exhaustive attention to patient characteristics to address confounds or alternative explanations of treatment effectiveness.
- Use of large samples and diverse sources of patients to improve sample representativeness, power, and external validity.
- Use of detailed standardized structured documentation of interventions with training and quality-control checks for the reliability of the measures of the actual process of care.
- Inclusion of frontline clinicians and patients in the design, execution, and analysis of studies and their data elements to improve ecological validity.

PBE studies require comprehensive data acquisition. By using bivariate and multivariate associations among patient characteristics, process steps, and outcomes can be identified. Concurrently, PBE study designs are structured to minimize the potential for false associations between treatments and outcomes. These studies focus on reducing the effects of potential alternative factors or explanations when estimating the complex associations between treatments and outcomes within a specific care context (Horn et al., 2005). However, the identified associations between treatment and outcome are not considered causal links. The associations still inform causal judgments to the extent that the research design can measure and statistically control for these confounders or alternative explanations.

The PBE approach does not infer causality directly like RCTs, but several sources indicate the strength of the evidence that a causal link exists. First, alternative hypotheses regarding possible causes are tested using a large number of available variables to identify additional potential variables that may influence outcomes. Results can be used to drill down to discover potential alternative causes and to generate additional specific hypotheses. Analyses continue until the project team is satisfied that they cannot think of any other variables to explain the outcomes. Second, one can test the predictive validity of significant PBE findings by introducing findings into clinical practice and assessing whether outcomes change when treatments change, as predicted by PBE models. Third, studies can be repeated in different healthcare settings and assessed to determine if the findings remain the same.

Underlying the common criticism of observational studies (that they demonstrate association but not causation) is an unchallenged assumption that the evidence for causation is dichotomous; that is, something either is or is not the cause. Instead, the evidence for causation should be viewed as a continuum that extends from mere association to undeniable causation. While observational studies cannot prove causation in some absolute sense, by chipping away at potential confounders and by testing for predictive validity in follow-up studies, we move upward on the continuum from mere association to causation. PBE studies offer a methodology for moving up this continuum.

Research design involves a balance of internal validity (the validity of the causal inference that the treatment is the "true" cause of the outcome) and external validity (the validity that the causal inference can be generalized to other subjects, forms of the treatment, measures of the outcome, practitioners, and settings). Essentially, PBE designs trade away the internal validity of RCTs for external validity (Mitchell & Jolley, 2001). PBE designs have high external validity (generalizability) because they include virtually all patients with or at risk for the condition under study, as well as potential confounders that could alter treatment responses. PBE designs attempt to minimize threats to internal validity by collecting information on all patient variables—demographic, medical, nursing, functional, and socioeconomic—that might account for differences in outcome. By doing so, PBE designs minimize the need for compensating statistical techniques such as instrumental variables and propensity scoring to mitigate selection bias effects, unknown sources of variance, and threats to internal validity.

PBE study designs attempt to capture the complexity of the healthcare process presented by patient and treatment differences in routine care; PBE studies do not alter or standardize treatment regimens to evaluate the efficacy of a specific intervention or combination of interventions, as one usually does in an RCT or other types of experimental designs (Horn & Gassaway, 2007, 2010). PBE studies measure multiple concurrent interventions, patient characteristics, and outcomes. This comprehensive framework provides for consequential analyses of significant associations between treatment combinations and outcomes, controlling for patient differences.

Steps in a Practice-Based Evidence Study

Table 11.6 outlines the steps involved in conducting a PBE study and gives a brief description of what each step involves. Once a clinical issue is identified, PBE methods by forming a multidisciplinary team, often with representatives of multiple sites. Participation of informaticians on the team is critical to ensuring that the electronic documentation facilitates data capture for the research and clinical practice without undue documentation burden.

Create a Multisite, Multidisciplinary Project Clinical Team

One factor that distinguishes PBE studies from most other observational studies is the extensive involvement of frontline clinicians and patients. Frontline clinicians and patients are engaged in *all* aspects of PBE projects; they identify data elements to be included in the PBE project based on initial study hypotheses, extensive literature review, and clinical experience and training, as well as patient experience. Many relevant details

TABLE 11.6	Steps in a Practice-Based Evidence Study
Step	**Description**
1. Create a multisite, multidisciplinary PCT	PCT (a) identifies outcomes of interest, (b) identifies individual components of the care process, (c) creates a common intervention vocabulary and dictionary, (d) identifies key patient characteristics and risk factors, (e) proposes hypotheses for testing, and (f) participates in data collection, analyses, and dissemination of findings. The PCT builds on theoretical understanding, research evidence to date, existing guidelines, and the clinical expertise and experience about factors that may influence outcomes.
2. Control for differences in patient severity, including comorbidities, treatment processes, and outcomes	Comprehensive severity measure should be in an age- and disease-specific measure of physiologic and psychosocial complexity. It is used to control for selection bias and confounding by indication. An example is the CSI that is disease- and age-specific and composed of more than 2200 clinical indicators.
3. Implement intensive data collection and check reliability	Capture data on patient characteristics, care processes, and outcomes drawn from medical records and study-specific data collection instruments. Data collectors are tested for interrater reliability.
4. Create a study database	The study database consists of merged, cleaned data and is suitable for statistical analyses.
5. Test hypotheses successively	Hypotheses are based on questions that motivated the study originally, previous studies, existing guidelines, and, above all, hypotheses proposed by the PCT. Bivariate and multivariate analysis approaches include multiple regression, analysis of variance, logistic and Cox proportional hazard regression, hierarchical mixed models, and other methods consistent with measurement properties of key variables.
6. Validate and implement study findings	Implement findings in practice to test predictive validity. In this step, findings from the first five steps are implemented and evaluated to determine whether the new or modified interventions replicate results identified in earlier phases and outcomes improve as predicted. After validating specific PBE findings, the findings are ready to be incorporated into routine care and clinical guidelines.

CSI, Comprehensive Severity Index; *PBE*, practice-based evidence; *PCT*, project clinical team.

about patients, treatments, and outcomes may be recorded in existing EHRs; however, the project clinical team (PCT) often identifies additional critical variables that must be collected in supplemental standardized documentation developed specifically for the PBE study. Clinicians and patients also participate in data analyses leading to publication. Front-to-back clinician and patient participation foster high levels of clinician and patient buy-in that contribute to data completeness and clinical ownership of study findings, even when findings challenge conventional wisdom and practice. Such ownership is essential to knowledge translation and best practice.

Control for Differences in Patient Severity of Illness

Controls for patient factors. PBE designs require the recording of each subject's treatment as determined by clinicians in practice rather than by randomizing subjects to neutralize the effect of patient differences. PBE studies address patient differences by *measuring* a wide variety of patient characteristics that go beyond race, gender, age, payer, and other variables that can be exported from administrative, registry, or EHR databases, and then accounting for patient differences through statistical control.

The goal is to measure all variables contributing to outcomes to have the information needed to control for patient differences. This is the primary reason for including frontline clinicians and patients in PBE study design and implementation. There always remains the possibility that some patient characteristic may be overlooked. Still, PBE's exhaustive patient characterization significantly minimizes the chances of not being able to resolve unknown sources of variance because of patient differences.

One critical component of the PBE study design is the use of tools for measuring the degree of illness, such as the Comprehensive Severity Index (CSI) ((Horn et al., 2005;

Horn et al., 2001; Averill et al., 1992; Clemmer et al., 1999; Horn et al., 2002; Willson et al., 2000; Ryser et al., 2005; Horn et al., 1991; Gassaway et al., 2005; Carter et al., 2009; Rosenbaum, 2002). In PBE studies, the CSI can be used to measure how ill a patient is at the time of presentation for care, as well as over time. *Degree of illness* is defined as the extent of deviation from "normal values." CSI is "physiologically-based, age- and disease-specific, independent of treatments, and provides an objective, consistent method to define patient severity of illness levels based on over 2,200 signs, symptoms, and physical findings related to a patient's disease(s), not just diagnostic information, such as ICD-9-CM coding alone."[67] The validity of CSI has been studied for over 30 years in various clinical settings and conditions such as inpatient adult and pediatric conditions, ambulatory care, rehabilitation care, hospice care, and long-term care settings (Averil et al., 1992; Carter et al., 2009). Patient diagnosis codes and data management rules are used to calculate severity scores for each patient overall and separately for each patient's disease (principal and each secondary diagnosis).

CSI and other measures of patient key characteristics, such as level and completeness of spinal cord injury, severity of stroke disability, or severity of traumatic brain injury, control for patient differences. Using these patient differences can help to account for treatment selection bias or confounding by indication in analyses.

Controls for treatment and process factors. Treatment in clinical settings is often determined by facility standards, regional differences, and clinician training. Therefore, like patient differences, treatment differences must be recorded during a PBE study. The goal is to find measurable factors that describe each treatment to be compared. Examples include the medications dispensed and their dosage; rehabilitation therapies performed and duration on each day of treatment; content, mode, and amount of patient education; and nutritional consumption.

PBE identifies better practices by examining how different approaches to care are associated with outcomes of care while controlling for patient variables. PBE does not require providers to follow treatment protocols or exclude certain treatment practices. However, characteristics of treatment, including timing and dose, require detailed documentation. These characteristics must be defined by the PBE team and measured in a structured, standard manner for all participating sites and their clinicians. Consistency is critical for minimizing variation in data collection and documentation (Horn et al., 2012).

The level of detail found in routine documentation of interventions may be insufficient. Each PBE team must assess the level of detail afforded by routine documentation and determine whether supplemental documentation is necessary (Horn et al., 2012). Further, point-of-care documentation or EHR data are pilot tested to ensure the complete representation of variables. Pilot testing ensures that point-of-care documentation or EHR data collection captures all elements that clinicians suggest may affect the outcomes of their patients. *If a variable is not measured, it cannot be used in subsequent analyses.*

Controls for outcome factors. Multiple outcomes can be addressed in a single PBE project; projects are not limited to one primary outcome, as in other study designs. In particular, PBE studies incorporate widely accepted, standard measures. For example, the Braden Scale for Risk of Pressure Ulcer Development is commonly collected in PBE studies, and it has been used as both a control and an outcome variable (Carter et al., 2009; Rosenbaum, 2002; Horn et al., 2012). Although PBE projects incorporate as many standard measures as possible, they also include outcome measures specific to the study topic. Additional patient outcomes commonly assessed in PBE studies are condition-specific complications, condition-specific long-term medical outcomes (based on clinician assessment or patient self-report), condition-specific patient-centered measures of activities and participation in society, patient satisfaction, quality of life, and cost (Deutscher et al., 2009).

Some outcomes (e.g., discharge destination [home, community, and institution], length of stay, or death) are commonly available in administrative databases. Other outcome variables (e.g., repeat stroke, deep vein thrombosis, pain, electrolyte imbalance, and anemia) are found in traditional paper charts or EHR documentation. However, they typically are available only up to discharge from the care setting.

Implement Intensive Data Collection and Check Reliability

Using the data elements identified in step 2, historical data are collected from the EHR. Direct care providers document the specific elements of treatment at the POC. For example, if the treatment includes physical therapy, the type, intensity, and duration are precisely recorded during each therapy session. If the healthcare provider offers patient counseling or education, the teaching methods, instructional materials, topical content, and duration of each teaching session are recorded. The informatics specialist is a critical partner in designing the data capture to prevent the need for parallel documentation.

If the documentation is too burdensome, clinicians will not comply with documentation requirements, and the data will be incomplete. Therefore, the design of the data collection is critical to the success of this research approach. The fact that the frontline clinicians define these data collection formats helps ensure that the data collection formats are specifically designed so that data can be documented easily and quickly.

Create a Study Database

The elements of data that are collected are compiled into a study-specific database with the assistance of informatics personnel. Data sources include existing or new clinician documentation of care delivered. Patients drop out of a PBE study if they leave the care setting before completion of treatment or drop out during follow-up (Deutscher et al., 2009). Patients who withdraw from a treatment do not distort the results of PBE study findings because PBE studies follow patients throughout the care process, taking date and time measurements on all therapies. Hence, if a patient withdraws from care of the study, investigators can use the existing data in the analyses, controlling for time in the study. PBE studies have an advantage because of their large sample size, number of information points, and complete comparison of those subjects who complete therapy and those who withdraw.

Successively Test Hypotheses

PBE studies use multivariable analyses to identify variables most strongly associated with outcomes. Detailed characterization of patients and treatments allows researchers to specify direct effects, indirect effects, and interactions that might not otherwise become apparent with less detailed data. CSI (overall, individual components, or individual severity indicators) can be used in data analysis to represent the role of comorbid and co-occurring conditions along with the principal diagnosis. Suppose a positive outcome is found to be associated with a specific treatment or combination of treatments. In that case, the subsequent methodological approach is to include confounding patient variables or combinations of variables in the analysis in an attempt to "disconfirm" the association. The association may remain robust, or variables may be identified that explain the outcome more adequately.

Data in PBE studies include many clinical and therapeutic variables, and a selection procedure is applied to decide on significant variables to retain in regressions. Only variables suggested by the team based on the literature and team members' education and clinical experience and with frequencies equal to or greater than 10 to 20 patients in the sample are usually allowed.

Analyses conducted using PBE databases are iterative. Counterintuitive findings are investigated thoroughly. In fact, counterintuitive and unexpected findings often lead to discoveries of important associations of treatments with outcomes.

Large numbers of patients (usually >1000 and often >2000) and considerable computing power are required to perform PBE analyses. When multiple outcomes are of interest, and there is little information on the effect size of each predictor variable, sample size is based on the project team's desire to find small, medium, or large effects of patient and process variables.

Validate and Implement Findings

See the exemplar in Box 11.10 showing how a PBE study of stroke rehabilitation culminated in validation studies and changes in the standard of care in a healthcare system. Because PBE studies are observational, the conclusions require prospective validation before being incorporated into clinical guidelines and standards of care. Validation of PBE findings can use a CQI approach consisting of the systematic implementation of those interventions that were found to be better, in conjunction

with monitoring their outcomes. If the findings from the outcome assessment replicate the findings of the initial retrospective stage in multiple settings and populations, the intervention would be a candidate for incorporation into clinical guidelines as a care process that has established efficacy and effectiveness. This is in contrast to interventions that only have RCT evidence, which generally indicates only efficacy.

Limitations and Strengths of Practice-Based Evidence Studies

PBE methods work best in situations where one wishes to study existing clinical practice. However, there are no limitations related to conditions or settings for the use of PBE study

---

BOX 11.10 Practice-Based Evidence Exemplar: Stroke Rehabilitation

An integrated healthcare system determined that outcomes were highly variable for patients following a stroke. Rehabilitation professionals in the geographic region were polled to determine the local standards of care, and the interventions were quite diverse. A regional task force was convened representing eight hospitals from 2 care-delivery systems, as well as an independent hospital. The task force was led by a rehabilitation nurse and a physical therapist. A practice-based evidence (PBE) study was initiated to determine what combinations of medical devices, therapies (e.g., physical therapy, occupational therapy, and speech therapy), medications, feeding, and nutritional approaches worked best for various subtypes of stroke patients in real-world practices. A multidisciplinary PCT was convened of physicians, nurses, social workers, psychologists, physical therapists, occupational therapists, recreational therapists, and speech-language therapists. Poststroke patients and caregivers were also invited to participate.

The first decisions of the group addressed the outcome variables, including the Functional Independence Measure (FIM) scale score, length of stay in rehabilitation, discharge disposition, mortality, and morbidity (contracture, deep vein thrombosis, major bleeding, pulmonary embolism, pressure ulcer, and pneumonia). Each profession identified possible interventions and developed documentation for the components of the intervention and the intensity (e.g., number of repetitions for each exercise maneuver and time required). Documentation was incorporated into the standard electronic health record documentation. Over a 2-year period, 1461 patients were studied, ranging from 18.4 to 95.6 years of age. Collected patient-related data included age, gender, race, payer, stroke risk factors, and FIM scores. Detailed process and outcome data were collected. The severity of illness was determined using the CSI scale. There were significant differences in the average severity of illness at the eight sites. There was heterogeneity in the intensity of therapies, use of tube feedings, and use of psychotropic and opioid medication. Following control for severity of illness, univariate and multivariate analysis of the data determined that factors were positively and negatively associated with the FIM scores at discharge.

Categories of Factors	Positive Association With FIM Score (↑ Independence)	Negative Association With FIM Score (↓ Independence)
Patient factors	Bed motility in first 3 h	Age
	Advanced gait activity in first 3 h	Severe motor and cognitive impairment at admission
	Home management by OT	
Therapy factors	Bed motility in first 3 h	Days until rehabilitation onset
	Advanced gait activity in first 3 h	
Nutrition	Enteral feeding	
Medications	Atypical antipsychotics	Tricyclic antidepressants
	Neurotropic pain treated with medications	Older SSRIs

OT, Occupational therapist; *SSRIs,* selective serotonin reuptake inhibitors.

Source: Horn, S. D., DeJong, G., Smout, R. J., Gassaway, J., James, R., & Conroy, B. (2005). Stroke rehabilitation patients, practice, and outcomes: Is earlier and more aggressive therapy better? *Archives of Physical Medicine and Rehabilitation, 86*(12 suppl 2), S101–S114.

After additional studies to replicate findings, the participating hospitals initiated the following policy changes in the treatment of stroke patients. Several of these are novel interventions that would not have been identified without the PBE study method. Continuous quality improvement monitoring was implemented to document adherence and outcomes:

- *Early rehabilitation admission:* patients are admitted to rehabilitation as soon as possible, and therapies begin in the intensive care unit if possible.
- *Early gait training by physical therapy:* patients are put in a harness on a treadmill for safety, but gait training is initiated as soon as possible, even in the most affected patients.
- *Early feeding:* if patients are not able to eat a full diet, early enteral feedings (nutritional supplements, tube feeding) are initiated.
- *Opioids for pain:* opioids are ordered at admission for any time the patient does not attend therapy because of pain.

methods. The technique can be time-consuming in terms of conducting the initial PBE steps, as well as data extraction. Although the relevant variables may change, PBE study designs have been found to work in various practice settings, including acute and ambulatory care, inpatient and outpatient rehabilitation, hospice, and long-term care, and for adult and pediatric patients.

INFORMATICS AND PRACTICE-BASED EVIDENCE

Challenges to Practice-Based Evidence Integration With Electronic Health Records

Data elements needed for PBE, and especially for CSI, can be captured in structured, exportable formats while also being used for clinical documentation of care EHR use in patient care as research expands. This concept is implemented already in health systems in Israel and various PBE studies in the United States (Deutscher et al., 2008). However, transitioning to EHRs presents its own challenges, especially for data-intensive PBE studies. EHRs can facilitate data acquisition, but they are not always research-friendly because many desired data elements are in text, such as clinical notes, and cannot be exported easily. If EHR data cannot be exported directly, they must be abstracted manually or alternatively, processed using Natural Language Processing (NLP) methods (Spyns, 1996). Whereas manual abstraction from EHR can be more labor-intensive than abstracting paper charts are, when relying on NLP methods, a bulk of the effort is spent on training the computer algorithms to extract the needed data elements. In addition, EHR modifications for optimizing point-of-care data documentation and abstraction are costly and time-consuming, potentially slowing down the planning and implementation of PBE studies based on routine electronic data capture. With HITECH, EHRs have become pervasive in clinical practice (Mennemeyer et al., 2016). Over time, new EHR exporting and reporting software are emerging, making EHR data abstraction less labor-intensive.

Examination of CSI elements themselves may show a reduced set that differentiates severity, as well as the full set. It is possible that two valid data elements would each contribute clinically unique information but be fully redundant with respect to their ability to differentiate severity in a population. For example, unresponsive neurological status and fever ≥ 104 degrees are clinically unique indicators of severity in pneumonia. If these indicators differentiate only the same most gravely ill pneumonia patients from the rest of the population, they provide redundant information with respect to the severity of pneumonia. In this case, it may be possible to use only one of the two indicators

in CSI scoring, reducing the information burden to compute a CSI score and increasing efficiency.

Comparative Effectiveness Research

PBE requires a multidisciplinary team approach for comparative effectiveness research and ensures inclusion of a wide spectrum of variables so that differences in patient characteristics and treatments are measured and controlled statistically (Horn et al., 2012).

The next step for comparative effectiveness research is to conduct more rigorous, prospective large-scale observational cohort studies. National efforts such as the Patient-Centered Outcomes Research Institute's (PCORI) Clinical Data Research Networks (CDRN) can enable comparative effectiveness research and PBE by providing informatics solutions for sharing data across multiple institutions (Amin et al., 2014). From a PBE perspective, rigor entails controlled measurement of outcomes related to multiple intervention combinations and a variety of patient characteristics in diverse clinical settings (Horn et al., 2012). PBE studies address questions in the real world where multiple variables and factors can affect the outcomes; they can fit seamlessly into everyday clinical documentation and, therefore, have the potential to influence and improve the evidence in EBP in the real-world clinical environment of patient care.

CONCLUSION AND FUTURE DIRECTIONS

Healthcare continues to be a dangerous experience for many patients. Moreover, many healthcare providers and other healthcare decision-makers continue to underuse interventions demonstrated to be effective at improving health outcomes (AHRQ, 2015; Stevens & Staley, 2006). The problem is not uncaring disinterested providers but a lack of organizational infrastructure and information systems designed to support the implementation of EBP and PBE within the LHS framework. Green is well recognized for asking the question, "If it is an EBP, where's the practice-based evidence?" (Green, 2008) In the future, only by creating well-designed healthcare information systems that present the evidence needed for providers to make best-practice decisions at the POC, and then capturing the patient-care data by which the effectiveness of those decisions can be measured will we have information systems that truly support high-quality, cost-effective care.

ACKNOWLEDGMENT

The authors wish to acknowledge the contributions of Kathleen R. Stevens, Susan D. Horn, Jacob Kean, Vikrant G. Deshmukh, Sandra A. Mitchell, and Ramona Nelson to the previous edition of this chapter.

DISCUSSION QUESTIONS

1. Review the three categories of EBP models and discuss how these models might be used to guide the development of EBP.
2. Discuss why computerization is required if EBP is to become a reality in clinical settings.
3. How can the design of a healthcare information system support or thwart the use of EBP guidelines at the point of care? Give examples from your own experience, if possible.
4. Explore the AHRQ Health Care Innovations Exchange at www.innovations.ahrq.gov/index.aspx. Discuss how automation and informatics-based tools could be used to bring resources from this site to the point of care.
5. Analyze the following statement and determine whether you do or do not support it: "With the development of a fully integrated national health information system, big data reflecting patient outcomes will replace the role of research studies in developing EBP guidelines."
6. Why is the informatician a critical member of the PBE team? What essential skills should this team member have?
7. You are a member of a PBE team that will study the prevention and management of ventilator-associated pneumonia. Describe how you would apply the steps of PBE to this problem.

EBP CASE STUDY

You are consulting with the education and practice development team in a large tertiary care hospital serving a region comprised primarily rural communities. The team is responsible for strengthening the implementation of evidence-based practice (EBP) based on outcomes. Over the next 2 years, it must set performance objectives to (1) strengthen screening for pain, depression, and adverse health behaviors (smoking, excess alcohol intake, and body mass index [BMI] >30) at intake for all adult admissions; (2) implement comprehensive geriatric assessment for all those over age 65 hospitalized for more than seven days or readmitted within less than 3 days following discharge; and (3) promote care-team performance.

The hospital has 200 adult admissions each week and has implemented an electronic health record. Guideline dissemination generally occurs through educational venues or via the electronic policy and procedure manual. The method of documentation for narrative notes is documentation by exception using subjective, objective, assessment, and plan (SOAP), and the hospital has made extensive use of checklists to complement the documentation system.

Discussion Questions

1. Using clinical guidelines and standards of care, identify what data elements should be included in the electronic health record assessment and evaluation screens if these goals are to be achieved.
2. Identify how information system defaults and alerts could be used to achieve these goals.
3. Once screening has been improved, what are the next steps in improving patient outcomes?
4. How could the electronic health record be designed to support these outcome-related goals?

PBE CASE STUDY

Pressure Ulcer Case Study[a]

A PBE study involving 95 long-term care facilities in the United States determined that nursing interventions for pressure ulcer (PrU) prevention and management were highly variable among facilities. Nearly 30% of patients at risk for developing a PrU developed an ulcer during the 12-week study. Characteristics and interventions associated with a higher and lower likelihood of PrU development are summarized in the following table.

Research findings were used to develop PrU prevention protocols that included standardized documentation of important data elements and CDS tools. Four long-term care facilities that participated in the study and shared a common electronic health record (all members of the same provider network) took the first step in changing practice by sharing study findings with clinical staff, who spend the most one-on-one treatment time with nursing home residents and thus are often the first members of the care team to observe changes in residents' nutritional intake, urinary incontinence, and mood state. Concurrently, local study leaders worked with their software vendor to incorporate standard documentation for nurses and the CDS tools for staff.

Negative Association With Likelihood of Developing a Pressure Ulcer (Less Likely)

Patient factors
  Patient new to long-term care
Treatment factors
  Use of disposable briefs for urinary incontinence for >14 days
Nutrition
  Use of oral medical nutritional supplements for >21 days
  Tube feeding for >21 days
  IV fluid supplementation
Medications
  Antidepressant medication
Facility Staffing Patterns
  RN hours ≥0.5 h/resident/day
  CNA hours ≥2.25 h/resident/day
  LPN turnover rate <25%

Positive Association With Likelihood of Developing a Pressure Ulcer (More Likely)

Patient factors

Higher admission severity of illness

History of PrU in previous 90 days

Significant weight loss

Oral eating problems

Treatment factors

Use of urinary catheter

Use of positioning devices

Discussion Questions

1. What are the steps of the PBE process related to this case study?

2. As the health professional or informatics specialist working with the clinical team in the four long-term care facilities, identify the following:

a. Elements to incorporate into the documentation that address factors identified in the original study.

b. CDS tools that could be incorporated into computer systems.

3. How can the cost-effectiveness of the new documentation requirements and standards of care be efficiently evaluated?

---

[a]This case study is fictional; factors are consistent with findings reported in Sharkey, S., Hudak, S., Horn, S. D., & Spector, W. (2011). Leveraging certified nursing assistant documentation and knowledge to improve clinical decision making: The on-time quality improvement program to prevent pressure ulcers. *Advances in Skin & Wound Care, 24*(4), 182–188.

CNA, Clinical nursing assistant; *CDS,* clinical decision support; *IV,* Intravenous; *LPN,* licensed practical nurse; *PBE,* practice-based evidence; *PrU,* pressure ulcer; *RN,* registered nurse.

REFERENCES

Abernethy, A. P., Etheredge, L. M., Ganz, P. A., Wallace, P., German, R. R., Neti, C., Murphy, S. B. (2010). Rapid-learning system for cancer care. *Journal of Clinical Oncology: Official Journal of the American Society of Clinical Oncology, 28*(27), 4268–4274. https://doi.org/10.1200/JCO.2010.28.5478.

Accreditation Council for Graduate, (2020). *Medical Education (ACGME). Common program requirements.* Chicago, IL: ACGME;.

Agency for Healthcare Quality and Research (AHRQ). AHRQ National scorecard on hospital-acquired conditions final results for 2014 through 2017; July 2020. shorturl.at/eqxJU.

Agency for Healthcare Research and Quality (AHRQ), (October 25, 2021).https://www.ahrq.gov/innovations/index.html /; *AHRQ Health Care Innovations Exchange.* AHRQ.

Agency for Healthcare Research and Quality (AHRQ), (2021). *National Quality Measures Clearinghouse (NQMC).* Bethesda, MD: Agency for Healthcare Research and Quality;.

Agency for Healthcare Research and Quality, (2015). *The 2014 National Healthcare Quality & Disparities Report.* Rockville, MD: Agency for Healthcare Research and Quality. http://www.ahrq.gov/research/findings/nhqrdr/nhqdr14/index.html.

American Association of Colleges of Nursing (AACN), (2021). *The essentials: Core competencies for Professional Nursing Education.* Washington, DC: AACN;.

Amin, W., Tsui, F. R., Borromeo, C., et al. (2014). PaTH: Towards a learning health system in the Mid-Atlantic region. *Journal of the American Medical Informatics Association, 21*(4), 633–636.

Anderson, J. G., & Abrahamson, K. (2017). Your health care may kill you: Medical errors. *Studies in Health Technology and Informatics, 234,* 13–17.

Anderson, K. M., Marsh, C. A., Flemming, A. C., Isenstein, H., & Reynolds, J. (2012). *Quality measurement enabled by health IT: Overview, possibilities, and challenges.* Rockville, MD: Agency for Healthcare Research and Quality. [AHRQ Publication No. 12–0061-EF].

Appraisal of Guidelines, Research, and Evaluation (AGREE). About the AGREE Enterprise AGREE; 2010. http://www.agreetrust.org/.

Armstrong, R., Waters, E., Roberts, H., et al. (2006). The role and theoretical evolution of knowledge translation and exchange in public health. *Journal of Public Health, 28*(4), 384–389.

Averill, R. F., McGuire, T. E., Manning, B. E., et al. (1992). A study of the relationship between severity of illness and hospital cost in New Jersey hospitals. *Health Services Research, 27,* 587–606. discussion 607–612.

Baumbusch, J. L., Kirkham, S. R., Khan, K. B., et al. (2008). Pursuing common agendas: A collaborative model for knowledge translation between research and practice in clinical settings. *Research in Nursing & Health, 31*(2), 130–140.

Bornmann, L., & Mutz, R. (2015). Growth rates of modern science: A bibliometric analysis based on the number of publications and cited references. *Journal of the Association for Information Science and Technology, 66,* 2215–2222. https://doi.org/10.1002/asi.23329.2015.

Brachanicc, M., Tillier, W., & Dell, F. (2006). The Institute of Musculoskeletal Health and Arthritis (IMHA) Knowledge Exchange Task Force: An innovative approach to knowledge translation. *The Journal of the Canadian Chiropractic Association, 50*(1), 8–13.

Caban, T.Z., Chaney, K., & Rucker, D. ONC Releases National Health IT Priorities for Research: A Policy and Development Agenda; 2020. shorturl.at/pqAP0.

Carter, M. J., Fife, C. E., Walker, D., & Thomson, B. (2009). Estimating the applicability of wound care randomized controlled trials to general wound-care populations by estimating the percentage of individuals excluded from a typical wound-care population in such trials. *Advances in Skin & Wound Care, 22*(7), 316–324.

Center for Evidence-Based Medicine (CEBM), (October 27, 2021). *The 2011 Oxford CEBM Levels of Evidence: Introductory Document.* CEBM. http://www.cebm.net/wp-content/uploads/2014/06/CEBM-Levels-of-Evidence-Introduction-2.1.pdf

Clancy, C. M., & Cronin, K. (2005). Evidence-based decision making: Global evidence, local decisions. *Health Affairs, 24*(1), 151–162.

Clarivate. EndNote;2021. https://endnote.com/.

Clemmer, T. P., Spuhler, V. J., Oniki, T. A., & Horn, S. D. (1999). Results of a collaborative quality improvement program on outcomes and costs in a tertiary critical care unit. *Critical Care Medicine, 27,* 1768–1774.

Collins, S., Dykes, P., Bates, D. W., Couture, B., Rozenblum, R., Prey, J., Dalal, A. K. (2018). An informatics research agenda to support patient and family empowerment and engagement in care and recovery during and after hospitalization. *Journal of the American Medical Informatics Association, 25*(2), 206–209. https://doi.org/10.1093/jamia/ocx054.

Deutscher, D., Hart, D. L., Dickstein, R., Horn, S. D., & Gutvirtz, M. (2008). Implementing an integrated electronic outcomes and electronic health record process to create a foundation for clinical practice improvement. *Physical Therapy, 88*(2), 270–285.

Deutscher, D., Horn, S. D., Dickstein, R., et al. (2009). Associations between treatment processes, patient characteristics, and outcomes in outpatient physical therapy practice. *Archives of Physical Medicine and Rehabilitation, 90*(8), 1349–1363.

Doran, D. M., & Sidani, S. (2007). Outcomes-focused knowledge translation: A framework for knowledge translation and patient outcomes improvement. *Worldviews on Evidence-Based Nursing, 4*(1), 3–13.

Duvall, S. L., Fraser, A. M., Rowe, K., Thomas, A., & Mineau, G. P. (2012). Evaluation of record linkage between a large healthcare provider and the Utah Population Database. *Journal of the American Medical Informatics Association, 19*(e1), e54–e59.

Gassaway, J. V., Horn, S. D., DeJong, G., Smout, R. J., & Clark, C. (2005). Applying the clinical practice improvement approach to stroke rehabilitation: Methods used and baseline results. *Archives of Physical Medicine and Rehabilitation, 86*(12 suppl 2), S16–S33.

Graham, I. D., & Tetroe, J. (2007). Some theoretical underpinnings of knowledge translation. *Academic Emergency Medicine, 14*(11), 936–941.

Graham, I. D., Logan, J., Harrison, M. B., et al. (2006). Lost in knowledge translation: Time for a map? *The Journal of Continuing Education in the Health Professions, 26*, 13–24.

Green, L. W. (2008). Making research relevant: If it is an evidence-based practice, where's the practice-based evidence? *Family Practice, 25*(suppl 1), i20–i24.

Guise, J. M., Savitz, L. A., & Friedman, C. P. (2018 Dec.). Mind the gap: Putting evidence into practice in the era of learning health systems. *Journal of General Internal Medicine, 33*(12), 2237–2239. https://doi.org/10.1007/s11606-018-4633-1.

Harris, R. P., Helfand, M., Woolf, S. H., et al. (2001). REPRINT OF: Current methods of the U.S. Preventive Services Task Force: A review of the process. *American Journal of Preventive Medicine, 20*(suppl 3), 21–35.

Higgins, J.P. T., & Thomas, J., eds. Cochrane handbook for systematic reviews of interventions version 6.2. The Cochrane Collaboration; 2021. https://training.cochrane.org/handbook/current.

Horn, S. D., DeJong, G., et al. (2012). Practice-based evidence research in rehabilitation: An alternative to randomized controlled trials and traditional observational studies. *Archives of Physical Medicine and Rehabilitation, 93*(suppl 8), S127–S137.

Horn, S. D., & Gassaway, J. (2010). Practice based evidence: Incorporating clinical heterogeneity and patient-reported outcomes for comparative effectiveness research. *Medical Care, 48*(6 suppl 1), S17–S22.

Horn, S. D., & Gassaway, J. (2007). Practice-based evidence study design for comparative effectiveness research. *Medical Care, 45*(suppl 2), S50–S57.

Horn, S. D., DeJong, G., Ryser, D. K., Veazie, P. J., & Teraoka, J. (2005). Another look at observational studies in rehabilitation research: Going beyond the holy grail of the randomized controlled trial. *Archives of Physical Medicine and Rehabilitation, 86*(12 suppl 2), S8–S15.

Horn, S. D., Sharkey, P. D., Buckle, J. M., Backofen, J. E., Averill, R. F., & Horn, R. A. (1991). The relationship between severity of illness and hospital length of stay and mortality. *Medical Care, 29*, 305–317.

Horn, S. D., Sharkey, P. D., Kelly, H. W., & Uden, D. L. (2001). Newness of drugs and use of HMO services by asthma patients. *The Annals of Pharmacotherapy, 35*, 990–996.

Horn, S. D., Torres, A., Jr., Willson, D., Dean, J. M., Gassaway, J., & Smout, R. (2002). Development of a pediatric age- and disease-specific severity measure. *The Journal of Pediatrics, 141*, 496–503.

Hu, H., Correll, M., Kvecher, L., et al. (2011). DW4TR: A data warehouse for translational research. *Journal of Biomedical Informatics, 44*(6), 1004–1019.

Institute of Medicine (IOM), (2011). *Clinical practice guidelines we can trust*. Washington, DC: National Academies Press.

Institute of Medicine, (2001). *Crossing the quality chasm: A new health system for the 21st century*. Washington, DC: National Academies Press.

Institute of Medicine, (2008). *Knowing what works in health care: A roadmap for the Nation*. Washington, DC: National Academies Press.

Institute of Medicine., (2010). *The future of nursing: Focus on scope of practice*. Washington, DC: National Academies Press.

Institute of Medicine, (2000). *To err is human: Building a safer health system*. Washington, DC: National Academies Press.

James, J. T. (2013). A new, evidence-based estimate of patient harms associated with hospital care. *Journal of Patient Safety, 9*(3), 122–128. (2013). http://journals.lww.com/journalpatientsafety/Fulltext/2013/09000/A_New,_Evidence_based_Estimate_of_Patient_Harms.2.aspx.

Jarry, J. (August 27, 2021). *Medical error is not the third leading cause of death*. McGill Office for Science and Society. https://www.mcgill.ca/oss/article/critical-thinking-health/medical-error-not-third-leading-cause-death.

Kharrazi, H., Lasser, E. C., Yasnoff, W. A., Loonsk, J., Advani, A., Lehmann, H. P., Weiner, J. P. (2017). A proposed national research and development agenda for population health informatics: Summary recommendations from a national expert workshop. *Journal of the American Medical Informatics Association, 24*(1), 2–12. https://doi.org/10.1093/jamia/ocv210.

Kitson, A. L., Rycroft-Malone, J., Harvey, G., McCormack, B., Seers, K., & Titchen, A. (2008). Evaluating the successful implementation of evidence into practice using the PARiHS framework: Theoretical and practical challenges. *Implementation Science., 3*, 1.

Logan, J., & Graham, I. D. (1998). Toward a comprehensive interdisciplinary model of health care research use. *Science Communication, 20*(2), 227–246.

Makary, M. A., & Daniel, M. (2016). Medical error—the third leading cause of death in the US. *BMJ, 353*, i2489.

McCann, E. (July 18, 2014). *Deaths by medical mistakes hit records*. Healthcare IT News. http://www.healthcareitnews.com/news/deaths-by-medical-mistakes-hit-records.

Melnyk, B. M., Fineout-Overholt, E., & Mays, M. Z. (2008). The evidence-based practice beliefs and implementation scales: Psychometric properties of two new instruments. *Worldviews on Evidence-Based Nursing, 5*(4), 208–216.

Mennemeyer, S. T., Menachemi, N., Rahurkar, S., & Ford, E. W. (2016). Impact of the HITECH act on physicians' adoption of electronic health records. *Journal of the American Medical Informatics Association, 23*(2), 375–379. https://doi.org/10.1093/jamia/ocv103.

Mitchell, M., & Jolley, J. (2001). *Research design explained* (4th ed.). New York, NY: Harcourt.

Mitchell, S. A., Beck, S. L., Hood, L. E., Moore, K., & Tanner, E. R. (2009). Putting evidence into practice: evidence-based interventions for fatigue during and following cancer and its treatment. *Clinical Journal of Oncology Nursing, 11*(1), 99–113.

Mitchell, S. A., Fisher, C. A., Hastings, C. E., Silverman, L. B., & Wallen, G. R. (2010). A thematic analysis of theoretical models for translational science in nursing: Mapping the field. *Nursing Outlook, 58*(6), 287–300.

Mitton, C., Adair, C. E., McKenzie, E., Patten, S. B., & Perry, B. W. (2007). Knowledge transfer and exchange: review and synthesis of the literature. *The Milbank Quarterly, 85*(4), 729–768.

National Quality Forum (NQF). http://www.qualityforum.org/Home. aspx. Accessed March 17, 2016.

Newhouse, R. P., Dearholt, S. L., Poe, S. S., Pugh, L. C., & White, K. M. (2007). *Johns Hopkins nursing evidence-based practice model and guidelines*. New York, NY: Sigma Theta Tau International Honor Society of Nursing.

Office of the National Coordinator for Health Information Technology Office of the Secretary. 2020-2025 Federal Health IT Strategic Plan; 2020. shorturl.at/mzGIJ.

Oncology Nursing Society (ONS), (June 19, 2015). *Putting evidence into practice*. ONS. https://www.ons.org/sites/default/files/Using%20the%20PEP%20website.pdf.

Rosenbaum, P. R. (2002). *Observational studies*. New York, NY: Springer.

Rycroft-Malone, J. (2004). The PARiHS framework—a framework for guiding the implementation of evidence-based practice. *Journal of Nursing Care Quality, 19*(4), 297–304.

Rycroft-Malone, J., Kitson, A., Harvey, G., et al. (2002). Ingredients for change: revisiting a conceptual framework. *Quality & Safety in Health Care, 11*(2), 174–180.

Ryser, D. K., Egger, M. J., Horn, S. D., Handrahan, D., Gandhi, P., & Bigler, E. D. (2005). Measuring medical complexity during inpatient rehabilitation after traumatic brain injury. *Archives of Physical Medicine and Rehabilitation, 86*, 1108–1117.

Shrank, W. H., Rogstad, T. L., & Parekh, N. (2019). Waste in the US health care system: Estimated costs and potential for savings. *JAMA, 322*(15), 1501–1509. https://doi.org/10.1001/jama.2019.13978.

Slattery, M. L., & Kerber, R. A. (1993). A comprehensive evaluation of family history and breast cancer risk. The Utah Population Database. *JAMA., 270*(13), 1563–1568.

Smoyer, W. E., Embi, P. J., & Moffatt-Bruce, S. (2016). Creating local learning health systems: Think globally, act locally. *JAMA, 316*(23), 2481–2482. https://doi.org/10.1001/jama.2016.16459.

Spyns, P. (1996). Natural language processing in medicine: An overview. *Methods of Information in Medicine, 35*(4), 285–301.

Stetler, C. B., Ritchie, J., Rycroft-Malone, J., Schultz, A., & Charns, M. (2007). Improving quality of care through routine, successful implementation of evidence-based practice at the bedside: An organizational case study protocol using the Pettigrew and Whipp model of strategic change. *Implementation Science, 2*(1), 3.

Stevens, K. R. (2015). *Stevens star model of EBP: Knowledge transformation*. San Antonio, TX: Academic Center for Evidence-Based Practice, University of Texas Health Science Center in San Antonio.

Stevens, K. R., & Staley, J. M. (2006). The Quality Chasm reports, evidence-based practice, and nursing's response to improve healthcare. *Nursing Outlook, 54*(2), 94–101.

Stevens, K. R., McDuffie, K., & Clutter, P. C. (2009). Research and the mandate for evidence-based practice, quality, and patient safety. In M. A. Mateo & K. T. Kirchhoff (Eds.), *Research for advanced practice nurses: From evidence to practice* (pp. 43–70). New York, NY: Springer Publishing Company. [Chapter 3].

Swinburn, B., Gill, T., & Kumanyika, S. (2005). Obesity prevention: A proposed framework for translating evidence into action. *Obesity Reviews, 6*(1), 23–33.

TeamSTEPPSfi, (April 2015). *National implementation*. Rockville, MD: Agency for Healthcare Research and Quality;. http://www.ahrq.gov/professionals/education/curriculum-tools/teamstepps/national-meeting/index.html.

The Cochrane Collaboration. The Cochrane Database of Systematic Reviews; 2016. http://www.cochranelibrary.com/cochrane-database-of-systematic-reviews/index.html.

Titler, M. G., Kleiber, C., Steelman, V. J., et al. (2001). The Iowa model of evidence-based practice to promote quality care. *Critical Care Nursing Clinics of North America, 13*(4), 497–509.

US Preventive Services Task Force (USPSTF). US Preventive Services Task Force ratings USPSTF; 2021. http://uspreventiveservicestaskforce.org/uspstf07/ratingsv2.htm.

Vratny, A., & Shriver, D. (2007). A conceptual model for growing evidence-based practice. *Nursing Administration Quarterly., 31*, 162–170.

Wandersman, A., Duffy, J., Flaspohler, P., et al. (2008). Bridging the gap between prevention research and practice: The interactive systems framework for dissemination and implementation. *American Journal of Community Psychology, 41*(3-4), 171–181.

Weiner, B. J., Lewis, M. A., & Linnan, L. A. (2009). Using organization theory to understand the determinants of effective implementation of worksite health promotion programs. *Health Education Research, 24*(2), 292–305.

Weir, C., Staggers, N., & Laukert, T. (2012). Reviewing the impact of computerized provider order entry on clinical outcomes: The quality of systematic reviews. *International Journal of Medical Informatics, 81*, 219–231.

Weir, C., Staggers, N., & Phansalkar, S. (2009). The state of the evidence for computerized provider order entry: A systematic review and analysis of the quality of the literature. *International Journal of Medical Informatics, 78*(6), 365–374.

Williams, M. S., Buchanan, A. H., Davis, F. D., et al. (2018 Mayy). Patient-centered precision health in a learning health care system: Geisinger's genomic medicine experience. *Health Affairs (Millwood), 37*(5), 757–764. https://doi.org/10.1377/hlthaff.2017.1557.

Willson, D. F., Horn, S. D., Smout, R., Gassaway, J., & Torres, A. (2000). Severity assessment in children hospitalized with bronchiolitis using the pediatric component of the Comprehensive Severity Index. *Pediatric Critical Care Medicine, 1*, 127–132.

Zayas-Cabán, T., Chaney, K. J., & Rucker, D. W. (2020). National health information technology priorities for research: A policy and development agenda. *Journal of the American Medical Informatics Association, 27*(4), 652–657. https://doi.org/10.1093/jamia/ocaa008.

12

Clinical Decision Support

Kensaku Kawamoto and Guilherme Del Fiol

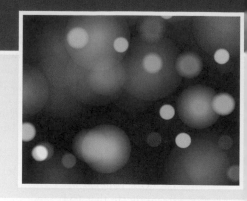

OBJECTIVES

At the completion of this chapter, the reader will be prepared to:
1. Summarize key components of clinical decision support.
2. Describe the history of clinical decision support.
3. Give examples of each type of clinical decision support.
4. Summarize the impact of clinical decision support.
5. Outline key considerations of widespread clinical decision support adoption.
6. Describe best practices for clinical decision support.
7. Outline recent progress toward disseminating clinical decision support on a national level.

KEY TERMS

Bayesian knowledge base, 189
clinical decision support (CDS), 188

decision-making, 188
expert system, 193

ABSTRACT ❖

Clinical decision support (CDS) is a key component of a variety of health information systems and a core component of electronic health record (EHR) systems. CDS systems can support effective clinical decision-making and improve clinical care by providing the right information to the right person at the right time and at the right location. CDS, encompassing various types of intervention modalities, has been shown to be effective for many decades. Important considerations in implementing CDS systems include the application of best practices and the incorporation of knowledge management capabilities. Despite its benefits, significant challenges limit the widespread adoption and impact of CDS. These challenges include a healthcare payment model that has traditionally rewarded volume over quality and the difficulty of scaling CDS capabilities across healthcare systems and their information systems. There has been significant progress in recent years on the development and adoption of standards-based approaches to enabling the deployment of advanced CDS at scale, that is, across a large number of clinical sites, health information technology (IT) platforms, and clinical domains. A future need exists to capitalize on these promising approaches to make advanced CDS available on a national scale.

INTRODUCTION

One original and central goal of leveraging IT in medicine has been to help clinicians in their **decision-making** process to prevent errors, maximize efficiency, enable evidence-based care, and ultimately to improve health and healthcare. Various cognitive limitations can lead to suboptimal clinical decision-making, but tools can be used to help overcome such limitations in human cognition (Morris, 2018). Tools that support the clinical decision-making process have been generally designated as **clinical decision support (CDS)** systems over time.

A systematic review concluded that approximately 22,000 preventable deaths occur each year in inpatient settings due to medical errors (Rodwin et al., 2020). Moreover, many more patients experience harm from preventable medical errors that do not lead to death (Panagioti et al., 2019). A landmark study by McGlynn et al. showed that, on average, patients in the United States receive only 54.9% of recommended medical care processes (McGlynn et al., 2003). More recent studies have shown that such care-quality issues persist (Levine et al., 2016).

Errors in healthcare are caused to a great extent by process errors, information overload, and knowledge gaps (Institute of

Medicine IOM, 1999; Leape et al., 1995). Several factors further aggravate this problem, including rapidly evolving domain knowledge, an aging population having multiple comorbidities, and an increasingly complex healthcare delivery system. Ultimately, this leads to a clinical information overload that significantly exceeds human cognitive capacity (Stead et al., 2011; Smith, 2010).

Many healthcare errors are preventable, particularly through process-improvement measures enabled by computerized information systems coupled with CDS tools. In fact, a large number of studies indicate that CDS tools help clinicians and patients adopt evidence-based care whenever applicable (Kawamoto & McDonald, 2020a). As a result, several relevant reports and regulations have called for the use of health IT to support healthcare decision-making, such as the report from the National Academy of Medicine (NAM) on *Crossing the Quality Chasm*, (Institute of Medicine [IOM], 2001) the National Quality Forum's (NQF's) *Driving Quality and Performance Measurement—A Foundation for Clinical Decision Support*, (National Quality Forum [NQF], 2010) the United States EHR Meaningful Use incentive program, (Jha, 2010) the IOM's *The Future of Nursing: Leading Change, Advancing Health*, (Institute of Medicine [IOM], 2010) and the NAM's report on optimizing strategies for CDS (Tcheng et al., 2017).

DEFINITION OF CLINICAL DECISION SUPPORT

Scope of Definitions

Multiple definitions of CDS have been proposed, but in general, these definitions have evolved from a narrow scope, typically focused on alerts and reminders, to a broader scope that encompasses a much wider set of tools that provide patient-specific information to support clinical decision-making. According to Osheroff, CDS comprises a variety of tools and interventions that "provide clinicians, staff, patients, or other individuals with knowledge and person-specific information, intelligently filtered or presented at appropriate times, to enhance health and health care." (Osheroff et al., 2007, p. 141). Similarly, the NQF defined CDS as "any tool or technique that enhances decision-making by clinicians, patients, or their surrogates in the delivery or management of health care." (National Quality Forum [NQF], 2010, p. 1).

Clinical Decision Support and Patient Care

In light of these definitions, CDS can support several aspects of patient care decision-making such as the following:
Passively reminding about a specific care need (e.g., patient due for an immunization or cancer screening).

Providing an interruptive alert about a specific care action that may impose risk to the patient (e.g., a drug interaction).

Providing intelligent views of a patient's record that help cultivate a better understanding of the patient's status and needed care (e.g., intensive care reports, chronic disease management dashboards).

Providing tools that assist in implementing and documenting decisions more efficiently and accurately (e.g., documentation tools, order sets, medication reconciliation tools).

Providing clinicians and patients with seamless access to patient-specific provider reference information and patient education available in online knowledge resources.

Providing access to information about similar patients in the population along with their treatments and outcomes.

Integrating information from nontraditional sources into the clinical workflow, such as patient self-reported outcomes, data collected via wearable sensors, and patient dietary information, as well as relevant data about the patient's environment, such as air pollution and infectious disease rates.

Applying advanced analytics to estimate risks for a specific individual, such as risk for hospital readmissions, risk for cardiovascular events, risk for falls, and risk for hereditary cancers.

HISTORY

The first studies demonstrating the impact of CDS were published in the early 1970s by groups at the Regenstrief Institute in Indiana and the Latter-Day Saints (LDS) Hospital in Salt Lake City. These early studies established CDS as one of the foundational components of health informatics. These examples of CDS, designed more than 4 to 5 decades ago, are still relevant and influence the design of today's CDS tools.

De Dombal Computer-Aided Diagnosis of Acute Abdominal Pain

According to a systematic review by Johnston et al., (Johnston et al., 1994) the first study to compare CDS with clinician performance was published in 1972 by de Dombal et al. on the diagnosis of acute abdominal pain (de Dombal et al., 1972). The system, comprised of a Bayesian knowledge base, provided diagnostic probabilities as output (Horrocks et al., 1972). The system was evaluated over the course of 11 months by comparing the diagnostic accuracy of a physician with that of a computer-aided diagnostic system for patients admitted with a diagnosis of acute abdominal pain (de Dombal et al., 1972). The system's overall diagnostic accuracy was significantly higher than the most senior member of the clinical team (91.8% vs. 79.6%). The results of this seminal study demonstrated the strong potential of using computers to assist decision-making for patient care.

Computer Reminders at Regenstrief Institute

A seminal randomized trial assessing the impact of a broad CDS intervention was published in 1976 by McDonald (1976). This study, conducted by physicians at the Regenstrief Institute, received patient-specific reminders about 390 patient management protocols on a myriad of clinical conditions. These reminders were computer-generated based on the patients' EHR and logic encoded in computable form. Applicable reminders were printed and attached to the patient's chart when a patient had a clinic visit. The study showed that physicians reacted to

51% of the events when exposed to reminders versus 21% when not exposed to reminders.

Clinical Decision Support Examples From the Health Evaluation Through Logical Processing System

A comprehensive set of CDS examples is provided by the Health Evaluation Through Logical Processing (HELP) System, a clinical information system developed in the late 1960s and used throughout the 21st century at the LDS Hospital in Salt Lake City, Utah (Haug et al., 1994). The HELP System included a broad range of CDS tools classified into the following four categories:

1. *Alerts* as a response to the presence of certain clinical data, such as life-threatening laboratory test results.
2. Tools that *critique* clinicians' decisions, such as the presence of drug interactions in medication orders.
3. Tools that provide on-demand diagnostic or therapeutic *suggestions*, such as computer protocols for ventilator management and antiinfective selection assistance.
4. *Retrospective* quality assurance tools.

Several of these CDS tools demonstrated a significant impact on clinicians' decisions and patient outcomes, such as appropriate use of perioperative antibiotics, reduced postoperative wound infections, reduced hospital length of stay when clinicians received alerts for life-threatening conditions, and increased survival rate in patients with acute respiratory distress syndrome (ARDS) when computer protocols were utilized for ventilator management. A compendium of the HELP CDS tools and a summary of the effects of these tools on clinicians' decisions and patient outcomes are available in an article by Haug et al. (1994).

CLINICAL DECISION SUPPORT TYPES AND EXAMPLES

Several taxonomies have been developed to systematically classify CDS systems. One taxonomy was developed by the NQF as an extension of a functional taxonomy developed by researchers affiliated with the Harvard Medical School (Wright et al., 2007). The taxonomy is composed of four functional categories: triggers, input data, interventions, and action steps. *Triggers* are the events that initiate a CDS rule (e.g., a drug prescription). According to the NQF taxonomy, CDS can be triggered by an explicit request from a user, updates to a patient's data, user interactions with an EHR system, or a specific time. *Input data* are the additional data used in the background to constrain or modify the CDS, such as patient conditions, medications, diagnostic tests, or the care plan. *Interventions* are the possible actions that result from the CDS system, such as sending a message to a clinician, displaying relevant clinical knowledge or patient information, and logging that a particular event took place. *Action steps* are actionable alternatives offered to the CDS user, such as collecting or documenting information (e.g., reason to override an alert, completion of care recommended by CDS), requesting an order, submitting a referral, or acknowledging a CDS

recommendation. The complete NQF taxonomy is available in the NQF consensus report, *Driving Quality and Performance Measurement—A Foundation for Clinical Decision Support* (National Quality Forum [NQF], 2010).

One of the most comprehensive taxonomies was developed by Wright et al. using a Delphi method with 11 CDS experts (Wright et al., 2011). The taxonomy classifies CDS types from the user ("front end") perspective into six overarching categories: medication dosing support, order facilitators, point-of-care alerts and reminders, relevant information display, expert systems, and workflow support. Each of these categories is broken down into subtypes, leading to a total of 53 CDS types. The following sections describe each of the six overarching categories and provide real-life examples. A brief summary of these CDS types and examples is provided in Table 12.1.

Medication Dosing Support

This category includes tools that assist clinicians in finding and monitoring the most appropriate doses for medication orders. Tools vary from simple "pick lists" with allowed dose options to more complex dose calculation algorithms (Ferranti et al., 2011) based on parameters such as patient weight, height, renal function, and hepatic function. Researchers at Brigham and Women's Hospital designed several medication dosing support tools for a broad range of medications within their computerized provider order entry (CPOE) system (Bates et al., 1999).

Order Facilitators

Order facilitators, which are broader than medication dosing support tools, are tools that assist clinicians in the order entry process in general. Order sets are perhaps the most common examples in this category (Del Fiol et al., 2005). They assist clinicians by providing a set of commonly used orders for a wide range of clinical situations such as a specific condition (e.g., community-acquired pneumonia) or service (e.g., internal medicine hospital admission orders, vascular surgery postoperative orders) (Miller

TABLE 12.1 Clinical Decision Support Types and Examples

CDS Type	Examples
Medication dosing support	Tool that facilitates dose calculation based on parameters such as patient weight, height, renal function, and hepatic function
Order facilitator	Order set for community-acquired pneumonia (see Fig. 12.1)
Point-of-care alerts and reminders	Patient care reminders (see Fig. 12.2) and drug-drug interaction alerts (see Fig. 12.3) provided within the her
Relevant information display	Disease management dashboard (see Fig. 12.4), Infobuttons with links to relevant information on medications (see Fig. 12.6)
Expert system	Diagnostic decision support system
Workflow support	EHR documentation template

CDS, Clinical decision support; *EHR*, electronic health record.

et al., 2020; Stilos et al., 2019; Cimic et al., 2020; Horton et al., 2020; Rubins et al., 2019; Muniga et al., 2020; Best et al., 2011; Bornstein et al., 2020). Order sets not only expedite the order entry process; they may also help reduce errors and promote evidence-based care (Muniga et al., 2020; Best et al., 2011) by reducing unnecessary variability, reducing inappropriate care, (Horton et al., 2020; Bornstein et al., 2020) enabling more complete orders, and reducing the need for verbal orders. Order sets are a commonly available form of Cherin EHR and CPOE systems (Wright et al., 2007; McGreevey, 2013). Fig. 12.1 depicts a sample community-acquired pneumonia order set from the HELP2 system at Intermountain Healthcare (Del Fiol et al., 2005).

Point-of-Care Alerts and Reminders

Point-of-care alerts and reminders raise the clinician's or patient's attention to important conditions or recommendations based on the patient's clinical data. One of the most common types of CDS, available for most EHR systems, is an alert that notifies clinicians when a drug being prescribed interacts with other drugs the patient is already receiving. Similar examples include duplicate therapy alerts, drug allergy alerts, and an alert when a patient's condition contraindicates the use of a particular drug. Reminders are similar to alerts and are designed to bring attention to a particular patient's need to receive certain care, such as immunizations, cancer screening, fall prevention, and pain assessment. Fig. 12.2 shows a set of patient care reminders generated by the VistA EHR system at the Veterans Health Administration (VHA).

Alerts have been shown to significantly reduce errors when designed appropriately (Bates et al., 1999). However, overuse of the alert mechanism may lead to a problem known as alert fatigue, where clinicians tend to ignore alerts because they trigger too frequently, are not relevant to the patient, are not displayed at the most appropriate time to influence a provider's decision, and do not provide clinically actionable information (Ash et al., 2007; McCoy et al., 2014). Fig. 12.3 illustrates one way in which drug-drug interaction alerts may be presented without interrupting clinicians' workflow as an attempt to minimize alert fatigue. Other approaches to reducing alert fatigue include prioritizing alerts deemed to be most important (Daniels et al., 2019); organizing alert display (Heringa et al., 2017); improving the precision of the alert logic through contextual information about the patient, healthcare provider, and care setting to prevent nonrelevant alerts (Duke & Bolchini, 2011; Chou et al., 2021); implementing institutional CDS governance (Kawamoto et al., 2018); and employing predictive analytics to filter out alerts that are likely to be ignored (Liu S et al., 2022).

Relevant Information Display

A different category of CDS addresses clinicians' information overload in the process of care with regard to both patient information

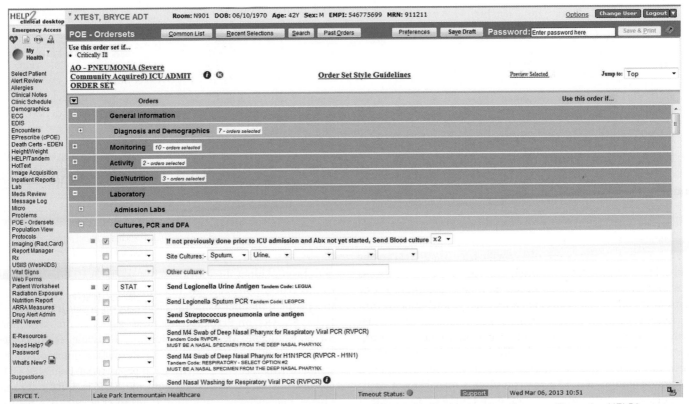

Fig. 12.1 Computerized provider order entry (CPOE) system with a community-acquired pneumonia order set. (From the HELP2 system at Intermountain Healthcare, Salt Lake City.)

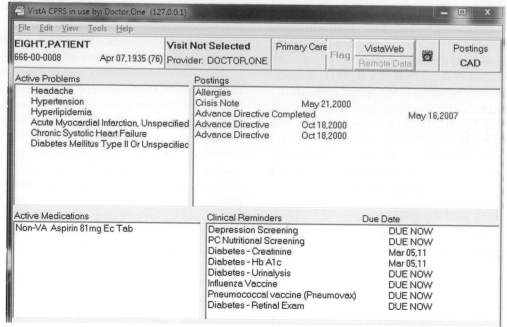

Fig. 12.2 A set of care reminders (bottom right of screen) presented within the VHA's VistA Computerized Patient Record System. (Copyright Veterans Health Administration. All Rights Reserved.)

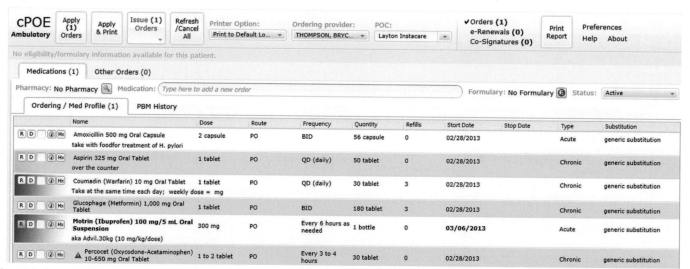

Fig. 12.3 A medication prescription system coupled with noninterruptive drug interaction checking. Pairs of interacting drugs are color-highlighted. Different colors denote different levels of interaction severity. The figure also shows Infobutton links adjacent to each drug that clinicians can click to retrieve context-specific information. *cPOE*, Computerized provider order entry. (From the HELP2 system at Intermountain Healthcare, Salt Lake City.)

and domain knowledge. This broad category includes CDS tools that provide seamless access to relevant patient information or summarize prominent aspects of a patient's record to help clinicians understand the patient's condition and status. Intensive care daily reports that assist clinicians in patient rounds are examples of such tools. Another example is that of disease management dashboards that summarize relevant data for managing a specific condition. Fig. 12.4 shows a disease management dashboard developed at Duke University to assist the management of patients with chronic conditions such as diabetes, hypertension,

and chronic kidney disease (Lobach et al., 2007). CDS applications of this type are increasingly implemented in an EHR platform-independent manner using the Health Level Seven International (HL7) SMART on FHIR (pronounced "smart on fire" and short for Substitutable Medical Applications Reusable Technologies on Fast Healthcare Interoperability Resources) interoperability standard (Mandel et al., 2016). Example SMART on FHIR CDS applications deeply integrated with the EHR include a chronic disease management application (Curran et al., 2020), a neonatal bilirubin management application (Kawamoto et al., 2019),

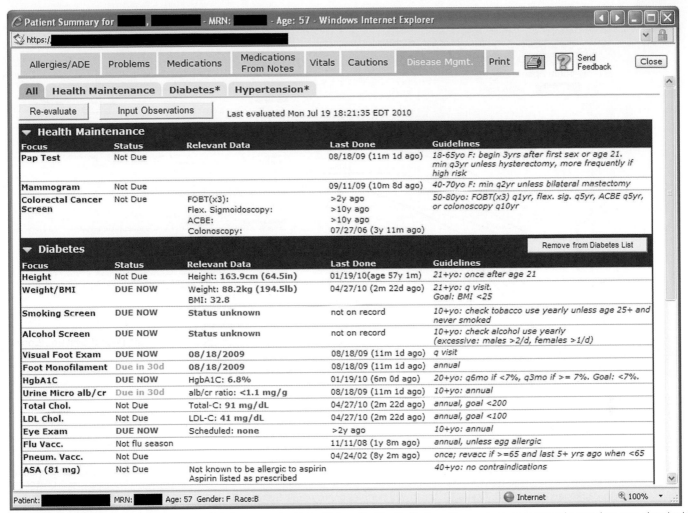

Fig. 12.4 Chronic disease management module in use at the Duke University Health System. The system presents relevant data associated with evidence-based care recommendations. (Copyright Duke University Health System. All Rights Reserved.)

and a pediatric patient summary to support the care of complex patients (Borbolla et al., 2021), all developed at the University of Utah. A screenshot from the bilirubin application is shown in Fig. 12.5 (Kawamoto et al., 2019).

In addition to the need for seamless access to relevant patient information, clinicians frequently raise domain knowledge questions when making patient care decisions. Research has shown that clinicians raise about two questions for every three patients seen and that more than half of these questions go unanswered (Covell et al., 1985; Del Fiol et al., 2014). Multiple online health knowledge resources are accessible through desktop and mobile devices. Although these resources provide answers to most of the clinicians' questions, significant barriers limit their use at the point of care, such as lack of time in busy clinical workflows, lack of seamless access to resources that directly address clinical questions, and the perception that a clinically useful answer is not available (Del Fiol et al., 2014). Researchers have been attempting to reduce barriers to accessing these resources within EHR systems through an approach to CDS known as "Infobuttons" (Cimino et al., 1997). Infobuttons leverage contextual attributes about the patient, clinician, care setting, and clinical task at hand within an EHR. They also anticipate clinicians' information

needs, and provide automated links to relevant online knowledge resources. For example, a physician prescribing a medication for a patient who has chronic kidney disease might want to know if the medication is contraindicated or if its dose needs to be adjusted based on the patient's condition. An Infobutton positioned beside the drug name within the EHR would provide access to this kind of information from an external drug knowledge resource. Fig. 12.6 shows an example of Infobuttons within the HELP2 drug prescription module deployed at Intermountain Healthcare (Del Fiol et al., 2008). A systematic review of studies reviewing the effect of infobuttons on providers found that Infobuttons answered clinicians' clinical questions in over 69% of infobutton sessions, leading to changes in patient care decisions, learning, and provider confidence (Cook et al., 2017).

Expert Systems

Expert systems provide diagnostic or therapeutic advice based on patient parameters. They typically contain more sophisticated computer logic than other forms of CDS and are less frequently found in commercial EHR systems (Wright et al., 2011). The term *expert system* within informatics is also used to classify computerized systems that go beyond decision support and

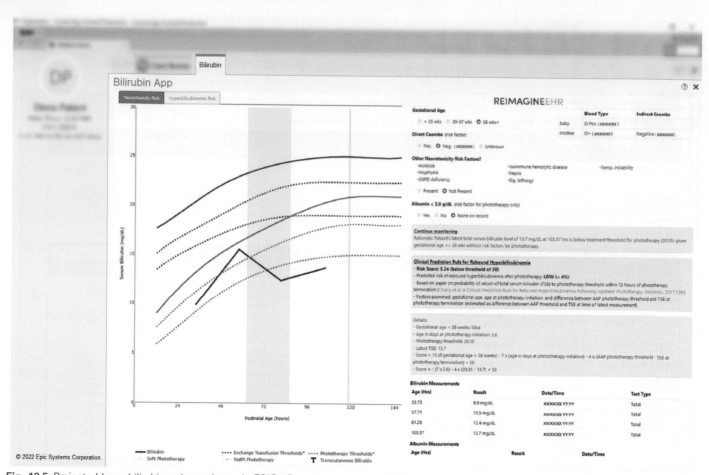

Fig. 12.5 Projected hyperbilirubinemia as shown in EPIC. (From Kawamoto, K., Kukhareva, P., & Shakib, J. H. [2019]. Association of an electronic health record add-on app for neonatal Bilirubin management with physician efficiency and care quality. *JAMA Network Open, 2*[11], e1915343. doi:10.1001/jamanetworkopen.2019.15343. Figure 1B. Used with permission from Epic Systems Corp.)

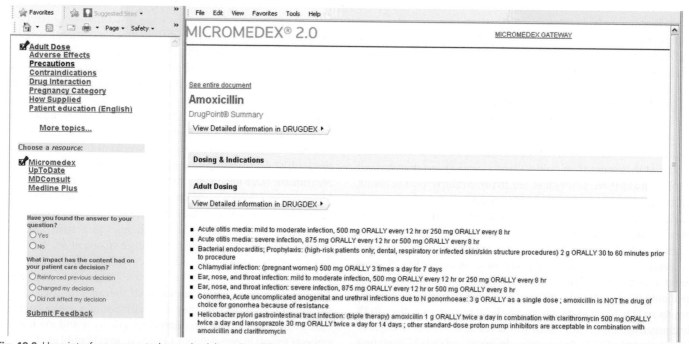

Fig. 12.6 User interface presented to a physician who clicks an Infobutton beside the drug amoxicillin, when prescribed to an adult patient. The left side has a navigation panel with automated context-specific links to relevant resources. The right side contains the content itself, which was retrieved from external online resources. (Truven Health Analytics Inc. and Intermountain Healthcare. All Rights Reserved.)

actually automate the decision-making process. This use of the term is described in Chapter 2.

The antibiotic assistant and ventilator management protocols described in the section titled "CDS Examples" from the HELP System are examples of this category of CDS. Another example is that of diagnostic decision support systems such as Iliad (Warner & Bouhaddou, 1994), Quick Medical Reference (QMR) (Bankowitz et al., 1989), and Dxplain (Barnett et al., 1987; Elkin et al., 2010). These systems propose a list of candidate diagnoses based on a patient's signs and symptoms. Although diagnostic CDS tools have achieved a quite reasonable level of diagnostic accuracy, especially for differential diagnoses (Berner et al., 1994), their use has often been limited to educational purposes (Lange et al., 1997; Miller & Masarie, 1989). More recently, advances in machine learning (ML) methods, especially deep learning, have enabled a different range of diagnostic CDS, particularly focused on imaging. Studies have shown ML-based methods to outperform other techniques and human experts on a wide range of image modalities and clinical scenarios such as diagnosis of melanoma, retinopathy, and differential diagnosis (Krittanawong et al., 2017; Liu et al., 2018; Levine et al., 2019; Balyen & Peto, 2019; Akkus et al., 2019).

Workflow Support

The last category of CDS tools comprises tools that aid in important steps of the patient care workflow, such as care transitions, patient documentation, and orders. These workflow steps are susceptible to various types of errors and inefficiencies that can be tackled with CDS. For example, medication errors in care transitions can be prevented with medication reconciliation tools (Bassi et al., 2010; Rungvivatjarus et al., 2020); structured documentation templates may facilitate consistent and efficient documentation (Rosenbloom et al., 2011); and automatic steps in the ordering workflow, such as order approval, routing, and termination, may improve the overall efficiency and safety of the ordering process (Buising et al., 2008; Topal et al., 2005; Youngerman et al., 2018).

CLINICAL DECISION SUPPORT IMPACT

Evidence of Effectiveness

Numerous research studies have evaluated the impact of CDS. Systematic reviews and meta-analyses of CDS clinical trials have found that CDS can improve care in a variety of areas, such as for performing preventive care (Bright et al., 2012), ordering clinical studies (Bright et al., 2012; Goldzweig et al., 2015), prescribing medications and other therapies (Bright et al., 2012; Page et al., 2017; Curtis et al., 2017), reducing morbidity and mortality (Curtis et al., 2017; Varghese et al., 2018), helping answer clinicians' clinical questions (Cook et al., 2017), and reducing life-threatening as well as non-life-threatening adverse events in the hospital (Varghese et al., 2018; Borab et al., 2017). Improved practitioner performance is not always associated with a statistically significant improvement in patient outcomes, at least in part because studies of CDS interventions often lack large sample sizes and the associated statistical power required to reliably identify improvements in patient outcome metrics (Kawamoto & McDonald, 2020b).

Examples of Clinical Decision Support Impact Studies

As one classic example of a CDS intervention resulting in positive outcomes, a study at Brigham and Women's Hospital in Boston found that a CPOE system with various CDS capabilities reduced nonintercepted serious medication errors by 86%, with increasing benefits seen with the introduction of additional CDS capabilities (Bates et al., 1999). In another classic example, also described in the section titled "CDS Examples" from the HELP System, the use of a rule-based CDS system for the mechanical ventilation of patients with ARDS resulted in a 60% survival rate, compared to an expected survival rate of approximately 35% (Thomsen et al., 1993). In another example, the impact of the antibiotic assistant developed by Evans et al. was assessed in a pre-post study. Use of the antibiotic assistant led to significant improvements in a variety of clinical measures, including antibiotic-susceptibility mismatches and adverse events caused by antiinfective agents (Evans et al., 1998). Moreover, patients who received antiinfective therapy according to the regimens recommended by the CDS system had a significantly reduced length of stay (10.0 days vs. 16.7 days, $P < .001$) and significantly lower total hospital costs ($26,315 vs. $44,865, $P < .001$) compared to patients who were not managed according to the CDS system's recommendations (Evans et al., 1998).

Not all CDS interventions result in the desired outcomes, however. For example, in a randomized controlled trial, involving 29 health centers, an external CDS system for diabetes management that was accessible through the EHR system did not result in any clinically significant changes in practitioner performance or patient outcomes (Hetlevik et al., 2000). In another example, a stand-alone CDS system designed to guide referrals for patients at increased risk for hereditary breast cancer was found to have limited impact in a randomized controlled trial involving 86 primary care practices, primarily due to the limited use of the tool by clinicians (Wilson et al., 2006). Last, a randomized controlled trial involving 60 primary care practices found no significant impact when a CDS system for asthma and angina management was made available to intervention clinicians as a separate path within their practices' EHR systems (Eccles et al., 2002). More recently, a systematic review of 236 evaluating the effects of health information technology interventions found mixed results, with 56% of the studies reporting consistently positive outcomes (Jones et al., 2014).

Financial Impact of Clinical Decision Support

Healthcare institutions should, as with any investment, consider the expected financial impact when making decisions related to CDS investment (Kawamoto & McDonald, 2020b). To the extent that CDS can facilitate desired changes in clinical practice patterns and patient outcomes, CDS can lead to positive returns on investment, for example, by reducing medical errors and lengths of stay. The VHA estimated that its health IT investments have resulted in more than $3 billion in net benefits, with CDS serving as an important catalyst for the return on investment (Byrne et al., 2010). CDS, in this analysis, provided a financial return on investment to the VHA in reduced costs related to preventable adverse drug events, avoided admissions, and redundant or unnecessary laboratory and radiology tests (Chaudhry et al., 2006). Conversely, several systematic reviews on CDS interventions for various clinical problems and healthcare domains have not been able to conclude whether CDS is cost-effective, both due to the paucity of and important limitations in studies that assess cost-effectiveness (Jacob et al., 2017; Mackintosh et al., 2016; Fillmore et al., 2013; Main et al., 2010; Roshanov et al., 2011).

It is important to recognize that the financial benefits of CDS may accrue to stakeholders other than those investing in CDS, when assessing the financial impact of CDS. For instance, if a healthcare delivery organization invests in CDS to support influenza and pneumococcal vaccinations and the rate of hospitalizations for these conditions decreases, the organization may lose money because of the decrease in revenue-generating hospitalizations, whereas society, patients, and health insurers would likely benefit from the investment. In another example, if a healthcare delivery organization invests in CDS systems to ensure that low back pain results in expensive diagnostic imaging and surgical procedures only when clearly warranted, it may lose money because of the decrease in revenue-generating radiologic exams and surgeries; again, society, patients, and health insurers would likely benefit from the investment. Thus, when assessing the financial impact of CDS, it is important to assess the impact in terms of the different stakeholders involved, particularly patients, healthcare delivery organizations, and health insurers.

The financial incentives of the major stakeholder groups may align well in the case of organizations such as the VHA that serve as both a healthcare delivery organization and a health insurer. Other health organizations' incentives do not align as well, but, as discussed later, healthcare payment models are increasingly changing toward models in which the financial incentives of the key stakeholders are better aligned. Currently, however, because of the healthcare payment models in the United States, the issue of misaligned financial incentives will likely continue to be an important issue in the financial case for CDS.

CLINICAL DECISION SUPPORT ADOPTION

Current Adoption Status

Despite five decades of substantial evidence demonstrating the ability of well-implemented CDS to improve practitioner performance and patient outcomes, along with almost universal adoption of EHR systems in the United States, (Henry et al., 2016) most commercial EHR systems and healthcare delivery organizations in the United States have implemented CDS for only a small fraction of the clinical decisions and care processes for which CDS could provide meaningful support (Tcheng et al., 2017). Hence, the broad dissemination of CDS remains one of the most significant challenges and prominent areas of research in healthcare informatics.

Challenges and Barriers to Clinical Decision Support Adoption

The dissemination of CDS is limited by a significant set of barriers, which collectively make CDS interventions not easily replicable. Some prominent barriers include the following:

- *Lack of incentives:* As discussed earlier, a key reason for the limited adoption of CDS is a healthcare payment model that often fails to reward the provision of higher quality care and, therefore, investments in quality-enhancing technologies such as CDS.

- *Implementation challenges:* Like with any healthcare quality improvement intervention, CDS requires a well-designed implementation approach to be successful. Insights from implementation science frameworks should be incorporated to help ensure successful CDS deployments. Potentially useful implementation science frameworks include the Exploration, Preparation, Implementation, Sustainment (EPIS) framework, (Moullin et al., 2019) and the Consolidated Framework for Implementation Research (CFIR) (Damschroder et al., 2009).

- *Challenges with sharing CDS logic and capabilities:* As discussed later in this chapter, despite progress (Middleton et al., 2016) in the past few decades, sharing of CDS across health information systems and healthcare organizations is still relatively limited (Tcheng et al., 2017). Historical reasons for this limited sharing have included the difficulties of establishing a business case for healthcare organizations to share their CDS logic and capabilities, lack of a clear legal framework covering potential liability implications associated with CDS recommendations, lack of a widely adopted formalism for representing and sharing CDS knowledge, and lack of widely available, standards-based CDS tools and infrastructure. Of note, there has been significant progress in the adoption of standards-based approaches to CDS, as described later.

CLINICAL DECISION SUPPORT BEST PRACTICES

While CDS interventions can profoundly impact clinical care, in a significant number of cases, they fail to result in meaningful improvements (Jones et al., 2014). There has been major interest in identifying best practices for CDS to help maximize the likelihood that a CDS initiative will lead to the desired outcomes, as implementing a CDS intervention can be associated with significant effort and cost. In other words, substantial work has been done to make CDS more of a science than an art. These best practices also aim at contributing to the replicability and wide dissemination of CDS interventions.

Guidelines for Clinical Decision Support Best Practices

As an important source of CDS best practices, seasoned experts have compiled guides for CDS best practices, two of which are discussed here. First, in 2003, Bates et al. published "Ten Commandments for Effective CDS: Making the Practice of

Evidence-Based Medicine a Reality" (Bates et al., 2003). These 10 commandments are as follows:

1. Speed is everything.
2. Anticipate needs and deliver in real time.
3. Fit into the user's workflow.
4. Little things can make a big difference.
5. Recognize that physicians will strongly resist stopping.
6. Changing direction is easier than stopping.
7. Simple interventions work best.
8. Ask for additional information only when you really need it.
9. Monitor impact, get feedback, and respond.
10. Manage and maintain your knowledge-based systems (Bates et al., 2003).

A second notable source of CDS best practices is *Improving Outcomes with CDS: An Implementer's Guide*, which was authored by experts in the field and published in 2011 by the Healthcare Information and Management Systems Society (HIMSS) (Osheroff et al., 2011). This book synthesizes best practices into worksheets to guide the reader through the CDS implementation and evaluation process. It also provides a practical framework for designing and implementing CDS interventions that follows the "CDS Five Rights," which refers to providing the right information to the right person using the right CDS intervention format, delivered through the right channel, and at the right point in the workflow.

Quantitative Analysis of Clinical Decision Support Features

As a complement to these best practice guides, some researchers have attempted to quantitatively analyze the features of CDS interventions that are strongly associated with, and therefore potentially explain, the success or failure of those interventions. In particular, a systematic review led by Kawamoto analyzed 70 randomized controlled trials of clinician-directed CDS interventions to assess the degree to which the trial outcomes correlated with the presence or absence of CDS intervention features suggested as important by domain experts (Kawamoto et al., 2005). This study found through a multiple logistic regression analysis that a single feature was, by far, the most critical: the automatic provision of CDS as a part of clinician workflow (adjusted odds ratio 112.1, $P < .00001$). Although there were CDS interventions that included this feature but had no impact, the CDS interventions that were not automatically part of the clinician's workflow failed to result in a significant improvement in clinical practice. This finding suggests that unless a CDS intervention is provided automatically to end users as a part of their routine workflow, there is a high likelihood that the CDS intervention will remain unused, and therefore, will not have an opportunity to affect patient care positively. In addition, this study found that providing CDS along with a recommendation at the time and location of decision-making, rather than just an assessment, were additional independent predictors of a positive outcome. A 2018 systematic review of CDS trials, directly comparing the impact of CDS with and without a given feature, confirmed the importance of providing CDS automatically as a part of regular workflows (Van de Velde et al., 2018). Additional

secondary success factors identified in this systematic review included making CDS more patient-specific and combining CDS with cointerventions aimed at professionals, patients, and staff.

As proposed earlier, another approach to help ensure the success of CDS is to use implementation science frameworks to guide the implementation and evaluation of CDS interventions (Haynes et al., 2020). In addition, more rigorous and standardized CDS evaluation methods, along with standard reporting, are needed to ensure comparability across CDS clinical trials (Kawamoto & McDonald, 2020a).

RECENT PROGRESS TOWARD DISSEMINATING CLINICAL DECISION SUPPORT ON A NATIONAL LEVEL

As noted throughout the chapter, CDS has the potential to significantly enhance the efficiency and effectiveness of healthcare delivery. Indeed, while CDS is not a silver bullet, it is a critical and largely underused resource for improving care and reducing costs, especially when implemented according to known best practices. Thus, disseminating comprehensive CDS on a national level is a critical challenge. A number of initiatives are being developed to tackle the challenges and barriers to CDS adoption. The following sections review a series of relevant initiatives and progress that should contribute to overall CDS adoption.

Value-Based Payment Models

The ongoing trend with perhaps the most significant potential to spur nationwide adoption of advanced CDS is the shift of healthcare payment from a fee-for-service model to approaches that reward the delivery of better quality and better outcomes at lower cost. Driven by the fundamental problem that the historical fee-for-service payment model leads to unsustainable and relentless increases in healthcare costs, health insurers are increasingly moving toward models of payment in which healthcare delivery organizations are reimbursed less for care volume and more for care value (outcomes relative to costs) (Burwell, 2015; Navathe et al., 2020; Ginsburg & Patel, 2017). This shift to value-based payment models will likely have a profound impact on the degree to which healthcare delivery organizations are motivated to implement CDS-supported process changes to improve care quality and reduce care costs.

Meaningful Use Incentives and Federal Regulations Promoting Electronic Health Record and Clinical Decision Support Adoption

In 2009, the U.S. federal government established a law providing approximately $30 billion in incentives for clinicians and hospitals to make "Meaningful Use" of EHR systems (Jha, 2010). In 2012, the regulations related to this law were relatively limited with respect to CDS, requiring only that compliant EHR systems implement a handful of CDS interventions and support a standard approach for integrating context-relevant information resources, typically referred to as Infobuttons

(Health Level Seven [HL7], 2010). With the exception of the Health Level Seven (HL7) Context-Aware Knowledge Retrieval Standard (also known as the "Infobutton Standard"), the 2015 Meaningful Use EHR certification requirements did not specify standards for the implementation of CDS capabilities. However, the Meaningful Use program provided powerful incentives for healthcare delivery organizations to adopt EHR systems, leading to near-universal adoption of EHRs in the United States (Office of the National Coordinator for Health Information Technology, 2017, 2016). As EHR systems are critical enablers of robust and widely distributable CDS, this federal program significantly increased the availability of a national base of EHR systems through which advanced CDS capabilities can be shared and widely used. More recently, the Office of the National Coordinator for Health IT published the 21st Century Cures Act Final Rule, which requires EHR systems to support the HL7 FHIR and SMART standards discussed below (Office of the National Coordinator for Health IT, 2021).

Statewide Health Information Exchanges

As noted in Chapter 6, health information exchanges (HIEs) enable the secure exchange of health information among healthcare providers in a defined region, often through secure web portals that enable authorized clinical access. Benefits of HIEs include fewer duplicated procedures, less imaging, lower costs, and improved patient safety (Menachemi et al., 2018). Moreover, HIEs can provide a platform beyond EHRs to deliver CDS to clinicians on a large scale, and HIEs can also help populate EHRs with relevant external data. As such, HIEs present an additional opportunity for enhancing the reach and capabilities of CDS on a national scale. Yet, despite progress in HIE adoption nationwide, especially among high-resource healthcare networks, low-resource community health centers still lag behind in advanced health IT capabilities such as HIE (Rittenhouse et al., 2017). Technical assistance and financial incentives are needed to help close this gap (Jones & Wittie, 2015).

Clinical Decision Support Standards

In general, there are two complementary approaches for sharing CDS across a large number of healthcare delivery organizations: (1) sharing structured CDS knowledge resources (e.g., order sets, alert definitions) and (2) sharing CDS capabilities over a secure internet connection (e.g., sending anonymous patient data to a secure web server, which returns evidence-based care recommendations) (Kawamoto, 2007). In both approaches, a critical element is that common standards are used by the various interacting health information systems so that the approach can scale widely and be implemented at a relatively low cost. A number of CDS standards that are required for a national approach to CDS have been developed and adopted by international standards development organizations such as HL7. Particularly exciting is the emergency of standards relevant for CDS that are aligned with the HL7 FHIR standard and are gaining increasing adoption among EHRs. These standards include the HL7 FHIR data interface standard; the HL7 SMART standard for app integration with health IT systems, including EHRs;

the HL7 CDS Hooks standard for integrating CDS Web services into the EHR; the HL7 Clinical Quality Language (CQL) standard for representing CDS and electronic clinical quality measurement logic; and the HL7 FHIR Clinical Reasoning standard for representing clinical knowledge. Interested readers can obtain further details regarding these CDS standards in a recent review article (Strasberg et al., 2021). In addition, other review articles identified CDS tools that use FHIR-based CDS standards, demonstrating increasing adoption of such standards (Taber et al., 2021; Kawamoto et al., 2021).

Federal Investment in Clinical Decision Support and Knowledge Management Initiatives

To underscore the degree to which the national dissemination of advanced CDS has become an explicit priority for many relevant stakeholder groups, federal agencies including the Office of the National Coordinator for Health IT, the Agency for Healthcare Research and Quality (AHRQ), the Centers for Medicare & Medicaid Services, the National Institutes of Health, and the Centers for Disease Control and Prevention have been investing in initiatives to move the country towards CDS and knowledge management at scale. As one example, the AHRQ supports an effort known as CDS Connect, which provides a repository for standards-based CDS knowledge artifacts and a forum for community discussion (Lomotan et al., 2020).

Open Source, Freely Available Resources

As a practical matter, the implementation of a common standards-based approach to CDS can be facilitated by resources that are freely available in the public domain. In recognition of this potential enabling role of open source, freely available CDS resources, several CDS stakeholders have launched efforts to collaboratively develop such resources. One such initiative is known as OpenInfobutton (www.openinfobutton.org), which was sponsored by the VHA to develop an open source solution for supporting context-sensitive information retrieval in a standards-compliant manner (Del Fiol et al., 2013; Jing et al., 2015). An additional initiative in this area is OpenCDS (www.opencds.org), which is a multistakeholder collaborative effort to develop standards-based, open source resources to enable CDS at scale (Del Fiol et al., 2011).

CONCLUSION AND FUTURE DIRECTIONS

As we look towards the future, there are a number of areas of opportunity for research to advance the capabilities and reach of CDS (Kawamoto & McDonald, 2020a). One area of research need is enhancing the specificity of CDS, such as by integrating data from HIEs, engaging patients to collect data directly from them, and leveraging data contained in free text through the use of natural-language processing. Other promising areas for continued CDS research include the incorporation of artificial intelligence into CDS, the optimization of the usability of CDS, economic analyses of CDS, and the continued development and deployment of standards to enable advanced CDS at scale.

Since shortly after computers were introduced into clinical settings in the 1960s and 1970s, CDS has been shown to be a powerful tool for positively affecting care delivery and patient outcomes. What has been lacking, however, is a business environment conducive to widespread CDS and technical approaches that enable large-scale CDS knowledge sharing. Today, there are a number of changes taking place that address both of these critical challenges. Therefore there is a real opportunity for relevant healthcare stakeholders to come together and realize the vision of an advanced CDS that is available ubiquitously and at low cost to support improved healthcare across the nation.

ACKNOWLEDGMENTS

Kensaku Kawamoto (KK) reports honoraria, consulting, sponsored research, writing assistance, licensing, or co-development in the past year with Hitachi, Pfizer, RTI International, Mayo Clinic, the University of California at San Francisco, Indiana University, MD Aware, and the U.S. Office of the National Coordinator for Health IT (via Security Risk Solutions) in the area of health information technology. KK was also an unpaid board member of the non-profit Health Level Seven International health IT standard development organization, he is an unpaid member of the U.S. Health Information Technology Advisory Committee, and he has helped develop a number of health IT tools which may be commercialized to enable wider impact.

DISCUSSION QUESTIONS

1. Describe examples of CDS that are available within your organization.
2. Identify the most important barriers to CDS adoption at your organization.
3. Explain how healthcare reimbursement reform will affect healthcare organizations' use of CDS moving forward.
4. What recommendations do you have for the use of CDS to improve care value at your organization?
5. What opportunities do you see for CDS to facilitate the work of healthcare professionals?
6. When implementing a CDS system, what should the appropriate relationship be between local values and standards and national standards?

CASE STUDY

Imagine that you have been appointed Director of Clinical Decision Support at a healthcare delivery system. This healthcare system consists of several large hospitals and multiple outpatient clinics and uses the same EHR system across the enterprise. There has been limited CDS activity at the institution prior to your arrival. Now, with the increasing need to provide increased care value, the appropriate use of CDS is an institutional priority. The current CDS available at your institution consists primarily of off-the-shelf drug-drug interaction and drug allergy alerting, which is the source of significant clinician complaints due to the rate of false-positive alerts. There is a strong sense within the institution's administration that IT in general, and CDS specifically, should be leveraged to improve care value and to enable the institution to influence its clinical practice patterns more systematically and more rapidly. You have a reasonable budget and adequate staff to make meaningful changes, and you do have support from key institutional stakeholders, including healthcare system executives, the nursing informatics officer, and the chief medical informatics officer. You have been asked to devise a strategic plan for CDS at your institution within 3 months of your arrival and to have concrete "wins" within 12 to 18 months.

Discussion Questions

1. Describe the approaches you would use to ensure that all aspects of patient care were considered when developing a CDS system. How would you prioritize the efforts of your CDS team? Potential areas on which to focus include areas in which payment rates are tied to national quality measures, CDS interventions that meet Meaningful Use requirements, readmissions for congestive heart failure and other care events for which payers are increasingly not reimbursing, and areas that have been identified as institutional priorities for clinical improvement.

2. How would you balance the need to deliver desired CDS capabilities quickly against the benefits of establishing a robust infrastructure to enable future deliverables to be implemented more quickly?

3. Identify one area for quality and value improvement. Define the CDS interventions that you would implement to address this area of need. Describe how your approach aligns with the best practices discussed in this chapter, such as the CDS Five Rights, the CDS 10 commandments, and the desire to use standards-based, scalable approaches. How would you systematically measure the impact of these CDS interventions?

REFERENCES

Akkus, Z., Cai, J., Boonrod, A., Zeinoddini, A., Weston, A. D., Philbrick, K. A., et al. (2019 Sep). A survey of deep-learning applications in ultrasound: artificial intelligence-powered ultrasound for improving clinical workflow. *Journal of the American College of Radiology, 16*(9 Pt B), 1318–1328.

Ash, J. S., Sittig, D. F., Campbell, E. M., Guappone, K. P., & Dykstra, R. H. (2007). Some unintended consequences of clinical decision support systems. *AMIA Annual Symposium Proceedings*, 26–30.

Balyen, L., & Peto, T. (May-Jun 2019). Promising artificial intelligence-machine learning-deep learning algorithms in ophthalmology. *The Asia-Pacific Journal of Ophthalmology, (Phila), 8*(3), 264–272.

Bankowitz, R. A., McNeil, M. A., Challinor, S. M., Parker, R. C., Kapoor, W. N., & Miller, R. A. (1989). A computer-assisted medical diagnostic consultation service: implementation and prospective evaluation of a prototype. *Annals of Internal Medicine, 110*(10), 824–832.

Barnett, G. O., Cimino, J. J., Hupp, J. A., & Hoffer, E. P. (1987). Dxplain: an evolving diagnostic decision-support system. *JAMA, 258*(1), 67–74.

Bassi, J., Lau, F., & Bardal, S. (2010). Use of information technology in medication reconciliation: a scoping review. *Annals of Pharmacotherapy, 44*(5), 885–897.

Bates, D. W., Kuperman, G. J., Wang, S., et al. (2003). Ten commandments for effective clinical decision support: making the practice of evidence-based medicine a reality. *Journal of the American Medical Informatics Association, 10*(6), 523–530.

Bates, D. W., Teich, J. M., Lee, J., Seger, D., Kuperman, G. J., Ma'Luf, N., et al. (1999). The impact of computerized physician order entry on medication error prevention. *Journal of the American Medical Informatics Association, 6*(4), 313–321.

Berner, E. S., Webster, G. D., Shugerman, A. A., Jackson, J. R., Algina, J., Baker, A. L., et al. (1994). Performance of four computer-based diagnostic systems. *New England Journal of Medicine, 330*(25), 1792–1796.

Best, J. T., Frith, K., Anderson, F., Rapp, C. G., Rioux, L., & Ciccarello, C. (2011 Novv). Implementation of an evidence-based order set to impact initial antibiotic time intervals in adult febrile neutropenia. *Oncology Nursing Forum, 38*(6), 661–668.

Borab, Z. M., Lanni, M. A., Tecce, M. G., Pannucci, C. J., & Fischer, J. P. (2017 Jul 01). Use of computerized clinical decision support systems to prevent venous thromboembolism in surgical patients: a systematic review and meta-analysis. *JAMA Surgery, 152*(7), 638–645.

Borbolla, D. A., Del Fiol, G., Norlin, C., Taft, T. E., Cornia, R., Warner, P., et al. (2021). Design and development of an electronic health record add-on app to support the care of children and youth with special health care needs. *Pediatrics, 147*(3_MeetingAbstract), 8–9.

Bornstein, E., Husk, G., Lenchner, E., Grunebaum, A., Gadomski, T., & Zottola, C. (2020 Dec 22). Implementation of a standardized post-cesarean delivery order set with multimodal combination analgesia reduces inpatient opioid usage. *J Clin Med, 10*(1), 7.

Bright, T. J., Wong, A., Dhurjati, R., Bristow, E., Bastian, L., Coeytaux, R. R., et al. (2012 Jul 03). Effect of clinical decision-support systems: a systematic review. *Annals of Internal Medicine, 157*(1), 29–43.

Buising, K. L., Thursky, K. A., Robertson, M. B., Black, J. F., Street, A. C., Richards, M. J., et al. (2008). Electronic antibiotic stewardship—reduced consumption of broad-spectrum antibiotics using a computerized antimicrobial approval system in a hospital setting. *Journal of Antimicrobial Chemotherapy, 62*(3), 608–616.

Burwell, S. M. (2015). Setting value-based payment goals—HHS efforts to improve U.S. health care. *New England Journal of Medicine, 372*(10), 897–899.

Byrne, C. M., Mercincavage, L. M., Pan, E. C., Vincent, A. G., Johnston, D. S., & Middleton, B. (2010). The value from investments in health information technology at the U.S. Department of Veterans Affairs. *Health Affairs, 29*(4), 629–638.

Chaudhry, B., Wang, J., Wu, S., Maglione, M., Mojica, W., Roth, E., et al. (2006). Systematic review: impact of health information technology on quality, efficiency, and costs of medical care. *Annals of Internal Medicine, 144*(10), 742–752.

Chou, E., Boyce, R. D., Balkan, B., Subbian, V., Romero, A., Hansten, P. D., et al. (2021 Mar 19). Designing and evaluating contextualized drug-drug interaction algorithms. *JAMIA Open, 4*(1), ooab023.

Cimic, A., Mironova, M., Karakash, S., & Sirintrapun, S. J. (2020 Aug 21). A synoptic electronic order set for placental pathology: a framework extensible to nonneoplastic pathology. *Journal of Pathology Informatics, 11*, 25.

Cimino, J. J., Elhanan, G., & Zeng, Q. (1997). Supporting Infobuttons with terminological knowledge. *Proc AMIA Annu Fall Symp*, 528–532.

Cook, D. A., Teixeira, M. T., Heale, B. S., et al. (2017 Mar 1). Context-sensitive decision support (infobuttons) in electronic health records: a systematic review. *Journal of the American Medical Informatics Association, 24*(2), 460–468.

Covell, D. G., Uman, G. C., & Manning, P. R. (1985). Information needs in office practice: are they being met? *Annals of Internal Medicine, 103*(4), 596–599.

Curran, R. L., Kukhareva, P. V., Taft, T., Weir, C. R., Reese, T. J., Nanjo, C., et al. (2020). Integrated displays to improve chronic disease management in ambulatory care: a SMART on FHIR application informed by mixed-methods user testing. *Journal of the American Medical Informatics Association, 27*(8), 1225–1234.

Curtis, C. E., Al Bahar, F., & Marriott, J. F. (2017). The effectiveness of computerised decision support on antibiotic use in hospitals: a systematic review. *PLoS One, 12*(8), e0183062.

Damschroder, L. J., Aron, D. C., Keith, R. E., Kirsh, S. R., Alexander, J. A., & Lowery, J. C. (2009). Fostering implementation of health services research findings into practice: a consolidated framework for advancing implementation science. *Implementation Science, 4*(1), 50. https://doi.org/10.1186/1748-5908-4-50.

Daniels, C. C., Burlison, J. D., Baker, D. K., Robertson, J., Sablauer, A., Flynn, P. M., et al. (2019 Mar). Optimizing drug–drug interaction alerts using a multidimensional approach. *Pediatrics, 143*(3), e20174111.

de Dombal, F. T., Leaper, D. J., Staniland, J. R., McCann, A. P., & Horrocks, J. C. (1972). Computer-aided diagnosis of acute abdominal pain. *British Medical Journal, 2*(5804), 9–13.

Del Fiol, G., Curtis, C., Cimino, J. J., Iskander, A., Kalluri, A. S., Jing, X., et al. (2013). Disseminating context-specific access to online knowledge resources within electronic health record systems. *Studies in Health Technology and Informatics, 192*, 672–676.

Del Fiol, G., Haug, P. J., Cimino, J. J., Narus, S. P., Norlin, C., & Mitchell, J. A. (2008). Effectiveness of topic-specific Infobuttons: a randomized controlled trial. *Journal of the American Medical Informatics Association, 15*(6), 752–759.

Del Fiol, G., Kawamoto, K., & Cimino, J. J. (2011). Open-source, standards-based software to enable decision support. *AMIA Annual Fall Symposium*, 2127.

Del Fiol, G., Rocha, R. A., Bradshaw, R. L., Hulse, N. C., & Roemer, L. K. (2005). An XML model that enables the development of complex order sets by clinical experts. *IEEE Transactions on Information Technology in Biomedicine, 9*(2), 216–228.

Del Fiol, G., Workman, E., & Gorman, P. N. (2014 May). Clinical questions raised by clinicians at the point of care: a systematic review. *JAMA Intern Med, 174*(5), 710–718.

Duke, J. D., & Bolchini, D. (2011). A successful model and visual design for creating context-aware drug-drug interaction alerts. *AMIA Annual Symposium Proceedings*, 339–348.

Eccles, M., McColl, E., Steen, N., Rousseau, N., Grimshaw, J., Parkin, D., et al. (2002). Effect of computerised evidence-based guidelines on management of asthma and angina in adults in primary care: cluster randomized controlled trial. *BMJ, 325*(7370), 941.

Elkin, P. L., Liebow, M., Bauer, B. A., Chaliki, S., Wahner-Roedler, D., Bundrick, J., et al. (2010 Nov). The introduction of a diagnostic decision support system (DXplain™) into the workflow of a teaching hospital service can decrease the cost of service for diagnostically challenging Diagnostic Related Groups (DRGs). *International Journal of Medical Informatics, 79*(11), 772–777.

Evans, R. S., Pestotnik, S. L., Classen, D. C., Morris, A. H., Kinder, A. T., Carlson, D. A., et al. (1998). A computer-assisted management program for antibiotics and other antiinfective agents. *New England Journal of Medicine, 338*(4), 232–238.

Ferranti, J. M., Horvath, M. M., Jansen, J., Schellenberger, P., Brown, T., DeRienzo, C. M., et al. (2011 Feb 21). Using a computerized provider order entry system to meet the unique prescribing needs of children: description of an advanced dosing model. *BMC Medical Informatics and Decision Making, 11*, 14.

Fillmore, C. L., Bray, B. E., & Kawamoto, K. (2013 Dec 17). Systematic review of clinical decision support interventions with potential for inpatient cost reduction. *BMC Medical Informatics and Decision Making, 13*, 135.

Ginsburg, P. B., & Patel, K. K. (2017 Jul 20). Physician payment reform—progress to date. *New England Journal of Medicine, 377*(3), 285–292.

Goldzweig, C. L., Orshansky, G., Paige, N. M., Miake-Lye, I. M., Beroes, J. M., Ewing, B. A., & Shekelle, P. G. (2015 Apr 21). Electronic health record-based interventions for improving appropriate diagnostic imaging: a systematic review and meta-analysis. *Annals of Internal Medicine, 162*(8), 557–565.

Haug, P. J., Gardner, R. M., Tate, K. E., Evans, R. S., East, T. D., Kuperman, G., et al. (1994). Decision support in medicine: examples from the HELP system. *Computers and Biomedical Research, 27*(5), 396–418.

Haynes, R. B., Del Fiol, G., Michelson, M., et al. (2020 Jun 2). Context and approach in reporting evaluations of electronic health record-based implementation projects. *Annals of Internal Medicine, 172*(11 Suppl), S73–S78.

Health Level Seven (HL7). *HL7 Context-Aware Information Retrieval (Infobutton) Standard HL7*; 2010. http://www.hl7.org/v3ballot2010may/html/domains/uvds/uvds_Context-awareKnowledgeRetrieval(Infobutton).htm.

Henry, J., Pylypchuk, Y., Searcy, T., et al. (May 2016). *Adoption of electronic health record systems among U.S. non-federal acute care hospitals: 2008–2015. ONC Data Brief, no.35.* Washington DC: Office of the National Coordinator for Health Information Technology.

Heringa, M., Siderius, H., Floor-Schreudering, A., De Smet, P. A., & Bouvy, M. L. (2017 Jan). Lower alert rates by clustering of related drug interaction alerts. *Journal of the American Medical Informatics Association, 24*(1), 54–59.

Hetlevik, I., Holmen, J., Krüger, Ø., Kristensen, P., Iverson, H., & Furuseth, K. (2000). Implementing clinical guidelines in the treatment of diabetes mellitus in general practice: evaluation of effort, process, and patient outcome related to implementation of a computer-based decision support system. *International Journal of Technology Assessment in Health Care, 16*(1), 210–227.

Horrocks, J. C., McCann, A. P., Staniland, J. R., Leaper, D. J., & de Dombal, F. T. (1972). Computer-aided diagnosis: description of an adaptable system, and operational experience with 2,034 cases. *British Medical Journal, 2*(5804), 5–9.

Horton, J. D., Corrigan, C., Patel, T., Schaffer, C., Cina, R. A., & White, D. R. (2020 Aug). Effect of a standardized electronic medical record order set on opioid prescribing after tonsillectomy. *Otolaryngology–Head and Neck Surgery, 163*(2), 216–220.

Institute of Medicine (IOM). (2001). *Crossing the quality chasm: A new health system for the 21st century.* Washington, DC: IOM.

Institute of Medicine (IOM), (2010). *The future of nursing: Leading change, advancing health.* Washington, DC: IOM;.

Institute of Medicine (IOM), (1999). *To err is human: Building a safer health system.* Washington, DC: IOM.

Jacob, V., Thota, A. B., Chattopadhyay, S. K., Njie, G. J., Proia, K. K., Hopkins, D. P., et al. (2017 May 1). Cost and economic benefit of clinical decision support systems for cardiovascular disease prevention: a community guide systematic review. *Journal of the American Medical Informatics Association, 24*(3), 669–676.

Jha, A. K. (2010). Meaningful use of electronic health records: the road ahead. *JAMA, 304*(15), 1709–1710.

Jing, X., Cimino, J. J., & Del Fiol, G. (2015). Usability and acceptance of the librarian infobutton tailoring environment: an open access online knowledge capture, management, and configuration tool for openinfobutton. *Journal of Medical Internet Research, 17*(11), e272.

Johnston, M. E., Langton, K. B., Haynes, R. B., & Mathieu, A. (1994). Effects of computer-based clinical decision support systems on clinician performance and patient outcome: a critical appraisal of research. *Annals of Internal Medicine, 120*(2), 135–142.

Jones, E., & Wittie, M. (Sep-Oct 2015). Accelerated adoption of advanced health information technology in Beacon community health centers. *The Journal of the American Board of Family Medicine, 28*(5), 565–575.

Jones, S. S., Rudin, R. S., Perry, T., & Shekelle, P. G. (2014 Jan 7). Health information technology: an updated systematic review with a focus on meaningful use. *Annals of Internal Medicine, 160*(1), 48–54.

Kawamoto, K., Flynn, M. C., Kukhareva, P. V., ElHalta, D., Hess, R., Gregory, T., et al. (2018). A pragmatic guide to establishing clinical decision support governance and addressing decision support fatigue: a case study. *AMIA Annual Symposium Proceedings, 2018*, 624–633.

Kawamoto, K., Houlihan, C. A., Balas, E. A., & Lobach, D. F. (2005). Improving clinical practice using clinical decision support systems: a systematic review of trials to identify features critical to success. *BMJ, 330*(7494), 765–768.

Kawamoto, K., Kukhareva, P., Shakib, J. H., Kramer, H., Rodriguez, S., Warner, P. B., et al. (2019). Association of an electronic health record add-on app for neonatal Bilirubin management with physician efficiency and care quality. *JAMA Network Open, 2*(11), e1915343.

Kawamoto, K., Kukhareva, P. V., Weir, C., Flynn, M. C., Nanjo, C. J., Martin, D. K., et al. (2021 Jul 31). Establishing a multidisciplinary initiative for interoperable electronic health record innovations at an academic medical center. *JAMIA Open, 4*(3), ooab041.

Kawamoto, K., & McDonald, C. J. (2020a). Designing, conducting, and reporting clinical decision support studies: recommendations and call to action. *Annals of Internal Medicine, 172*(11 Suppl), S101–S109.

Kawamoto, K., & McDonald, C. J. (2020b). Designing, conducting, and reporting clinical decision support studies: recommendations and call to action. *Annals of Internal Medicine, 172*(11 Suppl), S101–S109.

Kawamoto, K. (2007). Integration of knowledge resources into applications to enable clinical decision support: Architectural considerations. In: R. A. Greenes (Ed.), *Clinical decision support: The road ahead* (pp. 503–538). Boston, MA: Elsevier.

Krittanawong, C., Tunhasiriwet, A., Zhang, H., Wang, Z., Aydar, M., & Kitai, T. (2017 Apr 25). Deep learning with unsupervised feature in echocardiographic imaging. *Journal of the American College of Cardiology, 69*(16), 2100–2101.

Lange, L. L., Haak, S. W., Lincoln, M. J., Thompson, C. B., Turner, C. W., Weir, C., et al. (1997). Use of Iliad to improve diagnostic performance of nurse practitioner students. *Journal of Nursing Education, 36*(1), 36–45.

Leape, L. L., Bates, D. W., Cullen, D. J., Cooper, J., Demonaco, H. J., Gallivan, T., et al. (1995). Systems analysis of adverse drug events: ADE prevention study group. *Journal of the American Medical Association, 274*(1), 35–43.

Levine, A. B., Schlosser, C., Grewal, J., Coope, R., Jones, S. J., & Yip, S. (2019 Marr). Rise of the machines: advances in deep learning for cancer diagnosis. *Trends in Cancer, 5*(3), 157–169.

Levine, D. M., Linder, J. A., & Landon, B. E. (2016). The quality of outpatient care delivered to adults in the United States, 2002 to 2013. *JAMA Internal Medicine, 176*(12), 1778–1790.

Liu, F., Zhou, Z., Samsonov, A., Blankenbaker, D., Larison, W., Kanarek, A., et al. (2018 Octt). Deep learning approach for evaluating knee MR images: achieving high diagnostic performance for cartilage lesion detection. *Radiology, 289*(1), 160–169.

Liu S, Kawamoto K, Del Fiol G, Weir C, Malone DC, Reese TJ, Morgan K, ElHalta D, Abdelrahman S. The potential for leveraging machine learning to filter medication alerts. *Journal of the American Medical Informatics Association.* 2022 Apr 13;29(5): 891-899. doi: 10.1093/jamia/ocab292. PMID: 34990507; PMCID: PMC9006688

Lobach, D. F., Kawamoto, K., Anstrom, K. J., Russell, M. L., Woods, P., & Smith, D. (2007). Development, deployment and usability of a point-of- care decision support system for chronic disease management using the recently-approved HL7 decision support service standard. *Studies in Health Technology and Informatics, 129*(Pt 2), 861–865.

Lomotan, E. A., Meadows, G., Michaels, M., Michel, J. J., & Miller, K. (2020). To share is human! Advancing evidence into Practice through a National Repository of Interoperable Clinical Decision Support. *Applied Clinical Informatics, 11*(1), 112–121.

Mackintosh, N., Terblanche, M., Maharaj, R., Xyrichis, A., Franklin, K., Keddie, J., et al. (2016 Oct 18). Telemedicine with clinical decision support for critical care: A systematic review. *Systematic Reviews, 5*(1), 176.

Main, C., Moxham, T., Wyatt, J. C., Kay, J., Anderson, R., & Stein, K. (2010 Octt). Computerised decision support systems in order communication for diagnostic, screening or monitoring test ordering: Systematic reviews of the effects and cost-effectiveness of systems. *Health Technology Assessment, 14*(48), 1–227.

Mandel, J. C., Kreda, D. A., Mandl, K. D., Kohane, I. S., & Ramoni, R. B. (2016). SMART on FHIR: A standards-based, interoperable apps platform for electronic health records. *Journal of the American Medical Informatics Association, 23*(5), 899–908.

McCoy, A. B., Thomas, E. J., Krousel-Wood, M., & Sittig, D. F. (2014). Clinical decision support alert appropriateness: a review and proposal for improvement. *Ochsner Journal, 14*(2), 195–202.

McDonald, C. J. (1976). Protocol-based computer reminders, the quality of care and the non-perfectability of man. *New England Journal of Medicine, 295*(24), 1351–1355.

McGlynn, E. A., Asch, S. M., Adams, J., Keesey, J., Hicks, J., DeCristofaro, A., et al. (2003). The quality of health care delivered to adults in the United States. *New England Journal of Medicine, 348*(26), 2635–2645.

McGreevey, J. D., 3rd (2013). Order sets in electronic health records: Principles of good practice. *Chest, 143*(1), 228–235.

Menachemi, N., Rahurkar, S., Harle, C. A., & Vest, J. R. (2018). The benefits of health information exchange: An updated systematic review. *Journal of the American Medical Informatics Association, 25*(9), 1259–1265.

Middleton, B., Sittig, D. F., & Wright, A. (2016 Aug 2). Clinical decision support: A 25 year retrospective and a 25 year vision. *Yearbook of Medical Informatics, Suppl 1*(Suppl 1), S103–116.

Miller, R. A., & Masarie, F. E., Jr. (1989). Use of the Quick Medical Reference (QMR) program as a tool for medical education. *Methods of Information in Medicine, 28*(4), 340–345.

Miller, R. J. H., Bell, A., Aggarwal, S., Eisner, J., & Howlett, J. G. (2020 Jun 26). Computerized electronic order set: Use and outcomes for heart failure following hospitalization. *CJC Open, 2*(6), 497–505.

Morris, A. H. (2018 Febb). Human cognitive limitations. Broad, consistent, clinical application of physiological principles will require decision support. *Annals of the American Thoracic Society, 15*(Suppl 1), S53–S56.

Moullin, J. C., Dickson, K. S., Stadnick, N. A., Rabin, B., & Aarons, G. A. (2019). Systematic review of the exploration, preparation, implementation, sustainment (EPIS) framework. *Implementation Science, 14*(1), 1. https://doi.org/10.1186/s13012-018-0842-6.

Muniga, E. T., Walroth, T. A., & Washburn, N. C. (2020 Jan). The impact of changes to an electronic admission order set on prescribing and clinical outcomes in the intensive care unit. *Applied Clinical Informatics, 11*(1), 182–189.

National Quality Forum (NQF). (2010). *Driving quality and performance measurement—a foundation for clinical decision support: A consensus report. Washington,* DC: NQF. 2010. http://www.qualityforum.org/WorkArea/linkit.aspx?LinkIdentifier=id&ItemID=52608.

Navathe, A. S., Boyle, C. W., & Emanuel, E. J. (2020). Alternative payment models-victims of their own success? *Journal of the American Medical Association, 324*(3), 237–238.

Office of the National Coordinator for Health Information Technology. (2017). 'Non-federal acute care hospital electronic health record adoption,' Health IT Quick-Stat #47. https://dashboard.healthit.gov/quickstats/pages/FIG-Hospital-EHR-Adoption.php.

Office of the National Coordinator for Health Information Technology. (2016). 'Office-based physician electronic health record adoption,' Health IT Quick-Stat #50. https://dashboard.healthit.gov/quickstats/pages/physician-ehr-adoption-trends.php.

Office of the National Coordinator for Health IT. (2021). 21st Century Cures Act Final Rule. https://www.healthit.gov/curesrule/.

Osheroff, J. A., Teich, J. M., Levick, D., Saldana, L., Velasco, F. T., Sittig, D. F., et al. (2011). *Improving outcomes with clinical decision support: An implementer's guide* (2nd ed.). Chicago, IL: Health Information Management and Systems Society.

Osheroff, J. A., Teich, J. M., Middleton, B., Steen, E. B., Wright, A., & Detmer, D. E. (2007). A roadmap for national action on clinical decision support. *Journal of the American Medical Informatics Association, 14*(2), 141–145.

Page, N., Baysari, M. T., & Westbrook, J. I. (2017). A systematic review of the effectiveness of interruptive medication prescribing alerts in hospital CPOE systems to change prescriber behavior and improve patient safety. *International Journal of Medical Informatics, 09*(105), 22–30.

Panagioti, M., Khan, K., Keers, R. N., Abuzour, A., Phipps, D., Kontopantelis, E., et al. (2019). Prevalence, severity, and nature of preventable patient harm across medical care settings: systematic review and meta-analysis. *BMJ, 366*, l4185.

Rittenhouse, D. R., Ramsay, P. P., Casalino, L. P., et al. (2017). Increased health information technology adoption and use among small primary care physician practices over time: A national cohort study. *Annals of Family Medicine, 15*(1), 56–62.

Rodwin, B. A., Bilan, V. P., Merchant, N. B., Steffens, C. G., Grimshaw, A. A., Bastian, L. A., et al. (2020). Rate of preventable mortality in hospitalized patients: A systematic review and meta-analysis. *Journal of General Internal Medicine, 35*(7), 2099–2106.

Rosenbloom, S. T., Denny, J. C., Xu, H., Lorenzi, N., Stead, W. W., & Johnson, K. B. (2011). Data from clinical notes: A perspective on the tension between structure and flexible documentation. *Journal of the American Medical Informatics Association, 18*(2), 181–186.

Roshanov, P. S., Misra, S., Gerstein, H. C., Garg, A. X., Sebaldt, R. J., Mackay, J. A., et al. (2011 Aug 3). Computerized clinical decision support systems for chronic disease management: A decision-maker-researcher partnership systematic review. *Implementation Science., 6*, 92.

Rubins, D., Boxer, R., Landman, A., & Wright, A. (2019 Dec 1). Effect of default order set settings on telemetry ordering. *Journal of the American Medical Informatics Association, 26*(12), 1488–1492.

Rungvivatjarus, T., Kuelbs, C. L., Miller, L., Perham, J., Sanderson, K., Billman, G., et al. (2020 Jann). Medication reconciliation improvement utilizing process redesign and clinical decision support. *The Joint Commission Journal on Quality and Patient Safety, 46*(1), 27–36.

Smith, R. (2010). Strategies for coping with information overload. *BMJ, 341*, c7126.

Stead, W. W., Searle, J. R., Fessler, H. E., Smith, J. W., & Shortliffe, E. H. (2011). Biomedical informatics: Changing what physicians need to know and how they learn. *Academic Medicine, 86*(4), 429–434.

Stilos, K., Ford, B., Lilien, T., & Moore, J. (2019 Mar). The role of spiritual care with the introduction of an end of life order set. *Journal of Pastoral Care & Counseling, 73*(1), 41–48.

Strasberg, H. R., Rhodes, B., Del Fiol, G., Jenders, R. A., Haug, P. J., & Kawamoto, K. (2021). Contemporary clinical decision support standards using Health Level Seven International Fast Healthcare Interoperability Resources. *Journal of the American Medical Informatics Association, 28*(8), 1796–1806.

Taber, P., Radloff, C., Del Fiol, G., Staes, C., & Kawamoto, K. (2021 Aug). New standards for clinical decision support: A survey of the state of implementation. *Yearbook of Medical Informatics, 30*(1), 159–171.

Tcheng, J. E., Bakken, S., Bates, D. W., Bonner, H. I. I. I., Gandhi, T. K., Josephs, M., et al. (2017). *Optimizing strategies for clinical decision support: Summary of a meeting series.* Washington, D.C.: National Academy of Medicine.

Thomsen, G. E., Pope, D., East, T. D., et al. (1993). Clinical performance of a rule-based decision support system for mechanical ventilation of ARDS patients. *Proceedings of the Annual Symposium on Computer Application in Medical Care*, 339–343.

Topal, J., Conklin, S., Camp, K., Morris, V., Balcezak, T., & Herbert, P. (2005). Prevention of nosocomial catheter-associated urinary tract infections through computerized feedback to physicians and a nurse-directed protocol. *American Journal of Medical Quality, 20*(3), 121–126.

Van de Velde, S., Heselmans, A., Delvaux, N., Brandt, L., Marco-Ruiz, L., Spitaels, D., et al. (2018). A systematic review of trials evaluating success factors of interventions with computerised clinical decision support. *Implementation Science, 13*(1), 114.

Varghese, J., Kleine, M., Gessner, S. I., Sandmann, S., & Dugas, M. (2018 May 01). Effects of computerized decision support system implementations on patient outcomes in inpatient care: A systematic review. *Journal of the American Medical Informatics Association, 25*(5), 593–602.

Warner, H. R., Jr., & Bouhaddou, O. (1994). Innovation review: Iliad—a medical diagnostic support program. *Top Health Information Management, 14*(4), 51–58.

Wilson, B. J., Torrance, N., Mollison, J., Watson, M. S., Douglas, A., Miedzybrodzka, Z., et al. (2006). Cluster randomized trial of a multifaceted primary care decision-support intervention for inherited breast cancer risk. *Family Practice, 23*(5), 537–544.

Wright, A., Goldberg, H., Hongsermeier, T., & Middleton, B. (2007). A description and functional taxonomy of rule-based decision support content at a large integrated delivery network. *Journal of the American Medical Informatics Association, 14*(4), 489–496.

Wright, A., Sittig, D. F., Ash, J. S., Feblowitz, J., Meltzer, S., McMullen, C., et al. (2011). Development and evaluation of a comprehensive clinical decision support taxonomy: comparison of front-end tools in commercial and internally developed electronic health record systems. *Journal of the American Medical Informatics Association, 18*(3), 232–242.

Youngerman, B. E., Salmasian, H., Carter, E. J., Loftus, M. L., Perotte, R., Ross, B. G., et al. (2018 Aug). Reducing indwelling urinary catheter use through staged introduction of electronic clinical decision support in a multicenter hospital system. *Infection Control & Hospital Epidemiology, 39*(8), 902–908.

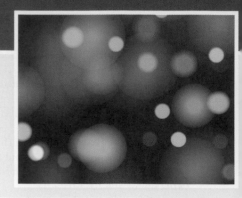

13

The Evolving ePatient

Sally Okun

The ePatient is, and will continue to be, a pivotal force in accelerating the healthcare system's adaptation to the ever-evolving world of technology, information management, and communication.

OBJECTIVES

At the completion of this chapter, the reader will be prepared to:
1. Summarize the driving forces behind the emergence of the ePatient movement.
2. Analyze the influence of online activity on patients' and caregivers' health experiences.
3. Summarize the opportunities and challenges digital health technologies bring to the clinician-patient relationship.
4. Outline how COVID-19 illuminated the need to increase inclusivity, equity and diversity in digital health engagement.

KEY TERMS

digital front door, 214
digital health, 213
eHealth, 205
ePatient, 205
ePatient movement, 205

guided discovery, 211
participatory healthcare, 211
patient-generated health data
   (PGHD), 213
quantified self, 208

virtual communities, 210
wearables, 207

ABSTRACT ❖

The term *ePatient* was coined long before the advent of the internet to describe patients who take an active role in their health and healthcare by being equipped, enabled, empowered, and engaged. Today, ePatients connect electronically to a vast array of digital health information and resources, such as traditional chat rooms, support sites, health-related social media, patient-to-patient research-based social networks, mobile devices, wearable sensors, and telehealth clinical visits. ePatients understand the value of engaging in a collaborative partnership with their healthcare providers and view the integration of participatory healthcare across the U.S. healthcare system as essential. The ePatient is, and will continue to be, a pivotal force in accelerating the healthcare system's adaptation to the ever-evolving world of technology, information management, and communication.

HISTORICAL BACKGROUND AND DRIVERS OF THE EPATIENT EVOLUTION

ePatient as a Pioneering Concept

As early as the 1960s, clinical researchers used emerging technology to test computer-based patient-driven medical interviews (Slack et al., 1966). Slack's philosophical view of "patient power," coupled with his belief that computers had a place in medical practice, were controversial at the time. Often asked, "Will your computer replace the doctor?" Slack's response was as true then as it is today: "Any doctor who can be replaced by a computer deserved to be" (Slack, 1999). Empowering patients with innovative tools is about fostering effective partnerships with their healthcare providers that lead to better outcomes. Empowering consumers with innovative health and wellness tracking tools is about giving individuals the opportunity to "lead more proactive and fulfilling lives" (Patient empowerment-who empowers whom, 2012).

The use of the term *ePatient* predates the availability of online medical resources. In 1975, another pioneering physician, author, and researcher, Thomas Ferguson, was interested in the empowered health consumer. Ferguson (2007) coined the term *ePatient* to describe people who take an active role in decisions about their healthcare and characterized as being:
- equipped
- enabled

- empowered
- engaged

By the early 1990s, with the rapid emergence of personal computers and the World Wide Web, Ferguson recognized the power and potential for consumer use of online health resources. In *Looking Ahead: Online Health & the Search for Sustainable Healthcare*, Ferguson (2002) wrote:

> *The 21st Century will be the Age of the Net-empowered epatient, and... the health resources of today will evolve into even more robust and capable medical guidance systems which will allow growing numbers of epatients to play an increasingly important role in medical care. Online patients will increasingly manage their own healthcare and will contribute to the care of others. Medical professionals will increasingly be called upon to serve as coaches, supporters, and coordinators of self-managed care.*

Ferguson's work is largely seen as the impetus of the **ePatient movement**, and his early observations, ideas, and recommendations continue to resonate. Today, an **ePatient** is characterized as one who uses technology to actively partake in his or her healthcare and manages the responsibility for his or her own health and wellness (Gee et al., 2012). ePatients are digitally enabled, seeking information, sharing their knowledge, and connecting with others. An ePatient manages health decisions regularly and uses the internet and digital technologies to supplement and enhance their health journey. The collection of data and knowledge from these sources helps to organize and support ePatients with highly personalized and contextualized information and medical vocabulary and concepts necessary for effective communications with their healthcare providers.

The first evolutionary phase of the connected ePatient movement occurred as access to health information and health-related services became increasingly available through electronic means. In late 1999, the term **eHealth** emerged in the lexicon to describe electronic communication and information technology (IT) related to health information and processes accessible through online means (Della Mea, 2001). eHealth has been defined as:

> *...an emerging field in the intersection of medical informatics, public health and business, referring to health services and information delivered or enhanced through the Internet and related characterizes not only a technical development, but also a state-of-mind, a way of thinking, an attitude, and a commitment for networked, global thinking, to improve health care locally, regionally, and worldwide by using information and communication technology (Eysenbach, 2001).*

Pagliaro et al. (2005) identified 36 different definitions of eHealth in publications and internet sources, suggesting a lack of consensus among various stakeholders. The term eHealth remains a broad concept used to describe internet or web-based activities that relate to healthcare (Belt et al., 2010).

As the ePatient movement evolved along with eHealth, the e-terms and context of use that characterize them evolved as well to include:

- Equipped. They have accessible digital technology.
- Enabled. They have the means, ability, and power to participate in their own health.
- Empowered. They seize opportunities to push traditional boundaries.
- Engaged. They take an active part in their care.
- Electronic. They use digital technologies to manage their health and healthcare.
- Equal. They are partners with providers in their care and decision-making.

Our Connected World

In addition to viewing eHealth as the delivery of health information to health professionals and consumers via the internet and telecommunications, the World Health Organization (2016) includes harnessing the power of the internet and e-commerce to improve public health services and business practices within healthcare. This global transformation must be considered in the context of the emergence of massive amounts of information on the World Wide Web, connected via the internet. Traversing the 20th and 21st centuries, the proliferation in the use of the internet has had unprecedented impact on access to information, sharing, and connectedness; moreover, it has been a driving force in the emergence of the 21st-century consumer.

The evolution of the internet is often characterized by a progression of functionality reflecting cumulative capabilities and emerging innovation with each new version building upon the previous version:

- Web 1.0—read-only web akin to a library where you could access loads of information but could not contribute anything.
- Web 2.0—social web with a community feel; a place where groups gather, where one exchanges information, and where one's contribution is included and even judged by others for its value.
- Web 3.0—semantic web with browsers and devices that behave more like personal assistants and search capabilities that harness user experience behavior to display content of interest including personally tailored advertising. integration of data from online and one's digital exhaust to deliver information to meet needs in the moment.
- Web 4.0—mobile web functionality transformed desktop and laptop experiences to an always on and always connected handheld experience that integrates data from online and digital experiences to deliver information that meet the user's needs in the moment.

Just as growth in the number of individuals using online resources continue, disparities between internet access "haves" and "have-nots" exist in large part due to cost, literacy, computer skills, language, and education. While some people voluntarily choose not to engage on-line the growth in the volume of those who do is staggering:

- In 1995 there were an estimated 16 million users.
- By 1998, when the search engine Google was launched, there were 147 million users.

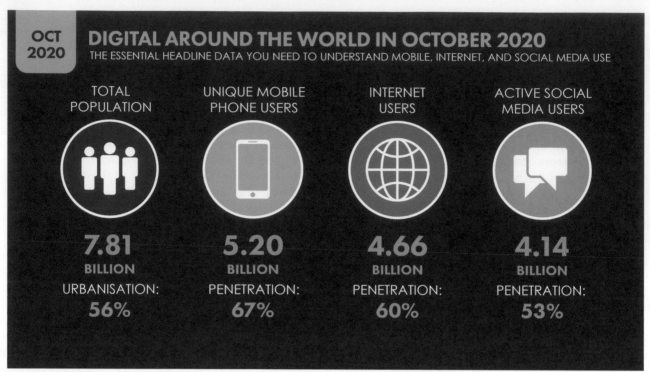

Fig. 13.1 Digital around the world. (Data from We Are Social's Digital Around the World in October 2020. Copyright 2020, We Are Social.)

- In 2001, only a decade after the graphic browser was conceived, 500 million users were online.
- By October 2020 the global digital landscape included 4.66 billion users representing nearly 60% of the world's population (Fig. 13.1) (We Are Social, 2020).

A report by Ericsson (2021), (Ericsson Mobility Report, 2021) a global communications technology company, suggests that by 2026 there will be 8.8 billion mobile subscriptions of which 91% will be for mobile broadband. Yet, despite this penetration the digital divide was laid bare by the COVID-19 pandemic when Americans nationwide were forced to manage their daily lives and educational needs primarily through the internet. In December 2020, Congress passed a stop gap measure to help families pay for the costs of on-line access. In August 2021, in recognition of the need for universal access and adoption of this essential resource the Senate passed the Infrastructure Investment and Jobs Act (IIJA) which would set policy and provide funding to support universal access and adoption of this essential resource (Levin, 2021).

Looking back the emergence of the internet as a valuable tool for health and healthcare became better understood at the turn of the century. In *The Future of the Internet in Health Care: Five-Year Forecast*, Mittman and Cain declared, "Health care has discovered the internet and the internet has discovered health care!" (Mittman & Cain, 1999). The National Academy of Medicine (2001) (previously known as the Institute of Medicine) report titled *Crossing the Quality Chasm: A New Health System for the 21st Century*, focused attention more broadly on the multiple dimensions of quality and safety concerns in need of fundamental change across the U.S. healthcare system. To narrow the quality chasm, the report provided "ten simple rules for the 21st century health

care system" that describe what patients should expect from their healthcare (Box 13.1), (National Academy of Medicine Institute of Medicine, 2001) Twenty years later, these future-focused reports continue to resonate and influence advances towards a more patient-centric learning health system where patient engagement and technology are highlighted as critical components for improving safety and quality. The Office of the National Coordinator (2015) for health IT released a report in 2015 that provides an interoperability roadmap and long-term vision for connecting health and care across the United States.

The recognition of safety and quality flaws in the U.S. healthcare system led many patients and those close to them to become vigilant advocates. Access to the internet, coupled with simplified search solutions offered by companies such as Alphabet Inc. (Google), made looking for health-related information online more feasible for an increasing number of people. Thus began the new generation of ePatients who started searching online for health information to learn more about their symptoms and conditions and to better understand the options available to treat and manage them.

The Pew Research Center's Internet & American Life Project began to monitor basic online activities in 1999 to understand who was using the internet and what people were doing while online. Susannah Fox, named Chief Technology Officer for Health and Human Services in 2015, previously led the Pew Internet & American Life Project, which explored the impact of the internet on families, communities, work and home, daily life, education, healthcare, and civic and political life (Fox and Jones, 2009). In subsequent research Fox (2011a, 2011b) found that 8 in 10 internet users look online for health information, making it the third most popular online activity at the time,

BOX 13.1	What Patients Should Expect From Their Healthcare

1. Beyond patient visits: You will have the care you need when you need it ... whenever you need it. You will find help in many forms, not just in face-to-face visits. You will find help on the Internet, on the telephone, from many sources, by many routes, in the form you want it.
2. Individualization: You will be known and respected as an individual. Your choices and preferences will be sought and honored. The usual system of care will meet most of your needs. When your needs are special, the care will adapt to meet you on your own terms.
3. Control: The care system will take control only if and when you freely give permission.
4. Information: You can know what you wish to know, when you wish to know it. Your medical record is yours to keep, to read, and to understand. The rule is: "Nothing about you without you."
5. Science: You will have care based on the best available scientific knowledge. The system promises you excellence as its standard. Your care will not vary illogically from doctor to doctor or from place to place. The system will promise you all the care that can help you, and will help you avoid care that cannot help you.
6. Safety: Errors in care will not harm you. You will be safe in the care system.
7. Transparency: Your care will be confidential, but the care system will not keep secrets from you. You can know whatever you wish to know about the care that affects you and your loved ones.
8. Anticipation: Your care will anticipate your needs and will help you find the help you need. You will experience proactive help, not just reactions, to help you restore and maintain your health.
9. Value: Your care will not waste your time or money. You will benefit from constant innovations, which will increase the value of care to you.
10. Cooperation: Those who provide care will cooperate and coordinate their work fully with each other and with you. The walls between professions and institutions will crumble, so that your experiences will become seamless. You will never feel lost.

From Institute of Medicine. 2001. Crossing the Quality Chasm: A New Health System for the 21st Century. https://doi.org/10.17226/10027. Reproduced with permission from the National Academy of Sciences, courtesy of the National Academies Press, Washington, D.C.

following e-mail and using a search engine. In *Health Online 2013*, Pew research found that the internet was being used as a diagnostic tool by one third of U.S. adults (Fox, 2013). In groundbreaking research conducted with teens and young adults, Fox and fellow researcher Victoria Rideout (Rideout & Fox, 2018) found that nearly 9 out of 10 (87%) say they have gone online for health information.

Health-related resources on the internet are constantly growing and becoming more innovative and complex. They provide ePatients with access to incredible resources and data previously unavailable, such as personal genetic information. To appreciate the power of rapidly changing technology, consider the Human Genome Project which began in 1990. It took 13 years and nearly $3 billion to complete the identification and sequencing of genes within human DNA (National Human Genome Research Institute, 2003). In contrast, 23andMe (2021) an internet company launched in 2007 offering direct-to-consumer kits, made it possible for anyone to access his or her personal genetic information quickly, simply, and for less than $500 (the 2021 price is as low as $99).

Another area of explosive growth has been in mobile technology or mHealth. Anyone with a smartphone can access more than 350,000 health- and fitness-related applications (IQVIA, 2021). Coupled with sensors and wearables digital technology is becoming more sophisticated and increasingly connected to all aspects of healthcare and research. Introduced by Apple in 2015, ResearchKit puts research opportunities in the palm of the hand. Tens of thousands of people, most of whom never participated in research of any kind, have enrolled in studies of Parkinson's disease, autism, and epilepsy (Bot et al., 2016; Egger et al., 2018; Johns Hopkins EpiWatch Project, 2021). mHealth technology bridges research and care by using real world data in real time to answer research questions, guide clinical decisions and importantly to engage study participants with personalized data visualized to highlight trends or patterns related to their health. The concept of mHealth is further explored in Chapter 14.

Policy and Legislative Influences

The economics of healthcare influenced the evolution of ePatients and their use of nontraditional and/or innovative sources for healthcare information. Patients with insurance saw their out-of-pocket expenses, including deductibles and copayments increase leading many to look for alternative ways to get answers and support for healthcare questions. The uninsured and underinsured are too often left trying to manage their own and their family members' healthcare needs to avoid incurring expenses associated with various services. Additionally, with changes in the healthcare reimbursement structure shifting care from the hospital to home, patients and caregivers are assuming more responsibility for increasingly complex care needs. The responsibilities of self-managing health and navigating the healthcare system motivated many to become ePatients, to find, connect with, and learn from others who may share similar experiences.

Policy and legislative actions in the United States have been important drivers in the ePatient movement. In 2009 the American Recovery and Reinvestment Act was signed into law. A hallmark of this legislation set specific objectives that eligible professionals and hospitals needed to achieve to qualify for incentive programs offered by the Centers for Medicare and Medicaid Services (CMS) for integrating electronic health records (EHRs) into their systems.

The focus on access to health information fueled the development of patient portals within EHR systems of large health systems, hospitals, physician practices, and other eligible healthcare providers. Another mechanism for ePatient health information access is personal health records (PHRs). PHR features vary from one system to another, but most support a menu of transactions including the ability to review test results, schedule appointments, refill prescriptions, and communicate via electronic messaging with healthcare providers. According to the U.S. Government Accountability Office, only 15% to 30% of patients use online patient portals despite their widespread availability of online patient portals. Other healthcare reform measures, including provisions in the Patient Protection and

Affordable Care Act (PPACA, 2020) and the Health Care and Education Reconciliation Act of 2010, which amended the PPACA and became law on March 30, 2010, impact healthcare coverage and care delivery. In 2015, Health and Human Services Secretary Burwell (2015) began to the shift of Medicare reimbursements from volume-based care, commonly known as fee-for-service, to value-based care. More recently HHS introduced other payment models intended to shift one-quarter of the country's primary care providers to outcomes-based payment models. Alternative payment models place increasing responsibility for managing cost and care to providers and patients, leading to the need for more collaboration and engagement at the actual point of care.

In 2016, the bipartisan bill known as the 21st Century Cures Act set expectations to increase choice and access for patients. Additionally, it established requirements to promote health information interoperability and to prohibit information blocking. In 2020, the CMS and the Office of the National Coordinator for Health Information Technology (ONC) released two rules and timelines for implementing these requirements empowering patients with access to their health data to support informed and shared decision making about their health. CMS and ONC have relaxed some early deadlines set for 2021 due to the COVID-19 pandemic.

CHARACTERISTICS OF DIGITAL HEALTHCARE CONSUMERS

Activists, Advocates and Innovators

Contemporary ePatients are information seekers and data gatherers. They take personal responsibility for researching online and offline resources to improve their health and well-being. The well ePatient is inclined to peruse a host of digital resources episodically to prepare for medical appointments, investigate intermittent family health questions, or search just out of curiosity (Cain et al., 2000). While activated ePatients (and their caregivers), including those newly diagnosed and those with chronic illnesses, are more invested in tracking their health with the use of online self-management tools and biosensors, such as heart rate monitors, seizure trackers, mood maps, sleep diaries, and glucose monitors. Although digital devices and wearables are becoming commonplace for monitoring mobility, medication adherence, and even for detecting behavioral changes, their use as part of routine clinical care remains nascent (Smuck et al., 2021). Empowered ePatients who are using these tools to track their health data digitally in conjunction with their online searches for information gain a sense of participation and ownership of their well-being, treatment options, and health.

In the ongoing evolution of ePatients some individuals have become well-known influencers. Dave deBronkart (2015a), also known as ePatient Dave, is a patient activist, blogger, international speaker at health and social media conferences, and health policy advocate for the ePatient movement. His call to action came in 2007 with the diagnosis of Stage IV renal cell carcinoma that had spread to his muscles, bones, and lungs and a median survival time of 24 weeks. Highly motivated to find an effective treatment deBronkart scoured the internet for viable options. With help from other patients on the Association of Cancer Online Resources (ACOR) website with a similar diagnosis, he learned about a promising clinical trial as well as tips on medications to avoid that could jeopardize his trial eligibility. Armed with this information, he engaged in meaningful discussions with his clinician about his options. Fortunately, deBronkart had a favorable outcome after the treatment regimen from the clinical trial led to his successful recovery. One year after his treatment ended, he began publicly sharing his story. deBronkart (2015b) believes that patients are the most underused resource within healthcare and champions the message of "Let Patients Help."

Other ePatients are called to activism because of their experiences with the healthcare system. Regina Holliday (2015) chose art as the medium to express her family's difficult experiences during her husband's illness and untimely death. Holliday shares her story in a powerful and provocative mural depicting the journey she and her family traveled through a fragmented and uncoordinated healthcare system. The journey was exemplified by her inability to access her husband's medical records in a timely way to ensure that he received needed care. The mural is titled *73 cents*, the price Holliday was told she would have to pay per page to make a copy of his medical record (Fig. 13.2). Holliday has continued to bring a voice to the patient and family experience through art. Since 2010, Holliday has painted hundreds of poignant and thematic paintings while on-site at healthcare conferences, events, and policy meetings, using them as an opportunity for public advocacy. She founded a movement called the Walking Gallery of Healthcare where she and other artists depict patients' stories or elements of medical advocacy on the back of jackets or lab coats for government employees, technology gurus, medical professionals, social media activists, executives of companies, patients, and artists. The Walking Gallery recently celebrated its 10th year with nearly 500 unique jackets now worn around the country and the world by their advocate owners.

A new type of health consumer emerged coined the *quantified self* (Quantified Self, 2021). Semantically, a quantified self may not consider themself to be an ePatient but rather someone whose goals are to achieve and maintain good health and who has an innate interest in tracking personal metrics. Quantified selfers capture health-related data such as blood pressure, exercise, activity, sleep, and dietary intake using personal informatics tools for self-monitoring to track their progress toward their goals. This type of tracking has the potential to identify health changes more quickly and may affect outcomes favorably, especially in circumstances when a nuanced change leads to an early diagnosis. This potential is exemplified by the experience of Steven Keating (Gallaher, 2019). While an undergraduate student, he participated in a brain study which showed a small abnormality near the smell center of his brain. Later, while a doctoral student at MIT's Media Lab, he collected and researched his own health data and symptoms including experiencing odd odors and headaches. Recalling the location of the small abnormality seen years before he sought medical attention and was found to have a low-grade glioma requiring immediate surgery. Relentless

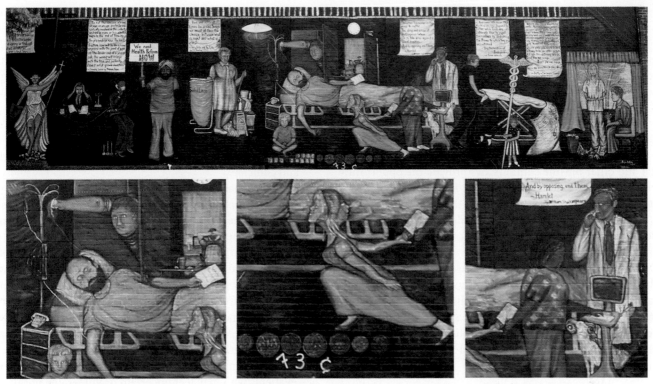

Fig. 13.2 73 cents. (Photograph 2011 Ted Eytan; adapted with permission of the copyright holder. Original image is available at www.flickr.com/photos/taedc/5680004634, under a CC BY-SA license.)

in the pursuit of his medical information he collected 200 gigabytes of his own medical data. He shared his journey freely on his website, including video of his surgical procedure and the printed 3-D model he developed of his own tumor. In a *New York Times* article, Keating stated, "there is a huge healing power to patients understanding and seeing the effects of treatments and medications" (Lohr, 2015). The aggregation of personal metrics, lifestyle factors, and real-world experiences has the potential to expand healthcare providers' understanding of patient responses to wellness and illness, both behaviorally and physiologically. In 2018 during a routine exam he was found to have glioblastoma. Steven continued to advocate for patient access to their medical data until succumbing to the disease in July 2019 at the age of 31. His legacy lives on through The Keating Memorial Self Research Group and website set up by is family.

ePatients innovators are using personalized data and informatics coupled with technology to create their own solutions rather than wait for the healthcare system to provide the solutions they need. Dana Lewis has been living with type I diabetes for more than 13 years. It is a disease invisible to others but monitoring and maintaining normal blood glucose levels is constant consideration. While advances in insulin pumps and continuous glucose monitors help manage daily fluctuations it is not a cure, and the technology is not perfect. When Dana was preparing to leave for college, she worried that without her mother's prompting at night she might sleep through a critical alert regarding her glucose level. Manufacturers were not responsive to Dana's requests to make the volume of alarms louder. Dana began thinking about how to rig a system that would allow her to customize the alarm on her glucose monitor which would require

access the data in her glucose monitor. This access was restricted by the manufacturer. Then, she spotted a tweet from a dad who had successfully accessed his son's real-time data from the same model continuous glucose monitor. He shared the code with Dana, and that was the tipping point for doing much more than simply gaining access to her own medical data. She launched her own design journey, creating a system that would allow her to take different actions based on the glucose monitoring data. Dana's n-of-1 device was created with commercially available components on nights and weekends. She and fellow innovators went on to develop Open Artificial Pancreas (OpenAPS), a full hybrid closed loop artificial pancreas system that auto-adjusts insulin pump levels. The innovators behind OpenAPS have published their reference design, documentation and code, and established a community to support those who are choosing to do similar n-of-1 implementation. As of July 2021, more than 2300 individuals have created their own DIY closed loop systems using data and code openly shared through the OpenAPS community. Most users of these n-of-1 innovators self-report less of glucose highs and lows, more time in their desired range, and reductions in hbA1c—not to mention the quality-of-life improvements associated with having a system that can auto-adjust basal rates (Litchman et al., 2019; Melmer et al., 2019).

Virtual Patient Communities and Research Networks

ePatients seeking health information and support increasingly turn to innovative tools and devices that include mHealth applications, comprehensive web-based content, interactive social networks, and wearable sensors that can seamlessly connect

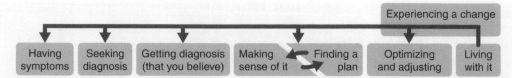

Fig. 13.3 The patient and caregiver journey. (Copyright 2017 The Authors. Learning Health Systems published by Wiley Periodicals, Inc. on behalf of the University of Michigan https://www.ncbi.nlm.nih.gov/pmc/articles/PMC6508568/figure/lrh210028-fig-0002/; 2012.)

data to online sites. As evidenced by the Open APS movement digital and other on-line communities provide the opportunity to reframe one's individual experience from "Why me?" to "Oh, you too? Tell me more." The interactions that occur provide support, validation, and a place to share ideas about how to live as well as possible with illness (Okun & Goodwin, 2017). This journey is depicted in Fig. 13.3.

One of the most transformative developments for ePatients has been the emergence of patient-focused virtual communities and research networks in which patients interact, sharing health-related data and learning from each other's experiences while unbounded by geographic limitations, social stigma, or other limiting characteristics. A virtual community has been defined as:

…a group of individuals with similar or common health related interests and predominately non-professional backgrounds (patients, healthy consumers, or informal caregivers) who interact and communicate publicly through a computer communication such as the internet, or through any other computer based tool (including non-text based systems such as voice bulletin board systems), allowing social networks to build over a distance (Eysenbach et al., 2004).

Health-related social networks and patient-powered research sites have become a rich resource for support, information, empowerment, and advocacy for ePatients and their caregivers. In an online environments ePatients exchange information, compare notes, learn about treatment options, and engage in discussions that may seem superfluous and deemed not within the purview of the medical professional. For example, they can exchange tips on where to purchase wigs in preparation for chemotherapy, advice on raising children, or advice on working while managing a chronic illness. Online communities can also function as a lifeline for those trying to manage the fear and uncertainty associated with illness. For many, including the uninsured, underinsured, and those with high-deductible plans, spending time online to explore ideas with others may be a reasonable first step in deciding what to do next about a health concern. Patients with rare diseases can search for specialists, researchers, and newly discovered information for their rare disease.

People seek out and find value in virtual health communities for different reasons. Researchers in the UK (Hodgkin et al., 2018) seeking to better understand the value of self-organizing online health communities found:

- They provide patients and caregivers with new resources.
- They offer new insights to non-patients.

- They challenge traditional power dynamics between patients and clinicians.
- They form part of a growing trend in data collection

Studies show that Americans are increasingly willing to share their health data if it improves their outcomes or the outcomes of others like them (Grajales et al., 2014).

Virtual communities share many of the characteristics of any social group and these characteristics may evolve and change as the community grows and matures. Most virtual communities can afford the user some degree of anonymity since engagement is not typically face to face. This can be both a benefit and a risk. Patients may feel more comfortable sharing sensitive information anonymously than they would in person.

Virtual communities may also carry risks, especially for novice ePatients who may feel uncertain or vulnerable in this environment. Many patient communities incorporate moderators as part of the experience, yet there is an inconsistent approach to how moderation is done in these communities (Huh et al., 2013). Organizations that create and support online communities should measure user input to gauge the perceived benefits, risks, and social health of the community from the patient's perspective. A study of six online communities for people living with chronic health conditions found that a fair balance between the risks and benefits of sharing can be achieved with active moderation (Green et al., 2020).

Yet, as with any online experience participants in health-related virtual communities should expect policies to be transparent and conveniently accessible on every page of the site. Following the report of the Cambridge Analytica data breach, Andrea Downing, an administrator for a private Facebook group helping women who have a gene mutation that puts them at risk for breast and ovarian cancer, discovered a security vulnerability affecting her closed Facebook group of over 10 thousand cancer patients (Prior, 2020). Along with other ePatients, privacy and cybersecurity experts Downing created The Light Collective (2021) to establish and advance safe data practices and digital rights for peer-to-peer on-line communities.

As insights and knowledge emerged from virtual communities the lines previously drawn between patients, care delivery, and health-related research blurred (Wicks & Hixson, 2013). Online and virtual health communities continue to be sources of novel patient experience data often unavailable for other health related data sources. Patient-powered research networks, including early innovators PatientsLikeMe and PCORnet developed data models, tools, and platforms for ePatients to securely contribute data with privacy protections in place (Fleurence et al., 2014). ePatients are participating in research, assisting in prioritizing research questions, and providing insight into best methods for sharing research findings and disseminating results. Data collection tools known as patient-reported outcome measures (PROMs) are increasingly of interest to academic and clinical researchers, government and regulatory agencies, and policy institutes. Data generated by patients themselves, either actively reported or passively gathered from wearable or sensor devices, are now an important part of the growing science of real-world data and real-world evidence generation.

CONVERGENCE OF PATIENTS, CLINICIANS, CARE AND DIGITAL HEALTH

Participatory Clinician-Patient Partnerships

The maxim of "doctors know best" is a statement of the past. Until the early 21st century, the old paradigm was a paternalistic model in which the healthcare provider was the exclusive source of medical knowledge. Deeply rooted cultural assumptions in this old medical model view the patient as the uninformed layperson and the medical professional as the keeper of all health knowledge. In a clinician-controlled environment the patient is the outsider with little ability to gather and access data about his or her condition and is expected to play the "good patient" role. This is changing with patient-centered care models.

As patient-centered care models evolved in the United States, questions emerge about who should direct the care: the patient or the healthcare provider (Scherger, 2009). Patient-centeredness promulgates a model in which the patient is not only at the center of care but also a full member and partner of the healthcare team. Patients know best when it comes to having the most intimate understanding of their personal circumstances, their preferences, and their bodies. Yet, for clinicians a model of team-based care, especially one that embraces patients as partners requires knowledge and skills not typically provided in clinical education (Wynia et al., 2012). New models of interprofessional education programs are needed to support a new generation of health professionals interested in and capable of developing effective and meaning partnerships with patients (Schoenbaum & Okun, 2015).

Importantly, the ePatient movement does not support displacing or replacing physicians and other healthcare providers. On the contrary, ePatients understand the value of collaborative patient-provider partnerships and seek healthcare providers who appreciate the value of engaging patients in their care and supporting participation in shared decision-making. ePatients appreciate the need for provider-directed care for certain types of situations such as trauma response, acute medical events, and surgical emergencies; however, the model of patient-centered care exists with the premise that patients are considered experts in their own care and self-management and must be allowed to exercise patient-driven controls. Patient-centered care is viewed as a critical component of achieving the Triple Aim—improving the experience of care, improving the health of populations, and reducing per capita costs of healthcare (Bisognano, 2018). For patient-centered care to succeed, patients and their clinicians must have respectful partnerships within which patients and clinicians mutually determine how care will be directed and managed to meet needs.

An unprecedented opportunity exists to fundamentally change the experience of healthcare encounters for both patients and their clinicians. ePatients have the tools and skills to elevate discussions with their healthcare providers and use limited office visit time engaged in a more constructive dialog. This can result in greater satisfaction for both stakeholders. This meaningful collaboration between the ePatient and the healthcare provider, known as participatory healthcare or participatory medicine, is defined as:

> …a cooperative model of healthcare that encourages and expects active involvement by all connected parties, including patients, caregivers, and healthcare professionals, as integral to the full continuum of care. The "participatory" concept may also be applied to fitness, nutrition, mental health, end-of-life care, and all issues broadly related to an individual's health (Society of Participatory Medicine, 2021).

While opportunities for health professionals' growth in participatory healthcare exist, it is equally important to acknowledge the challenges. Current care models may not be structured to support patient-centeredness and even well-intentioned clinicians may find it difficult to allocate sufficient time and resources to fully engage with ePatients who come with a well-prepared agenda. However, there is no doubt that ePatients will continue to push and advocate for their place in the healthcare system.

Many ePatients want to integrate empirical knowledge into their understanding of their health conditions. Therefore, clinicians should engage these ePatients in developing a shared hypothesis based on data and patient-reported experiences to help explain symptoms and other findings. Developing a shared hypothesis and including the ePatient in creating a plan to manage care initiates a process known in teaching as guided discovery. Guided discovery includes integrating open-ended questions in the medical encounter, pre-identifying data collection parameters that have meaning to the ePatient, planning time for analysis of collected information, completing an evaluation of outcomes, and recognizing that those results may require experimentation to achieve shared goals. Clinicians can take a proactive role in educating and supporting to use internet-based resources safely and effectively. Examples of key points to consider in this education are included in Box 13.2.

Clinicians involved in informatics are uniquely positioned to participate in system changes that support ePatients' desire for data driven learning and engagement by helping to build data collection models that support connection, partnership, and guided discovery (Sarasohn-Kahn, 2008). Patients and healthcare providers need the right tools at the right time to collect data to support their need to investigate and hypothesize health issues to create a shared plan. Clinicians may need to learn new skills and gain new knowledge to serve as a "guide" for ePatients as they integrate information and data from multiple sources while navigating their healthcare experience. It is within this culture of partnership that guided discovery of

---

BOX 13.2   Key Points for Teaching Patients Safe and Effective Use of Social Media Sites

- Take the time to read the *Conditions of Use* and *Privacy Statement*. The website should be designed in such a way that you can read these documents before establishing an account.
- Read the *About* section to determine who has established the site and the mission or purpose of the site.
- Spend time learning how to navigate the site and set privacy/security setting before participating on the site.
- Lurk on the site until you learn the names and characteristics of frequent participants on the site as well as the personality of the social media group as a whole.
- If you are unclear about a comment that has been posted, ask questions. Other people in the group might have some of the same questions.

- Treat people with respect and kindness. If you think something that has been posted is incorrect, point out that it is different than your previous knowledge or experience and ask for more information or clarification.
- If you are feeling strong emotion such as angry, excitement and anxiety it is often helpful, to compose your comments and let them set for a bit of time before posting. Remember, once it is posted it is permanent.
- Carefully evaluate the information posted by others. Listen/read the whole conversation. Information may be accurate but not apply to your situation or case. The first answer to a question is not always the best answer and group consensus is not always correct.

Sources used include: Joos, I., Nelson, R., & Smith, M. (2014). *Introduction to computers for health professionals*. Burlington, MA: Jones & Bartlett., Box 12.1 and Nelson, R., Joos, I., & Wolf, D. M. (2012). *Social media for nurses*. New York, NY: Springer Publishing Company., Table 1.4.

---

the ePatient's health and well-being can be fully realized (Dill & Gumpert, 2012). Healthcare providers must be flexible and open to the possibility that patients may be more intimately adept at the experience of their own illness and that clinicians should not be expected to have all the answers. However, ePatients do expect their clinicians to use timely technology, including online and digital sources, to build their own knowledge and expertise and to support meaningful partnerships.

Data Access, Transparency, and Interoperability

ePatients are staunch advocates for data access, transparency and interoperability of medical data. Regina Holliday, mentioned earlier, believes that no patient or family should ever have to struggle, as she did, to gain timely access to health records. Importantly, on April 5, 2021, federal rules implemented the bipartisan 21st Century Cures Act specifying that eight types of clinical notes are among electronic information that must not be blocked and must be made available free of charge to patients. Under the Interoperability and Information Blocking Rule all health systems in the United States must provide medical record data access to patients and with third-party applications of the patient's choosing (Office of the National Coordinator Cures Act Final Rule, 2021).

Increasing transparency of medical documentation to patients offers new opportunities for patient engagement. Consider the OpenNotes project, which began in 2010, to share clinical encounter notes from primary care providers with patients. Early concerns by nonparticipating providers indicated worry over the increased demand on their time and lengthier visits as well as an inability to record their thoughts candidly about sensitive issues regarding mental health, obesity, cancer, and substance abuse. In addition, nonparticipating providers believed transparency of the notes would negatively affect their practices and have minimal positive effect on patients. Research a decade later describes how clinician perspective changed after participating in sharing notes with their patients. Prior to implementation of Open Notes in their practice, less than one-third (29%) of physicians thought sharing notes was beneficial overall. After implementation 71% of physicians believed sharing notes was beneficial overall (Ralston et al., 2021).

For patients, Open Notes is an empowering experience. Early research suggested that giving patients access to their provider's notes may improve communication and efficiency of care and may lead to patients becoming more involved with their health and healthcare (Delbanco et al., 2010). This has been borne out as evidenced by the benefits reported by patients from reading their clinical notes online including:

- Being better prepared for clinic visits,
- Being better able to take medications as prescribed,
- Having better understanding of health conditions, and the plan of care, and
- Feeling more in control of their care (Nazi et al., 2015; Delbanco et al., 2012; Walker et al., 2019).

By 2020 more than 250 health organizations were participating in Open Notes representing more than 50 million patients registered via their patient portals (Blok et al., 2021).

Access and transparency in research are especially important to ePatients. Many seek out to studies on their chronic illnesses, only to find paywalls to access research papers constrains their efforts. In addition, closed access prohibits patients who participated in studies from reviewing study outcomes. Not only are patients often limited in their access to research results from studies in which they participated, they are often denied access to their own health data collected as part of the research study. This practice within the research and publishing world creates a roadblock for patients and an imbalanced dissemination of knowledge. Open access to research literature has gained traction through coalitions such as the Open Access Scholarly Publishing Association (OASPA) and the Scholarly Publishing and Academic Resources Coalition (SPARC) (Redhead, 2014; SPARC, 2021). The Patient Centered Outcomes Research Institute (PCORI) and patient-powered research networks such as PatientsLikeMe embraced open access as essential for all of their publications. In early 2019 leading medical journals set expectations for authors to disclose plans for sharing deidentified raw data from participants in clinical trials. Researchers wishing to publish in these journals must use a public registry, such as ClinicalTrials.gov to declare their data sharing plans (Li, 2019).

ePatients have inherent knowledge of their sense of self and encourage those in the healthcare field to recognize and support their interest in continuous and shared learning. ePatients look to clinicians not only for their clinical expertise but also for their willingness to effectively communicate using various modalities to offer information and guidance. Enabled by increased transparency, data access, and interoperability participatory patient-centric care models and patient powered research will continue to mature making effective and empowering clinician-patient partnerships even more essential.

Digital Health

ePatients are uniquely positioned to advance the acceleration of transformative innovation in health care through the explosive growth of digital health technology. ePatients have long used technology to engage in various health-related activities and to influence the experiences of others on a global scale. It is therefore no surprise that ePatients continue to adopt emerging technologies supported by data driven algorithms to track, monitor and measure life-style, behavior, sleep, mobility, function, and many other indicators of health, wellness and illness. Yet, most are unable to share their data with clinicians as the data architecture to support the integration of meaningful and relevant patient-generated health data (PGHD) at the point of care is nascent (Deering, 2013). PGHD, defined as health-related data that is created, recorded, or gathered by patients, family members, and caregivers to address a health concern, is an integral component of digital health technologies (HealthIT.Gov, 2021).

As capabilities in data science and engineering matured wireless, interrelated, and connected digital devices can now collect, send, and store data over integrated networks making remote monitoring and real time communication a reality. Connecting health-related devices, monitors and sensors offer opportunities to reimagine information and data sharing within clinician-patient relationships and partnerships—both of which depend on effective and efficient communication tools. No longer limited to voice messaging, texting, and email ePatients can communicate real time data such as blood pressure via connected apps and using smartphone video conferencing could "see" their doctor virtually. Yet, integrating digital tools and real time data flow presented untested challenges to clinicians and health systems. Most lacked the processes, infrastructure, and policies to support real time response and decision-making safely and ethically for health data abnormalities or to engage patients in virtual clinical visits.

INFLUENCE OF COVID-19 AND FUTURE DIRECTIONS FOR THE DIGITALLY ENGAGED PATIENT

Technology and COVID-19

The challenges to widespread integration of digital technology and PGHD into routine care were severely tested in early 2020 as the implications of the COVID-19 pandemic became clear. Digital health technologies including telehealth visits, video conferencing, self-reported data sharing and remote monitoring of health-related data became a necessity to avoid unnecessary exposure to the novel corona virus. ePatients already well equipped to manage digital technologies adapted to the convenience and

efficiency of digital health tools and solutions. For those patients most vulnerable to the virus, including those living with chronic and serious health conditions, digital tools became a lifeline to essential care needs when routine health care visits, elective procedures and use of emergency services were largely eliminated or severely curtailed for anything unrelated to COVID-19.

As the pandemic prompted payment and coverage mechanisms for digital tools no longer viewed as a novelty but as a necessity investment in digital health skyrocketed. And, while the gap between the "haves" and "have-nots" had begun to narrow the pandemic made obvious that there are far too many who cannot access or afford broadband and smartphones even if clinicians, health systems and payers were ready to offer them. This digital divide has both individual and public health implications since those lacking access are unable to benefit from the wisdom of collective knowledge to improve health outcomes, whether in real time or longitudinally, especially during a public health crisis.

As technology, policy, legislation, patient-centered reform, and patients' interests in personal health data converge the capacity to support the long desired learning health system becomes possible (National Academy of Medicine, 2011). Clinician-patient participation, engagement and collaboration are critical components of a learning health system where data, informatics and digital technologies align scientific knowledge, biomedical informatics, value-added incentives, and cultural norms converge to ensure that continuous improvement and innovation become natural by-products of the experience of healthcare.

The Digitally Engaged Patient

Over the years the evolution of ePatients has moved in fits and starts often with patients themselves accelerating its growth made possible by the global connectivity of the internet. This has been apparent in the mobilization of ePatients during the COVID-19 pandemic. ePatients recognized the critical need to share and learn from the experiences of others to better understand the impact of the virus from those living with and managing it. They launched support groups, created patient registries, and initiated clinical studies to gather data from people experiencing what has come to be known as long COVID-19, a term coined by patients (Greenhalgh et al., 2020).

The experience of a pandemic forced people across the globe to think about and react to changes in their health and health-care needs. Many, who might not previously identify as ePatients, were nonetheless empowered digital consumers simply by virtue of their generational identity. Consider a generation of computer users born after 1993. They have grown up with immediate access to information and knowledge sources that were previously unavailable. This generation is also called the Net generation, the Google generation, digital natives, and millennials. They are very skilled at navigating internet and digital resources and are accustomed to sharing data in real time in online environments (British Library and the Joint Information Systems Committee, 2008). Insight into this generation of users is important because they have little or no recollection of life without the internet. They are now adults, taking jobs, starting families, and are increasingly engaged in decisions about their health and the health of their families. These are today's

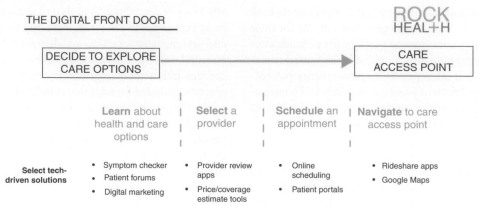

Fig. 13.4 Digital Front Door. (Copyright Rock Health, 2021.)

ePatients and their appetite for immediacy and responsiveness from online and digital tools drive innovation across all consumer interactions including healthcare. Not far behind is Generation Z, also known as iGen or Digitarians. These ePatients of the future only know a world of access powered by the internet, having been raised with touch-enabled devices and the ability to connect to anyone globally (Levit, 2015). Yet, even with the proliferation of savvy digital consumers and many newly identified ePatients there is no escaping the fact that COVID-19 has disproportionately impacted racial and ethnic populations, many of whom are not well represented among ePatients, bringing into stark reality the critical need to address systemic inequities that have long existed across health and healthcare.

What does this mean for health and healthcare? Topol (2011) described technological advances in medical devices and other diagnostic tools emerging in practice. Just 4 years later, Topol (2015) said that patients hold the future of medicine in their hands—literally, in the form of a smartphone suggesting that the digitalization of medicine has now democratized it, calling this digitization medicine's "Guttenberg moment." Today, we recognize that much remains to be done to ensure that patients across the spectrum of race, ethnicity and socioeconomic status can benefit from the increased application of digital technology, as evidenced during the COVID-19 pandemic (Whitelaw et al., 2020).

The internet and digital technologies are now evolving within the emerging environment of Web 5.0 characterized by intelligent systems that have the capacity to measure individual's emotions, wants and desires based on detection and predictive algorithms. There is much interest in applying these data driven digital technologies to health and healthcare as evidenced by the scope and scale of investments being made however, whether these tools translate into innovative, inclusive, and diverse models of health and healthcare is yet to be demonstrated (Chiu et al., 2020).

CONCLUSION AND FUTURE DIRECTIONS

Surveys indicate that U.S. consumers are showing increased interest in broader virtual health tools beyond simple telehealth visits (Bestsennyy et al., 2021). And, to give perspective on the impact of COVID-19 on health consumer preferences, a 2019 study found that about one-quarter of those queried considered changing their primary care provider to access virtual care options. By August 2020 that number rose to 75% (Cordina et al., 2021).

Considering these shifts in consumer preferences and the continued digital advances being made it seems feasible to imagine innovative models of care characterized by well-integrated clinician-patient partnerships and continuously learning technology solutions where the "digital front door" offers all patients an ePatient-like journey (Fig. 13.4) (Day & Zweig, 2021).

As the evolution of the digitally enabled ePatient continues where does the responsibility for achieving inclusiveness, diversity and equity reside? Might ePatients themselves be best suited to set expectations that demand accountability within health care, research and policy to ensure that the benefits they experience as ePatients become the norm for all patients—in essence, making the term *ePatients* irrelevant.

ACKNOWLEDGMENT

The author wishes to acknowledge the contribution of Christine A. Caligtan to the previous edition of this chapter.

DISCUSSION QUESTIONS

1. Discuss reasons why clinicians may be reluctant to change their current practice to accommodate the principles of participatory medicine.
2. What ethical concerns do you have about the sharing of health data online?
3. Considering today's privacy rules, how can you be expected to maintain confidentiality when patients are sharing data so freely? How might privacy rules evolve?
4. Defend or refute the following: Patients should have real-time access to all information in their health records, including narrative notes.

5. How can we narrow the gap between technology "haves" and "have-nots"?

6. Develop strategies for working with ePatients and using patient-generated health data in your personal practice and consider if those strategies would be acceptable in your work setting.

7. Debate this statement: Employers who contribute to the cost of employee health insurance can require employees to monitor certain health parameters or pay a higher premium to maintain coverage.

8. If you believe that participatory healthcare should become the standard of care, what policy and legislative changes are needed to make that a reality?

9. Create a vision for the model of healthcare you want in place by 2025. What is the single most important characteristic of your vision on which you are unwilling to compromise?

10. In the interest of public health, shouldn't all capable patients be expected to monitor their health using accessible tools? What, if any, are the unintended consequences of that expectation?

CASE STUDY

A few weeks ago you were hired as Director of Patient Education for a regional medical center located in the Midwest. The medical center includes three community hospitals ranging from 175 to 321 beds, four outpatient clinics, and five centers of excellence. The five centers of excellence are located at two of the hospitals and focus on heart disease, cancer care, care of the aging, neuromuscular disorders, and women's health. Two hospitals serve a large population of Hmong people.

In your position you are responsible for coordinating patient education across the medical center, including all programs and print materials. Your staff includes three BSN-prepared nurses, one located at each of the hospitals. As one of your initial steps in this new position, you have completed an assessment of the current educational offerings and staff satisfaction with the quality of the current programs. One area of need stands out: The professional staff report that a growing number of patients have been joining online social networking sites. One staff member said, "It seems patients are helping each other get access to these online groups where they share lots of information about their conditions." These connected patients are now raising new and sometimes challenging questions about treatment options. Few among the staff has explored the online sites, and they express concern that by joining the site they could be at risk of violating the Health Insurance Portability and Accountability Act (HIPAA).

Discussion Questions

1. Describe how you would develop a staff education program and create an outline of key points that you would include.

2. Discuss how partnering with patients might influence the content of the educational materials created for both patients and staff.

3. Develop patient information materials in languages relevant to each hospital's local community that are accessible in print and via the patient portal, that the staff can make available to patients regarding the effective use of online resources.

REFERENCES

23andMe. (2021). Retrieved from https://www.23andme.com/

Belt, T. H. V. D., Engelen, L. J., Berben, S., & Schoonhoven, L. (2010). Definition of health 2.0 and medicine 2.0: A systematic review. *Journal of Medical Internet Research, 12*(2), e18. https://doi.org/10.2196/jmir.1350.

Bestsennyy, O., Gilbert, G., & Harris, A. (2021). Telehealth: A quarter trillion dollar post covid-19 reality? *McKinsey.* Retrieved from https://www.mckinsey.com/industries/healthcare-systems-and-services/our-insights/telehealth-a-quarter-trillion-dollar-post-covid-19-reality.

Bisognano, M. (2018). Unleashing patient's power in improving health and care. *Health Catalyst.* Retrieved from https://www.healthcatalyst.com/insights/patient-engagement-triple-aim-healthcare-improvement/.

Blok, A., Amante, D., Hogan, T., Sadasivam, R., Shimada, S., Woods, S., et al. (2021). Impact of patient access to online VA notes on healthcare utilization and clinician documentation: A retrospective cohort study. *Journal of General Internal Medicine, 36,* 592–599. https://doi.org/10.1007/s11606-020-06304-0.

Bot, B., Suver, C., Neto, E., Kellen, M., Klein, A., Bare, C., et al. (2016). The mPower study, Parkinson disease mobile data collected using ResearchKit. *Scientific Data, 3,* 160011. https://doi.org/10.1038/sdata.2016.11.

British Library and the Joint Information Systems Committee. (2008). *Information behaviour of the researcher of the future.* Retrieved from htttps://library.educause.edu/resources/2008/1/information-behaviour-of-the-researcher-of-the-future.

Burwell, S. (2015). Setting value-based payment goals—HHS efforts to improve U.S. health care. *New England Journal of Medicine, 372,* 897–899. https://doi.org/10.1056/NEJMp1500445.

Cain, M., Sarasohn-Kahn, J., & Wayne, J. (2000). *Health e-people: The online consumer experience.* California HealthCare Foundation. Retrieved from https://www.chcf.org/publication/health-e-people-the-online-consumer-experience/.

Chiu, N., Kramer, A., & Shah, A. (2020, July). 2020 midyear digital health market update: Unprecedented funding in an unprecedented time. *Rock Health* Retrieved from https://rockhealth.com/reports/2020-midyear-digital-health-market-update-unprecedented-funding-in-an-unprecedented-time/.

Cordina, J., Levin, E., Ramish, A., & Seshan, N. (2021). How COVID-19 has changed the way US consumers think about healthcare. *McKinsey.* Retrieved from https://www.mckinsey.com/industries/healthcare-systems-and-services/our-insights/how-covid-19-has-changed-the-way-us-consumers-think-about-healthcare.

Day, S., & Zweig, M. (2021). Winning at the digital front door. *Rock Health.* Retrieved from https://rockhealth.com/reports/winning-at-the-digital-front-door/.

deBronkart D. (2015a). *About Dave.* e-Patient Dave. Retrieved from http://epatientdave.com/about-dave/

deBronkart, D. (2015b). From patient centered to people powered: Autonomy on the rise. *BMJ, 350*, h148. https://doi.org/10.1136/bmj.h148.

Deering, M. (2013). *Issue brief: Patient generated health data and health IT.* Washington, D.C: Office of the National Coordinator for Health Information Technology. Retrieved from https://www.healthit.gov/sites/default/files/pghd_brief_final122013.pdf.

Delbanco, T., Walker, J., Bell, S., Darer, J., Elmore, J., Farag, N., et al. (2012). Inviting patients to read their doctors' notes: A quasi-experimental study and a look ahead. *Annals of Internal Medicine, 157*(7), 461–470. https://doi.org/10.7326/0003-4819-157-7-201210020-00002.

Delbanco, T., Walker, J., Darer, J., Elmore, J., Feldman, H., Leveille, S., et al. (2010). Open notes: Doctors and patients signing on. *Annals of Internal Medicine, 153*(2), 121–125. https://doi.org/10.7326/0003-4819-153-2-201007200-00008.

Della Mea, V. (2001). What is ehealth (2): the death of telemedicine? *Journal of Medical Internet Research, 3*(2), e22. https://doi.org/10.2196/jmir.3.2.e22.

Dill, D., & Gumpert, P. (2012). What is the heart of health care? Advocating for and defining the clinical relationship in patient-centered care. *Journal of Participatory Medicine, 4*, e10. http://www.jopm.org/evidence/reviews/2012/04/25/what-is-the-heart-of-health-care-advocating-for-and-defining- the-clinical-relationship-in-patient-centered-care/#footnote_82.

Egger, H. L., Dawson, G., Hashemi, J., Carpenter, K., Espinosa, S., Campbell, K., et al. (2018). Automatic emotion and attention analysis of young children at home: A ResearchKit autism feasibility study. *NPJ Digital Medicine, 1*, 20. https://doi.org/10.1038/s41746-018-0024-6.

Ericsson Mobility Report. (2021): *5G on the road to mass market.* Retrieved from https://www.ericsson.com/4a03c2/assets/local/mobility-report/documents/2021/june-2021-ericsson-mobility-report.pdf

Eysenbach, G. (2001). What is ehealth? *Journal of Medical Internet Research, 3*(2). https://doi.org/10.2196/jmir.3.2.e20.

Eysenbach, G., Powell, J., Englesakis, M., Rizo, C., & Stern, A. (2004). Health related virtual communities and electronic support groups: Systematic review of the effects of online peer to peer interactions. *BMJ, 328*(7449), 1166. https://doi.org/10.1136/bmj.328.7449.1166.

Ferguson T. (2002). *Looking ahead: Online health & the search for sustainable healthcare* [online exclusive]. Ferguson Report. Retrieved from http://www.fergusonreport.com/articles/fr00901.htm

Ferguson T. (2007). *ePatients: How they can help us heal healthcare* [white paper]. Retrieved from http://e-patients.net/e-Patient_White_Paper_2015.pdf

Fleurence, R. L., Beal, A., Sheridan, S., Johnson, L., & Selby, J. (2014). Patient-powered research networks aim to improve patient care and health research. *Health Affairs, 33*(7), 1212–1219. https://doi.org/10.1377/hlthaff.2014.0113.

Fox, S. (2011a). *The social life of health information.* Washington, DC: Pew Internet & American Life Project. Retrieved from https://www.pewresearch.org/internet/2011/05/12/the-social-life-of-health-information-2011/.

Fox, S. (2011b). *Health topics.* Washington, DC: Pew Internet & American Life Project. Retrieved from https://www.pewresearch.org/internet/2011/05/12/health-topics/.

Fox, S. (2013). *Health Online 2013.* Washington, DC: Pew Internet & American Life Project. Retrieved from https://www.pewresearch.org/internet/2013/01/15/health-online-2013/.

Fox, S., & Jones, S. (2009). *The social life of health information: Americans' pursuit of health takes place within a widening network of both online and offline sources.* Washington, DC: Pew Internet & American Life Project. Retrieved from https://www.pewresearch.org/internet/2009/06/11/the-social-life-of-health-information/.

Gallaher, M. B. (2019). Celebrating a curious mind: Steven Keating 1988–2019. *MIT News* July 22, 2019. Retrieved from https://news.mit.edu/2019/celebrating-curious-mind-steven-keating-0722.

Gee, P., Greenwood, D., Kim, K., Perez, S., Staggers, N., & Devon, H. (2012). Exploration of the epatient phenomenon in nursing informatics. *Nursing Outlook, 60*(4), e9–e16.

Grajales, F., Clifford, D., Loupos, P., Okun, S., Quattrone, S., Simon, M., et al. (2014). *Social networking sites and the continuously learning health system: A survey.* Washington, DC: NAM Perspectives. Discussion Paper, National Academy of Medicine. https://doi.org/10.31478/201401d.

Green, B., Van Horn, K., Gupte, K., Evans, M., Hayes, S., & Bhowmick, A. (2020). Assessment of adaptive engagement and support model for people with chronic health conditions in online health communities: Combined content analysis. *Journal of Medical Internet Research, 22*(7), e17338. https://doi.org/10.2196/17338. Jul 7.

Greenhalgh, T., Knight, M., Buxton, M., & Husain, L. (2020). Management of post-acute COVID-19 in primary care. *BMJ, 370*, m3026.

HealthIT.Gov. (2021). Consumer eHealth: Patient-generated health data. Retrieved from https://www.healthit.gov/policy-researchers-implementers/patient-generated-health-data

Hodgkin, P., Horsley, L., & Metz, B. (2018). The emerging world of online health communities. *Stanford Social Innovation Review* April 10, 2018. Retrieved from https://ssir.org/articles/entry/the_emerging_world_of_online_health_communities.

Holliday R. (2015). *The Walking Gallery.* Regina Holliday's medical advocacy blog. Retrieved from http://reginaholliday.blogspot.com/2011/04/walking-gallery.html

Huh, J., McDonald, D., Hartzler, A., & Pratt, W. (2013). Patient moderator interaction in online health communities. *AMIA Annual Symposium Proceedings*, 627–636. Retrieved from https://www.ncbi.nlm.nih.gov/pmc/articles/PMC3900205/.

IQVIA. (2021). *Digital health trends 2021: Innovation, evidence, regulation and adoption.* Retrieved from https://www.iqvia.com/-/media/iqvia/pdfs/institute-reports/digital-health-trends-2021/iqvia-institute-digital-health-trends-2021.pdf?_=1629576029025

Johns Hopkins EpiWatch Project. (2021). Retrieved from https://tic.jh.edu/work/epiwatch

Levin, B. (2021). *The Senate infrastructure bill's four interconnected broadband components.* The Brookings Institution. Retrieved from https://www.brookings.edu/blog/the-avenue/2021/08/13/the-senate-infrastructure-bills-four-interconnected-broadband-components/.

Levit, A. (2015). Make way for generation Z. *The New York Times.* Retrieved from http://nyti.ms/1G2FPXD.

Li, R. (2019). Move clinical trial data sharing from an option to an imperative. *STAT* February 19, 2019. Retrieved from https://www.statnews.com/2019/02/19/data-sharing-imperative-clinical-trials/.

Litchman, M. L., Lewis, D., Kelly, L., & Gee, P. (2019). Twitter analysis of #OpenAPS DIY artificial pancreas technology use suggests improved A1C and quality of life. *Journal of Diabetes Science and Technology, 13*(2), 164–170. https://doi.org/10.1177/1932296818795705.

Lohr, S. (2015). The healing power your own medical records. *The New York Times.* Retrieved from http://nyti.ms/1DmQsEj.

Melmer, A., Zuger, T., Lewis, D., Leibrand, S., Stettler, C., & Laimer, M. (2019). Glycaemic control in individuals with type 1 diabetes using an open source artificial pancreas system (OpenAPS). *Diabetes, Obesity and Metabolism*, *21*, 10. https://doi.org/10.1111/dom.13810.

Mittman, R., & Cain, M. (1999). *The future of the internet in health care: Five-year forecast*. California HealthCare Foundation. Retrieved from http://www.chcf.org/publications/1999/01/the-future-of-the-internet-in-health-care-fiveyear-forecast.

National Academy of Medicine (Institute of Medicine). (2001). *Crossing the quality chasm: A new health system for the 21st century*. Washington, DC: The National Academies Press. https://doi.org/10.17226/10027.

National Academy of Medicine. (2011). *The learning health system series*. Washington, DC: The National Academies Press.

National Human Genome Research Institute. (2003). *The Human Genome Project Completion: Frequently Asked Questions*. Retrieved from http://www.genome.gov/11006943.

Nazi, K., Turvey, C., Klein, D., Hogan, T., & Woods, S. (2015). VA OpenNotes: Exploring the experiences of early patient adopters with access to clinical notes. *Journal of the American Medical Informatics Association*, *22*(2), 380–389. https://doi.org/10.1136/amiajnl-2014-003144.

Office of the National Coordinator Cures Act Final Rule. (2021). Empowering patients in the U.S. health care system. Retrieved from https://www.healthit.gov/curesrule/final-rule-policy/empowering-patients-us hcalth-care-system

Office of the National Coordinator for Health Information Technology. (2015). *Connecting health and care for the nation: A shared nationwide interoperability roadmap*. Retrieved from https://www.healthit.gov/sites/default/files/nationwide-interoperability-roadmap-draft-version-1.0.pdf.

Okun, S., & Goodwin, K. (2017). Building a learning health community: By the people, for the people. *Learning Health Systems*, *1*(3), e10028. https://doi.org/10.1002/lrh2.10028.

Pagliaro, C., Sloan, D., Gregor, P., Sullivan, F., Detmer, D., Kahan, J. P., et al. (2005). What is ehealth (4): A scoping exercise to map the field. *Journal of Medical Internet Research*, *7*(1). https://doi.org/10.2196/jmir.7.1.e9.

Patient empowerment-who empowers whom? (2012). *Lancet* *379*(9827), 1677. https://doi.org/10.1016/S0140-6736(12)60699-0

PPACA (2020) Patient Protection and Affordable Care Act: Interoperability and patient access for Medicare Advantage Organization and Medicaid Managed Care plans, state Medicaid agencies, CHIP agencies and CHIP managed care entities, issuers of qualified health plans on the federally facilitated exchanges, and health care providers. 85, Fed. Reg. 25510 (May 1, 2020) (to be codified at 45 C.F.R. 156). Retrieved from https://www.govinfo.gov/content/pkg/FR-2020-05-01/pdf/2020-05050.pdf

Prior, R. (2020). This breast cancer advocate says she discovered a Facebook flaw that put the health data of millions at risk. *CNN Health*. Retrieved from https://www.cnn.com/2020/02/29/health/andrea-downing-facebook-data-breach-wellness-trnd/index.html.

Quantified Self. (2021). Retrieved from https://quantifiedself.com/

Ralston, J., Yu, O., Penfold, R., Gunderson, G., Ramaprasan, A., & Schartz, E. (2021). Changes in clinician attitudes toward sharing visit notes: surveys pre-and post-implementation. *Journal of General Internal Medicine* https://doi.org/10.1007/s11606-021-06729-1.

Redhead, C. (2014, October 20). Second release of HowOpenIsIt? Guide now available. *OASPA blog* Retrieved from https://oaspa.org/second-release-howopenisit-guide-now-available/.

Rideout, V., & Fox, S. (2018). Digital health practices, social media use, and mental well-being among teens and young adults in the U.S. *Articles, Abstracts, and Reports*, *1093* Retrieved from https://digitalcommons.psjhealth.org/publications/109323.

Sarasohn-Kahn, J. (2008). The wisdom of patients: health care meets online social media. *California HealthCare Foundation* Retrieved from http://www.chcf.org/publications/2008/04/the-wisdom-of-patients-health-care-meets-online-social-media.

Scherger, J. (2009). Future vision: Is family medicine ready for patient-directed care? *Family Medicine*, *41*(4), 285–288.

Schoenbaum, S., & Okun, S. (2015). High performance team-based care for persons with chronic conditions. *Israel Journal of Health Policy Research*, *4*, 8. https://doi.org/10.1186/s13584-015-0003-1.

Slack, W. (1999). The patient online. *American Journal of Preventive Medicine*, *16*(1), 43–45. https://doi.org/10.1016/s0749-3797(98)00109-3.

Slack, W., Hicks, G., Reed, C., & Van Cura, L. (1966). A computer-based medical-history system. *New England Journal of Medicine*, *274*(4), 194–198. https://doi.org/10.1056/NEJM196601272740406.

Smuck, M., Odonkor, C., Wilt, J., Schmidt, N., & Swiernik, M. (2021). The emerging clinical role of wearables: Factors for successful implementation in healthcare. *NPJ Digital Medicine*, *4*, 45. https://doi.org/10.1038/s41746-021-00418-3.

Society of Participatory Medicine. (2021). Retrieved from http://participatorymedicine.org

SPARC Scholarly Publishing and Academic Resources Coalition. (2021). https://sparcopen.org/open-access/

The Light Collective. (2021). Retrieved from https://lightcollective.org/

Topol, E. (2011). *The creative destruction of medicine: How the digital revolution will create better health care*. New York, NY: Perseus Books Group.

Topol, E. (2015). *The patient will see you now: The future of medicine*. New York, NY: Perseus Books Group.

Walker, J., Leveille, S., Bell, S., Chimowitz, H., Dong, Z., Elmore, J., et al. (2019). OpenNotes after 7 years: Patient experiences with ongoing access to their clinicians' outpatient visit notes. *Journal of Medical Internet Research*, *21*(5), e13876. https://doi.org/10.2196/13876.

We Are Social. (2020). *Digital 2020: Global overview report*. Retrieved from https://datareportal.com/reports/digital-2020-october-global-statshot

Whitelaw, S., Mamas, M., Topol, E., & Van Spall, H. (2020). Applications of digital technology in COVID-19 pandemic planning and response. *The Lancet. Digital Health*, *2*(8), e435–e440. https://doi.org/10.1016/S2589-7500(20)30142-4.

Wicks, P., & Hixson, J. (2013, February 7). The patient engagement pill: Lessons from epilepsy. *Health Affairs Blog* https://doi.org/10.1377/hblog20130207.027850.

World Health Organization. (2016). *Atlas of eHealth country profiles: The use of eHealth in support of universal health coverage: Based on the findings of the Third Global Survey on eHealth 2015*. Retrieved from https://www.who.int/publications/i/item/9789241565219

Wynia, M., Von Kohorn, I., & Mitchell, P. (2012). Challenges at the intersection of team-based and patient-centered health care. *JAMA*, *308*(13), 1327–1328. https://doi.org/10.1001/jama.2012.12601.

14

Digital Health: Managing Health and Wellness

Sarah J. Iribarren and Rebecca Schnall

There are now more mobile phones than people.
—*ITU-International Telecommunication Union (2020).*

OBJECTIVES

At the completion of this chapter, the reader will be prepared to:
1. Describe key components of digital health's evolution over time.
2. Describe common mobile health (mHealth) application domains.
3. Outline the driving forces that have informed the field of digital health.
4. Summarize evidence identifying the benefits and challenges to widespread use of mHealth.
5. Describe future directions of digital health.

KEY TERMS

connected health, 218	eHealth, 218	mobile applications, 219
digital health, 218	mHealth tools, 219	sensors, 219

ABSTRACT ❖

This chapter analyzes digital health technologies and their potential to transform the access, management, and delivery of healthcare services and to restructure patient–provider relationships in the US and global contexts. Topics discussed include the emergence and driving forces leading to vast mobile health (mHealth) activities, examples of the range of ecosystems where an array of mHealth technologies are used, and benefits and barriers to its implementation. Potential directions and emerging trends are described.

INTRODUCTION

WHAT IS DIGITAL HEALTH?

Terms and Categories

The terms and categories to describe the transformative field of information technology to support health care have expanded, changed, and adapted. HIMSS, a leading nonprofit professional organization, presented a definition to help clarify an often-ambiguous term of digital health. The definition proposed by HIMSS is "Digital health connects and empowers people and populations to manage health and wellness, augmented by accessible and supportive provider teams working within flexible, integrated, interoperable, and digitally-enabled care environments that strategically leverage digital tools, technologies and services to transform care delivery" (Snowdon, 2020). For example, digital health includes concepts of mobile health (mHealth), telehealth, and telemedicine. Mobile health, commonly referred to as **mHealth**, m-Health, and

more recently as "connected health," is described as a catalyst for healthcare change (Klotz, 2015; Kvedar et al., 2014). Widespread recognition exists for mHealth technologies' potential to address and overcome disparities in health services access, health inequities, shortage of healthcare providers, and high costs for healthcare (Mendoza et al., 2013). mHealth falls under the umbrella of digital health or the broad use of information and communication technologies (ICT) to support health and health-related fields. The World Health Organization's (WHO's) Global Observatory for eHealth (GOe) defines mHealth as "medical and public health practice supported by mobile devices, such as mobile phones, patient monitoring devices, personal digital assistants (PDAs), and other wireless devices" (World Health Organization, 2011). Simply put, it is the use of mobile devices or wireless technology to achieve health objectives (Lee et al., 2013). Before discussing examples from the nascent field of mHealth, this chapter explores what makes it unique from other health ICT.

mHealth Evolution

mHealth, initially a term used interchangeably with telehealth (healthcare at a distance), emerged during the 21st century as its own field with distinct characteristics different from telehealth. In 2000, the movement toward mobile and wireless was defined as "unwired e-med" (Laxminarayan & Istepanian, 2000). Later in 2006, Istepanian et al. (2006) indicated that mHealth "represents the evolution of e-health systems from traditional desktop "telemedicine" platforms to wireless and mobile configurations" (Istepanian & Pattichis, 2006). mHealth has redefined the original definition and concept of telemedicine as medicine practiced at a distance to include the new mobility and invisible communication technologies.

Using Istepanian's definition, mHealth was recognized as a new field of study more broadly by 2010. The Federal Health Information Technology (IT) Strategic Plan 2015–2020, produced by the U.S. Office of the National Coordinator for Health Information Technology (ONC), noted telehealth and mHealth as separate technologies and services (The Office of the National Coordinator for Health Information Technology [ONC], 2021). Unlike telehealth, often requiring more advanced tools, mHealth uses consumer-grade hardware and allows for using technology with greater mobility. In a review of technologies and strategies to improve patient care with telemedicine and telehealth, Kvedar et al. stated that mHealth has increased consumer access to telehealth services and suggests the term "connected health" be used to encompass the entire family of technologies and services (Kvedar et al., 2014). Although the delineation between mHealth and telehealth may be more nuanced within the larger umbrella of eHealth, mHealth tools, such as mobile phones with video capability, can be used for telehealth to deliver care at a distance. One example is the use of video conferencing on mobile devices rather than desktop computers. One thing is clear—the focus of mHealth is maximizing a ubiquitous tool carried and used by most people in their daily lives. The rapid proliferation of mobile technologies and recognition of their inherent potential for improving health has resulted in major reports and global surveys, dedicated conferences and journals, and centers of expertise focused on the field of mHealth.

MOBILE HEALTH TOOLS, APPLICATIONS, AND EXAMPLES OF USES

Labrique et al. (2013a) developed a taxonomy of 12 common mHealth applications/domains and recommended mHealth strategies be viewed as integratable systems fitting into existing health systems rather than stand-alone solutions (Labrique et al., 2013b). Table 14.1 lists the 12 common mHealth application domains, describes the functions of mobile devices used within each domain, and provides examples of applications in healthcare settings.

Short Messaging Service

mHealth technologies comprise a wide range of tools with various technical capabilities and functionalities to support health-related programs. For example, short messaging service (SMS),

or texting, is a core mobile phone function enabling one- and/or two-way communication commonly employed in mHealth initiatives. Globally, over 350 billion text messages are sent monthly, exemplifying its extensive use (Mobile Marketing Association, 2014). Rationale for the frequent use in mHealth programs are: (1) it is more economical than a phone call; (2) SMS is versatile, as it can be sent, stored, or answered; (3) it is retrieved at the user's convenience; and (4) SMS is available on all phone types (ITU-International Telecommunication Union, 2013).

Mobile Applications

Smartphones, on a more functionally advanced level, combine features of a personal computer operating system with other features useful for mobile or handheld use. More complex functionalities include general packet radio service (GPRS), now fifth-generation mobile telecommunications (5 G systems), global positioning systems (GPS), and Bluetooth technology (World Health Organization, 2011). Additional smartphone tools include cameras, calendars, mobile applications (apps), multimedia messaging with pictures or video, gaming, educational tools, mobile internet access, and wearable devices and sensors Before describing examples of mHealth programs, it is helpful to understand the features offered by various mobile devices. Table 14.2 provides a list of the main characteristics/features for common mHealth devices.

Mobile apps are important mHealth tools for smartphone and tablet mobile devices. In the past few years, the number of health-related apps based on the two leading platforms, iOS and Android, that are available to consumers has more than doubled (Research2guidance, 2014). A 2015 study by the IMS Institute for Healthcare Informatics identified over 165,000 health-related apps, (IMS-Institute for Healthcare Informatics, 2015) compared to about 40,000 in their 2013 report (IMS-Institute for Healthcare Informatics, 2013). From 2015 to 2018, the number of mHealth apps again nearly doubled to over 318,000 apps available in the top app stores with more than 200 apps added each day (Digital Health, 2018). Fig. 14.1 provides the categories of apps available to consumers based on the IMS study. Of the 26,864 downloaded apps selected for their evaluation, two-thirds targeted wellness management (e.g., fitness, lifestyle and stress, and diet and nutrition), and one quarter were for disease treatment and management, medication reminders and information, women's health and pregnancy, and disease-specific (IMS-Institute for Healthcare Informatics, 2015). For disease-specific apps, 29% focused on mental health. However, the majority of the apps had simple functionality, with over half only providing information, thereby limiting their role in healthcare. About 10% included the capacity to link to a sensor or a device (IMS-Institute for Healthcare Informatics, 2015).

Client Education and Behavior Change

The mHealth domain of client education and behavior change largely focuses on the client to improve knowledge, modify attitudes, and support behavior change (Labrique et al., 2013b). Many examples of mHealth interventions exist in this domain. MomConnect, an initiative in South Africa, is an example of a program providing pregnant women with tailored information

TABLE 14.3	Leading Mobile Health Organizations, Key Resources, and Databases	
Resource/Report	**Aim**	**Link**
K4health	Key considerations, planning, and evaluation of mHealth interventions	https://www.k4health.org/toolkits/mhealth-planning-guide
Nine Principles of Digital Development	Established to support integration of best practices into technology-enabled programs	http://digitalprinciples.org/
mHealth Compendium	Focuses on mHealth strategies, best practices, and technical capacities for health in Africa	https://www.msh.org/sites/msh.org/files/mhealth_compendium_volume_3_a4_small.pdf
Healthcare Information and Management Systems Society (HIMSS)	mHealth Roadmap	http://www.himss.org/ResourceLibrary/mHimssRoadmapLanding.aspx?ItemNumber=30480&navItemNumber=30479
John's Hopkins Global mHealth Initiative	Resources, mHealth news, webinars	http://www.jhumhealth.org/
mHealth Evidence, mHealth Knowledge	Database of literature demonstrating the feasibility, usability, and efficacy of mobile technologies in healthcare	https://www.mhealthevidence.org/
mHealth Registry	Register projects with the World Health Organization to synergize the added advantage in the space.	https://www.miregistry.org
NIH	mHealth information from the National Institutes of Health	https://obssr.od.nih.gov/scientific_areas/methodology/mhealth/
Global Health Learning Center	mHealth Basics: Introduction to Mobile Technology for Health. United States Agency for International Development (USAID).	http://www.globalhealthlearning.org/course/mhealth-basics-introduction-mobile-technology-health
Apple research kit	An open-source framework for developing health apps	http://www.apple.com/researchkit/
mHealth working group	Community to share resources and ideas on mHealth challenges and successes and project inventory	https://www.mhealthworkinggroup.org/project
The Groupe Speciale Mobile Association (GSMA) mHealth Tracker	Database of programs	http://www.m4dimpact.com/data/products-services
Center for Health Market Innovations	Learn about and connect with programs to improve the health of the world's poor	http://healthmarketinnovations.org/programs
Federal Health IT Strategic Plan 2015–2020 (The Office of the National Coordinator for Health Information Technology ONC, 2015)	U.S.-based health IT plan that includes mHealth as a tactic	https://www.healthit.gov/sites/default/files/federal-healthIT-strategic-plan-2014.pdf
SDG ICT Playbook: From Innovation to Impact (Stern, 2015)	Recommendations for investments in e-health. Produced in collaboration across leading organizations, e.g., United Nations, Microsoft, NetHope	http://www.knowledgefordevelopmentwithoutborders.org/2016/01/07/sdg-ict-playbook-from-innovation-to-impact/
Health Organization's Global Observatory for eHealth (GOe)	Report on a 64-country survey on broad applications of information and communications technology	http://www.who.int/goe/en/

ICT, Information and communication technologies; *NIH*, National Institutes of Health; *SDG*, sustainable development goals.

networks and hardware to software and services (World Bank, 2012). The next generation of mHealth apps using 5 G is likely to revolutionize and transform healthcare, with its projected speeds 100 times faster than today that can support billions of simultaneously connected devices. This level of connectivity will enable reaction times that can support the precise control of autonomous vehicles, improve network reliability, and reduce energy use by a factor of 1000 (Kohlenberger, 2015).

Connectivity

The future points to the connectivity of anything and everything. Multiple forms of sensors monitoring physiological responses will capture tremendous amounts of data over extended periods and will likely change what we know about our bodies. By 2020,

over 78.5 million consumers globally are estimated to use home health technologies and remote monitoring tools, up from 14.3 million in 2014 (Tractica, 2015). This revolution of data-gathering sensors monitoring everything is called the Internet of Things (IoT) and is mobile, virtual, and instantaneous (Burrus, 2015).

Wearable technology such as the Apple Watch (an "intelligent health and fitness companion"), Jawbone, and Smart Scale (monitoring body fat) exists and is widely used. Smartphones are being fitted for testing blood, saliva, and sweat, and breath tests (Klotz, 2015). The challenge will be how to analyze and respond to the growing databases of information. The fields of big data and personalized medicine will likely integrate to allow better understanding of the impacts and capacities of mHealth data.

Major players in the area of data and technology integration include Apple's HealthKit and GoogleFit, which were both released in 2014. These are central platforms to aggregate healthcare information, collect fitness and health data, access personal medical information (diagnoses, lab tests), develop tools such as apps or integrate existing ones used by healthcare facilities, and allow users to choose what will be shared with healthcare teams. According to a Reuters poll, 14 of 23 top hospitals in the United States have rolled out programs using Apple's HealthKit service (Farr, 2015). In addition, the Apple ResearchKit, an open-source software framework, has the potential to transform how individuals or patients become involved to advance medical research.

Another example is Emerald, a touchless sensor and machine learning platform for health analytics. Emerald has been successfully used in a number of important clinical contexts, including monitoring medication self-administration (Zhao et al., 2021), assessing postoperative recovery from endometriosis surgery (Loring et al., 2021), and monitoring Parkinson's patients in their home (Tarolli et al., 2020). This is especially notable because this technology can allow remote observation of a patient's gait, which is a technological achievement (Hsu et al., 2017). Most recently, Emerald was reportedly used to remotely monitor a COVID-19 patient's breathing, movement, and sleep patterns using wireless signals (Wiggers, 2020). This has important implications since this can potentially minimize health workers' exposure while potentially improving health outcomes, which was especially challenging at the onset of the COVID-19 pandemic when there were extreme shortages in personal protective equipment.

CONCLUSIONS

mHealth is changing the delivery of healthcare, though its continued role in the future of global healthcare delivery seems certain. It is uncertain how mHealth will evolve in response to the challenges outlined above. mHealth has the potential to empower patients, allowing them to take control of their health; healthcare may become more personalized and responsive to individual needs. The ideal would be for integrated systems to shift from the current reactive, disease treatment focus to a proactive, disease prevention focus, including problem detection at early stages outside healthcare structures. A tighter integration of mHealth into health systems will allow even greater results than today. The future focus on mHealth and its health impacts is assured in part because the National Institutes of Health (NIH) included mHealth as one of its main goals in its NIH-wide 2016–2020 strategic plan (National Institutes of Health [NIH], 2015).

■ DISCUSSION QUESTIONS

1. Describe the components of an mHealth intervention to support a patient with a chronic condition.
2. What are the strengths of using mHealth technologies in clinical practice?
3. What are the barriers to using mHealth technologies in clinical practice?
4. Explain risks involved in using mHealth technology.
5. How can mHealth technologies be used to support patient care?
6. How might mHealth change the patient–provider relationship?

■ CASE STUDY

Henry Brown is a 67-year-old American living in the rural central United States. He is prescribed multiple medications for hypertension, depression, diabetes mellitus type 2, and a recent bacterial infection. Henry is not alone. In fact, estimates suggest at least 70% of the US aging population is prescribed multiple medications due to the rapid increase of chronic diseases. This presents a major challenge for our healthcare system. Most medications require consistent adherence to the prescribed regimen for them to achieve therapeutic effect. Yet, it is known that adherence rates remain suboptimal across populations and disease states. Because Henry uses a smartphone, his primary healthcare provider might recommend a mobile app called the Medication Tracker to help him manage his complicated medication regimen. Henry's primary healthcare provider recognizes apps have the potential to address the specific needs of patients in a manner that is timely, cost-effective, informative, and engaging. This app can be configured to deliver automated, personalized messaging to remind Henry to take his medication; can help Henry reinforce good self-management behaviors; can provide education on his chronic diseases; and can provide information about his medications, such as black box warnings, side effects, and contraindications for use.

Discussion Questions
1. Describe the factors that Henry's primary healthcare provider should consider when selecting an app for him.
2. Identify the features most important to facilitate the primary treatment goals of Henry and his primary provider.
3. Describe how Henry should communicate his activities with the app to his primary healthcare provider.
4. List some risks for Henry associated with using this app.

REFERENCES

Anderson, M. (2015). Racial and ethnic differences in how people use mobile technology. Retrieved from https://www.pewresearch.org/fact-tank/2015/04/30/racial-and-ethnic-differences-in-how-people-use-mobile-technology/

Anglada-Martinez, H., Riu-Viladoms, G., Martin-Conde, M., Rovira-Illamola, M., Sotoca-Momblona, J. M., & Codina-Jane, C. (2015). Does mHealth increase adherence to medication? Results of a systematic review. *International Journal of Clinical Practice*, 69(1), 9–32. https://doi.org/10.1111/ijcp.12582.

Armstrong, K. A., Semple, J. L., & Coyte, P. C. (2014). Replacing ambulatory surgical follow-up visits with mobile app home monitoring: Modeling cost-effective scenarios. *Journal of Medical Internet Research*, 16(9), e213. https://doi.org/10.2196/jmir.3528.

Bailey, S. C., Belter, L. T., Pandit, A. U., Carpenter, D. M., Carlos, E., & Wolf, M. S. (2014). The availability, functionality, and quality of mobile applications supporting medication self-management. *Journal of the American Medical Informatics Association*, 21(3), 542–546. https://doi.org/10.1136/amiajnl-2013-002232.

Baquero, G. A., Banchs, J. E., Ahmed, S., Naccarelli, G. V., & Luck, J. C. (2015). Surface 12 lead electrocardiogram recordings using smart phone technology. *Journal of Electrocardiology*, 48(1), 1–7. https://doi.org/10.1016/j.jelectrocard.2014.09.006.

Beauchemin, M., Gradilla, M., Baik, D., Cho, H., & Schnall, R. (2019). A multi-step usability evaluation of a self-management app to support medication adherence in persons living with HIV. *International Journal of Medical Informatics*, 122, 37–44. https://doi.org/10.1016/j.ijmedinf.2018.11.012.

Becker, S., Kribben, A., Meister, S., Diamantidis, C. J., Unger, N., & Mitchell, A. (2013). User profiles of a smartphone application to support drug adherence—experiences from the iNephro project. *PLoS ONE*, 8(10), e78547. https://doi.org/10.1371/journal.pone.0078547.

Bender, J. L., Yue, R. Y., To, M. J., Deacken, L., & Jadad, A. R. (2013). A lot of action, but not in the right direction: Systematic review and content analysis of smartphone applications for the prevention, detection, and management of cancer. *Journal of Medical Internet Research*, 15(12), e287. https://doi.org/10.2196/jmir.2661.

Ben-Zeev, D., Kaiser, S. M., Brenner, C. J., Begale, M., Duffecy, J., & Mohr, D. C. (2013). Development and usability testing of FOCUS: A smartphone system for self-management of schizophrenia. *Psychiatric Rehabilitation Journal*, 36(4), 289–296. https://doi.org/10.1037/prj0000019.

BinDhim, N. F., Hawkey, A., & Trevena, L. (2015). A systematic review of quality assessment methods for smartphone health apps. *Telemedicine Journal and e-Health: The Official Journal of the American Telemedicine Association*, 21(2), 97–104. https://doi.org/10.1089/tmj.2014.0088.

Boulos, M. N., Wheeler, S., Tavares, C., & Jones, R. (2011). How smartphones are changing the face of mobile and participatory healthcare: An overview, with example from eCAALYX. *Biomedical Engineering Online*, 10, 24. https://doi.org/10.1186/1475-925x-10-24.

Burns, M. N., Montague, E., & Mohr, D. C. (2013). Initial design of culturally informed behavioral intervention technologies: Developing an mHealth intervention for young sexual minority men with generalized anxiety disorder and major depression. *Journal of Medical Internet Research*, 15(12), e271. https://doi.org/10.2196/jmir.2826.

Burrus, D. (2015). The internet of things is far bigger than anyone realizes. Retrieved from https://www.wired.com/insights/2014/11/the-internet-of-things-bigger/

Car, J., Gurol-Urganci, I., de Jongh, T., Vodopivec-Jamsek, V., & Atun, R. (2012). Mobile phone messaging reminders for attendance at healthcare appointments. *Cochrane Database of Systematic Reviews*, 7, Cd007458. https://doi.org/10.1002/14651858.CD007458.pub2.

ClinicalTrials.gov. (2014). Paper-based and electronic partogram systems to safe lives at birth (PartoMa). Retrieved from https://clinicaltrials.gov/ct2/show/NCT02318420

Crocker, P. (2013). Converged-mobile-messaging analysis and forecasts. Retrieved from http://www.smithspointanalytics.com/Converged_Mobile_Messaging.pdf

Dan, L. (2013). The rise of third party mhealth app stores. Retrieved from http://histalkmobile.com/the-riseof-third-party-mhealth-app-stores

de Jongh, T., Gurol-Urganci, I., Vodopivec-Jamsek, V., Car, J., & Atun, R. (2012). Mobile phone messaging for facilitating self-management of long-term illnesses. *Cochrane Database of Systematic Reviews*, 12(12), Cd007459. https://doi.org/10.1002/14651858.CD007459.pub2.

de la Vega, R., & Miró, J. (2014). mHealth: A strategic field without a solid scientific soul. A systematic review of pain-related apps. *PLoS ONE*, 9(7), e101312. https://doi.org/10.1371/journal.pone.0101312.

Digital Development Principles Working Group. (2015). Principles for digital development. Retrieved from https://digitalprinciples.org/about/

Digital Health. (2018). The Rise of mHealth Apps: A Market Snapshot. Retrieved from https://liquid-state.com/mhealth-apps-market-snapshot/

Farr, C. (2015). Apple's health tech takes early lead among top hospitals. Retrieved from https://www.reuters.com/article/us-apple-hospitals-exclusive/exclusive-apples-health-tech-takes-early-lead-among-top-hospitals-idINKBN0L90G920150205

Fazen, L. E., Chemwolo, B. T., Songok, J. J., Ruhl, L. J., Kipkoech, C., Green, J. M., & Christoffersen-Deb, A. (2013). AccessMRS: Integrating OpenMRS with smart forms on Android. *Studies in Health Technology and Informatics*, 192, 866–870.

Fiordelli, M., Diviani, N., & Schulz, P. J. (2013). Mapping mHealth research: A decade of evolution. *Journal of Medical Internet Research*, 15(5), e95. https://doi.org/10.2196/jmir.2430.

Flynn, G., Jia, H., Reynolds, N. R., Mohr, D. C., & Schnall, R. (2020). Protocol of the randomized control trial: The WiseApp trial for improving health outcomes in PLWH (WiseApp). *BMC Public Health*, 20(1), 1775. https://doi.org/10.1186/s12889-020-09688-0.

Free, C., Phillips, G., Galli, L., Watson, L., Felix, L., Edwards, P., & Haines, A. (2013a). The effectiveness of mobile-health technology-based health behaviour change or disease management interventions for health care consumers: A systematic review. *PLoS Medicine*, 10(1), e1001362. https://doi.org/10.1371/journal.pmed.1001362.

Free, C., Phillips, G., Watson, L., Galli, L., Felix, L., Edwards, P., & Haines, A. (2013b). The effectiveness of mobile-health technologies to improve health care service delivery processes: A systematic review and meta-analysis. *PLoS Medicine*, 10(1), e1001363. https://doi.org/10.1371/journal.pmed.1001363.

GSMA. (2013a). Socio-economic impact of mHealth: An assessment report for Brazil and Mexico. Retrieved from https://www.gsma.com/iot/wp-content/uploads/2013/06/Socio-economic_impact-of-mHealth_BrazilnMexico_14062013V2.pdf

GSMA. (2013b). Socio-economic impact of mHealth: An assessment report for the European Union. Retrieved from https://www.gsma.com/iot/wp-content/uploads/2013/06/Socio-economic_impact-of-mHealth_EU_14062013V2.pdf

Gurupur, V., & Wan, T. T. H. (2020). Inherent bias in artificial intelligence-based decision support systems for healthcare. *Medicina, 56*(3), 141. Retrieved from. https://www.mdpi.com/1648-9144/56/3/141.

Hale, K., Capra, S., & Bauer, J. (2015). A framework to assist health professionals in recommending high-quality apps for supporting chronic disease self-management: Illustrative assessment of type 2 diabetes apps. *JMIR mHealth and uHealth, 3*(3), e87. https://doi.org/10.2196/mhealth.4532.

HealthTap. (2015). Doctors are making house calls again. Retrieved from https://www.healthtap.com/

Horvath, T., Azman, H., Kennedy, G. E., & Rutherford, G. W. (2012). Mobile phone text messaging for promoting adherence to antiretroviral therapy in patients with HIV infection. *Cochrane Database of Systematic Reviews, 2012*(3). https://doi.org/10.1002/14651858.Cd009756. Cd009756.

Hsu, C.-Y., Liu, Y., Kabelac, Z., Hristov, R., Katabi, D., & Liu, C. (2017). Extracting gait velocity and stride length from surrounding radio signals. Paper presented at the *Proceedings of the 2017 CHI Conference on Human Factors in Computing Systems*, Denver, Colorado, USA. https://doi.org/10.1145/3025453.3025937

IMS-Institute for Healthcare Informatics. (2013). Patient apps for improved healthcare: From novelty to mainstream. Retrieved from http://ignacioriesgo.es/wp-content/uploads/2014/03/iihi_patient_apps_report_editora_39_2_1.pdf

IMS-Institute for Healthcare Informatics. (2015). Patient adoption of mhealth. Use, evidence and remaining barriers to mainstream acceptance. Retrieved from https://www.iqvia.com/-/media/iqvia/pdfs/institute-reports/patient-adoption-of-mhealth.pdf

Iribarren, S. J., Schnall, R., Stone, P. W., & Carballo-Diéguez, A. (2016). Smartphone applications to support tuberculosis prevention and treatment: Review and evaluation. *JMIR mHealth and uHealth, 4*(2), e25. https://doi.org/10.2196/mhealth.5022.

Istepanian R, L, S., & Pattichis, C. E. (2006). *M-Health: Emerging mobile health systems*. New York, NY: Springer.

ITU-International Telecommunication Union. (2009). The world in 2009: ICT facts and figures. Retrieved from https://www.itu.int/net/TELECOM/World/2009/newsroom/pdf/stats_ict200910.pdf

ITU-International Telecommunication Union. (2013). The world in 2013: ICT facts and figures. Retrieved from https://www.itu.int/en/ITU-D/Statistics/Documents/facts/ICTFactsFigures2013-e.pdf

ITU-International Telecommunication Union. (2015). The World in 2015: ICT facts & figures. Retrieved from https://www.itu.int/en/ITU-D/Statistics/Documents/facts/ICTFactsFigures2015.pdf

ITU-International Telecommunication Union. (2020). Measuring digital development: Facts and figures 2020. Retrieved from https://www.itu.int/en/ITU-D/Statistics/Pages/facts/default.aspx

Ivatury G, M. J., & Bloch, A. (2009). A doctor in your pocket: Health hotlines in developing countries. *Innovations: Technology, Governance, Globalization, 4*(1), 119–153.

Jandoo, T. (2020). WHO guidance for digital health: What it means for researchers. *Digital Health, 6* https://doi.org/10.1177/2055207619898984. 2055207619898984.

Kiberu, V. M., Matovu, J. K., Makumbi, F., Kyozira, C., Mukooyo, E., & Wanyenze, R. K. (2014). Strengthening district-based health reporting through the district health management information software system: The Ugandan experience. *BMC Medical Informatics and Decision Making, 14*, 40. https://doi.org/10.1186/1472-6947-14-40.

Klotz, F. (2015). How mobile is transforming healthcare. Retrieved from https://impact.economist.com/perspectives/healthcare/how-mobile-transforming-healthcare

Kohlenberger, J. (2015). Mobilizing America: Accelerating next generation wireless opportunities everywhere. Retrieved from https://www.interdigital.com/post/mobilizing-america-making-5g-an-opportunity-for-broadbased-progress-

Kuehn, B. M. (2015). Is there an app to solve app overload? *The Journal of the American Medical Association, 313*(14), 1405–1407. https://doi.org/10.1001/jama.2015.2381.

Kuhns, L. M., Garofalo, R., Hidalgo, M., Hirshfield, S., Pearson, C., Bruce, J., et al. (2020). A randomized controlled efficacy trial of an mHealth HIV prevention intervention for sexual minority young men: MyPEEPS mobile study protocol. *BMC public health, 20*(1), 65. https://doi.org/10.1186/s12889-020-8180-4.

Kvedar, J., Coye, M. J., & Everett, W. (2014). Connected health: A review of technologies and strategies to improve patient care with telemedicine and telehealth. *Health Affairs (Millwood), 33*(2), 194–199. https://doi.org/10.1377/hlthaff.2013.0992.

Labrique, A. B., Vasudevan, L., Kochi, E., Fabricant, R., & Mehl, G. (2013b). mHealth innovations as health system strengthening tools: 12 common applications and a visual framework. *Global Health: Science and Practice, 1*(2), 160–171. https://doi.org/10.9745/ghsp-d-13-00031.

Labrique, A., Vasudevan, L., Chang, L. W., & Mehl, G. (2013a). Hope for mHealth: More "y" or "o" on the horizon? *International Journal of Medical Informatics, 82*(5), 467–469. https://doi.org/10.1016/j.ijmedinf.2012.11.016.

Laxminarayan, S., & Istepanian, R. S. (2000). UNWIRED E-MED: The next generation of wireless and internet telemedicine systems. *IEEE Transactions on Information Technology in Biomedicine, 4*(3), 189–193. https://doi.org/10.1109/titb.2000.5956074.

Lee, C., Raney, L., & L'Engle, K. (2013). mHealth Basics: Introduction to Mobile Technology for Health. Retrieved from https://www.globalhealthlearning.org/course/mhealth

Lee, N.-J., Chen, E. S., Currie, L. M., Donovan, M., Hall, E. K., Jia, H., & Bakken, S. (2009). The effect of a mobile clinical decision support system on the diagnosis of obesity and overweight in acute and primary care encounters. *Advances in Nursing Science, 32*(3), 211–221. https://doi.org/10.1097/ANS.0b013e3181b0d6bf.

Leo B, Morello R., & Ramachandran, V. (2015). The face of African infrastructure: Service availability and citizens' demands. *CGD Working Paper, 393* Retrieved from. https://www.cgdev.org/sites/default/files/CGD-Working-Paper-393-Leo-Morello-Ramachandran-African-Infrastructure-Citizens-Demands_1.pdf.

Lester, R. T., Ritvo, P., Mills, E. J., Kariri, A., Karanja, S., Chung, M. H., et al. (2010). Effects of a mobile phone short message service on antiretroviral treatment adherence in Kenya (WelTel Kenya1): A randomised trial. *Lancet, 376*(9755), 1838–1845. https://doi.org/10.1016/s0140-6736(10)61997-6.

Levine R, Corbacio A., & Konopka S., et al. (2015). African strategies for health, management sciences for health. Retrieved from http://www.africanstrategies4health.org/

Loring, M., Kabelac, Z., Munir, U., Yue, S., Ephraim, H. Y., Rahul, H., & Katabi, D. (2021). Novel technology to capture objective data from patients' recovery from laparoscopic endometriosis surgery. *Journal of Minimally Invasive Gynecology, 28*(2), 325–331.

Macleod, B., Phillips, J., Stone, A. E., Walji, A., & Awoonor-Williams, J. K. (2012). The architecture of a software system for supporting community-based primary health care with mobile technology: The Mobile Technology for Community Health (MoTeCH) initiative in Ghana. *Online Journal of Public Health Informatics, 4*(1). https://doi.org/10.5210/ojphi.v4i1.3910.

Marcano Belisario, J. S., Huckvale, K., Greenfield, G., Car, J., & Gunn, L. H. (2013). Smartphone and tablet self-management apps for asthma. *Cochrane Database of Systematic Reviews, 2013*(11), Cd010013. https://doi.org/10.1002/14651858.CD010013.pub2.

Martínez-Pérez, B., de la Torre-Díez, I., López-Coronado, M., & Sainz-De-Abajo, B. (2014). Comparison of mobile apps for the leading causes of death among different income zones: A review of the literature and app stores. *JMIR mHealth and uHealth, 2*(1), e1. https://doi.org/10.2196/mhealth.2779.

Masterson Creber, R. M., Maurer, M. S., Reading, M., Hiraldo, G., Hickey, K. T., & Iribarren, S. (2016). Review and analysis of existing mobile phone apps to support heart failure symptom monitoring and self-care management using the mobile application rating scale (MARS. *JMIR mHealth and uHealth, 4*(2), e74. https://doi.org/10.2196/mhealth.5882.

McNeil-PPC Inc. (2015). Allergy forecast tools and apps. Retrieved from https://www.zyrtec.com/allergy-forecast

Mendoza, G., Okoko, L., Konopka, S., & Jonas, E. (2013). African Strategies for Health Project, management sciences for health *mHealth Compendium, Volume Three*. Retrieved from http://www.africanstrategies4health.org/uploads/1/3/5/3/13538666/mhealth_compendium_volume_3_a4_english.pdf

Mitchell, M., Hedt-Gauthier, B. L., Msellemu, D., Nkaka, M., & Lesh, N. (2013). Using electronic technology to improve clinical care—results from a before-after cluster trial to evaluate assessment and classification of sick children according to Integrated Management of Childhood Illness (IMCI) protocol in Tanzania. *BMC Medical Informatics and Decision Making, 13*, 95. https://doi.org/10.1186/1472-6947-13-95.

Mobile Marketing Association. (2014). Industry overview. Retrieved from https://www.mmaglobal.com/about/industry-overview

Moore, J. O., Marshall, M. A., Judge, D. C., Moss, F. H., Gilroy, S. J., Crocker, J. B., et al. (2014). Technology-supported apprenticeship in the management of hypertension: A randomized controlled trial. *Journal of Clinical Outcomes Management, 21*. Retrieved from. https://www.mdedge.com/jcomjournal/article/147123/practice-management/technology-supported-apprenticeship-management.

Mungai, C. (2015). The mobile phone comes first in Africa; before electricity, water, toilets or even food. *17*(10). Retrieved from http://www.afriem.org/2015/03/mobile-phone-comes-first-africa-electricity-water-toilets-even-food/

National Institutes of Health (NIH). (2015). NIH-wide strategic plan, fiscal years 2016–2020. Retrieved from https://www.nih.gov/sites/default/files/about-nih/strategic-plan-fy2016-2020-508.pdf

NetHope. (2015). SDG ICT playbook. From innovation to impact. retrieved from https://digitalprinciples.org/resource/nethope-sdg-ict-playbook-from-innovation-to-impact/

NHS England. (2014). TECS CASE STUDY 002: Florence text messaging to monitor a range of conditions. Retrieved from https://www.england.nhs.uk/wp-content/uploads/2014/12/tecs-flo.pdf

Nicholas, J., Larsen, M. E., Proudfoot, J., & Christensen, H. (2015). Mobile apps for bipolar disorder: A systematic review of features and content quality. *Journal of Medical Internet Research, 17*(8), e198. https://doi.org/10.2196/jmir.4581.

O'Donovan, J., Bersin, A., & O'Donovan, C. (2015). The effectiveness of mobile health (mHealth) technologies to train healthcare professionals in developing countries: A review of the literature. *BMJ Innovations, 1*(1), 33–36. https://doi.org/10.1136/bmjinnov-2014-000013.

Patel V, Barker W., Siminerio E. (2014). Individuals' access and use of their online medical record nationwide. *ONC Data in Brief, No. 20*. Retrieved from https://www.healthit.gov/sites/default/files/consumeraccessdatabrief_9_10_14.pdf

Patrick, J. R. (2015). How mHealth will spur consumer-led healthcare. *mHealth, 1*, 14. https://doi.org/10.3978/j.issn.2306-9740.2015.07.01.

Pew Research Center. (2014). Mobile technology fact sheet. retrieved from https://www.pewresearch.org/internet/fact-sheet/mobile/

Philips Survey. (2012). Consumer attitudes towards healthcare technology. Retrieved from https://www.usa.philips.com/a-w/about/news/archive/standard/news/press/2012/20121212_Philips_Survey_Health_Info_Tech.html

Research2guidance, (2014). *mHealth app developer economics* (4th ed.). The State of the Art of mHealth App Publishing. Retrieved from: https://research2guidance.com/product/mhealth-app-developer-economics-2014/.

Rowland, S. P., Fitzgerald, J. E., Holme, T., Powell, J., & McGregor, A. (2020). What is the clinical value of mHealth for patients? *NPJournal Digital Medicine, 3*, 4. https://doi.org/10.1038/s41746-019-0206-x.

Sage Bionetworks. (2015). mPower: Mobile Parkinson Disease study. retrieved from https://parkinsonmpower.org/your-story

Salgado, T., Tavares, J., & Oliveira, T. (2020). Drivers of mobile health acceptance and use from the patient perspective: Survey study and quantitative model development. *JMIR mHealth and uHealth, 8*(7), e17588. https://doi.org/10.2196/17588.

Sanabria, G., Scherr, T., Garofalo, R., Kuhns, L. M., Bushover, B., Nash, N., et al. (2021). Usability evaluation of the mLab App for improving home HIV testing behaviors in youth at risk of HIV infection. *AIDS Education and Prevention, 33*(4), 312–324. https://doi.org/10.1521/aeap.2021.33.4.312.

Schnall, R., & Iribarren, S. J. (2015). Review and analysis of existing mobile phone applications for health care-associated infection prevention. *American Journal of Infection Control, 43*(6), 572–576. https://doi.org/10.1016/j.ajic.2015.01.021.

Schnall, R., Bakken, S., Rojas, M., Travers, J., & Carballo-Dieguez, A. (2015a). mHealth technology as a persuasive tool for treatment, care and management of persons living with HIV. *AIDS and Behavior, 19*(Suppl 2), 81–89. https://doi.org/10.1007/s10461-014-0984-8. (0 2).

Schnall, R., Cho, H., Mangone, A., Pichon, A., & Jia, H. (2018). Mobile health technology for improving symptom management in low income persons living with HIV. *AIDS and Behavior, 22*(10), 3373–3383. https://doi.org/10.1007/s10461-017-2014-0.

Schnall, R., Higgins, T., Brown, W., Carballo-Dieguez, A., & Bakken, S. (2015b). Trust, perceived risk, perceived ease of use and perceived usefulness as factors related to mHealth technology use. *Studies in Health Technology and Informatics, 216*, 467–471.

Sheehan, B., Nigrovic, L. E., Dayan, P. S., Kuppermann, N., Ballard, D. W., Alessandrini, E., Bakken, S., et al. (2013). Informing the design of clinical decision support services for evaluation of children with minor blunt head trauma in the emergency department: A sociotechnical analysis. *Journal of Biomedical Informatics, 46*(5), 905–913. https://doi.org/10.1016/j.jbi.2013.07.005.

Shen, N., Levitan, M. -J., Johnson, A., Bender, J. L., Hamilton-Page, M., Jadad, A. A., & Wiljer, D. (2015). Finding a depression app: A review and content analysis of the depression app marketplace. *JMIR mHealth and uHealth, 3*(1), e16. https://doi.org/10.2196/mhealth.3713.

Snowdon, A. (2020). HIMSS defines digital health for the global healthcare industry. Retrieved from https://www.himss.org/news/himss-defines-digital-health-global-healthcare-industry

SNS Research. (2014). The mobile healthcare (mHealth) bible: 2015–2020. SNS Research Marketing Intelligence & Consultancy Solutions.

Staggers, N., McCasky, T., Brazelton, N., & Kennedy, R. (2008). Nanotechnology: The coming revolution and its implications for consumers, clinicians, and informatics. *Nursing Outlook, 56*(5), 268–274. https://doi.org/10.1016/j.outlook.2008.06.004.

Statista. (2015a). Cumulative number of apps downloaded from the Apple App Store from July 2008 to June 2015 (in billions). *The Statistics Portal*. Retrieved from https://www.statista.com/statistics/263794/number-of-downloads-from-the-apple-app-store/

Statista. (2015b). Global smartphone penetration from 2008 to 2014 (in percent of new handset sales). Retrieved from https://www.statista.com/statistics/203734/global-smartphone-penetration-per-capita-since-2005/

Stern, C. (2015). Goldman Sachs says a digital healthcare revolution is coming—and it could save America $300 billion. Retrieved from https://www.businessinsider.com/goldman-digital-healthcare-is-coming-2015-6

Stoyanov, S. R., Hides, L., Kavanagh, D. J., Zelenko, O., Tjondronegoro, D., & Mani, M. (2015). Mobile app rating scale: A new tool for assessing the quality of health mobile apps. *JMIR mHealth and uHealth, 3*(1), e27. https://doi.org/10.2196/mhealth.3422.

Tarolli, C., Kabelac, Z., Myers, T., Waddell, E., Rahul, H., Hristov, R., & Ellis, T. (2020). A day in the life of Parkinson's: Using passive monitoring to characterize the disease at home: 1433. In. *Movement Disorders, Vol. 35*

The IQVIA Institute. (2017). The growing value of digital health. Retrieved from https://www.iqvia.com/insights/the-iqvia-institute/reports/the-growing-value-of-digital-health

The Office of the National Coordinator for Health Information Technology (ONC). (2021). Federal health IT strategic plan 2020–2025. Retrieved from https://www.healthit.gov/topic/2020-2025-federal-health-it-strategic-plan

The Office of the National Coordinator for Health Information Technology (ONC). (2015). Federal health IT strategic plan 2015–2020. Retrieved from https://www.healthit.gov/topic/about-onc/health-it-strategic-planning

Tractica. (2015). Home Health Technologies. Medical monitoring and management, remote consultations, eldercare, and health and wellness applications: Global market analysis and forecasts.

Tripp, N., Hainey, K., Liu, A., Poulton, A., Peek, M., Kim, J., & Nanan, R. (2014). An emerging model of maternity care: Smartphone, midwife, doctor? *Women and Birth: Journal of the Australian College of Midwives, 27*(1), 64–67. https://doi.org/10.1016/j.wombi.2013.11.001.

Turner, A. (2021). How many smartphones are in the world? Retrieved from https://www.bankmycell.com/blog/how-many-phones-are-in-the-world

US Food and Drug Administration. (2013). FDA issues final guidance on mobile medical apps. Retrieved from http://www.fda.gov/NewsEvents/Newsroom/PressAnnouncements/ucm369431.htm

US Food and Drug Administration. (2014). Device approvals, denials and clearances. Retrieved from http://www.fda.gov/medicaldevices/productsandmedicalprocedures/deviceapprovalsandclearances/default.htm

US Food and Drug Administration. (2015). Mobile medical applications. Guidance for Industry and Food and Drug Administration Staff. Retrieved from https://www.fda.gov/media/80958/download

USAID-United States Agency for International Development. (2015). The mHealth planning guide: Key considerations for integrating mobile technology into health programs. Retrieved from https://www.thecompassforsbc.org/sbcc-tools/mhealth-planning-guide-key-considerations-integrating-mobile-technology-health-programs-0

Vodopivec-Jamsek, V., de Jongh, T., Gurol-Urganci, I., Atun, R., & Car, J. (2012). Mobile phone messaging for preventive health care. *Cochrane Database of Systematic Reviews, 12*(12), Cd007457. https://doi.org/10.1002/14651858.CD007457.pub2.

Wakadha, H., Chandir, S., Were, E. V., Rubin, A., Obor, D., Levine, O. S., et al. (2013). The feasibility of using mobile-phone based SMS reminders and conditional cash transfers to improve timely immunization in rural Kenya. *Vaccine, 31*(6), 987–993. https://doi.org/10.1016/j.vaccine.2012.11.093.

Wallace, L. S., & Dhingra, L. K. (2014). A systematic review of smartphone applications for chronic pain available for download in the United States. *Journal of Opioid Management, 10*(1), 63–68. https://doi.org/10.5055/jom.2014.0193.

Waltz, E. (2014). BlueStar, the first prescription-only app. Doctors start prescribing the BlueStar app for diabetes management. Retrieved from https://spectrum.ieee.org/bluestar-the-first-prescriptiononly-app

Watterson, J. L., Walsh, J., & Madeka, I. (2015). Using mHealth to improve usage of antenatal care, postnatal care, and immunization: A systematic review of the literature. *BioMedical Research International, 2015*, 153402. https://doi.org/10.1155/2015/153402.

Whittaker, R. (2012). Issues in mHealth: Findings from key informant interviews. *Journal of Medical Internet Research, 14*(5), e129. https://doi.org/10.2196/jmir.1989.

Wiggers, K. (2020). A clinical team used MIT CSAIL's AI to remotely monitor a COVID-19 patient. Retrieved from https://venturebeat.com/2020/04/14/a-clinical-team-used-mit-csails-ai-to-remotely-monitor-a-covid-19-patient/

World Bank. (2012). Information and communications for development 2012: Maximizing mobile. Retrieved from https://www.worldbank.org/en/topic/digitaldevelopment/publication/ic4d-2012

World Bank. (2013). Mobile usage at the base of the pyramid: Research findings from Kenya and South Africa. Retrieved from https://openknowledge.worldbank.org/handle/10986/17623

World Health Organization. (2011). mHealth: New horizons for health through mobile technologies: Second global survey on eHealth. Retrieved from https://www.who.int/goe/publications/goe_mhealth_web.pdf

World Health Organization. (2019). WHO guideline: Recommendations on digital interventions for health system strengthening. Retrieved from https://www.who.int/reproductivehealth/publications/digital-interventions-health-system-strengthening/en/

Zhao, M., Hoti, K., Wang, H., Raghu, A., & Katabi, D. (2021). Assessment of medication self-administration using artificial intelligence. *Nature Medicine, 27*(4), 727–735. https://doi.org/10.1038/s41591-021-01273-1.

15

Personal Health Records

Matthew Sakumoto, Jessica M. Ruff, and David A. Pearson

> *If trends in adoption and expansion of the functionality of personal health records (PHRs) persist, PHRs have the potential to become the platform for a more efficient, effective, and personalized healthcare system.*

OBJECTIVES

At the completion of this chapter, the reader will be prepared to:

1. Describe key components of personal health records (PHRs).
2. Describe key factors leading to the widespread adoption of electronic PHRs.
3. Outline the technical implementation considerations for PHRs.
4. Summarize the challenges of adoption for PHRs.
5. Describe the impact of current evidence regarding how the effectiveness of PHRs improves healthcare in the context of the quadruple aim.
6. Discuss the future of PHRs.

KEY TERMS

connected personal health record, 236

digital divide, 242

Fast Healthcare Interoperability Resources (FHIR), 239

interoperability, 243

patient-generated health data (PGHD), 239

standalone personal health record, 236

ABSTRACT ❖

This chapter begins with a definition of the electronic personal health record (PHR) and a description of the types of PHRs. This is followed by a discussion of its development, evolution, and current use. Technical implementation considerations are explored, including data sources, interoperability, and privacy/security concerns. Challenges and barriers in PHR adoption are discussed, especially awareness, provider engagement, and the digital divide. Next, in the context of the quadruple aim for healthcare (enhancing the patient's care experience, improving the health of populations, reducing costs, and improving the work-life balance of healthcare providers), the growing body of evidence supporting the benefits of PHRs is reviewed. The chapter concludes with an exploration of the future of PHRs.

INTRODUCTION

The digitization of medical information and increasing ubiquity of web-enabled devices has increased patient access to their own health information via personal health records (PHRs). With increasing complexity of medical care and increased care coordination needs, PHRs have the potential to consolidate, coordinate, and empower patients in their healthcare journey.

PERSONAL HEALTH RECORDS

Essential Aspects of Personal Health Records

Although no single description is universally agreed upon, organizations have developed a definition for PHR. A joint definition by the PHR Task Force of the Medical Library Association and the National Library of Medicine stated the following:

> *Electronic personal health record [is]: a private, secure application through which an individual may access,*

manage, and share his or her health information. The PHR can include information that is entered by the consumer and/or data from other sources such as pharmacies, labs, and health care providers. The PHR may or may not include information from the electronic health record (EHR) that is maintained by the health care provider and is not synonymous with the EHR. PHR sponsors include vendors who may or may not charge a fee, health care organizations such as hospitals, health insurance companies, or employers (Jones, Shipman, Plaut, & Selden, 2010).

Other organizations, including the Markle Foundation, American Health Information Management Association, and American Medical Informatics Association, have published definitions of a PHR (AHIMA e-HIM Personal Health Record Work Group 2005; Koskinen & Rantanen 2020; Markle Foundation 2006; Vincent, et al. 2008).

The definitions from these groups emphasize three essential aspects of the PHR: the first is that the PHR serves as an information aggregator and storage system. The second is that the PHR is a tool or suite of tools that individuals or their delegates may use to manage their health (Tang, Ash, Bates, Overhage, & Sands, 2006). Third, the intentional avoidance of the word "patient" in the definitions highlight that these tools are to be used for health and wellness and not only during illness.

Types of Personal Health Records

There are multiple proposed classifications of PHRs based on the data sources, the direction of data flow, and the functionality (Vincent, et al. 2008; Tang, et al. 2006). For this chapter, we will use the taxonomy from ONC/HealthIT.gov based on data source and method of entry: (1) standalone (or untethered) and (2) connected (Are there different types of personal health records [PHRs] 2021). Fig. 15.1 demonstrates the PHR dependence and complexity in various approaches to PHRs.

Standalone Personal Health Record

Standalone (untethered) PHRs store health information on an individual's electronic device (e.g., computer, smartphone, flash memory drive) or are commercial web-based applications. These systems might be of use in particular cases (e.g., the capacity for emergency medical providers to access the person's USB stored data or they might collect information related to a specific disease). Early examples of standalone PHRs include Microsoft Word or Excel templates. These were not widely adopted, likely

because they require manual data entry by the user and lack interoperability with other systems such as EHRs (Tang, et al. 2006). Another form of standalone PHRs, often called untethered PHRs, are web-based systems separate from an EHR. The advantage of web-based systems is they are accessible anytime and can aggregate data from multiple sources. The drawback is that they do not link to healthcare providers; thus, users cannot e-mail their doctors, request medication refills, view their medical records, or schedule appointments. Despite these deficits, proponents of untethered and standalone systems suggest that these formats offer users maximum control over the content included in their PHR (Simons, Mandl, & Kohane, 2005).

Examples of untethered commercial PHRs include the initial Google Health (2008–12) platform, Microsoft HealthVault (2007–19), and Apple Health. The Google and Microsoft products were web-based PHR platforms, while Apple's product is a mobile app. These systems integrate data from multiple sources: individuals can upload documents and images, connect their wearable device, and/or have their medical records added directly to the PHR. One of the strengths of these platforms is the ability to automatically capture data using compatible self-monitoring devices such as pedometers, glucometers, and blood pressure monitors. A second strength is that when users allow access, app developers can leverage data for research. Google discontinued their first PHR in 2012, and HealthVault ended in 2019, with the primary reason being lack of widespread adoption (An update on Google Health and Google PowerMeter 2021; mHealthIntelligence 2018). Apple's PHR launched in 2018 and Google is currently making a second attempt (Google is exploring 2021; What the failure of Microsoft's 2019; Mullin 2011).

Connected Personal Health Record

A connected (tethered) PHR is typically linked to a single clinic or healthcare system. Because these systems enable the user to view EHR data via the PHR, they are often called a *patient portal* (i.e., the system provides a portal into the person's medical information within the EHR). The benefits of patient portals include direct communication with healthcare providers, the ability to request medication refills, and appointment self-scheduling. Furthermore, their linkage to the EHR reduces the manual data entry required in standalone PHRs. The main disadvantage of the patient portal is that the information is linked only to one specific healthcare provider or system, making it challenging to create a single PHR reference source for patients with clinicians in different healthcare systems. Fortunately, EHR vendors are beginning to allow patients to link PHRs to more than one entity, wearable devices, and sensors. When a connected PHR integrates data from multiple sources, from different healthcare providers, health plans, or laboratories, it is referred to as a networked PHR. The data are integrated through access services that conduct user authentication before allowing the patient or proxy access to data. Ideally, this allows users single sign on (SSO) access to comprehensive, integrated personal health data. As with EHRs, the development of comprehensive, integrated PHRs is dependent on the wide implementation of data representation and data exchange standards that are still needed to create interoperable records. Fig. 15.2 illustrates the relationships between EHRs and PHRs and interfaces between personal and organizational domains.

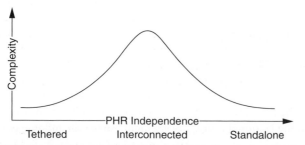

Fig. 15.1 Range of complexity in various approaches to personal health records *(PHRs)*. (From Tang, P. C., Ash, J. S., Bates, D. W., Overhage, J. M., & Sands, D. Z. [2006]. Personal health records: Definitions, benefits, and strategies for overcoming barriers to adoption. JAMIA, *13*[2], 121–126.)

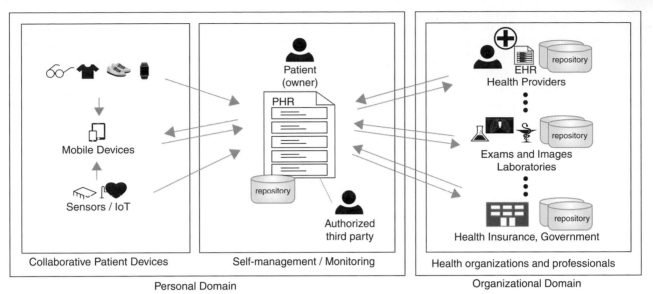

Fig. 15.2 Personal health records *(PHR)* and electronic health record *(EHR)* relationships. (From Roehrs, A., da Costa, C.A., da Rosa Righi, R., & de Oliveira, K.S.F. [2017]. Personal health records: a systematic literature review. *J Med Internet Res, 19*[1], e13.)

One of the earliest examples of a patient portal is the Veterans Health Affairs' (VHA's) MyHealthyVet (MHV) from 2003 (Nazi & Woods 2008). MHV has two levels of use. The first level allows anyone to create an account online and use the system as a stand-alone web-based PHR. The second level is for individuals receiving care through the VHA. Veterans can take full advantage of MHV's functionality, including exchanging secure e-mails with their healthcare providers, viewing portions of their EHRs, viewing upcoming appointments, and receiving wellness reminders.

Both standalone and connected PHRs represent a rapid area of development and deployment among start-up entrepreneurial ventures, technology companies, and healthcare systems, with more examples available and being updated for the future.

THE EVOLUTION OF THE ELECTRONIC PERSONAL HEALTH RECORD

Individuals have long kept paper records of their healthcare as adjuncts to their medical records. Common examples include paper records of immunizations and lists of prescription medications or medical problems that people may keep in their personal files or printed out and stored in their wallet. A Harris Interactive poll (Harris Interactive, 2007) in the early 2000s found that most people thought it was a positive approach to keep PHRs; 46% of those surveyed kept records, and of those who did keep records, 86% of them had them on paper. The evolution from paper to digital health records continues today as patients obtain the tools to ease the transition, healthcare systems push EHR data into PHRs for patient care coordination and communication, and the US government policies seek to increase EHR and PHR adoption.

Consumer Evolution

In 2000, an estimated 52% of Americans had access to the internet, and this has grown to 93% today (Pew Research Center n.d.a, n.d.b). In February 2021, The Pew Foundation estimated that 85% of US adults owned smartphones, and this percentage is increasing steadily (Pew Research Center n.d.a, n.d.b). Over

time, improved electronic information access in other industries (especially finance and banking), as well as the growth in internet access and mobile device ownership, has paved the way for PHRs and other personal health technologies. Fig. 15.3 presents the trends in ownership of mobile phones in the United States from 2002 to 2021.

Health System Evolution

While the widespread adoption and use of personal computing devices and the internet provide the infrastructure that makes PHRs possible, EHRs serve as the primary source of data populating the PHR. Large-scale implementation of EHRs began in the early 1990s at several integrated health systems, such as the VHA (Timson 2021). Intermountain Healthcare in Utah, and the Regenstrief Institute in Indiana (Duke, et al. 2014; McDonald, et al. 1999). Early efforts to make EHRs available to patients resulted in wide variation in both content and presentation. An early example of allowing patients to access their EHR was the Blue Button. The idea for Blue Button was developed during a meeting of the Markle Connecting for Health workgroup in 2010 (Markle Foundation 2015). With a single click of the Blue Button, the vision was for patients to access their records in human-readable or machine-readable format. The initial deployment of the Blue Button was at the Veteran's Administration in August 2010, and continues to expand into other governmental agencies and private enterprises today (Healthit.gov 2021; US Department of Veteran Affairs 2018). As health systems also seek to expand their digital front doors, improve the digital patient experience, and provide more efficient care, reaching their patients via connected PHRs is an increasing priority.

Evolving Government Policies

In recent years, the U.S. government implemented policies specifically intended to increase the adoption of both EHRs and PHRs. In this chapter, we will only provide a brief overview of these policies and their relation to PHR adoption. The Health Information Portability and Accountability Act (HIPAA) of

North, F., Hanna, B. K., Crane, S. J., Smith, S. A., Tulledge-Scheitel, S. M., & Stroebel, R. J. (2011). Patient portal doldrums: Does an exam room promotional video during an office visit increase patient portal registrations and portal use? *Journal of the American Medical Informatics Association: JAMIA, 18*(Suppl 1), i24–i27. https://doi.org/10.1136/amiajnl-2011-000381.

Ontario Shores' HealthCheck Patient Portal benefits evaluation report Canada Health Infoway. (n.d.). Retrieved August 7, 2021, from https://www.infoway-inforoute.ca/en/component/edocman/resources/reports/benefits-evaluation/3174-ontario-shores-healthcheck-patient-portal-benefits-evaluation-report

Onyeaka, H. K., Romero, P., Healy, B. C., & Celano, C. M. (2021). Age differences in the use of health information technology among adults in the United States: An analysis of the health information national trends survey. *Journal of Aging and Health, 33*(1–2), 147–154. https://doi.org/10.1177/0898264320966266.

OpenNotes: Research repository. (n.d.). Retrieved August 7, 2021, from https://www.opennotes.org/research/

Osborn, C. Y., Mayberry, L. S., Mulvaney, S. A., & Hess, R. (2010). Patient web portals to improve diabetes outcomes: A systematic review. *Current Diabetes Reports, 10*(6), 422–435. https://doi.org/10.1007/s11892-010-0151-1.

Paccoud, I., Baumann, M., Le Bihan, E., Pétré, B., Breinbauer, M., Böhme, P., Leist, A. K. (2021). Socioeconomic and behavioural factors associated with access to and use of personal health records. *BMC Medical Informatics and Decision Making, 21*, 18. https://doi.org/10.1186/s12911-020-01383-9.

Pan, C.-C., Sivo, S. A., & Graham, J. A. (2019). Demographics, learner characteristics, and use of wearable devices. *Journal of Hispanic Higher Education, 20*, 422–437. https://doi.org/10.1177/1538192719877622.

Patel, V., & Johnson, C. (2018). *Individuals' use of online medical records and technology for health needs* (ONC Data Brief No. 40; ONC Data Brief, pp. 1–17).

Patel, V., & Johnson, C. (2019). Trends in individuals' access, viewing and use of online medical records and other technology for health needs: 2017–2018 | HealthIT.gov (No. 48; ONC Data Brief, pp. 1–13). https://www.healthit.gov/data/data-briefs/trends-individuals-access-viewing-and-use-online-medical-records-and-other

Patel, V., Barker, W., & Siminerio, E. (2015). Trends in consumer access and use of electronic health information. *ONC Data Brief, 30*.

PatientEngagementHIT. (2019, May 3). *Can Apple Health Records become healthcare's data access solution?* PatientEngagementHIT. https://patientengagementhit.com/features/can-apple-health-records-become-healthcares-data-access-solution

Paton, C., Hansen, M., Fernandez-Luque, L., & Lau, A. Y. S. (2012). Self-tracking, social media and personal health records for patient empowered self-care. Contribution of the IMIA Social Media Working Group. *Yearbook of Medical Informatics, 7*, 16–24.

Pew Research Center. (June 2021). Mobile Fact Sheet. Pew Research Center. Retrieved July 19, 2021, from https://www.pewresearch.org/internet/fact-sheet/mobile/.

Pew Research Center. (June 2021). Internet/Broadband Fact Sheet. Pew Research Center. Retrieved August 12, 2021, from https://www.pewresearch.org/internet/fact-sheet/internet-broadband.

Portz, J. D., Powers, J. D., Casillas, A., Baldwin, M., Bekelman, D. B., Palen, T. E., Bayliss, E. (2021). Characteristics of patients and proxy caregivers using patient portals in the setting of serious illness and end of life. *Journal of Palliative Medicine* https://doi.org/10.1089/jpm.2020.0667.

Ralston, J. D., Carrell, D., Reid, R., Anderson, M., Moran, M., & Hereford, J. (2007). Patient web services integrated with a shared medical record: Patient use and satisfaction. *Journal of the American Medical Informatics Association: JAMIA, 14*(6), 798–806. https://doi.org/10.1197/jamia.M2302.

Ralston, J. D., Hereford, J., Carrell, D., & Moran, M. (2006). Use and satisfaction of a patient web portal with a shared medical record between patients and providers. *AMIA Annual Symposium Proceedings, 2006*, 1070.

Rights (O.C.R.), O. for C. (2008, May 7). *Your rights under HIPAA [Text]*. HHS.Gov. https://www.hhs.gov/hipaa/for-individuals/guidance-materials-for-consumers/index.html

Roblin, D. W., Houston, T. K., II, Allison, J. J., Joski, P. J., & Becker, E. R. (2009). Disparities in use of a personal health record in a managed care organization. *Journal of the American Medical Informatics Association, 16*(5), 683–689. https://doi.org/10.1197/jamia.M3169.

Russ, A. L., & Saleem, J. J. (2018). Ten factors to consider when developing usability scenarios and tasks for health information technology. *Journal of Biomedical Informatics, 78*, 123–133. https://doi.org/10.1016/j.jbi.2018.01.001.

Saparova, D. (2012). Motivating, influencing, and persuading patients through personal health records: A scoping review. *Perspectives in Health Information Management / AHIMA, American Health Information Management Association, 9*(Summer), 1f.

Saripalle, R., Runyan, C., & Russell, M. (2019). Using HL7 FHIR to achieve interoperability in patient health record. *Journal of Biomedical Informatics, 94*, 103188. https://doi.org/10.1016/j.jbi.2019.103188.

Schnipper, J. L., Gandhi, T. K., Wald, J. S., Grant, R. W., Poon, E. G., Volk, L. A., Middleton, B. (2008). Design and implementation of a web-based patient portal linked to an electronic health record designed to improve medication safety: The Patient Gateway medications module. *Journal of Innovation in Health Informatics, 16*(2), 147–155. https://doi.org/10.14236/jhi.v16i2.686.

Schooley, B. L., Horan, T. A., Lee, P. W., & West, P. A. (2010). Rural veteran access to healthcare services: Investigating the role of information and communication technologies in overcoming spatial barriers. *Perspectives in Health Information Management / AHIMA, American Health Information Management Association, 7* (Spring), 1f.

Sharko, M., Wilcox, L., Hong, M. K., & Ancker, J. S. (2018). Variability in adolescent portal privacy features: How the unique privacy needs of the adolescent patient create a complex decision-making process. *Journal of the American Medical Informatics Association, 25*(8), 1008–1017. https://doi.org/10.1093/jamia/ocy042.

Simborg, D. W. (2008). Promoting electronic health record adoption. Is it the correct focus. *Journal of the American Medical Informatics Association: JAMIA, 15*(2), 127–129. https://doi.org/10.1197/jamia.M2573.

Simons, W. W., Mandl, K. D., & Kohane, I. S. (2005). The PING personally controlled electronic medical record system: Technical architecture. *Journal of the American Medical Informatics Association, 12*(1), 47–54. https://doi.org/10.1197/jamia.M1592.

State of California. (2021). *Digital COVID-19 Vaccine Record*. https://myvaccinerecord.cdph.ca.gov/

Taha, J., Czaja, S. J., Sharit, J., & Morrow, D. G. (2013). Factors affecting usage of a personal health record (PHR) to manage health. *Psychology and Aging, 28*(4), 1124–1139. https://doi.org/10.1037/a0033911.

Talmadge, T. (2019). Views on the Apple Health application from future health science professionals. *Health Sciences Student Work.* https://scholarworks.merrimack.edu/hsc_studentpub/19

Tang, P. C., Ash, J. S., Bates, D. W., Overhage, J. M., & Sands, D. Z. (2006). Personal health records: Definitions, benefits, and strategies for overcoming barriers to adoption. *Journal of the American Medical Informatics Association : JAMIA, 13*(2), 121–126. https://doi.org/10.1197/jamia.M2025.

Tarabichi, Y., Goyden, J., Liu, R., Lewis, S., Sudano, J., & Kaelber, D. C. (2020). A step closer to nationwide electronic health record-based chronic disease surveillance: Characterizing asthma prevalence and emergency department utilization from 100 million patient records through a novel multisite collaboration. *Journal of the American Medical Informatics Association: JAMIA, 27*(1), 127–135. https://doi.org/10.1093/jamia/ocz172.

The future of health *is cognitive* (Point of View, pp. 1–12). (2016). IBM Healthcare and Life Sciences.

Timson, G. (2021). *The history of the Hardhats.* Hardhats. https://www.hardhats.org/history/hardhats.html

Topaloglu, U., & Palchuk, M. B. (2018). Using a federated network of real-world data to optimize clinical trials operations. *JCO Clinical Cancer Informatics*, 2. https://doi.org/10.1200/CCI.17.00067. CCI.17.00067.

Trends and disparities in patient portal use (No. 45; HINTS Briefs). (2021). National Cancer Institute. https://hints.cancer.gov/docs/Briefs/HINTS_Brief_45.pdf

Turner, K., Clary, A., Hong, Y.-R., Tabriz, A. A., & Shea, C. M. (2020). Patient portal barriers and group differences: Cross-sectional national survey study. *Journal of Medical Internet Research, 22*(9), e18870. https://doi.org/10.2196/18870.

US Department of Veteran Affairs. (2018, December 3). *Blue Button Home* [Program Homepage]. https://www.va.gov/bluebutton/

Vincent, A., Kaelber, D. C., Pan, E., Shah, S., Johnston, D., & Middleton, B. (2008). A patient-centric taxonomy for personal health records (PHRs). *AMIA Annual Symposium Proceedings, 2008*, 763–767.

Vogels, E.A. (2020, January 9). About one-in-five Americans use a smart watch or fitness tracker. *Pew Research Center.* https://www.pewresearch.org/fact-tank/2020/01/09/about-one-in-five-americans-use-a-smart-watch-or-fitness-tracker/

Wang, Q., Su, M., Zhang, M., & Li, R. (2021). Integrating digital technologies and public health to fight Covid-19 pandemic: Key technologies, applications, challenges and outlook of digital healthcare. *International Journal of Environmental Research and Public Health, 18*(11), 6053. https://doi.org/10.3390/ijerph18116053.

Wang, S., Ding, S., & Xiong, L. (2020). A new system for surveillance and digital contact tracing for COVID-19: Spatiotemporal reporting over network and GPS. *JMIR MHealth and UHealth, 8*(6), e19457. https://doi.org/10.2196/19457.

What the failure of Microsoft's HealthVault means for the future of EHRs. (2019, April 19). https://hitconsultant.net/2019/04/19/what-the-failure-of-microsofts-healthvault-means-for-the-future-of-ehrs/

Willis, J. M., Macri, J. M., Simo, J., Anstrom, K. J., & Lobach, D. F. (2006). Perceptions about use of a patient internet portal among Medicaid beneficiaries. *AMIA. Annual Symposium Proceedings. AMIA Symposium, 2006*, 1145.

Yamin, C. K., Emani, S., Williams, D. H., Lipsitz, S. R., Karson, A. S., Wald, J. S., & Bates, D. W. (2011). The digital divide in adoption and use of a personal health record. *Archives of Internal Medicine, 171*(6), 568–574. https://doi.org/10.1001/archinternmed.2011.34.

Zhou, Y. Y., Leith, W. M., Li, H., & Tom, J. O. (2015). Personal health record use for children and health care utilization: Propensity score-matched cohort analysis. *Journal of the American Medical Informatics Association, 22*(4), 748–754. https://doi.org/10.1093/jamia/ocu018.

Zulman, D. M., Nazi, K. M., Turvey, C. L., Wagner, T. H., Woods, S. S., & An, L. C. (2011). Patient interest in sharing personal health record information: A web-based survey. *Annals of Internal Medicine, 155*(12), 805–810. https://doi.org/10.7326/0003-4819-155-12-201112200-00002.

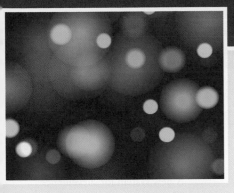

16

Social Media Tools for Health Informatics

Heather Carter-Templeton and Tiffany Kelley

Peer-to-peer healthcare is a way for people to do what they have always done—lend a hand, lend an ear, lend advice—but at internet speed and at internet scale.

Susannah Fox

OBJECTIVES

At the completion of this chapter, the reader will be prepared to:
1. Summarize key considerations of using social media for health-related purposes.
2. Outline the issues and challenges associated with the use of social media in healthcare and healthcare education.
3. Discuss the guidance for writing social media policies.

KEY TERMS

microblogging, 251   social media, 249   social networks, 251

ABSTRACT ❖

This chapter begins with defining the concept of social media and describing tools that operationalize this concept to better understand the concept of social media. Additionally, this chapter explores ways that healthcare professionals and healthcare consumers can leverage such social media tools. Social media is not without challenges that include *(but are not limited to)* privacy, confidentiality, inappropriate behavior, security, regulatory issues, and market pressure. To help address these challenges, the chapter provides a comprehensive overview related to the development of social media policies in healthcare, as well as the implications of social media during a national healthcare public health crisis.

SOCIAL MEDIA

Social Media Versus Other Media

What is social media? Social media (a term first used in 2004) is a type of digital communication where users create their own information content to post online and share, relating to their areas of personal or professional interests (Merriam-Webster, 2021).

Six core principles differentiate social media from other forms of communication and collaboration:
1. Participation
2. Collective
3. Transparency
4. Independence
5. Persistence
6. Emergence

These characteristics collectively describe social media as a digital environment allowing for mass collaboration among users (Kaplan & Haenlein, 2010).

Today, the most popular social media platforms are those allowing an individual to make and maintain social digital connections with other users. These social media platforms offer user-friendly and easy-to-use methods for maintaining relationships with colleagues, family, friends, and/or create and develop new connections and relationships. Many personal and professional relationships have been maintained or strengthened by social media platforms. Additionally, these personal and professional relationships may not exist without the development of these social media platforms. The impact of social media on individuals, groups, populations, and communities is often overlooked, despite the easy-to-use nature of these platforms in establishing and maintaining relationships (American Psychological Association [APA], 2019).

Social media platforms are transforming how individuals and groups collect and communicate data and information with others who have similar interests. Additionally, social media platforms are becoming increasingly powerful for data- and information-sharing to persuade and influence others. The healthcare industry recognizes the potential for social media platforms to increase the awareness of healthcare services, disseminate health promotion and preventative education, recruit new clients, connect patients to others with similar experiences, and increase access to health services through the use of user accounts. Social media platforms offer an alternative form of marketing that is different from the traditional print, radio, and one-way internet mass communication. Instead, social media platforms provide healthcare with a novel venue for fast and efficient information sharing, such as new services, health-promotion programs, and advances in patient care (Surani et al., 2017). Table 16.1 demonstrates the evolving nature of social media applications using several well-recognized names. Box 16.1 offers information about the most popular social media networks.

Many consumers turn to resources found in social media platforms to assist in answering their healthcare questions. Reports examining the future transformation of healthcare noted the use of social media platforms as a viable method to meet the widespread information needs of consumer and/or patient populations. The conclusion was that social media platforms can

BOX 16.1 Top 10 Most Popular Social Media Networks, as of July 2021

1. Facebook
2. YouTube
3. WhatsApp
4. Instagram
5. Facebook Messenger
6. WeChat
7. TikTok
8. QQ
9. Douyin
10. Telegram

Information retrieved from Statista. Available at: https://www.statista.com/statistics/272014/global-social-networks-ranked-by-number-of-users/

facilitate the promotion of both health and wellness (Bipartisan Policy Center, 2019).

Social Media Tools

People use one or more social media platforms daily. Users' social media behaviors may routinely include accessing news outlets, connecting with friends and/or family, locating services, and/or professional networking to build necessary connections (Hale, 2021). More specifically, a recent study revealed that social media usage among healthcare providers is common. However, there is considerable variation in how social media is perceived and used by nurses (Lefebvre et al., 2020).

Social media platforms facilitate interaction and networking among their communities through web- and/or app- (application) based tools. Multiple social media platform types exist, including networking, media sharing, blogs, wikis, video blogs, microblogs, and more. These platforms form the foundation for an ever-growing list of tools. There are ways to classify these social media tools. One method is a classification (Fox, 2011) system based on social theories (social presence (Short et al., 1976) and media richness (Daft & Lengel, 1986) and two key social-process elements (self-presentation and self-disclosure). This system is particularly useful for researchers examining the impact of social media tools. Another way to categorize the use of social media tools is to understand that the structure of a social media site is dependent on its purpose and the exchange of information. A simpler method of organizing social media tools is to classify them by their type (see Box 13.1 for more information) (Shellenbarger & Robb, 2013; Eckler et al., 2010).

For example, social media tools can commonly be divided into these five categories:

1. Social networking (e.g., Facebook, LinkedIn);
2. Blogging (http://thehealthcareblog.com) and wikis (http://wikidoc.org);
3. Microblogging (e.g., Twitter);
4. Social bookmarking or pinning (e.g., Pinterest) and social sharing news (Digg, Reddit); and
5. Video or image sharing (e.g., YouTube, Instagram, TikTok, SnapChat).

TABLE 16.1 Development of Social Media Applications and/or Devices

Year	Device and/or Application
1978	Computerized bulletin board
1992	First smartphone released
1998	Blogger
2000	Friendster
2002	MySpace
2003	LinkedIn and Facebook
2005	YouTube
2007	iPhone
2009	Twitter
2010	iPad and Pinterest
2010	Instagram
2011	Snapchat
2014	Learnist
The future	Interactions within an augmented virtual reality

Adapted from Nelson, R., Joos, I., & Wolf, D. (2013). *Social media for nurses.* New York, NY: Springer Publishing Company.

Social Networking

Social networks are online platforms that enable individuals and groups to connect with others who share similar interests. These social networking platforms transcend time and geographic restrictions, opening lines of communication and allowing users to share text, photographs, and videos, and even a combination of all three. The notion is that social networks build on the wisdom of the crowd (Surowiecki, 2005). Social networks have changed the way individuals, businesses, and organizations experience and interact with the world of healthcare. Examples of health-related services provided by social networks include information-sharing, social support, and self-care promotion (Jackson et al., 2014).

An infinite number of health-related social networking sites have been developed by for-profit and not-for-profit groups, including healthcare institutions, professional groups, voluntary associations, and healthcare consumers. An example of a not-for-profit health social networking site is CaringBridge (www.caringbridge.org). CaringBridge allows patients, their family, and/or friends to create their own private and personal websites to facilitate health status information exchange and encourage support during health crises. PatientsLikeMe, CureTogether, and Inspire are examples of for-profit social health networking sites. These social health networking sites offer the opportunity to link and facilitate data- and information-sharing among patients with similar diagnoses.

General consumer social media sites also facilitate important aspects of health-related networking. Facebook, one of the more well-known social networking sites, is an example. A wide range of individuals, businesses, healthcare institutions, companies, special interest groups, and health organizations have Facebook pages and groups. Although not exclusively designed as a forum for healthcare, these Facebook pages and groups are often accessed to gather healthcare information and to market practices or institutions to patients (Duquesne University, 2020).

Blogging and Wikis

Blogs represent a web-based, chronological journal of an individual author's thoughts. Blogs allow for asynchronous conversations and invite readers to comment and join the discussion. Blogs contain a variety of media types beyond simple text, including links to other websites, videos, images, publications, and more. Blogs that engage individuals and create a sense of community through the expertise of the author on a specific topic of interest are poised for growth in interest (Sparks et al., 2011). Medical journals, healthcare facilities, nursing organizations, healthcare provider networks, and educational institutions commonly maintain blogs to relay the latest information and facilitate discussion.

Wikis are collaborative, web-based tools designed to compile information on a particular topic or group of topics and differ from blogs. Wikis provide a platform for the creation of a flexible document by allowing many authors to add and edit content, rather than just one or a few dedicated authors. It is important to note that wikis are edited by users, and they are not peer-reviewed. In addition, tracking of edits by users is usually limited. Wikis should not be considered primary sources on a topic of interest.

Microblogging (Twitter)

Microblogging is a form of blogging in which entries are kept brief using character limitations. Twitter, the primary microblogging site, restricts blog threads, known as "tweets," to 280 characters. These posts are delineated with a hashtag (#) symbol to organize tweets of a particular topic. Examples of health-related hashtags used on Twitter can be seen at The Healthcare Hashtag Project (symplur.com). Twitter has emerged as an increasingly popular site for public health research and is used in many studies to track trends and behaviors related to illnesses and conditions (Hart et al., 2017). Twitter is also a useful tool for instant communication of vital information during crises or disasters, such as the coronavirus pandemic that started in March 2020. Authors have suggested that standard hashtags could be used to create a national conversation within and across disciplines. For example, a recent publication called for nursing leaders in Canada to consider the need for a national social media hashtag or series of hashtags that could be utilized to unify and extend professional messaging for registered nurses (RNs) (Resling, 2016).

Phil Baumann, in 2009, provided a multipurpose overview of different healthcare uses of Twitter, which continues to be a useful resource more than a decade later.

Social Bookmarking

Social bookmarking is a method to organize and store online resources. Unlike saving bookmarks to your individual computer browser, the bookmarks are tagged on a third-party website, such as Pocket, Digg, or Pinterest. Social bookmarking offers three primary advantages: convenience, labeling, and partnerships (Barton, 2009). Accessibility means that users' bookmarks are accessible from any computer. The bookmarks are no longer tied to a particular computer; instead, the social-bookmarking service allows users to connect and access all saved bookmarks. Second, labeling or tagging allows the creation of established tags that are meaningful to the user and not just those established by a computer algorithm. Users can share their tags with others in their network or join other networks to view their tags. In the spirit of social media, these tools facilitate collaboration within specific or general networks. Negative aspects include great variability in labelling or tagging, as there is a lack of standardization with taxonomies resulting in spelling errors and personal tags. Consequently, searching challenges may ensue (Barton, 2009).

Video- and Image-Sharing Content

Another method for sharing health information is through video. A commonly used website for video sharing is YouTube. This social media channel that began in 2005 allows visitors to view and share videos posted by individuals, businesses, and organizations. YouTube, started by three employees from eCommerce company PayPal, began as a platform for people to share "home videos." It quickly grew, and, in just over a year, more than 20,000 new videos were being uploaded to YouTube daily. YouTube, recently acquired by Google, offers a space for both professional and amateur videographers to share content. Videos can be "liked" or "disliked." Credibility and accuracy of the videos vary because end users are uploading content.

YouTube can provide benefits to students in presenting visual instruction for hands-on nursing skills, such as changing a tracheotomy dressing or giving an insulin injection. Thus, YouTube has a unique advantage for providing nursing and health education to students, patients, and providers. Possible examples of easily accessible and deliverable video content includes health-promoting exercise instructions, computer-generated depictions of how a condition, such as diabetes, affects internal organs, as well as general educational content on diseases. Podcasts are asynchronous recordings designed to provide healthcare information and current events announcements. YouTube has also worked to promote factual and credible information about the COVID-19 pandemic. They have partnered with authoritative groups to assist in delivering important education about COVID-19 vaccines.

Flickr is a public photo-sharing site that offers a forum for sharing photos and encouraging conversation and dialog. Medical facilities are actively using these social media tools to interact with clients, promote facility activities, and open alternate means of communication. Foursquare, a social media tool designed specifically for mobile applications, allows users to "check in" at various venues, instantly communicating with friends and, at times, receiving discounts at "checked-in" locations (Foursquare—Independent Location Data Platform). Medical facilities that use mobile platforms are creating the opportunity for visitors to comment on their hospital experience.

Other healthcare sectors are turning to Second Life (Second Life), a multiuser virtual environment (MUVE), or virtual, world that allows users to create a three-dimensional arena with graphics and sound simulation for education and socialization purposes. The disabled community has embraced Second Life and has created the Virtual Ability Island; 20 several schools of nursing use this tool for educational purposes (Skiba, 2009). Both Second Life and Virtual Ability Island allow those with disabilities to thrive in online virtual worlds.

Social Media Statistics

Use of social media statistics, while constantly changing, are in an upward trend. In 2021, 70% of Americans use some type of social media, which is up from 65% in 2015 (Pew Research Center, 2021). YouTube and Facebook remain the dominant forms of social media being used by adults in the United States. Adults under 30 report using Instagram, TikTok, and Snapchat more than other age groups. This increased use of social media is also seen in healthcare.

Healthcare consumers turn to these resources to learn more about their conditions or to connect with others. The number of health-related institutions of with social media policies is also becoming more standard. Scholarly journals and professional organizations are using social media to promote and share content, and healthcare organizations are creating and expanding social media pages. Social media platforms may in fact increase dissemination of some scholarly works with some nursing journals (31%) using a journal-specific social media account (Waldrop & Dunlap, 2021). Furthermore, some journals use a coordinated strategy to share new content. Likewise, clinicians may share helpful research-based information found in scholarly works through social media platforms. Research has been done to assess the impact of social media on increasing the number of citations in health-related research (Bardus et al., 2020).

A recent report by PricewaterhouseCoopers Health Research Institute noted that one-third of healthcare consumers now use social media to find out more about their medical condition and symptoms and to share their thoughts about their doctors, medications, and insurance companies with others (ReferralMD, 2021). Social media reviews may also offer new opportunities to merge consumer perspectives into existing quality appraisals of services in care such areas as nursing homes (Li et al., 2019). The following social medical–related statistics were also compiled by Referral MD:

- Greater than 40% of healthcare consumers are influenced by social media that inform them about health-related matters.
- Social media platforms inform users about experiences in healthcare settings. At least 32% of US social media users share information about their friends' and families' healthcare experiences, with 29% of these users viewing health information and the experiences of others with their disease.
- Engaged users on social media are those coping with a chronic condition or disability.
- Only 26% of hospitals in the United States are using social media. Hospitals in California, New York, and Texas use social media more than hospitals in other states.
- At least 53% of physicians have a Facebook page for their office.
- There are 165,000 health and medical apps available. About two-thirds of these are focused on general wellness, such as lifestyle, stress, fitness, and diet.
- At least 60% of people surveyed said they trust a doctor's social media post versus a pharma post (ReferralMD, 2021).

Health-related social network use is expanding rapidly. Specific social networks, such as PatientsLikeMe and MedHelp, present membership and daily usage statistics on their web pages demonstrate an impressive number of members. Additionally, professional workforce sites, such as LinkedIn, allow healthcare professionals to connect with others in their field.

Many major healthcare systems have realized the positive influence of social media and committed to the use of social networking tools to support the delivery of healthcare information, describe their services, recruit employees, and communicate their mission (Nelson & Wolf, 2013). The U.S. Department of Veterans Affairs (VA) recognized the power of social media and is aggressively incorporating social media tools into its agenda. The VA has its own YouTube channel, Twitter feeds, and a veteran-run blog. The VA's *Directive 6515: Use of Web-Based Collaboration Technologies* not only highly encourages the use of social media but also "endorses the secure use of

Web-based collaboration and social media tools to enhance communication, stakeholder outreach collaboration, and information exchange; streamline processes; and foster productivity improvements to achieve seamless access to information" (Department of Veterans Affairs, 2011) The VA believes that the use of social media technologies will support the organization's mission effectiveness through the benefits of speed, broad reach, targeted reach, collaboration, a medium for dialog, and expansion of real-time, sensitive communications (Department of Veterans Affairs, 2011).

Healthcare insurance companies are joining the trend of using social media tools to promote well-being. Blue Cross and Blue Shield (BCBS) maintains a social media site for its members that allows for individual profiles, blogs, discussion threads, and access to experts in nutrition, cooking, and health coaching. Pharmaceutical companies are using social media tools to provide customers and physicians with educational materials. Input from physicians facilitates a relationship with pharmaceutical companies for improved patient outcomes. These sites also offer customer and patient services, opening channels for medication users to discuss experiences and needs.

Benefits of Social Media Platforms

There are benefits associated with the use of social media. Social media benefits in healthcare can be seen in talent recruitment, networking among colleagues, and collaboration with other disciplines (Hale, 2021). Another benefit may be the opportunity to improve provider-to-provider communication as well as a bidirectional provider-to-patient communication. Social media offers a means of communication between provider and patient that is more personable; however, it can also have unintended consequences that impact the patient's experience. By improving communication and facilitating the swift transfer of information, the use of social media may correlate with a positive influence on patient outcomes. These tools go beyond simple one-way communication, creating an engaging form of conversation between patient and provider.

Another benefit is in research. A growing number of studies describe potential benefits of social media. Social media in healthcare has been studied since the early 2000s. However, evidence of the effectiveness of social media about healthcare is inconclusive. A recent systematic review provides a summary to date of research in medicine and may help identify the appropriate application of social media (Giustini et al., 2018).

Challenges of Social Media Platforms

The world of social media is not free of challenges and opposition. The strengths of social media's open platform and networking capabilities are also its greatest weaknesses. Social media can enhance the healthcare experience but it also has the potential to undermine optimal healthcare (American Nurses Association [ANA], 2011a). The uptake of new technology requires a careful appraisal and informed risk analysis. Unfortunately, many are not exploring the benefits of social media due to prolonged discussion and debate often stalled by skepticism and by those who are risk averse (Chretien & Kind, 2013). While social media

connections are facilitated through technology, the technology should not necessarily be the focal point, but it should serve as the medium used to connect with others. Apprehension exists about using social media platforms to communicate with others, including reasons such as:

- It takes too much time to learn;
- Participation may be seen as unprofessional by other healthcare providers;
- It is too easy to make a mistake and post something that is prohibited by an employer's social media policy; and
- It is too easy to make a mistake and post something that compromises patient confidentiality.

Social media has quickly developed into an acceptable form of mass communication. However, managing the stakes associated with social media communication channels requires professionals that learn to effectively use these tools, work to share quality information, engage other stakeholders, and respond to feedback from others. Health professionals should be aware of the dangers associated with social media use prior to engaging in its activities (ANA, 2011a). The primary principle influencing the use of social media in healthcare is the obligation to serve the best needs of the public. However, clinicians are bound by laws, practice ethics, and professional codes of conduct governing how and when to use social media applications. The digital environment is not isolated from the real world, (American Nurses Association [ANA], 2011b) and professional standards that exist in one realm should carry over to the other. Moreover, naïve and negligent social media practices bring about security vulnerabilities that can compromise professional integrity and consumer confidence (ANA, 2011a). Private and professional organizations recognizing these issues have provided guidance regarding appropriate social media practices. Table 16.2 provides information pertaining to health-related professional guidelines and social media. Each of these issues will be explored in more detail in the sections that follow.

Privacy and Confidentiality

The most significant challenge for healthcare providers who use social media is to maintain privacy and confidentiality. Healthcare organizations and all their employees must follow patient privacy laws in addition to any unique laws at the state level (Hale, 2021). There is an innate relationship between privacy and sharing many aspects of a personal or professional situation. Digital social media tools have brought these challenges to the forefront. Prior to social media, with its open access, individuals and organizations had more control over what information was shared and who had access to that shared information. With online, real-time capabilities, that control is much more limited. This loss of control requires more attention and awareness about personal information that can be quickly and easily shared within online social environments. Each social media application offers options, often referred to as settings, related to privacy. It is not easy to find and determine how these options function. However, it is important to invest the time and effort necessary to understand these options. The advantages that social media offers for professionals and scholars in terms of

Resling, T. (2016). Social media and nursing leadership: Unifying professional voice and presence. *Nursing Leadership, 28*(4), 48–57.

Ritter, A. Z., Aronowitz, S., Leininger, L., et al. (2021). Dear Pandemic: Nurses as key partners in fighting the COVID-19 infodemic. *Public Health Nursing, 38*(4), 603–609.

Ross, P., & Cross, R. (2019). Rise of the e-nurse: The power of social media in nursing. *Contemporary Nurse, 55*(2-3), 211–220.

Shellenbarger, T., & Robb, M. (2013). Pinstructive ideas. *Nurse Educator, 38*(5), 206–209.

Short, J., Williams, E., & Christie, B. (1976). *The social psychology of telecommunications.* Hoboken, New Jersey: John Wiley & Sons.

Skiba, D. (2009). Nursing education 2.0: A second look at Second Life. *Nursing Education Perspectives, 30*(2), 129–131.

Sparks, M. A., O'Seaghdha, C. M., Sethi, S. K., & Jhaveri, K. D. (2011). Embracing the internet as a means of enhancing medical education in nephrology. *American Journal of Kidney Diseases, 58*(4), 512–518.

Surani, Z., Hirani, R., Elias, A., et al. (2017). Social media usage among health care providers. *BMC Res Notes, 10*, 654.

Surowiecki, J. (2005). *The wisdom of crowds.* New York: Anchor Books.

Symantec, Internet Security Threat Report. 2014.

Tunick, R. A., Mednick, L., & Conroy, C. (2011). A snapshot of child psychologists' social media activity: Professional and ethical practice implications and recommendations. *Professional Psychology: Research and Practice, 42*(6), 440–447.

U.S. Department of Health and Human Services. (2013). *Summary of the HIPAA privacy rule.* Available from: https://www.hhs.gov/hipaa/for-professionals/privacy/laws-regulations/index.html#:~:text=The%20U.S.%20Department%20of%20Health%20and%20Human%20Services,and%20control%20how%20their%20health%20information%20is%20used.

U.S. Food and Drug Administration (FDA). (2021). *What does FDA regulate?* https://www.fda.gov/about-fda/fda-basics/what-does-fda-regulate.

Ventola, C. L. (2014). Social media and health care professionals: Benefits and best practices. *PT, 39*(7), 491–520.

Waldrop, J., & Dunlap, J. J. (2021). Analysis of tweeting on journal usage and identification of nursing journals using social media. *CIN: Computers, Informatics, Nursing, 39*(6), 291–295.

Wang, Z., Wang, S., Zhang, Y., & Jiang, X. (2019). Social media usage and online professionalism among registered nurses: A cross-sectional survey. *International Journal of Nursing Studies, 98*, 19–26.

Westrick, S. J. (2016). Nursing Students' Use of Electronic and Social Media. *Nursing Education Perspectives, 37*(1), 16–22.

Wilson, B. (2017). Using social media to fight fraud. *Risk Management, 64*(2), 10–11.

Young, S.D. (2011). Recommendations for using online social networking technolgoes to reduce innacurate online health information. *Journal of Health and Allied Sciences, 10*(2), 2.

17

Project Management Principles

Michele Mills

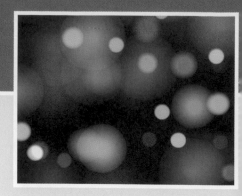

As costs continue to increase and more government regulations are mandated, healthcare professionals need to approach strategic initiatives and projects in a proven, methodical way by using formal project management principles. Use of project and portfolio management principles, processes and tools extends well beyond health information technology (IT).

OBJECTIVES

At the completion of this chapter, the reader will be prepared to:
1. Describe the organizational need for project management.
2. Describe commonly used healthcare project management terms.
3. Describe the purpose of portfolio management.
4. Distinguish skills needed for project, program, and portfolio managers.
5. Summarize the functions of commonly used project management tools.

KEY TERMS

ABSTRACT ❖

The increased demand for effectiveness and efficiency in healthcare delivery forced leaders at all levels to determine the best way to use available resources whether these are human, physical, or monetary. Project management, a systematic approach to planning and guiding project processes from start to finish, is a proven way to improve outcomes that can directly and positively affect costs through the efficient and effective use of limited resources for health information technology. Fundamental project management practices allow organizations to reach strategic goals within a planned timeline within cost parameters. A strong project management discipline includes high degrees of communication, organization, interpersonal leadership, cross-functional team coordination and negotiations, problem-solving, attentiveness to detail, technical and business domain knowledge, and the ability to methodically guide the project processes through organizational governance parameters using these formal steps:

- Initiation or pre-planning
- Formal planning with the creation of a project plan
- Implementation and execution of that project plan with measurement of progress and performance
- Project closure through delivery of value through project objectives

INTRODUCTION

Dr. Armstrong started a small ear nose and throat (ENT) clinical practice recently acquired by a large local hospital network. Each morning he meets with his clinic's nurses and staff to review a list of patients treated the day before to ensure information in their files is complete and correct. Up to now, he has not been able to fully expand his office capabilities to include a full electronic health record (EHR) system. Instead, he and his office staff spend time reviewing paper patient forms. He was just informed that hospital administration found his clinic to be losing revenue because they are not accurately capturing all the patient data needed for efficient billing. He understands the importance of optimization for the patient experience and efficiency of cost, which a streamlined electronic patient documentation process would provide. He and the hospital would like a solution within three months. He has proposed that they select key patient paper forms they could convert into electronic forms that would integrate into the hospital system.

Later that week, Dr. Armstrong had conversations with hospital administration and the information technology (IT) department about making his forms electronic. He found a larger hospital initiative already underway for an enterprise document management system that would integrate departmental documentation into the larger hospital EHR system. That initiative had an expected timeline of 18 months. Under his current timeline constraints, Dr. Armstrong negotiated a small capital budget to get a temporary electronic solution in place for his critical ENT patient forms until the larger solution was available. The biggest question on his mind at this point was "How in the world am I going to get this all done in three months?"

In a complex organization like a hospital where clinics and physicians have competing priorities and demands, healthcare providers are responsible for ensuring that the tools, processes, infrastructure, and capabilities are in place to meet the demand for superior patient care. The project management role can be indispensable in health IT as it employs a structured approach to help ensure effective implementations of healthcare initiatives. A strong project management process should include initiation or pre-planning, formal planning, creation and implementation of a project plan, measurement of progress, and performance (PMI, 2014). A health IT project might focus on the implementation of a single application or initiative within a short timeline, such as supplying a temporary electronic documentation solution for Dr. Armstrong's clinic.

Program management involves larger implementations, like a large-scale hospital document management application or an organizational wide EHR system. With program management there are multiple, aligned projects affecting teams or departments that are coordinated and managed in concert.

Portfolio management is even more complex and involves the creation of common programs and projects that are not necessarily related but are important to combine and view. One example would be managing a clinical portfolio where all projects and programs that directly affect patient care are in a common category. Other portfolios might be a financial or a technology infrastructure portfolio. Effective management of portfolios is essential for a healthcare organization to prioritize and approve new project requests, and to work strategically on projects throughout the years. Portfolio management provides an essential foundation for decisions and discussions in governance committees as projects are prioritized and funded (Rajegopal, 2012).

THE NEED FOR PROJECT MANAGEMENT IN HEALTHCARE ORGANIZATIONS

Influence of Project Management

The project manager can improve the quality of health IT project outcomes, provide accountability of expenses, and reduce inefficiencies through structured change control processes. The PMI, an association created to improve organizational success and further mature the profession of project management through its globally recognized standards, has conducted studies related to the impact of project management. These studies revealed that 80% of all projects fail to meet their objectives if they do not have a structured project methodology (Project Management Institute [PMI], 2006).

Applying proper processes, methodologies, and tools within a hospital setting can have multi-dimensional benefits by reducing variability across processes, providing standardization across projects, and increasing the overall project success rate. This is important in any industry but even more critical in a healthcare environment where multiple stakeholders, departments, clinics, and providers functioning under a single hospital umbrella must coordinate between competing priorities, budgets, capital expenses, and large enterprise initiatives. Many healthcare projects across departments can overlap or even clash. This is because departments are often regarded as separate entities or *silos* where clinical projects and initiatives are often done independently at the discretion of a leader and at times without aligning project goals with the larger organizational objectives. In the case of Dr. Armstrong, without a coordinated and structured project management approach at the hospital, his ENT clinic might implement a software solution for his electronic patient forms that may be incompatible with the hospital document management system. This could result in rework for interoperability/integration and a waste of valuable resources in the longer term although it may provide a short-term solution for his area.

Project Management Methodologies

Healthcare practitioners implement projects with the best intent, but providers are seldom trained in formal project management methodologies. They may lack the skillset and knowledge base to properly mitigate project risks, define the scope of the project, develop realistic schedules, or manage resource issues throughout a given project timeline. Without these requisite skills, organizations may have projects with inconsistent outcomes, including cost over-runs, time delays, and/or poor-quality deliverables. At the macro level of hospital administration, this can often create conflicts where differences in project implementations from department to department result in an inability to estimate annual costs and departmental performance. Without a standardized approach it is difficult to gather and measure organizational performance metrics, prepare performance reports, forecast financial data, and understand financial impacts and human capital costs of organizational initiatives. Standardized and consistent project management is necessary throughout the organization at all levels to perfect the process and project outcomes across all entities. The most effective organizations have formal strategic plans showing what they can and will do, so there is a clear understanding of the expectations across organizational departments and levels. Project management best practices can help create transparency and visibility within the organization and helps reduce these issues (Bhide, 2011).

Effective use of project management techniques can help align key areas and ensure skills and tools are consistently

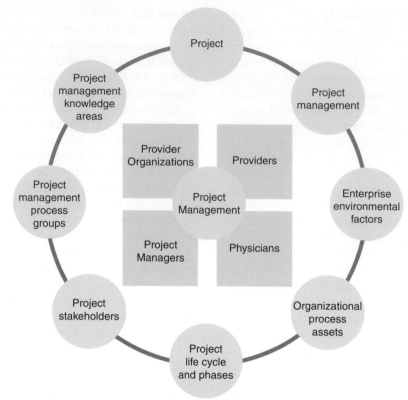

Fig. 17.1 Coordination areas of project management.

applied to health IT. This is important because healthcare must generate revenue while in a competitive landscape, control costs, operate within government regulations and not compromise quality, patient care or satisfaction. Project management can help ensure delivery of initiatives and projects on-time, within budget and provide well-defined value requirements that positively affect the organization's financial performance, productivity, and delivery of patient services. It can also enhance patient satisfaction either directly or indirectly (Bhide, 2011).

Project management serves as an effective way to bring all these concepts together to more efficiently appropriate resources in support of an organization's goals (see Fig. 17.1). The figure shows project management areas surrounded by typical stakeholders. A PMI Pulse of the Profession study showed that projects within high performing organizations can meet planned goals two-and-a-half times more frequently than those in low performing organizations. Additionally, high-performing organizations waste about 13 times less money than low performers. The need for strong project management skills and a solid understanding of the process has never been more important in healthcare (Stang et al., 2021).

PROJECT, PROGRAM, AND PORTFOLIO MANAGEMENT

As defined earlier, project, program and portfolio management are three levels of focus in formal project management. The following section explores each level and their interrelationships.

Project Management

A project refers to an undertaking that is time-bound and delivers a particular product or service. It is a temporary undertaking ending after achieving a set of goals and involving the application of knowledge, ideas, and skills to execute a plan of action (PMI, 2014). More specifically, a project consists of goals, activities, a timeline, projected risks, and mitigation plans. Each project has an appointed manager who leads the effort. An example of a project is the purchase of a peri-natal clinical system that needs to integrate with the current EHR.

To follow project management best practices, project processes, documentation, and procedures must follow a methodical approach through a series of defined phases that each have a specific set of deliverables and steps that must be completed before the next phase should begin. These project phases include Initiation, Planning, Execution, and Closure (see Fig. 17.2).

Project Process Groups

The PMI provides various process groups (or steps) and knowledge areas critical to the success of a project or program (Rajegopal, 2012). These process groups and associated activities form the primary foundation for the life cycle of a project (see Table 17.1).

Initiating Activities

Initiating activities is the most important activity and yet often the most rushed or under-valued. The initiation phase of a project requires a project manager to gather initial information and resource estimates to assess the viability of the

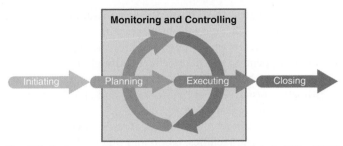

Fig. 17.2 Project management phases. (Copyright Michele Mills, 2021.)

TABLE 17.1 Project Management Process Groups (Steps)

Process Group	Description	Activities and Steps
Initiation	Project Managers collect sufficient data to decide about the viability of a project and assess what is necessary	• Define objectives • Define scope • Define purpose • Define deliverables • Provide financial and human capital estimates • Obtain necessary approvals and funding • Create project proposals
Planning	Project Managers collaborate with domain and subject matter experts to create a detailed plan to guide the project team throughout project execution and closure	• Create project charters • Break down deliverables into workable tasks • Create project plan • Identify critical work path and schedule • Assign resources • Create communication plan • Identify risks and create risk mitigation plans • Create testing plans • Create quality assurance plans • Create release management plans
Execution	Staff and vendors begin building the project deliverables and provide them to customers for testing and signoff. Monitoring and control of the project are significant to ensure the executed plan does not deviate from the original purpose or scope.	• Complete project tasks • Monitor and control time, cost, quality, change, risks, issues, procurements, customer acceptance, communications, etc. • Adhere to plans established in Planning phase
Closure	Delivery of the project, and communication and hand-off to operations and maintenance teams	• Create ongoing support models for operations and maintenance • Document Lessons learned

project. This includes activities like submission of a formal project proposal or business case for approval from leadership teams, prioritization of competing projects at the program or portfolio governance levels, approvals for capital funding and operational budget from hospital administration. Initial project scope and timelines should be established so leaders can balance the impact on resources and existing workloads. Projects should have organization visibility so larger risks and changes on architecture and existing initiatives can be mitigated across efforts. This can help mitigate unnecessary spending and ensure solid alignment, organization, and strategic goals and objectives. Once projects are approved, funded, and resourced, formal project planning can begin.

Planning Activities

Planning activities lays the foundation for the project life cycle and tracks future project performance. Planning is where projects are formally defined by project teams and subject matter experts who decompose project deliverables into workable tasks as part of the overall project plan. The plan will help project leaders with time management, cost estimation, quality, change, risk, and issues throughout the life of a project. Often this step is where healthcare project advocates struggle because there is a constant need to deliver "quicker, better, faster" in the rush to implement a product or solution. Key risks may not be fully planned for or even considered and tasks affecting the scope or the timeline may not be identified early enough to mitigate them. Steps may be left out completely. Defining the project through planning helps team members achieve defined goals and objectives and serves as a basis for effective communication and evaluation for managing project staff and external vendors about timelines and budget. Skipping this step or even inadequately completing this step typically hinders progress throughout the life of a project and affects long-term results stakeholders seek. The formal project is ready for execution with its completion, resourcing, and scheduling.

Execution Activities

Execution activities often take the most time and resources to complete. The execution phase defines the success of a project. This is where the build of project deliverables and customer testing and approval occurs. Use of solid management processes, including effective monitoring and control of all elements of a project including time, cost, quality, change, risk, issues, procurement, customer acceptance, and communications can help assure success at the execution phase (Matthews, 2013). The project manager monitors for challenges encountered during development, mitigates risks using well thought-out risk plans, and controls the changes to project scope and issues to keep the project on schedule and avoid derailment. Project closure begins once this phase has its goals met.

Closing Activities

Closing activities include release management, project delivery, documentation of lessons learned, and formal hand-off to operational and maintenance teams (PMI, 2014). This is critical

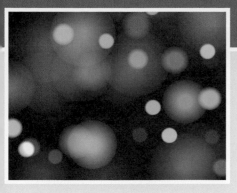

18

Strategic Planning and Information System Selection

Thomas H. Payne

OBJECTIVES

At the completion of this chapter, the reader will be prepared to:
1. Summarize organizational health information technology values and cost considerations.
2. Summarize processes required for project/system initiation.
3. Explain methods of system or project team formation.
4. Summarize key aspects for system security.
5. Outline overall needed system functionality based upon organizational needs and complexities.
6. Discuss trends in using vendors and locally developed EHRs.
7. Give examples of steps commonly used in selecting a system.
8. Discuss the final steps in choosing a system.

KEY TERMS

mission statement, 278	request for proposals, 284	strategic plan, 278
request for information, 284	scope creep, 282	strong authentication, 280

ABSTRACT ❖

Leveraging electronic health record and other information systems to improve care begins with a clear understanding of the health care organization's mission and strategic objectives. Matching what is available in the electronic health record (EHR) marketplace with your needs requires careful and meticulous assessment of the needs of clinicians and others in the organization, and then determining what vendor systems can meet those needs. This chapter describes the process of creating a strategic plan, performing needs assessment, determining if a formal Request for Proposals is warranted, and then using vendor proposals to select the best match for the organization. The next step is to begin a relationship with the vendor by creating a contract that is most likely to lead to a successful, long-term relationship and serves as the foundation for implementation and use of the system to benefit patients and providers. There are many questions provided as fodder for thought as you consider information system strategic planning.

INTRODUCTION

Healthcare organizations depend on information technology more than ever. Healthcare organizations are influenced and supported by information systems. Efficiency is extremely important, and efficiency depends upon optimizing information flow and patient care management given the narrow financial margin most organizations operate under. There are overwhelming demands for reporting and conformance to regulatory requirements that are impossible to manage without information systems; there are incentives to use health IT and penalties if you do not. An important use of health information technology is that it provides opportunities to measure and improve the quality and safety of healthcare.

The largest and most used health information technology system in most healthcare organizations is the electronic health record (EHR) which will serve as an example system for this chapter. Most healthcare organizations already use an EHR because of previous Meaningful Use incentives that were part of the American Recovery and Reinvestment Act (ARRA). For this reason, an EHR implementation project is more likely to be a replacement of one EHR with another than a transition from paper medical records to an EHR. These two transitions—paper to EHR or one EHR to another—have similar characteristics, but

TABLE 18.1   How Does Switching From One Electronic Health Record to Another Differ From Switching From a Paper Record to an Electronic Health Record?

	Paper EHR	One EHR to another
Training	How does the electronic workflow differ from paper?	How does accomplishing tasks in the new EHR differ from the old EHR?
		Will users familiar with the new EHR from experience elsewhere receive the same training as everyone else?
Data	Are paper documents scanned?	What data are imported from the old EHR to the new one?
	Will paper records be available at the point of care?	Will providers be required to use a legacy data viewer, or will lab, imaging, pathology, and notes all be available in the new EHR?
Underlying models	Is there a single paper chart used in clinics and hospitals?	Is the definition of encounter the same?
	If so, do they have common elements such as problem list?	Are there any big differences in orders and documentation?
Infrastructure	Are there workstations and devices at the point of care?	Does the existing EHR infrastructure support the new EHR?
Policy development	What happens during a downtime?	Have downtime procedures been reviewed and refreshed?
	Does everyone have a password?	Any changes in authentication?
Patient experience	Are patients familiar with using electronic messaging, requesting appointments, viewing notes?	Will the patient portal change?
		Will there be a change in patient viewing of results and notes?

EHR, Electronic health record.

also differ (Table 18.1). Both rely on an understanding of the organization's strategic objectives and its mission and financial state. Both should be regarded as clinical projects and deep involvement clinician users.

System replacement or implementation should be undertaken with the understanding we have learned about clinician burnout. Clinician burnout, defined by AHRQ as "long-term stress reaction marked by emotional exhaustion, depersonalization, and a lack of sense of personal accomplishment" (https://www.ahrq.gov/prevention/clinician/ahrq-works/burnout/index.html) is a widely recognized problem to which EHRs are known to contribute. When implementing an EHR, it is wise to plan from the start to do everything possible to reduce the contribution of EHR to burnout, such as reducing time required for documentation, reducing data entry tasks, and reducing unnecessary between-visit tasks such as EHR inbox management. Because workforce members have widely varying aptitudes and interest in using an EHR and find EHRs to be burdensome and that their workday is longer as a result, EHR contribution to burnout should be well understood and addressed in the organization's project.

Implementing or standing up an EHR is best undertaken with understanding of basic principles such as the following:
1. Implementing an EHR is a clinical project. Clinicians should be heavily involved and should be project leaders. Those leaders are best chosen from existing clinical opinion leaders, not just from those who are technically minded and facile with technology.
2. Implementing any EHR is a complex project with many facets. We've learned over the years that the discipline of project management is extremely helpful in managing all the aspects of the project in the resources required to successfully conclude the project.
3. Although it seems useful to make a distinction between implementing an EHR and operating one, there really is no sharp line. Implementation starts with functionality that is essential

to meet the objectives of the project but certainly not all functionality is included initially, and may be implemented over time. This occurs at the same time when some functionality is also heavily used, and so it occurs in the time traditionally labeled as "operations." In fact, a new phrase has been coined—"optimization"—a term used by consultants who assist organizations with the transition to EHRs. Optimization really means that there are opportunities for more extensive use of any EHR features to meet organizational objectives, and workflow is refined to best use the capabilities of the electronic health records.

KNOW YOUR ORGANIZATION

Mission Statements and Strategic Planning and Their Value in Successful Use of Health Information Technology

Successful projects start with a goal. The goal of a health IT project is likely to support your organization achieve its purpose and objectives. Start by asking simple questions, like "What is the purpose of your organization?" Information technology (IT) initiatives should support that purpose. The organizational purpose is often laid out in a simple statement, sometimes called a Mission Statement. What is your organizational mission? Do people who work with you know the mission? What are the organization's strategic objectives? Is there a strategic plan, and if so, has it been updated recently? The strategic plan offers a view into what leaders and involved workforce members feel are guideposts to the future of the organization. Mission achievement and support requires challenging work, a strategy, and a plan. Your strategy is to create clinics to serve healthcare needs of a geographic region, or to generate return to stockholders while delivering high quality healthcare. The mission and the strategy should inform the health IT project.

Many organizations develop a formal process to create a mission statement and a strategic plan. This very likely has occurred in advance of the IT project you are preparing for and is used to guide all aspects of the organization. A senior leader typically leads the strategic planning process, usually projects 3 to 5 years into the future, involves vision and mission statements, objectives, and strategies for achieving them. It may involve SWOT analysis where Strengths, Weaknesses, Opportunities and Threats are considered. Because the strategic planning process is involved, critically important, and involves time from busy, important people, often a consulting firm with experience in strategic planning is engaged to assist with this process. The strategic planning process includes understanding the external environment, the organizational mission and business strategy, and how IT fits into and supports these.

A full strategic planning process that may require 4 to 6 months or more may benefit from shorter strategic planning activities focused on specific needs or to update the current strategic plan may also be helpful. As the name implies, to be strategic, and for the organization to plan its future, the project should not drift or simply react to outside events. IT systems are key elements to support the organization by supporting the work the organization performs, and by leveraging the important data that arise from organizational activities. In fact, organizations consider information to be one of the most important organizational assets.

It takes more than understanding a few paragraphs in the mission statement and strategic plan to implement an IT system. We need to have a broad and deep organizational understanding before beginning an information system. An understanding of who works here, who comes to the organization for care, and for what reasons. It is essential to know how the organization generates revenue to keep the doors open and generate a positive margin (the difference between what you take and what you spend), and it helps to know the history of the organization. Deep understanding of the culture and the perspectives of the leaders and workers is key to success as we will see. Additionally, while you are learning about this organizational information, you should reflect on how the mission resonates with you personally. Life is short and if you are reading this book, you have skills organizations would love to have. Work in a place that you will be proud to tell your grandchildren about.

The strategic planning process is key to the success of an information system project because it is important to align large IT initiatives with clinical and financial strategy and integration of service delivery.

EHR Cost Considerations

Carefully consider the financial aspects of this project from the beginning. Know how much it will cost, and how it will be financed/paid for. EHR implementation costs vary widely, but the Office of the National Coordinator (ONC) has resources to help estimate the costs. Costs will include hardware, licensing EHR software, implementation assistance including configuration and support, training (that includes the cost of having an orthopedic suheron in EHR training instead of in the operating room) and most importantly ongoing maintenance costs. Large,

complex projects such as implhernting an EHR are very expensive. Many organizations do not have funds for capital projects of this scale readily available and may need to borrow or "float a bond" to finance it. Remember that many of the benefits of the EHR accrue to payers and others outside of the organization. Expect at least a temporary drop in physician productivity. These costs are born by the organization, not by federal incentive programs.

WHERE TO START?

Clayton's Framework

Starting a large and complex project may seem overwhelming. Implementing an EHR is an enormous effort from the time and effort required by everyone in the organization and the financial costs that are incurred, therefore, the decision to implement a large system such as an EHR often involves the highest levels of organizational leadership. You may be the leader, part of the leadership group, or a team member, but it is helpful to break the project into pieces and to have a framework on which to hang the pieces. Here is a framework based on what I learned from Paul Clayton, a national leader in health IT, whose career included Intermountain Health and Columbia Presbyterian Medical Center informatics projects (pay careful attention to the order of the elements of this framework).

Components of Clayton's Framework

1. Institutional commitment

    Implementing an IT system is one of the biggest projects the organization will undertake, involves nearly everyone and requires substantial amounts of time and money. The organization must be committed to maximize the chances of success. How do you measure commitment? One useful proxy for commitment is project budget. The first mistake to avoid is underestimating (low-balling) what it will take and the length of time it will take to be successful. If there is wavering in institutional commitment, then this may not be the time for this large project. If there is clear commitment, meaning that funding and staffing of other projects is reduced or placed on hold as necessary, and if the senior leader publicly commits to making this project successful, then you are off to a good start.

    Many organizations borrow money to pay for EHR implementations, incurring debt that may limit borrowing for other reasons. The word *commitment* is important in this context: It requires commitment for EHR projects to reach a successful conclusion.

2. Leadership

    Big projects need a leader who is known by all and where total responsibility lies. The leader requires the ability to make challenging decisions, accountability, and commitment even when things are grim, in addition to genuine talent for inspiring and leading people. A leader is not always recognized when the project is going well; you may find out when seemingly impossible problems arise, which they likely will.

3. People

    No leader can do this alone. It takes people whose time and energy are devoted to making the EHR project a success.

One of the first tasks of a good leader is to assemble a team of talented, engaging people. But there is a catch: Because they are acknowledged to be talented, they may already have an important job or role within the organization that will need to be put on hold. These valued individuals may discover that they would like to continue in this new role as a new aspect of their career.

4. Infrastructure

The last thing clinicians should be concerned about when switching to or implementing a new EHR is the dependability of the network, availability of workstations, or the reliability of the data center. This clinical computing infrastructure underlies the EHR and departmental systems, and should be a firm, reliable foundation maintained by experienced IT professionals. Be certain this is true within your organization or wait until it is before switching thousands of clinicians to workflows that are dependent on an EHR for care delivery.

5. Software

Last on this list is the software system used, not because it isn't important (it is critical to success that the best system with the best fit to the organization is licensed) but because even the best system will not be successfully used without the previous four framework elements.

The Clayton framework is useful for many reasons—most notably because it focuses on what are the most important aspects of the project and lead to its success. It does not begin with technical considerations but with the commitment of the organization.

Also consider using the Quadruple Aim to guide your project. The four elements of the Quadruple Aim, formulated initially by Don Berwick and extended by others, are: improving the individual experience of care, improving the health of populations, reducing the per capita cost of healthcare, and improving the experience of providing care. Keeping these objectives in mind throughout the project can provide a refreshing reference point when important decisions are made.

FORMING YOUR TEAM

Key Decisionmakers

EHR projects benefit from varied skills, and the composition of the project team should reflect this. A notable key is that this is a clinical project and that clinicians lead and contribute to it at all levels. The choice of "suits or scrubs" is an easy one: there should be ample representation by the health professionals who will be the heaviest users of EHRs: nurses, physicians, pharmacists, and the many other professions that directly care for patients. It is best that business and administrative experts do not make key decisions about features, functionality, and workflow unless they also provide care to patients. Reasons that EHR projects fail, either small or national-level initiatives, can often be traced to decisions to separate clinician-users with their deep knowledge of clinical workflow, from project decision-making.

Role of Project Management

Given the scope and complexity of these projects, the team also benefits from project management expertise, and from experience in organizing similar large projects successfully. Sometimes that means people who have prior experience, and sometimes those people will work for consulting firms. Care should be taken that consultants do not dominate the project team, because just as they came from elsewhere to help you, they will usually leave to help in another organization, taking their expertise with them. They also usually charge a premium and this has an important and sometimes significant impact on your project budget.

When forming the team, remember who will be using the system. It will be mostly clinicians who are focused on patient care rather than on EHR technology. It is best to include respected clinician opinion leaders rather than technically avid individuals, though interest in the potential of technology to solve real-world problems is an important attribute.

It is essential to plan for the interaction between project professionals and outside consultants with your clinician workforce. Organizations have learned, sometimes at great cost, that there should be a very close connection between the project team (including any consultants) and the clinician user community so that real-world needs and workflow are considered. Clinical workflow is complex, and understanding it often makes the difference between clinical computing projects that are an enormous success and those that are not (Fig. 18.1).

SYSTEM SECURITY

Security Concerns

Security should be considered and built in from the beginning. Security of the EHR and conformance with federal and state law is of the utmost importance in the world of electronic health records. Security should be a consideration from the outset, and involves everyone, not just the security team and Chief Information Security Officer. Questions should be posed regarding who will access the EHR, and how they will be authenticated. Consideration should also be addressed related to the of use 2- (or 3-) factor authentication. Security issues must be considered related to the safety of the system and data with offsite users. There should be an established security education program for the organizational workforce, and measurements to determine its effectiveness.

Ensuring System Security

EHR security breaches are more common as they are in other sectors of society. One of the most common methods used by perpetrators is *phishing*, which often leverages social relationships to trick a user into disclosing credentials they then use to access an information system. This is one reason, among others, EHR user training should include provisions to improve security at all levels: from awareness of likely methods used to breach security including phishing, use of strong passwords and **strong authentication** ("something you know, something you have"), use of encryption of protected health information in transit and at rest, physical security of data centers, and all other security measures appropriate to the high value of EHR records.

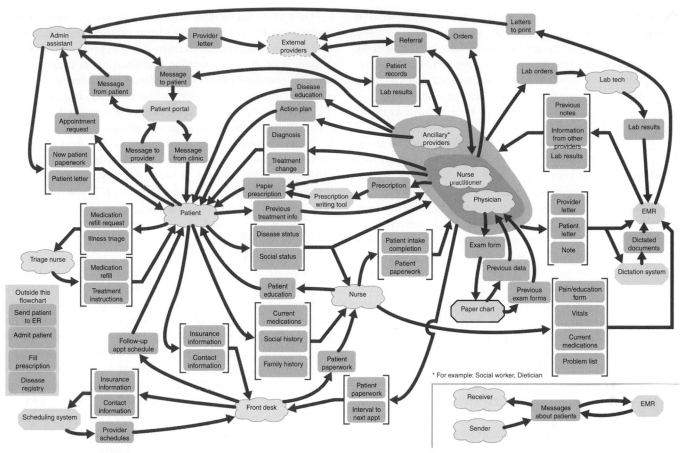

Fig. 18.1 Information flow in chronic disease care. *Admin*, Administration; *appt*, appointment; *EMR*, electronic medical record; *ER*, emergency room. (From Unertl, K. M., Weinger, M. B., Johnson, K. B., & Lorenzi, N. M. [2009]. Describing and modeling workflow and information flow in chronic disease care. *Journal of the American Medical Informatics Association, 16*, 832. With permission from BMJ Publishing Group Ltd.)

WHAT IS THE "HERE" IN GETTING THERE FROM HERE?

Understanding Organizational Needs

Though people and healthcare organizations are fundamentally like each other, every organization differs in some ways, and you should have a deep understanding of the current state of the organization.

Some considerations include:

- Do you have an EHR or as is often the case, do you have more than one?
- What does your current EHR do well, and what do clinicians like and dislike about it?
- Has your organization changed by adding new service lines, merging, or aligning with other organizations?

It is also a suitable time to reflect on your prior experience with EHR projects and what you have learned from them. For example, was the type and level of user support you used the last time adequate, or (as is the case with many organizations) would you do it differently next time? Do you have an engaged patient advisory council or community board? What about collective bargaining units who should be involved in EHR planning if appropriate? Do you have a strong relationship with an EHR vendor with whom you are very satisfied, or do you wish to part ways and begin

anew? You can see that many questions should be considered from the beginning and throughout the institution of any IT system.

What are Your Needs?

When considering your needs, begin with the reasons you are embarking on this project. What are they? Is your current EHR vendor going out of business, or have you outgrown its capabilities? Are you trying to reduce operational costs by consolidating your IT systems? Is your organization joining with other organizations, resulting in the fragmentation of the patient experience and provider workflow?

It is essential to know what you need. You have a distinct advantage if you have an existing system, but consideration should be given to what has changed. You may have partner organizations, new service lines, and the regulatory world may have changed. Patient engagement in use of EHRs is strong and growing rapidly. Therefore, needs are different than they were when your existing system was acquired. The choice may have been made for you if you have decided to use the same system as partners or your parent organization. Still there are choices to be made: Will you be an extension of their 'instance' of the EHR? Will you tailor it to your own specific needs? Consideration is needed to determine where the IT system will be hosted (remotely host or locally).

Next, an understanding is needed to determine what is required to meet the project mission, strategic objectives, and day-to-day operational requirements. Documenting specific needs is often referred to as defining *requirements*. But *requirement* also includes things that are desired but not required. Being certain that needs are met is key, or some aspects of patient care will not be supported or benefit from available system functionality. It is worth reflecting on what is wanted and needed, which are the drivers for launching this enormous project. There is a wide range of functionality in EHRs, much of which can benefit your organization and some that are not needed. There may be items you need that the vendor cannot provide. Do not rely solely on the personal experience of the project team to figure this out. A systematic method for a needs assessment is necessary for everyone who works in your organization—needs of those who clean operating rooms, of executives who plan new relationships with other organizations, of physical therapists, mental health professionals and all the others who contribute to your mission. This needs assessment must be thoroughly performed and cataloged. Build on the team's experience with your current EHR if you have one, and on the processes that were developed, whether or not a current EHR is in place.

Your process for defining requirements may include many complementary approaches: direct observation of workflow, mapping interviews, focus groups and expert interviews. Sometimes this results in large diagrams showing workflow and transfer of information during the process of care. One example of a clinical scenario is how a patient with abdominal pain is evaluated in the emergency room, how test results are conveyed back to the ordering clinician (Fig. 18.2), the sequence of steps leading to admission to the hospital and the scheduling of an urgent operation, and the transfer of the patient to an intensive care unit postoperatively. This example is one of many complex workflows that need to be supported by the EHR. Gathering these requirements is aided by involving clinicians who perform these tasks daily, yet these clinicians may be busy in their duties, so scheduling these sessions may be difficult.

In a large organization, the process of defining requirements may require significant time, effort and people, but the alternative is to discover later that important needs were not addressed or that the newly installed system lacks the needed functionality. Technical organizational aspects must also be considered, like workstation availability, adequacy of point of care devices and wireless coverage, and leverage your current infrastructure (data center or remote hosting) and expertise of your IT team.

Other Considerations

Other entities (hospitals or clinics) in your organization may have already implemented an EHR from a vendor, and by using the same vendor you can leverage the experience and workforce familiarity with that vendor. This is an important consideration. Another important consideration is the vendors used by other organizations within the area you serve. Some vendors may have a larger set of customers in your area, and with EHR market trends, this is more likely to be the case now than in the past.

Data exchange is often easier if you use the same vendor's software. (Ideally it shouldn't matter—patient data should flow just as easily between EHRs from different vendors and between instances of the same vendor, but alas, that is usually not the case.) If you share patients, either because of referrals or specialized services that your organization or others in your community offer, then using that same vendor may make it easier to get the patient's information when you need it.

There are trends in EHR vendor market share. Occasionally, vendors appear to be everyone's choice, but the choice then drifts to another vendor. A sense that "everyone is their customer" is the modern equivalent of the 1970s catch phrase, "no one ever got fired for choosing IBM."

Project Scope

Clearly define the project's scope. Determine if the project includes the EHR only or if other systems will be involved. Most healthcare organizations depend on many information systems. Some are specialized and used primarily by a single department, such as laboratory information systems, pharmacy systems, radiology systems and others. These are collectively referred to as "departmental systems." Others can be regarded as infrastructure (discussed in Chapter 6), such as admission/discharge/transfer (ADT) systems, patient registration systems, and others. Financial systems were among the first to be adopted in healthcare, and now there are many varieties such as hospital billing, professional fee billing, financial analytics, and others. Data analytics is an area of tremendous growth reflecting the value of data. Negotiating "at risk" contracts hinges on understanding the finances of caring for groups of patients. Patterns in resource use—especially labor and supplies—gives opportunity for efficiency. Is your intent to replace some or all these systems at the same time?

The system seen by most clinicians lies on top of most of these departmental, infrastructure and financial systems: the EHR. Vendors can supply some or all of these systems, but a decision should be made related to how many systems will be replaced or implemented in the current project. There are benefits and costs to using one vendor for many systems or using many specialized vendors for departments. This is the "best of breed" versus integrated system discussion. The secular trend is for dominant health care IT vendors to supply a greater percentage of the departmental and other systems that health care organizations need. This makes most sense when there are key advantages to close integration, for example between an inpatient pharmacy system and computerized practitioner order entry (CPOE). In other cases, such close integration is not as critical: messages can be sent between systems created by different vendors using standard protocols such as HL7 2.4.

The decision of scope—what systems to use in the project—is key and should be made early on, by organizational leadership. There may be strong opinions about moving away from a long-used departmental system toward one provided by an EHR vendor, and the discussion can be heated. Conversely, expanding the scope of the project after planning and budgeting has occurred ("scope creep") should be avoided by developing and using processes to keep to the plan and on budget.

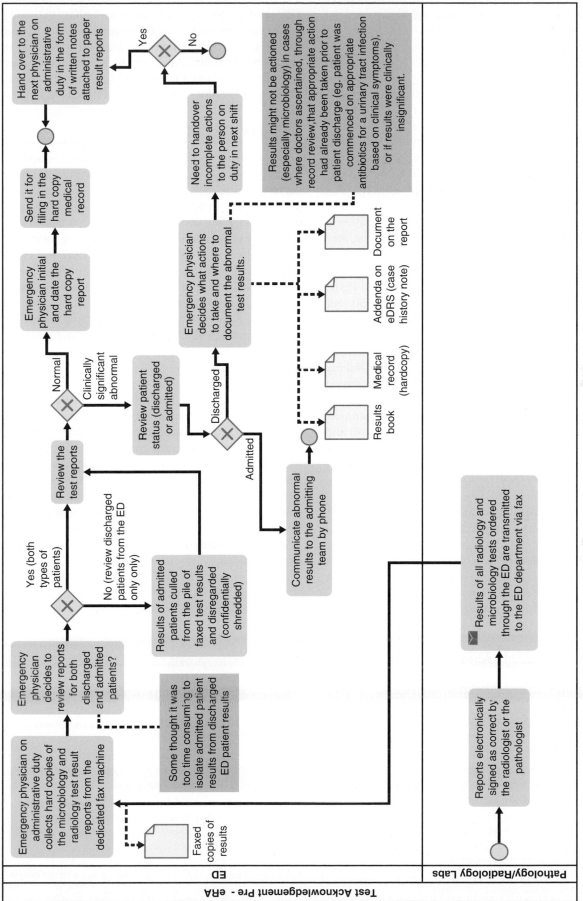

Fig. 18.2 Example of workflow for receiving and acknowledging test results in the emergency department. (From Georgiou, A., McCaughey, E. J., Tariq, A., Walter, S. R., Li, J., Callen, J., et al. [2017, March]. What is the impact of an electronic test result acknowledgement system on Emergency Department physicians' work processes? A mixed-method pre-post observational study. *International Journal of Medical Informatics, 99,* 29–36.)

This can all be brought together in a requirements document that is the foundation for your next step—understanding the EHR marketplace.

OPTIONS FOR ACQUIRING AN EHR

Consider the following questions when looking for EHR options:
- How do you figure all this out?
- Do you begin with a blank sheet of paper or by using someone else's wheel that you don't need to reinvent?

Begin by determining project needs, informed by what you learn in the investigation phase of your project. Your organization very likely has experience with EHRs from past use.

Developing Custom EHRs

Though 30 years ago the buy/build decision was on this list, very few organizations now develop their own EHRs; nearly all of them license EHR software from a vendor since the list of vendors used is smaller than in the past. Locally developed EHRs were the source of research supporting the value of EHRs, but one by one they have been supplanted by commercial systems. The buy/build decision is now much easier to make and commercial EHRs are the norm and locally developed EHRs the rare exception. There is room for local innovation by linking locally developed applications to the EHR, and in development if smaller systems used in conjunction with a commercial EHR. A future hope is that commercial EHRs will increase interoperability and thereby increasing patient benefits, such as cost and quality.

What Can EHR Vendors Offer? And What They Cannot

Communicating your needs and requirements is important, and your organization may have a structured method for this. You may require a formal request for proposal (RFP) process (Boxes 18.1 and 18.2) for projects of this size, or for smaller organizations fewer formal means may be appropriate. Either way, it is important to remember that "You are buying what they are selling"—putting something in an RFP doesn't magically cause it to exist. Be careful to pay attention to tense in what enthusiastic vendor representatives say: Is something in broad production use at many sites today or is it envisioned for the long-term, and subject to competition with other priorities the vendor is considering? Clarity is required to determine if functionality is essential to your organization and to let vendors know this, so you can find products that are a good match for your needs.

SYSTEM SELECTION

The options for EHRs are becoming fewer—most organizations choose from a smaller pool and almost none have locally developed EHRs. But even within this smaller set of choices it is necessary to understand how the choice is made. Begin by educating yourself and your team. One place to start is by contacting colleagues at an organization like yours and finding out how the system they use meets their needs. Leverage your contacts, but remember that a single individual may not accurately reflect opinions of everyone in the organization. Your professional society may have resources on EHR selection. Attending a national meeting of your professional society or HIMSS can be an efficient way to understand what the market offers.

RFP? or Not?

A **Request for Proposals** (RFP) (Boxes 18.1 and 18.2) is a formal process for soliciting proposals from vendors to meet your project needs. Your organization may require an RFP for projects over a certain size and may also specify the structure of the RFP. It includes a description of your organization—now familiar to you because of the work you have done—your current information technology environment, and clearly describes your needs. This can be very detailed so that there is no confusion about what you must have and what you would like to have, and represents the result of your needs assessment process from throughout your organization. Be clear about project timing: when you must begin your project and start using the new system. Your financial constraints should also be specified so a realistic proposal will be offered to you.

BOX 18.1   RFI, RFP, RFQ

RFI: **Request for information**. Request made typically during the project planning phase where a buyer cannot clearly identify product requirements, specifications, and purchase options. RFIs clearly indicate that award of a contract will not automatically follow.

RFP: Request for proposal. A document that an organization posts to elicit bids from potential vendors for a product or service. A weighted point assignment method of evaluation may be used if considered appropriate.

RFQ: Request for quotation. Used when requirements are clear-cut.

BOX 18.2   Contents of a Request for Proposal

- *Background:* The description of the institution, including mission size and number and type of patients treated.
- *Qualifications:* Any specific qualifications required by the vendor. For example, does it need to have been in business for 5 or more years?
- *Information requested:* A list of specific elements that should be answered. For example:
  - Size, history, and financial status of the company

- Basic system architecture and software configuration
- Number of installations and selected names of customers
- Describe your needs—functional, technical, business requirements
- Timing and implementation requirements
- Financial constraints
- Lay out the vendor selection process, timeline, and selection criteria
- Conform to organizational requirements

Selection Criteria

The RFP should also describe the rules that will govern your selection of one or more vendors. What criteria will you use to choose a vendor, and how are those criteria weighted? You should describe the timeline for the process: exactly when the proposals are due, what happens if they are late, and when you will make your choice. The formality of the RFP is there for a reason: sometimes large contracts are legally disputed by a vendor that isn't chosen, and this can result in legal proceedings. The RFP can be helpful in resolving these disputes. Leave time to send out or post the RFP and publicize its availability. There may be rules within your organization on how this is done.

You can see that an RFP process can be very complex and therefore expensive, and it is not needed for every contract or for every organization. Other methods of soliciting vendor proposals might be a better fit for smaller organizations, and even in the biggest organizations there are reasons for not using an RFP.

Evaluating and Scoring Proposals

Once your RFP has been posted and received within the allotted time, begin evaluating the proposals you receive to identify those vendors to move forward in the consideration process. Your RFP had a scoring system within it—if you are reading this before creating your RFP, then strongly consider this—so your next step is to carefully read and score the proposals. Some criteria are clear-cut, and others are subject to your judgement, so the scoring process may be time-consuming. It is best to have a group participate in scoring proposals. Of course, the financial portion is critical and is included in the evaluation of proposals.

Site visits and Reference Calls

Once you have educated yourself and have scored proposals in hand, there are ways to sort between the options. Here are some approaches:

Visiting an organization that is using the system you are considering can be extremely helpful. Best are visits you organize rather than visits arranged by your vendor—vendors may choose sites that are happy with their product, and have incentives to conduct visits rather than a more typical site. Talk to busy clinicians on the wards and in clinics and avoid boardroom PowerPoint demonstrations. Five minutes talking with a tired clinician in scrubs can yield more information than an hour with an executive from the same organization.

Reference calls are not as helpful as a site visit, but they are logistically simpler to arrange, less expensive, and extend your reach. Calling people in an organization like your own—or someone you know to have good judgment—is better than relying on the vendor to arrange a call.

Vendor User Group Meetings

User group meeting attendees present a very biased sample, usually in favor of the true believers and long-term customers. (If everyone were as happy with the EHR as those attending the user group meeting, why are there articles titled "Why Doctors Hate Their Computers"?) But you can get a sense of the enthusiasm of the user community, see presentations on what is coming, and network with colleagues from across the country whom you may wish to contact about site visits or conference calls.

The ONC has excellent resources on www.healthit.gov. Lastly, consulting firms would love to help you, for a (usually large) price.

Demonstrations

Vendors will come on to your campus and show how their system works. Using one or more scenarios (admitting and caring for an ICU patient, registering and conducting a well-child visit) can be helpful when comparing one system with another. Leave lots of time for questions from members of our community. Demonstrations have the advantage of involving more of your community in the search for a vendor.

Involving your larger community of potential users is key and can help in pointing out strengths and weaknesses, and to continue engaging them in the project.

Financial Evaluation

Due diligence is another key, noting whether the vendor is likely to remain in the EHR business or phase it out, and whether they are financially healthy. Engage your Chief Financial Officer or other financial experts to help make this judgement. Other questions to ask are:

- Will the vendor remain in business or not?
- How long have they been in business?
- Are they privately or publicly held?
- Are they likely to be acquired?
- What does their balance sheet tell you about their likely future?

The answers to these questions will aid the success of your project. It would be disappointing and difficult for your organization if the EHR vendor you select and implement is acquired by another organization with another focus, and your vendor does not devote enough resources to upgrading and supporting the EHR as you had expected and hoped.

FINAL CONSIDERATIONS

Who Makes the Choice

The day comes when you must make your choice, or choices. It may be to your advantage to have two options: A first choice and a backup. How this choice is made varies between organizations: A selection committee identified by the project team, senior clinical leaders from all disciplines and executives, a vote of those who have participated in the selection process, or in other ways that fit with your organization's culture. Even in very large organizations a single individual may make the choice. Remember that you will very likely be using the system you choose for longer than many of your senior leaders will be in their position. Because the switch cost is so high for EHRs, organizations may stick with that vendor for a decade or more, and will have a long-term, close relationship for that long. So, this is a critical choice.

Contract Negotiations

Implementing and operating an EHR is a long-term commitment, and the contract governs a very important part of this commitment: Your relationship with the EHR vendor. Technically you do not buy an EHR—you license it. Part of licensing include regular maintenance payments which are the lion's share of what is paid to the EHR vendor. What you get for the initial capital outlay, implementation and maintenance payments is an important part of your contract. If you rendered an RFP and the vendor responded to it, then the vendor's written proposal should be included in the contract, so that if they responded in their proposal that they have a certain functionality, then it becomes a part of the contract. You should have legal help in the negotiation and contracting process—you can be sure the vendor will. Contract negotiations should not be rushed. The choice of more than one vendor, with one the "apparently successful" vendor and another as backup so you have an alternative during contract negotiations gives you a Best Alternative To Negotiated Agreement (BATNA) rather than having to start from nothing if the sticking points are too large to overcome.

Things to include in the contract are implementation service scope and costs, software licensing and hardware costs, annual maintenance payments, what constitutes acceptance of the system, performance clauses and failure to perform clauses. Some organizations do not pay on a schedule but when milestones are met, so that if there is an unexpected problem with the vendor's software or implementation, they are not paid until it is resolved. Remember that over long term, most money is in support payments, which are governed by the contract. And what you pay to the vendor is only a fraction of the cost of the entire project, so delays may harm you more than your vendor.

The legal considerations in the contract are a fact of modern life and include a large list of items. Who is liable if a patient is harmed because of a software problem? What remedy does the organization have if the vendor misconfigures the EHR system and downtime results? Does the vendor ask for "hold harmless cases" that protect them from liability for software errors? Your legal team (if you have one or hired counsel if not) can make sure that these topics and others are addressed in this important contract. The Office of the National Coordinator has resources that review legal considerations at the elevated level. Legal considerations related to contract negotiations and software licensing can be found in Chapter 19. Chapter 20 provides additional information related to implementing and upgrading an IT system.

CONCLUSION AND FUTURE DIRECTIONS

Information technology and EHRs are key to the delivery of healthcare, and account for a large and growing part of the healthcare organization's budget. Investing time in understanding your organizational mission, strategic plan, and information technology needs and matching licensed EHR software to your needs is an investment in your future. Though you are itching to get started, leveraging the latest and best system to help deliver care, the process of understanding the marketplace, finding the best fit for you and your organization, and coming to agreement with your vendor in a signed contract should not be rushed.

ACKNOWLEDGMENTS

The author wishes to acknowledge the contributions of Cynthia M. Mascara and Mical Debrow to the previous edition of this chapter.

DISCUSSION QUESTIONS

1. How do strategic vision and alignment affect decisions made in your organization?
2. What is the role of healthcare providers in the identification and selection of a healthcare information system?
3. The selection team should be an interdisciplinary team, but how should the chair of the committee be selected?
4. What is the impact of a well-defined and complete RFI and RFP process on identification and selection of a healthcare information system?
5. What are the key roles and functions in identification of system requirements?
6. Why are vendor relationships with management essential? Brainstorm ideas for maintaining good site–vendor relationships.

CASE STUDY

You have been chosen to be part of the selection team for a new electronic health record to be licensed from a vendor and implemented at the community hospital where you are a staff nurse, to replace the electronic record you currently use. The selection team has been asked to develop an initial list of requirements that they would like to use for the evaluation of potential systems in relation to documentation of assessments for interprofessional use, including nursing, physicians, and other departments such as physical therapy and occupational therapy. The selection team has decided to group the requirements that they identify into the following categories:

- Patient care objectives
- Usability
- IT technical requirements
- Organization objectives

Your task for this case study is to use the key considerations listed below to develop a list of system requirements for electronic documentation in a clinical information system, grouping the requirements into the four categories listed above. The key considerations include information that the selection team has gathered in anticipation of developing system requirements.

Key Considerations for System Selection
Findings From Inventory of Current Systems and Functionality

- Electronic laboratory and radiology report results are produced by departmental (laboratory and radiology) systems.

- The intensive care units (ICUs) have a separate ICU information system where documentation is done electronically, including vital signs, intake and output, and some interfaced data from monitoring systems.

Findings From Inventory of Functionality From the Two EHRs Currently in Use

- Nursing notes and care planning currently are documented in a combination of flowsheets and narrative text in different formats in acute care and intensive care.
- Physician progress notes currently are documented electronically using templates and dictation.
- Orders are entered using EHR functionality (Box 18.3) that differs between ICU and acute care, using order sets that have been reviewed and varying times in the past. Some no longer utilize the most current evidence.

Findings From Staff Interviews and Observations

Direct observation studies were conducted in the ICU, medical/surgical units, and pediatric unit. Observations and interviews also were conducted in various other clinical departments including physical therapy (PT), occupational therapy (OT), and wound care. The study revealed that all these practitioners feel they spend too much time documenting and that this detracts from time at the bedside. Key findings included the following:

- Need to be able to document using the best fit for the need, utilizing narrative text and structured data entered when necessary.
- Need to be able to enter free-text comments.
- Entry of an electronic assessment must include the user's electronic signature and the current date and time.
- All entries must have the capability to be edited, and changes to the document must be tracked by the system.

SWOT Analysis

A SWOT analysis of the current documentation was conducted with the following findings:

- *Strengths.* Structured electronic data in the ICU facilitates accurate and timely data collection.
- *Weaknesses.* Time required for documentation and order entry is contributing to clinician burnout.
- *Opportunities.* New documentation methods may decrease time requirements and increase expressivity in a way that supports professional practice.
- *Threats.* Vendor functionality and usability may continue clinician dissatisfaction with EHRs.

BOX 18.3   Electronic Health Record Functionality (Partial List)

1. Clinical Features
   a. Message box
   b. Problem and medication lists
   c. Results review
   d. Documentation
   e. Order Management
   f. Medication Administration Record
   g. Patient summary displays
   h. Documentation
   i. Clinical Summary
   j. Medication Reconciliation Documentation
   k. Patient lists/schedule
   l. Rounding/handoff tools
   m. Informed Consent Documentation
   n. Evidence-based resources and CDS
   o. Electronic communication, with team and with patients
2. Data Management, Data Mining
3. Population Health Management Reporting
4. Patient portal including messaging
5. External educational resources
6. Professional fee billing
7. Health Information Management Requirements
8. Account Management and Billing

REFERENCES

Agency for Healthcare Research and Quality. Physician burnout. https://www.ahrq.gov/prevention/clinician/ahrq-works/burnout/index.html Accessed August 31, 2021

Brigl, B., Ammenwerth, E., Dujat, C., Gräber, S., Grosse, A., Häber, A., Jostes, C., & Winter, A. (2005, Jan). Preparing strategic information management plans for hospitals: A practical guideline SIM plans for hospitals: a guideline. *International Journal of Medical Informatics*, 74(1), 51–65. https://doi.org/10.1016/j.ijmedinf.2004.09.002. PMID: 15626636.

Dymek, C., Kim, B., Melton, G. B., Payne, T. H., Singh, H., & Hsiao, C. J. (2020). Building the evidence-base to reduce EHR-related clinician burden. *Journal of the American Medical Informatics Association* ocaa238. doi:10.1093/jamia/ocaa238.

Fletcher, G. S., & Payne, T. H. (2017). Selection and implementation of an electronic health record. *PM&R Journal*, 9(5S), S4–S12.

Gawande, A. (2018). Why doctors hate their computers. *The New Yorker.* https://www.newyorker.com/magazine/2018/11/12/why-doctors-hate-their-computers (accessed June 2020).

Grisim, L. M., & Longhurst, C. A. (2011, Dec). An evidence-based approach to activating your EMR. *Healthcare Informatics*, 28, 47–50.

Kelly, K. F. (1999). Contract negotiations: Guidelines for the acquisition of EHR and clinical systems. In G. Murphy, M. Hanken, & K. Waters (Eds.), *Electronic health records: Changing the vision.* Philadelphia: W.B. Saunders.

McEvoy, D., Barnett, M. L., Sittig, D. F., Aaron, S., Mehrotra, A., & Wright, A. (2018, May 1). Changes in hospital bond ratings after the transition to a new electronic health record. *Journal of the American Medical Informatics Association*, 25(5), 572–574. https://doi.org/10.1093/jamia/ocy007.

Payne, T. H. (2008). Architecture of clinical computing systems. In T. H. Payne (Ed.), *Practical guide to clinical computing systems. Design, operations, and infrastructure.* Oxford: Elsevier.

19

Contract Negotiations and Software Licensing

Craig B. Monsen, Elizabeth G. Olson, and John D. Manning

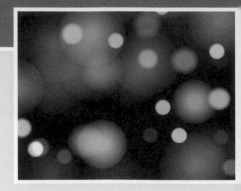

Never underestimate the leverage that a healthcare organization has to contractually protect itself.

OBJECTIVES

At the completion of this chapter, the reader will be prepared to:
- Discuss a software licensing contract.
- Describe the people, processes, and key provisions involved in negotiating a contract.
- Describe components of the licensing agreement.
- Give examples of special clauses that may be included in an agreement (contract).

KEY TERMS

cloud licensing, 290
derivative works, 289
limitations and exclusions of liability, 301

open-source software, 290
service level agreement (SLA), 295
software as a service (SaaS), 290
software escrow, 294

software license agreements, 288
software warranty, 295

ABSTRACT ❖

Healthcare organizations (HCOs) need a negotiating team with the expertise and knowledge to properly assess and negotiate software license agreements with vendors. This team will need to represent different interests, including user, technical, finance, and legal interests of the HCO. The agreements provided by software vendors tend to be one-sided and do not adequately protect HCOs or address all HCO needs. "Legalese," the legal terms and language of contracts, is not harmless and in many respects affects technical, business, and financial issues, including business continuity, data protection, return on investment, and other value propositions. HCOs should not underestimate their leverage to negotiate for better terms in their software license agreement with vendors. This chapter describes a process for health information technology (IT), contract negotiation, and provides a description of contract terms, related issues, and negotiation compromises.

INTRODUCTION

Healthcare organizations (HCOs) depend on computer software for the delivery of healthcare services to patients and for most, if not all, of their business operations. It is unimaginable today that an HCO could function without the use of software for a wide variety of applications and purposes, including clinical care, billing, security, compliance, research, and operations. Software vendors who provide the software are diverse in size, expertise, resources, ability, and the solutions they offer, but one practice they have in common is their insistence on software license agreements (also referred to as contracts) as a prerequisite to using their software. The term "vendor" refers to the licensor, service provider, or other company that licenses or provides the software to the HCO. The term *HCO* is used generically in this chapter to mean not only the HCO itself but also, when the context allows, the HCO's leadership or the designated representatives on a team doing the contract negotiations.

A negotiating team for a software agreement may be at the executive level or composed of other designated team members who first work with the vendor on the terms and conditions of the agreement. Then, the agreement is signed by an authorized signatory such as the chief executive officer (CEO), chief financial officer (CFO), or the chief information officer (CIO) who is authorized to sign purchases or contracts and make financial commitments. A negotiating team's typical composition is listed in Box 19.1.

Although this chapter does not address Stark, anti-kickback, Health Information Portability and Accountability Act (HIPAA), and other regulatory issues, those issues must always be carefully considered and accounted for by the HCO. Details about legal issues may be found in Chapter 27. HIPAA is discussed in Chapter 28, and regulatory issues such as Health Information Technology for Economic Clinical Health (HITECH) and Meaningful Use are in Chapter 29.

This chapter focuses on commercial software license agreements rather than open-source software licenses. It is written primarily to address traditional "on-premises" software licenses, but much of what is said about "on-premises" licenses also applies to cloud-based services. The chapter includes a discussion of cloud-based services (e.g., software as a service [SaaS] licenses) and is written from the perspective of informing healthcare professionals and informaticians who are expected to take a leadership role in understanding the implications of these types of agreements. It is not written for attorneys but rather for others responsible for understanding and approving software license agreements and ensuring that the HCO complies with those agreements. By necessity, the chapter is not completely comprehensive (i.e., any given software license agreement is likely to include additional provisions not mentioned here and may not include some provisions that are mentioned). However, the chapter provides a description of the topics and contractual provisions deemed the most relevant to the intended reader.

When purchasing a license for software that is mission critical or highly important, the HCO should be sure to understand what it is agreeing to and should make sure that the agreement makes sense in the context of which the HCO will use the software. Software license agreements can be relatively simple, but more often they are lengthy and complex and even confusing. They include provisions that address significant business and technical issues often in legalese or "boilerplate." These provisions should never be dismissed or overlooked as routine or harmless, as they may lead to surprises with business, technical, financial, and/or patient care consequences.

There are three key points to always remember when dealing with these types of agreements (Box 19.2).

OVERVIEW OF LICENSING AGREEMENTS

Intellectual Property Concepts Relevant to Software

Software is a "work of authorship" under the copyright laws. There is always a copyright to any software that is original (i.e., not copied from someone else). Copyrights only protect "expression" and not ideas, methods, facts, concepts, inventions, or systems. Writing computer software is analogous to writing a book. Both are expressions protected by copyright, but the concepts and ideas in them are not. Therefore, copyrights can protect software against copying and even against other derivative works.

A copyright is different from a patent. Whereas copyright is a form of protection provided to the authors of original works, a patent protects the invention of an inventor (Section 2016). Sometimes, software includes or represents a patentable invention, or the use of the software may be or involve a patentable method. Software that is involved in a patentable invention creates additional considerations and potential liabilities for HCOs. A software vendor might have one or more patents applicable to its software, some of which may be owned by a competing company. In this case, the HCO licensing the software may be unintentionally infringing on a patent and be liable for damages payable to the owner of the patent.

Trade secrets are a third form of intellectual property applicable to software. A trade secret is information that is not generally known to others and not readily ascertainable by others (Uniform Trade Secrets Act Definition, 2016). Trade secrets are protected against misappropriation (e.g., taking by improper means). Software can include trade secrets. The source code to commercial software is often held by the owner of the software as a trade secret. Open-source software is not a trade secret, as the software and its source code are typically made available to the public and therefore are generally known to the public. Typically, when commercial software is distributed, it is the object code or executable code version of the software that is distributed, and the source code is withheld from distribution. In such cases, the source code may be a trade secret.

Why Are Contracts Used for Software Licensing?

In general, a contract represents an agreement between parties that creates legally enforceable obligations. A contract may represent an exchange of value, such as a service where one party pays the other. Alternatively, there may be no charge at all, such as a nondisclosure agreement for software sustained by selling advertisements.

Software vendors will insist on using a binding contract, such as a software license agreement, when licensing commercial software to an HCO. License agreements provide the vendor with contractual protection of its software in addition to intellectual property protection. They create payment obligations and restrictions on use and limitations of liability and disclaimers that protect the vendor. However, a license agreement can also protect HCOs by including obligations and warranties binding on the vendor that give the HCO assurance as to the software and its functionality, performance, and compatibility, as well as other protections (e.g., indemnification against claims that the software infringes another person's intellectual property).

It may not always be obvious that a license agreement has been agreed upon. Many licensing agreements will be called "Software Licensing Agreement" or "Master Agreement"; however, sometimes they take different names. It is not uncommon for vendors to create a "Purchase Order" or "Sales Order" that references a separate software licensing agreement. End User License Agreements requiring users to acknowledge "I Accept" are commonly agreed upon as "click through" agreements that create obligations for the user and may also create uncomfortable obligations for their employer. Finally, depending on the maturity and approach of a vendor, "Letter of Agreements," "Term Sheets," "Memorandum of Understanding," "Amendment," and "Letter of Intent" may all represent contracts with software licensing terms.

The Concept of Licensing Versus Sale

Software is typically not sold when distributed to customers. Instead, vendors will often sell licenses to use the software rather than the software itself. If the software were sold, this generally would give ownership in the form of copyright or other intellectual property (IP) protection to the customer, which is often unacceptable to a vendor wanting to license the software to others. A license is, in effect, permission to use the software.

The media (e.g., DVDs) on which the software resides and is distributed to an HCO (1) may be owned by the HCO as a purchaser, or (2) may be leased or loaned to the HCO (i.e., the

vendor owns the media). Ownership of the media is not an issue when software is downloaded by the HCO via the internet from the vendor or is remotely accessed and used by the HCO via the internet as in a software as a service (SaaS) agreement. SaaS is a software distribution model where applications are hosted by a vendor and made available to customers over a network, typically the internet.

"On-Premises" Licensing Versus Licensing Through the "Cloud"

Traditionally, software licenses have been "on-premises" licenses, meaning that the software (usually the executable code but not the source code) is installed and runs on a computer or network located at the facility of the licensee (e.g., the HCO). (See Table 19.1 for definitions of the terms source code, executable code, and interpretive code.) Cloud licensing takes a different approach. The software resides and runs on the vendor's server(s), and the licensee (e.g., the HCO) remotely accesses and uses the software through the internet (e.g., via a web browser).

An example of cloud licensing is SaaS licensing. SaaS can be characterized by a single instance of the software running on the vendor's server that is accessed and used by multiple licensees (i.e., "multitenant"). This maximizes some of the benefits of a SaaS solution (e.g., the cost of hosting, running, maintaining, and supporting a single instance of the same version of the software reduces costs when those costs can be shared by multiple licensees). The term *SaaS* can also apply to solutions that are not single instance or are multitenant.

Other cloud services include hosting, managed services, on-demand services, and application service provider (ASP) services. Some agreements are structured as a hybrid of an on-premises license and a cloud license. For example, some vendors will license the software through an on-premises license but then offer hosting services through a services agreement (e.g., a hosting or managed services agreement). In such cases, the HCO is licensed to use the software under the license but engages the vendor through a services agreement to host and run the software for the HCO on the vendor's servers. If the services agreement were to terminate, it remains possible for the HCO to run and use the software on its own computers or network under the terms of the on-premises license agreement.

TABLE 19.1	Definition of Terms
Term	**Definition**
Source code	Software written in a programming language such as C++. The source code is understandable to the human programmer.
Executable code (machine code or object code)	Source code compiled into a format understandable by computers (machine code).
Interpretive code	Source code written in a specific language that is "interpreted" on the fly when the software is run to produce code that the computer can execute.

The Vendor's Contract: Healthcare Organizations, Beware!

Typically, the vendor has a standard template for a license agreement. However, it is often possible to negotiate the terms of any software license. The vendor's version should be viewed by the HCO as only a starting point. The vendor's form of agreement is mostly designed to protect the vendor and not the HCO. The agreement usually includes legalese that can mislead or surprise an HCO. It often fails to include many protections and assurances important to the HCO that must be sought through negotiation. Health providers and informaticians involved in contract negotiations should not be distracted by the "friendliness" of a vendor or with the developing informatics-vendor relationship, but rather they should focus on gaining a clear and objective understanding of what is in the agreement. HCOs should not hesitate to negotiate aggressively for the needs of the healthcare institution. Vendors can be persuaded to change their agreements, but they will not do so without a request from the HCO. *HCOs should not underestimate their leverage.* While HCOs should negotiate firmly and aggressively for the needs of the institution, a collegial, professional manner is always the most effective way to reach an acceptable agreement. The HCO and its representatives should maintain an amicable and a professional relationship with the vendor at all times, and contract negotiations are no exception.

SOFTWARE LICENSE CONTRACT NEGOTIATION

Although situations will vary, the progression of a negotiated agreement is likely to include a process similar to the one outlined in Box 19.3. As is illustrated, the process involves numerous cycles.

The reason for having the vendor prepare a second draft is that this allows the agreement to move closer to what the HCO needs and wants in an agreement before the HCO starts to change the agreement. Assuming that the vendor accommodates some of the changes requested by the HCO in the first teleconference or meeting, there will be fewer changes that the HCO needs to make in its final draft. In the process, there should be shared control of the agreement document, by taking turns in preparing response drafts that are redlined to show

changes to the prior draft. Two major tips for version control are listed in Box 19.4.

Before the Agreement Is Signed: Due Diligence

Even the best agreement is not a substitute for due diligence (see also Chapter 18 on system selection processes). The HCO should check formally and informally with other users and obtain references from existing customers via conversations and site visits for larger purchases. The HCO can ask who has recently discontinued use of the vendor's software and why. References provided by the vendor are not likely to include customers with bad experiences or complaints that the HCO might need to know. Sometimes vendors are asked to provide financial statements so that the financial stability of the vendor can be assessed. Suddenly losing support and maintenance services from a vendor in bankruptcy or buyouts can place HCOs in a difficult position.

Key to the due diligence process is to perform it on several alternative vendors. This can provide a greater perspective on desired functionality, and it strengthens negotiating leverage with several backup options should negotiations with the preferred vendor stall. The HCO needs to know its requirements and must clearly communicate those requirements to the vendor. Document the responses from the vendor to these requirements, including those presented during demonstrations of the software. Outside consultants/experts engaged by the HCO may be useful to it in the due diligence and negotiating process.

The Request for Proposal Process

Request for proposal (RFP) or request for information (RFI) processes are worth the effort, time, and expense for larger software purchases. The RFP process, outlined in Chapter 18, sets

---

BOX 19.3   Typical Negotiating Process for an Agreement

1. Vendor's standard form of agreement—Draft #1.
2. HCO reviews Draft #1.
3. Telephone conference or meeting with the vendor to discuss Draft #1.
4. Vendor prepares Draft #2.
5. HCO reviews Draft #2.
6. HCO prepares Draft #3.
7. Vendor reviews Draft #3.
8. Telephone conference or meeting with the vendor.
9. Vendor prepares Draft #4.
10. Repeat as necessary to reach final agreement.

HCO, Healthcare organization.

BOX 19.4   Tips on How to Control the Versions of a Draft Contract

1. **Tip #1:** If a vendor insists that it must control all drafting and refuses to provide an editable draft that is not locked or protected, simply inform the vendor (especially its salespeople) that this will greatly delay the negotiating process, as the HCO must then retype (or convert from a locked PDF) the entire agreement from the uneditable draft provided by the vendor to create an editable draft so that changes can be tracked and then sent to the vendor in an editable form. Given the complexity and length of license agreements, this is not a trivial issue, as the HCO's representatives responsible for the agreement and negotiating process will incur much more review time if they cannot rely on document comparison and tracking functionality in word processing software that can be used on editable documents. Also, manual typing, text readers, and other conversions can introduce errors. In any event, a careful comparison of the final version of the agreement against prior versions is critical before it is signed. This will ensure no provisions in the contract were changed during the numerous steps without the HCO knowing the changes.
2. **Tip #2:** Whenever there is a teleconference or meeting to negotiate the agreement, it is always advantageous to the HCO if the then-most-recent draft on the negotiating table (other than the first draft) is a draft provided by the HCO, even if that means reducing the frequency of the calls or meetings to negotiate.

HCO, Healthcare organization.

forth the HCO's requirements and expectations for the software, including its functionality, performance, compatibility, and maintenance. The RFP should also be used to ask relevant questions of prospective vendors, including costs. The more comprehensive the RFP, the more comprehensive the response should be from the vendor. This will reduce the likelihood of misunderstandings and surprises later. Traditionally, an RFP is used with multiple vendors and is the basis for a bidding, comparison, and selection process, but can be a great tool to learn even from a single vendor.

The vendor's response to the RFP should be made a part of the license agreement. For example, the license agreement can reference the vendor's response and state that the vendor stands behind its response (i.e., that the response is accurate and that any promise or assurance in the response will be met by the vendor). Because of the nature of "Entire Agreement" clauses (see the next section), the response will be of no effect if not incorporated into the license agreement.

If the vendor objects to the inclusion of its response to the RFP in the license agreement, then the HCO should insist that the HCO relied on the vendor's response in the selection of the vendor. If the vendor still objects, the HCO should offer to allow the vendor to correct or clarify its response, and then the corrected or clarified response should be added to the agreement. If the corrections reveal some unpleasant surprises, it is better for the HCO to know before rather than after signing the agreement.

Although it is not common to do so, the RFP should be used to address the tough contract issues (including legal issues) that inevitably arise in contract negotiations (e.g., limitations of liability, termination, and scope of use). Negotiating these is much more difficult after the vendor knows that it has been selected, so early in the selection process is a good time to solidify these terms. This approach can reduce the amount of time spent negotiating the agreement and can lead to a better result for the HCO.

The "Entire Agreement" Clause: Know What This Means!

An "Entire Agreement" clause, also known to attorneys as an integration clause, might read as follows:

> *Entire Agreement. This Agreement is the entire agreement between the parties with regard to the subject matter of this Agreement and supersedes and incorporates all prior or contemporaneous representations, understandings or agreements, and may not be modified or amended except by an agreement in writing signed by the parties hereto.*

This means the HCO must put everything it is relying on in the agreement. Exhibits, addendums, appendices, and documents that are incorporated by reference into the agreement can be used for this purpose. Statements made by salespersons, demonstrations, marketing materials, and other peripheral statements and documents do not count unless they are incorporated into the agreement. The agreement should identify what the HCO is paying for (Box 19.5).

BOX 19.5 Elements in an Agreement Typically Paid for by Healthcare Organizations

- Licensed software/databases
- Hardware
- Third-party software
- Technical and end user documentation
- Customizations
- Interfaces
- Implementation services
- Support
- Maintenance
- Other services (e.g., data migration)

SPECIFIC COMPONENTS OF THE LICENSING AGREEMENT

Licensing Agreement Terms or Definitions

Definitions of terms is often one of the first major components of a licensing agreement listed in Box 19.6. The agreement should include definitions of all vendor-specific terms and concepts, as mentioned in Chapter 18. The system selection team, negotiating team, or designated representatives should review these to ensure they are consistent with the HCOs use of the terms and for clarity. Though it may be tempting to consider definitions boilerplate or mutually understood, this section often includes important content such as the definition of a Licensed User that impacts the pricing model.

Implementation Time Schedule

Although there is significant variation, a mission-critical license agreement might include the steps and stages listed in Box 19.7. Expectations for progressing through these stages in a timely fashion is often reflected on a time schedule to keep the vendor on track. The contract should contain a good estimate of

---

BOX 19.6 Main Components of a Licensing Agreement

- Definition of terms
- Time schedule
- Scope of the license
- Scope of use
- Derivation works
- Software and SaaS escrow
- Specifications
- Software warranties
- Service level agreements
- Acceptance
- Maintenance and support, other services (e.g., implementation support)
- Revenue recognition and payments
- Dispute resolution
- Termination
- Limitations and exclusions of liability
- Special clauses—confidentiality, intellectual property infringement

SaaS, Software as a service.

> **BOX 19.7   Steps in the Performance of a Mission Critical License Agreement**
>
> - Create specifications (before or after signing of the agreement).
> - Develop customized components and interfaces, if needed.
> - Deliver the defined software and documentation (the "deliverables").
> - Install and implement the software.
> - Train HCO personnel.
> - Conduct acceptance testing of the software and then accept the software if it passes the testing.
> - Determine when the warranty period begins.
> - Determine when the maintenance and support phases begin.
> - Conduct future phases and projects, if applicable.

HCO, Healthcare organization.

the initial project from start to go-live, including purchasing hardware, installation, customization, interfaces, training, testing, and user acceptance testing. For example, a community hospital may project an 18-month timeline that is broken into discrete events representing a project plan. (For more information about project management, see Chapter 17.) Generally, vendors resist contractual time commitments, but usually, an HCO can get some meaningful time commitments or at least good faith estimates. Even if the estimates are nonbinding, they create expectations and increase the probability that the project will be completed within an expected time frame. Furthermore, payments or monetary incentives can be tied to milestones, even if the dates associated with the milestones are nonbinding estimates. For example, the vendor would not be in breach of the agreement for failing to meet an estimated date for a given milestone, but if that milestone is also a payment, then payment may be delayed until the milestone is met.

Assuming that the vendor is committed to a time schedule, the agreement should indicate the consequences of a failure to meet the schedule. Such consequences may include liquidated damages, credits, discounts, or delay in payments. For example, if a go-live date is missed by more than a week, the contract may specify that the license fee will be reduced by a specified amount. In response, some vendors may seek financial incentives for early or timely performance of the schedule. Assuming the vendor accepts the concept of a binding time schedule, the HCO should expect the vendor to insist on exceptions for delay or non-performance caused by the HCO, another supplier, or a *force majeure* (disruptions caused by causes beyond the control of the vendor such as natural disasters or other unforeseeable circumstances beyond the control of a group). The vendor may also insist on building a margin for error into the time schedule.

Scope of the License

Who Are the Users?

Fundamentally, the license is permission from the vendor for the HCO to use the software. The license agreement needs to define who may access and use the software. Obviously, this includes the HCO and its employees, but a broader scope may be needed. Contractors acting on behalf of the HCO or other affiliated organizations may need to use the software as well.

Examples of users may also include (1) independent physicians having admitting privileges at the HCO's hospitals; (2) independent healthcare providers and clinics (e.g., to share medical records or perform billing); (3) patients or their family members who will see screen displays or output generated by the software; (4) consultants, other independent contractors (e.g., programmers), and volunteers; and (5) in some cases affiliated foundations or staff and students from affiliated institutions of higher learning. For example, the emergency department may contract with an outside billing agency. This outside agency needs to be mentioned as a user. Otherwise, billing and reimbursements will be negatively affected. The HCO needs to anticipate who the users will be and then make sure that the license agreement allows for those users.

Rights

- The basic rights to software under a license are permissions to:
  - Use the software
  - Copy the software as needed for licensed use
  - Generate and use the output of the software (e.g., screen displays and reports)
- Additional rights in a software license may include permission to:
  - Disclose the software or its output or screen displays to others
  - Distribute the software to others (in special cases)
  - Modify the software and create derivative works based on it

Restrictions and License Metrics

The scope of the license will often be subject to "internal use" or "permitted use" restrictions. The language may vary, but the HCO should be comfortable that these types of restrictions do not prohibit the intended use of the software. For example, a simple restriction that the software may only be used for internal purposes might prohibit use of the software that benefits or involves others outside of the HCO. The scope of a software license is often defined or limited by various license metrics, such as those listed in Box 19.8.

HCOs should anticipate that applicable license metrics (e.g., licensed users) might be exceeded at some time in the future and to provide for the same discounted pricing originally negotiated to cover the excess. This is often covered through an annual reconciliation or "true up" of the license. In other words, the agreement should allow for a review of the license volume annually and for the payment of additional license fees if needed to cover

> **BOX 19.8   Typical License Metrics in a Software License**
>
> - Number of "named" users (either by specific name or by category such as physician, nurse, or pharmacist)
> - Number of "concurrent" users
> - Number of computers, servers, or workstations
> - Number of processors or other measure of processing power
> - Number of procedures, images, reports, etc.
> - Specific site or facilities
> - Entire enterprise

the excess. With this approach, the HCO will not be in breach of the agreement for exceeding a license metric provided.

Scope of Use

Number of Copies

The license might include limits on the number of copies of the software. An extreme example might be the following clause: *Vendor grants to HCO a license to use one copy of the software and to have and maintain one backup copy of the software.* This is a problem because multiple copies of the software can be found in the areas listed in Box 19.9.

An HCO will certainly exceed a one-copy limit because the software held in the computer's memory (e.g., random access memory, or RAM) is legally considered under the copyright laws as a copy of the software, and there will be a copy of the software on the hard drive. Any limitation on the number of copies should reflect the reality of the technology and use.

Environments and Instances

Sometimes, a license is limited to certain numbers and types of environments and instances. The HCO will need to be licensed to use the software in a "production environment" at a minimum. The HCO's technical advisors should review this wording carefully to be sure that it is adequate in the context of expected use. Often, the HCO will want the right to use the software in more than one production environment or in other environments, such as testing, training, development, and recovery environments. The same is true if this concept is expressed in terms of "instances" or some other technical terminology.

Derivative Works

Normally, a software license will prohibit the HCO from modifying the software or creating derivative works based on the software. If the HCO needs to maintain, customize, or enhance the software, then the HCO will need to expand the license to include permission to modify and create derivative works. In such a case and at a minimum, the agreement needs to require the vendor to provide the materials listed in Box 19.10 to the HCO. The HCO will also need programmers, employees, or contractors with the necessary abilities to use the source code to maintain, customize, and enhance the software.

Software and Software as a Service Escrows

For mission-critical or highly important software, an escrow may be included with the license agreement for business

---

> **BOX 19.9   Where Copies of Software Might Exist**
>
> - The master copy provided by the vendor
> - Updates of the software
> - Memory (e.g., RAM)
> - Storage devices (e.g., hard drives)
> - Backups (and other archive and disaster recovery storage)
> - Nonproduction (non-live) environments used for testing, training, development, etc.

> **BOX 19.10   Materials to be Provided to the Healthcare Organization if Derivative Work Rights Are Granted**
>
> - Source code and comments (if not already delivered as part of the software)
> - Development environment (to the extent not commercially available)
> - Programming documentation (e.g., compilation and build instructions)
> - Updates to the foregoing to keep current with the software used by the HCO
> - Anything needed by developers to understand the source code

HCO, Healthcare organization.

---

continuity purposes. For instance, if the vendor goes out of business or otherwise ceases to provide maintenance of the software (e.g., to fix programming errors or to update the software), the HCO may be left in an untenable position. A software escrow is a means to provide protection of the HCO if such an event arises. For a software escrow, a neutral third-party escrow company holds the source code, programming documentation, and other items needed for maintenance and modification of the software. The escrow agreement includes release conditions, release procedures, and terms addressing intellectual property and bankruptcy law issues. A release condition is typically the bankruptcy or insolvency of the vendor, the vendor's breach of maintenance or other obligations, the discontinuation of support by the vendor, the vendor going out of business, or the vendor disrupting use of the software in any other manner. The occurrence of a release condition entitles the HCO to receive the escrowed materials from the escrow company.

A SaaS escrow is an escrow for a SaaS or other cloud-based software solutions. It is similar to the typical software escrow described previously, but also includes having the escrow company maintain a mirror or similar solution on its own server. The SaaS escrow must be in a condition that can be brought live and online for the HCO's use if a release condition occurs or the HCO's access to the software is terminated by the vendor. The frequency of data updates to the escrow's server is just one of many details to be addressed in the escrow agreement. How "hot," "warm," or "cold" the escrowed materials may affect cost and how quickly the escrowed solution can be brought live for the HCO.

Specifications

The HCO should seek detailed specifications, as these define the software that the HCO expects to receive. Specifications may apply to warranties, acceptance, payment milestones, and maintenance obligations of the vendor. The initial draft of the license agreement from the vendor will likely include few or no specifications. The HCO should negotiate for meaningful specifications and preferably create and negotiate them prior to the signing of the agreement. Sometimes, the specifications need to be created after signing. If so, then stage 1 of the agreement can focus on the creation of the specifications. If parties agree on the specifications (which is almost always the case), then they proceed to subsequent stages of the agreement. If they do not agree, then the agreement is terminated.

Many types of specifications can be included in the agreement, such as those in Box 19.11. If the agreement includes custom development or if the development is "agile," then few if any specifications may exist. Agile software development (What is Agile Software Development, 2021) has its advantages that may outweigh the protections that an HCO may otherwise seek in an agreement.

Software Warranties and Exclusions

Sometimes, the vendor offers no warranty (i.e., software is provided "as is" without any guarantee). The HCO should refuse to accept such an agreement. A good software warranty addresses most or all components in Box 19.12. The vendor is likely to have in its draft of the license agreement disclaimers or protections listed in Box 19.13. There may be other disclaimers or limitations. For example, a clause may state that the software is not intended or licensed for high-risk uses or applications. The HCO should seek clarification that those high-risk uses or applications do not apply to healthcare or the specific purposes the HCO intends for its use of the software.

Service Level Agreements

When the license agreement is a SaaS agreement, a service level agreement (SLA) is often included as part of, or in addition to, the SaaS agreement. The SLA is intended to define certain service levels and the consequences of failure to meet those levels. Typically, the service levels are not commitments of the vendor. Therefore, the vendor is not in breach of contract for failure to meet those levels, but rather is only obligated to provide the specified remedy (e.g., service credits). The most common service levels address uptime versus downtime (i.e., availability of the software to the HCO), performance, resolution time, and remedies.

Uptime

There can be disagreement about what "uptime" means. Does it simply mean that the HCO is able to access the software? What if some critical functionality of the software is producing errors or is not functioning but 90% of the functionality is available? Health professionals and informaticians need to understand that 100% uptime is typically not feasible. For each increment toward 100% uptime, expenses can increase dramatically and be unaffordable.

In the end, the agreement should be clear. *A very favorable clause for the HCO would define "uptime" as the time during which the software, including all functionality and without material error, is available for access and use by the HCO.*

What is considered downtime typically has several carve-outs. Scheduled downtime for maintenance and updates is commonly not considered downtime. Downtime caused by the HCO is often not included in a calculation of downtime (e.g., connectivity issues or failure to meet the vendor's requirements). *Force majeure* events (i.e., disruptions beyond the control of the vendor such as natural disasters such as floods, war, or lightning strikes) are also often excluded from uptime calculations. The HCO should ensure that the vendor is obligated to maintain disaster recovery solutions sufficient to overcome many *force majeure* events (see Chapter 21 on downtime and disaster recovery). Because of these adjustments to uptime calculations, an uptime service level of 99.999% is not likely to reflect true uptime and availability of the software.

The appropriate uptime percentage should be based on several factors, including the criticality of the software and impact

---

> **BOX 19.11 Types of Specifications in Agreements**
>
> - Features and functionality
> - Reports, forms, screen displays, output, input
> - Compatibility with hardware, operating system, third-party software, etc.
> - Communications and networking
> - Minimum system requirements
>   - System software (e.g., operating system)
>   - Other third-party software
>   - Hardware and peripheral devices
>   - Communications, networking, interfaces, etc.
> - Performance (e.g., response time, and latency in the case of a SaaS solution)
> - Interfaces

SaaS, software as a service.

> **BOX 19.12 Components of a Software Warranty**
>
> - A good software warranty addresses most or all of the following:
>   - Programming errors (a "No Error" warranty is not realistic)
>   - Compliance with specifications
>   - Compliance with documentation
>   - Performance problems
>   - Output or input problems or errors
>   - Interface, network, or communications problems
>   - Compatibility
>   - Minimum system configuration
> - Other warranties may address:
>   - No self-help code or termination triggers
>   - No viruses or harmful code
>   - Compliance of the software with applicable laws and government regulations (e.g., Health Information Portability and Accountability Act [HIPAA])
>   - Appropriate certification (such as for certified Electronic Health Record Technology [cEHRT])
>   - Vendor owns software or has right to license
>   - No conflict with other contracts or rights of others
>   - Non-infringement of intellectual property
>   - Compliance with privacy, security, and information technology (IT) policies

---

> **BOX 19.13 License Agreement Disclaimers or Protections**
>
> - No warranties clause or "as is" approach (you get only what you get)
> - A clause requiring the healthcare organization (HCO) to agree that there are no warranties that are not expressly included in agreement
> - A clause disclaiming all implied warranties, including the following implied warranties:
>   - Merchantability
>   - Fitness for a particular purpose
>   - Non-infringement

that downtime would have on the HCO. An uptime of 99.999% is generally considered the gold standard, but lesser uptimes may be appropriate for certain contexts. For example, software needed for monitoring in an ICU may need the gold standard, whereas business software used during business hours can have lower uptime, thus reducing costs. Even if an uptime percentage of near 100% is achieved, there can still be other issues, such as network bottlenecks, poor latency, and other performance problems.

Performance

In the context of a SaaS agreement, users will not tolerate a solution that performs slowly, and the SLA should be drafted to address this. Sometimes this type of performance is described as response time (i.e., the time for the computer running the software to respond to the user's input of a command). These performance issues can be very complex and difficult to precisely define in an SLA, and slow performance is not necessarily the fault of the vendor or the software. A simpler solution, but often unacceptable to the vendor, is to use general wording to define a service level in terms of reasonableness (e.g., response time will not be unreasonable).

Resolution Time

Another type of response time is the time it takes for the vendor to respond to a notice of a problem. It is easy to draft this type of response time in an SLA. Resolution time is much more difficult. Vendors vary on their contractual commitments to fix a problem. The range of commitments include those listed in Box 19.14. Without knowing what the problem is, the vendor will be hesitant to commit to a resolution time or even to guarantee that the problem will be resolved. Nonetheless, the HCO should attempt to build these concepts into the SLA or into warranties elsewhere in the agreement. The HCO should note that a "response" is not a solution. A response time of 30 minutes may only mean that the vendor's support personnel will acknowledge receipt of a support ticket. One compromise is to have good response times coupled with an assurance by the HCO that diagnosis or troubleshooting of the problem will begin within the response period and that efforts to resolve the problem will be diligently pursued to completion as soon as reasonably possible. This should also include a promise to provide a workaround solution, if practicable, while the permanent resolution is being worked on. This compromise may be better expressed as a warranty or contractual promise outside of the SLA.

Problem Severity

An SLA commonly defines different categories of problem severity. Simplistically, categories will range from critical to nothing

---

> ### BOX 19.14   The Range of Vendor Commitments to Fix Problems
>
> - Absolute commitment that errors will be fixed
> - Best efforts to fix
> - Commercially reasonable efforts to fix
> - "You get what you get"—which may be a late fix or no fix

---

more than a minor fix or a change request. The agreement may spell out response times and severity levels in simple terms or in complex detail. The HCO should carefully review the actual wording used by the vendor to define severity categories, because a lesser category may result in a long and unacceptable resolution time. For example, the resolution time for a low-severity category might be nothing more than a promise by the vendor to include a fix in the next release of the software without any assurance as to if and when the next release will take place. The HCO should insist that a patient safety issue is critical and should be addressed within a few hours.

Remedies

The usual remedy for a failure to meet an SLA level is a credit to be applied against future payments to the vendor. For uptime, the credit may be defined as a percentage of a monthly fee for the level of uptime achieved during that month. As the level of uptime decreases, the credit increases. Remedies other than credits can be used in an SLA, but vendors are typically reluctant to use anything other than credits. The HCO should make sure that the SLA allows for use of the credit to pay for any obligation to the vendor, not just as a credit against future payments of a specific service. For example, the HCO should be allowed to apply credits toward training, consulting, custom development, data migration, and additional software products. It should also allow for the HCO to collect cash for the credit if the credit still exists at the time the agreement terminates.

Vendors often include a clause in SLAs to the effect that the credit or other remedy is the sole and exclusive remedy for a failure to meet an SLA level. The HCO should be leery about this. For example, this should never apply to a breach by the vendor of an obligation to provide maintenance of the software. As a more extreme example, if the credit for uptime is capped at 25% of the SaaS fee, then literally, the SLA would still require the HCO to pay the remaining 75% of the SaaS fee even if uptime were 0%. Of course, that would be outrageous, but the literal wording of many SLAs means this. As ultimate protection, the HCO should insist on the right to terminate the SaaS agreement if the SLA levels are significantly or continuously not met. This termination right is typically considered separate from other remedies.

Acceptance of the Software

After implementation, the HCO should have the right to test and then accept (or reject) the software. Acceptance should be based on conformance of the software to the acceptance criteria. Acceptance criteria can include those listed in Box 19.15.

If a problem (i.e., nonconformance with any acceptance criterion) is discovered through testing, then the HCO should reject the software and the vendor should be required to fix the problem and redeliver the software for retesting. When no problem is discovered, then the HCO should accept the software. The process may be repeated as necessary.

In many situations, HCOs will do pre-production testing of the software before it is used and tested live in a production environment. With this approach, the HCO does not risk using the software on live data and at the risk of patients' well-being

---

BOX 19.15 Typical Acceptance Criteria in an Agreement

- Relevant provisions in the agreement (such as functionality or software performance once installed)
- Warranties
- Response to RFP or RFI issues
- Specifications exhibit
- Free of known errors
- End user documentation and other documentation
- Specifications published by the vendor

RFP, Request for proposal; *RFI*, request for information.

BOX 19.16 Possible Remedies if Software Fails Acceptance Testing

1. Final rejection of the software by the HCO
   - Software is deinstalled and erased or destroyed or, if this is a SaaS solution, access to the software is terminated.
   - The HCO receives a complete refund, including some or all of the following:
     - License fees
     - Hardware payments
     - Third-party software fees
     - Fees for customization
     - Implementation and development
2. Acceptance of the software "as is" with compensation for the nonconformance with the acceptance criteria.
   - Compensation can be a partial refund, credit, some free services, or additional software licenses.
   - This acceptance should not excuse the vendor's obligation to maintain the software.
3. Some other solution that the vendor and HCO agree to.

HCO, Healthcare organization; *SaaS*, software as a service.

---

until after it is accepted through pre-production testing. Testing in a live environment is still important because live testing can reveal problems not discovered in a pre-live environment. In effect, the testing and acceptance (or rejection) process is repeated for the live environment.

Sometimes vendors want separate acceptance testing of software components, applications, and interfaces. This is often called unit testing. If done separately, this might not reveal problems that arise when the whole system (all components, applications, and interfaces) is used together. This is called integrated testing. An HCO should not accept unit testing alone for acceptance. A possible compromise is to have preliminary acceptance of each unit followed later by final acceptance testing of the integrated system.

For a multisite solution, testing of the software at one site may not reveal all problems when the software goes live for all sites, especially if there is transmission or sharing of data between sites or other interactions between sites. Final testing and acceptance for all sites is advisable.

Software acceptance ideally may be incorporated as a payment milestone on which a portion of the license fee is conditioned.

Remedies for Rejection

The HCO's right to reject the software if acceptance criteria are not met should be expressly stated in agreement. The vendor should be obligated to fix problems and redeliver for a repeat of acceptance testing. The entire software should be retested, not just the corrected portion of the software because correcting one problem may lead to a new one.

Often a difficult issue to negotiate with the vendor is the concept of an absolute obligation to fix versus an effort to use "best efforts" or "commercially reasonable efforts" to try to fix. There may be pre-specified limits on the time allotted to complete a fix or to provide a workaround solution. Such obligations may specify what happens if acceptance testing still fails after repeated attempts to correct the problem, or if the vendor exceeds the defined time limit.

In case of failure, vendors may say that the HCO will get a refund of the license fee, but only for the software components or applications that fail. There is no refund for other software components and applications that pass and are accepted and no refund for services (e.g., installation, implementation, training). This should be unacceptable to the HCO. For example, if some

of the accepted software components require an unaccepted component, then the HCO should be able to reject everything. (As a reminder, for more detail on downtime and disaster recovery, see Chapter 21.) The HCO should have the option to elect one of the following remedies in Box 19.16 if the software ultimately fails to pass acceptance testing.

Maintenance and Support

Maintenance and support by the vendor of the software are essential in most license agreements to ensure HCOs have a reliable system in place for continuous use. Maintenance and support include some or all of the components listed in Box 19.17. HCOs may employ various tactics to reduce maintenance and support costs. The HCO may create its own help desk to discount or reduce fees payable for support. Through the HCO's help desk, support personnel provide frontline or "first-tier" support to HCO users of the software. The vendor's support personnel provide backup or second-tier support to the HCO's support personnel as needed, helping to avoid additional support fees incurred if users were to reach out to the vendor directly.

The agreement should clearly indicate the support hours of the vendor. The nature of the software and the HCO's reliance on it will dictate whether 24/7 support should be requested from the vendor (at higher cost), if business hours are appropriate, or if something in between is needed.

Maintenance Fees

Fees for maintenance and support are typically between 15% and 22% of the initial license fee per year but may range from 10% to 40%. Under a SaaS agreement, the maintenance and support cost is typically included in recurring SaaS fees.

Vendors will often include a term permitting annual increases in fees such as a 3% increase per year in the contract. HCOs should aim to cap increases on fees. The cap may be based on a percentage or CPI (a specified customer price index) or other limit. The HCO should also consider negotiating for multi-year fixed prices to facilitate budget planning and to preserve discounts.

A significant issue is how long the vendor will commit to providing support and maintenance. This should be at least 5 years and preferably a longer period sufficient to cover the expected return on the investment. However, HCOs should not be locked to use the services for that same number of years as they should preserve a termination right if they choose to discontinue use of the software. It would be costly (and embarrassing!) to pay for support and maintenance of software no longer being used.

Payment for support and maintenance should also entitle the HCO to updates and new releases of the software. The fine print in the agreement may make exceptions to this obligation or charge extra fees in some cases.

Supported Software Versions

The agreement should indicate how far back versions of the software will be supported and maintained. For example, an agreement may indicate that only the most current version of the software will be supported and maintained, but the HCO may want to continue to use prior versions. Upgrading to a new version may be costly, time consuming, and inconvenient. Security issues may arise when a new version is implemented. On the other hand, upgrading eventually becomes necessary, as security patches may require major upgrades and the HCO cannot reasonably expect the vendor to continue to support and maintain versions with dependencies on hardware or operating systems that are many years old. Compromises on this issue often include support and maintenance for one or two of the most recent prior versions or giving the HCO a transition period to upgrade. Sometimes the vendor may support "out-of-support" versions if the HCO is willing to pay a premium in maintenance fees.

If the overall software solution includes third-party software, then support of the third-party software may not be covered by the support and maintenance obligations in the agreement and may instead depend on the support and maintenance provided by the third party. In general, understanding the roles and obligations of third parties is important prior to signing the agreement.

Other Services

The license agreement should include, often via attached Scope of Work, other vendor services that the HCO needs or may want, such as installation and implementation, training, data conversion, interfaces, or custom development.

System Implementation or Installation Support

Agreements often include services in support of system implementation, as listed in Box 19.18.

A significant issue can be determining if services are purchased for time versus results. Typically, it is favorable to pay for results since paying by the hour or day is no assurance as to how many hours or days it may take to complete a project. This approach gives certainty in budgeting and a greater chance that the results will be obtained without cost overruns. However, if the HCO insists on a fixed-fee approach, the quote from the vendor is likely to build in a healthy margin for error, possibly resulting in a higher cost to the HCO. If paying for time, the HCO should also include in the agreement the number of hours that the vendor estimates in good faith is needed for completion. The estimate can help the HCO negotiate if the vendor exceeds the estimated hours and asks for more.

Since it is rare for all needs to be anticipated upfront, the HCO should include in the agreement an open-ended obligation for the vendor to provide additional services at the option of the HCO. Needs may occur for additional assistance on installation, implementation, data conversion, training, customization and interfaces, or consultation.

Outsourcing to Data Centers for Hosting and Software Management Services

A typical license agreement includes restrictions that prohibit transferring or disclosing the software to any third party, and these restrictions would prohibit the HCO's use of third-party data centers to host the software for the HCO. Therefore, for any on-premises solution HCOs may want to deliver to users from a third-party data center, HCOs will need to include the right to have a third-party data center host the software and provide data center services. Here is a sample clause that gives the HCO the right to use a third-party data center and other vendors for other purposes:

HCO may outsource to other vendors any of HCO's needs or requirements for information technology equipment, resources, or services, including, without limitation, hosting, co-location, application management, and data center services. If and to the extent that any such outsourcing is applicable to any of the licensed software licensed to HCO under this Agreement, then this Agreement and the licenses granted to HCO will be reasonably expanded, if and as necessary, to allow such outsourcing, including, without limitation, the right for the licensed software to be run on servers, computers or processors of such vendors, or at their data centers for HCO. Any such vendor must agree in writing that it will not store, run, or use the licensed software for any purpose other than services for HCO and to protect the licensed software from any unauthorized copying, use, or access by others.

Revenue Recognition and Payments

From the vendor's perspective, revenue recognition issues—the timing with which they get paid for or in anticipation of services—affect many key provisions in the agreement. These issues may arise from:

1. Conditions on payment
2. Delivery of software not existing at the time the agreement is signed
3. Payment milestones (e.g., acceptance)
4. Possible refunds or other elements

Do not be caught by surprise—this is a huge issue to many vendors, especially those that are public companies. The HCO should expect pressure to commit or finalize the agreement by the end of the quarter or end of the year, but the negotiating team should work together to recognize and avoid this pressure. Vendors will always be happy for the business, and the urgency can return at the end of the next quarter, for example. Often, discounts are conditioned by the vendor on a signing of the agreement by a certain deadline, with the expectation that the HCO will concede on important points of negotiation to meet the deadline. However, HCOs are usually in a strong negotiating position to ignore this urgency and receive the discount in the next quarter.

Shopping enterprise agreements is very different from retail shopping. Prices are frequently considered confidential information of the vendor subject to nondisclosure. For this reason, a confidential RFI/RFP process can be a helpful way to obtain a broad swath of pricing quotes and better enable shopping for value. In general, an HCO should not have to pay list price for a software license, and any discounts should have a long-term life for future purchases. Sometimes, HCOs and other customers ask for "most favored nations" pricing and terms for newer products looking to gain a market foothold, but this is not typically accepted by established vendors who stand to alienate prior customers or risk significant revenue opportunity.

In many cases, vendors are willing to offer discounts for "strategic accounts." This can mean many different things such as HCOs sharing hard-to-find expertise, participating in case studies, or providing specific feedback that informs future development. This is not charity from the vendor, and they will often need some reassurance that there is value to the HCO's participation as a strategic or beta customer. Discounts can be deep (e.g., 75% of the cost of the software) if vendors perceive this will enable subsequent sales at the purchasing HCO or similar HCOs that are not yet customers.

When negotiating the agreement, HCOs may seek opportunities to lock in prices or discounts on optional software, expansions, or future projects. *The HCO has the most leverage before signing the agreement and loses that leverage after signing.* The HCO should negotiate for a payment schedule that ties some payments to milestones and acceptance. This is a good way to motivate a vendor to stay on schedule. The agreement will often provide that the HCO pay for the vendor's expenses and other charges, especially with respect to some services. This should not apply to support and maintenance services. For other services, expenses should be reasonable, capped, and documented.

The HCO should consider credits, refunds, or other financial consequences for delays, breaches, or other failures by the vendor. If custom development or lengthy and complicated implementations and rollouts are involved, this can be important. For legal reasons, these credits, refunds, and other financial consequences should not be characterized as "penalties," even though non-attorneys tend to do so. In some cases, it may be appropriate to characterize them as "liquidated damages." When faced with the prospect of credits, refunds, or other financial consequences, a vendor may respond by asking for incentives (e.g., additional payment) if time schedules or other performances are overachieved by the vendor. The HCO should be prepared for this response by the vendor and can usually reject it.

The HCO should make sure that everything is covered. The vendor should provide line-by-line pricing for the system selection and/or the negotiating team to review to avoid unpleasant surprises. Open-ended obligations to pay for services (e.g., implementation) may lead to unexpected budget overruns.

Overview of Termination

It is tempting to expect an implementation and software solution to work as advertised. However, the sales process typically inflates the ease of implementation and use. When things do not meet initial expectations, the termination provisions may be the most important part of the license agreement and represent a key source of negotiating leverage. On one hand, the agreement may be terminated simply because its term expires or because both parties amicably agree to an early termination. On the other hand, breach of the agreement by the HCO or vendor is usually defined as a cause for termination. Sometimes, the agreement includes a clause giving the HCO the right to terminate for convenience—with great reluctance from vendors—or for dissatisfaction. For example, failure of the vendor to meet a nonbinding time schedule or an SLA performance level might not be a breach of the agreement but could trigger a right on the part of the HCO to terminate the agreement if this right is sought prior to signing. HCOs should not give this right to a vendor. Other termination rights may include termination for bankruptcy or insolvency.

Multiyear agreements are often written with an annual auto-renewal term. This indicates that the HCO and vendor intend to work together for several years but offers an annual frequency with which the HCO can terminate the contract for convenience. Vendors typically require 30-, 60-, or 90-days' notice prior to the renewal date if terminating a contract with auto-renewal.

It should be noted that a license agreement usually includes a survival clause that indicates that certain provisions of the agreement will continue in effect after termination of the agreement. Confidentiality provisions, data storage, and auditing rights are a few such examples. Rarely, the license itself can survive, but other provisions, such as maintenance and support, will terminate.

Termination for Breach

Nearly every license agreement includes a clause giving each party the right to terminate the agreement if the other party breaches the agreement. Sometimes, one-sided license agreements only give the vendor this right, but in such cases, it is typically easy for the HCO to successfully negotiate for reciprocity.

From the perspective of the HCO, termination, even for a breach by the HCO, can be much more dangerous and unreasonable than meets the eye. If the software is mission critical, it is not practical or realistic to expect the HCO to suddenly stop using the software being relied upon. For example, if the electronic health record (EHR) of the HCO is reliant on the software, the HCO could not possibly stop use of it without severe consequences to patients and operations. Typically, provisions are included that obligate the HCO to stop using the software upon termination. Without a license, continued use of the software would be an infringement of the copyright and other intellectual property of the vendor.

An agreement includes many provisions that can potentially be breached by the HCO. For example, confidentiality provisions could be inadvertently or carelessly breached. Other restrictions, such as a prohibition against benchmark testing, may be breached without realizing that the agreement includes this prohibition. Exceeding the scope of the license is also a breach and can be done unintentionally. In a payment dispute, the vendor can claim a breach and threaten termination if the HCO does not concede and pay the disputed amount. Examining the agreement will reveal many provisions that might be breached.

In the case of an "on-premises" license, the HCO might ignore a notice of termination for breach by the vendor and continue to use the software running on the HCO's computers to provide continuity of patient care operations. The HCO would do so without support and maintenance from the vendor. The vendor would then be forced to seek an injunction from a court to order the HCO to stop use. Hopefully, a court would not issue such an order if patient safety were jeopardized, but it may be hard to explain to the court why the HCO agreed that it would stop use upon termination for breach and now refuses to do so. The situation is riskier in the case of a SaaS license because the SaaS vendor can more easily terminate HCO access

to the software running on the vendor's servers. Hopefully, the vendor would not do this, but it is particularly unwise for the HCO to agree to breach termination provisions for SaaS. In any event, the vendor is likely to use the threat of termination to extract concessions to its advantage.

At the very least, the HCO should insist that the agreement include provisions that require (1) the breach be "material" to justify termination and (2) the vendor give the HCO notice of the breach and an opportunity to cure the breach before termination (typically 30 days). If the breach is timely cured, then no right exists for the vendor to terminate. Sometimes, more than 30 days is needed to complete a cure, so the HCO should request a clause that allows for an extension of the 30 days if the cure begins within the 30-day period and is diligently pursued to completion.

The ultimate protection for an HCO is to include in the agreement a provision to the effect that the license will survive termination of the agreement even if there is a breach of the agreement. This does not excuse the breach, as the HCO remains liable for damages caused by the breach. The vendor can still obtain injunctive relief to stop the breach, but it is very difficult to get vendors to agree to such a provision. Their attorneys are often adamant that termination of the license is essential for protection of the vendor's software and intellectual property. This concern is somewhat overstated because (1) the HCO is only seeking the right to continue to use the software within the scope of a license that the HCO has already paid for, and (2) the vendor can always obtain injunctive relief against any use, disclosure, distribution, or copying beyond the scope of that license.

If the HCO cannot get the ultimate protection described previously, the following clause or a variation is reasonable despite the vendor's dislike for it. It will as often as not be accepted by the vendor:

In view of the mission critical nature of the Licensed Software to HCO and HCO's reliance on it and of the responsibility of HCO to protect the safety, health, and well-being of patients, Vendor may not suspend or terminate the License [or any services or rights of HCO under this Agreement or any access to or use of the Licensed Software by HCO or its users] unless this Agreement is terminated in accordance with this Section. The vendor may terminate this Agreement only upon a material breach of this Agreement by HCO that is not cured by HCO within 30 days after receiving written notice from the vendor of such breach. The notice must specifically identify the provisions of this Agreement that are breached and must state the actions that the vendor believes are necessary for HCO to cure the breach and must give notice of the vendor's intention to terminate the Agreement if the breach is not cured. If more than 30 days are needed to cure the breach, then HCO will be allowed such additional time as is reasonably required for the cure, provided that HCO gives notice of the need and begins the cure within the 30-day period and that HCO is thereafter diligent in pursuing the cure to completion. If the breach is not curable, then for the purposes of this Section, the breach will be deemed cured if HCO takes reasonable steps to prevent a repeat of the breach. HCO remains liable for damages caused by its breach and nothing in this Section excuses monetary liability for those damages, but damages are subject to the agreed upon limitations of liability. If HCO disputes in good faith that a material breach has occurred, then the issue must first be decided through the dispute resolution provisions and, if necessary, litigation in accordance with governing law and forum provisions of this Agreement. If a court holds that a material breach occurred, then HCO shall have an opportunity to cure the breach as described above (or to address an incurable breach as described above) to preserve its license and rights and to avoid termination of the Agreement by the vendor. The 30-day cure period will begin when HCO receives notice of the final decision of the court in writing and such 30-day cure period is subject to extension as described above. Nothing herein permits HCO to use, distribute, or copy the Licensed Software outside the scope of the License and rights granted to HCO. Nothing prohibits or delays Vendor from obtaining an injunction to stop HCO from using, distributing, or copying the Licensed Software outside of such license and rights or from otherwise infringing or misappropriating any intellectual property or confidentiality information of Vendor.

Do not think that the nightmare of termination cannot happen. It does and can happen, although rarely. Even if a vendor is very unlikely to abuse termination rights in the agreement if the HCO acts in good faith and is repentant, the HCO is still exposed to the "termination blackmail" threat when the HCO disputes the existence of a breach or disputes what the remedy should be for the breach.

As a final comment on the issue of termination, the importance of this issue is proportional to the significance of the HCO's reliance on the software and the ease of transitioning to a substitute solution in the event of termination. Many situations exist where the HCO can, with relative safety, ignore the issue because the risk or downside of termination is so low that negotiating with the vendor is not justified. If the software is mission critical to the HCO, then the risk can be summed up as follows: (1) the probability of a serious termination issue occurring is very low, but (2) in the unlikely event that it does occur, the consequences can be very serious. In a worst-case scenario, it may be difficult for the HCO's representatives responsible for approving the agreement to explain to management why the HCO agreed to allow the vendor to terminate or threaten to terminate the use of mission critical software.

Transition and Transition Period

As an additional protection in case of termination, the HCO may want to add a clause entitling it to transition rights and a transition period. A clause of this nature might read as follows:

If the Agreement is terminated for any reason or expires and if the safety, health, or well-being of any patients or healthcare or business operations of the HCO are jeopardized or compromised by such termination or expiration,

then the HCO will be entitled to a reasonable transition period to transition to computer programs, products, services, and solutions from another vendor that are a substitute for the Licensed Software, Services, and Solution of this Agreement. During this transition period, HCO may continue to use and exercise the License and rights with respect to the Licensed Software, Services, and Solution pursuant to this Agreement and subject to this Agreement. In effect, the transition period is an extension of the term of this Agreement and delays termination or expiration until the end of the transition period. The transition period must be sufficient in duration to allow for an orderly transition to substitute computer programs, products, services, and solutions, but HCO may not extend the transition period beyond one year. HCO will give notice to Vendor after the transition period ends.

Sometimes, especially for an SaaS license, the transition clause will require the vendor to provide transition services at the vendor's current standard fees plus expenses.

Exclusive Remedy Clauses

License agreements frequently include exclusive remedy clauses that state that the HCO's sole and exclusive remedy for a breach is limited to one specific remedy and not others. For example, a section may state that if the services are not performed in accordance with the warranties, then the exclusive remedy is that the services will be re-performed. Even if performed properly later, there is no compensation to the HCO for the delay. The agreement may even include a provision stating the exclusive remedy still applies even if the remedy "fails of its essential purpose." The provision then leaves the HCO without a meaningful remedy.

No other damages or remedies can be recovered if the exclusive remedy clause is enforced. Usually, an exclusive remedy clause is applied to warranties, but they can be applied to any obligation in the agreement. Sometimes, vendors are overly aggressive and broad in the language of an exclusive remedy clause and incorrectly (or unfairly) apply it to any breach of the agreement. For example, an exclusive remedy may mention having a vendor re-perform an activity as the sole remedy for any breach of the agreement. However, this action would be illogical for a security or confidentiality breach by a vendor. The exclusive remedy should make sense in the context of the specific breach to which it applies and should only apply to specific breach of contract claims, not to other claims such as negligence or damage to property.

Limitations and Exclusions of Liability

A license agreement will almost always include clauses on limitations and exclusions of liability (EHR contracts untangled, 2016). The HCO should understand these clauses and impacts to the business if invoked.

Limitation of Liability

A limitation of liability clause limits the HCO's liability to an amount or cap that cannot be exceeded. For example, "In no event shall Vendor's aggregate liability exceed an amount equal to the license fee paid to Vendor under this Agreement." The consequence of an HCO agreeing that the vendor's liability is limited means that the HCO cannot recover damages from the vendor more than the cap, even if the HCO can prove a higher amount of damages. Vendors will typically defend this clause during negotiation, so an HCO strategy may be to require that the limitation instead be a multiple of the license fee (e.g., 300%, 500% of the license fee). It may be better to increase the cap to all amounts paid under the Agreement (e.g., to include support, maintenance, training, implementation, and other service fees in addition to the license fee). Carve-outs on limitations of liability are also common. For example, if Protected Health Information is necessary to use the service, breaches of patient privacy and confidentiality are often carved out and handled elsewhere in an agreement (e.g., a business associate agreement) with higher caps.

Exclusion of Liability

An exclusion of liability clause totally excludes certain types of damages from recovery. For example, "In no event shall Vendor be liable for any consequential, indirect, special, punitive, or incidental damages, or for any loss of business, opportunity, profits, revenue, data, or programs." The consequence of the HCO agreeing to this means that the HCO recovers nothing for these types of damages, even if the HCO can prove that it suffered the damages. Only direct damages remain recoverable, subject to the limitation of liability cap described previously.

Reciprocity and Exceptions

The HCO should insist these clauses are reciprocal, so they benefit the HCO, not just the vendor. When these clauses are made reciprocal, the vendor will often insist on exceptions for infringement of its intellectual property, breach of confidentiality, indemnification, and possibly some other clauses. The HCO should negotiate for other exceptions, such as breach of a business associate agreement or data security agreement, intentional breaches, willful misconduct, and wrongful suspension or termination. For example, if the vendor were to wrongfully suspend or terminate a SaaS license and access to the software, the HCO would have little or no monetary recourse against the vendor because the limitation and exclusion of liabilities would prevent recovery of the most significant damages, including loss of revenue and disruption of business. Having these exceptions in the agreement will make a SaaS vendor leery about being too quick to suspend or terminate services for fear of being exposed to unlimited liability for doing so wrongfully.

Liability Insurance

The vendor should agree to maintain adequate liability insurance, including cyber liability insurance governing data privacy, security breaches, and business continuity. The HCO may need recourse against the insurance for negligence and other covered faults of the vendor, or the HCO may need to be additionally protected. The HCO should carefully consider whether it should be named as an additional insured party in the vendor's insurance policy, because existing insurance policies may not cover claims against another insured (e.g., the HCO). The limitations

and exclusions of liability should not limit or exclude any losses and liabilities covered by the vendor's insurance policies. The HCO insurance advisor or risk management officer should work with the HCO's negotiating team in deciding on adequate insurance requirements expected of the vendor.

Dispute Resolution

Some license agreements require a dispute resolution process before litigation or arbitration. There is no single standard for what a contractual dispute resolution process looks like, but a reasonable example may be to hold a meeting to discuss and attempt to resolve the dispute. If that meeting is unsuccessful, the dispute must be escalated to a higher level of management of both parties for discussion and resolution. In some cases, there are even joint steering boards with explicit voting rights as a final step prior to arbitration or litigation. It is often easier to agree to a process for dispute resolution rather than an outcome of a dispute, so having a process defined upfront is a good approach for HCOs, especially as a prerequisite to termination.

SPECIAL CLAUSES

Confidentiality

The license agreement typically includes confidentiality protections for the parties and their confidential information. The HCO's confidential information may include RFPs, plans, financial information, and anything that can be learned by the vendor's access to any networks or computer systems of the HCO. The party receiving the other party's confidential information should agree not only to keep the information confidential but also to not use it for any purpose other than performing obligations or exercising rights under the agreement.

The HCO should expect to see some or all of the following exceptions in Box 19.19 to the confidentiality provisions. The HCO should make sure that these exceptions do not apply to protected health information or other personally identifiable information, or to any obligation under a business associate agreement or data security agreement. The confidentiality provisions should not prohibit a disclosure required by law, regulation, or court or government order, but a protective order or similar protection should be sought.

An important issue is the duration of the confidentiality obligations. The confidentiality obligations may be indefinite or may expire a certain number of years after the date of the agreement or after the date of first disclosure.

BOX 19.19   Exceptions to Confidentiality Provisions

- Information that is or becomes (through no fault of the receiving party) publicly known or generally known in the industry or profession of either party
- Information known to the receiving party prior to first disclosure by the other party
- Information that is lawfully disclosed on a nonconfidential basis by third parties to the receiving party
- Information that is independently created by or for the receiving party

The vendor will include provisions that specifically protect the software and documentation against disclosure or transfer to others. It is not always clear if and to what extent protections apply to screen displays and output (e.g., reports). Because of the broad and restrictive nature of confidentiality provisions, the HCO may want to include an exception for incidental disclosures. For example:

Nothing in this Confidentiality Section or any other confidentiality provisions of this Agreement prohibits any disclosure that reasonably or inherently occurs as part of the licensed use of the Licensed Software or the servicing by contractors of hardware or systems for the HCO. By way of non-limiting examples, screen displays, interfaces and reports generated by the Licensed Software may be visible to visitors to HCO's facilities and reports and other output generated by the Licensed Software may be given to others in the ordinary course of business.

Data Security

If the vendor, especially a SaaS vendor, holds or stores any of the HCO's data, then data security provisions will be needed in addition to the confidentiality provisions of the agreement. These provisions may include absolute restrictions from disclosing certain confidential information to third parties or, more likely, disclosure without written approval of the HCO. Commonly, vendors are asked to complete a Security Risk Assessment document that includes questions for the vendor to complete about compliance with security principles, process for reviewing personnel and avoidance of "bad actors," use of contracted third parties, network security practices, system security practices, and use of third-party applications. Software security breaches can expose an enterprise to fraud, ransomware, or other threats, so it is advisable to include an IT security review as a part of any software licensing review.

Data Usage and Data Ownership

HCO data can confer important strategic advantages to the organization and involves additional considerations and protection under HIPAA in the case of patient data. To the extent patient data are involved, the HCO may want to go beyond the protections afforded by a business associate agreement. Vendors will often include a provision to de-identify patient data to support product development or other commercial purposes. Once appropriately de-identified, the data are no longer protected by HIPAA, essentially offering the vendor a license to use the data as it sees fit. HCOs should seek provisions that specifically protect patient data even if de-identified and aggregated. Furthermore, the agreement should specify data ownership, especially for aggregated data generated through use of the vendor's software. The HCO will want to consider carefully how population health data will be managed, define who owns the resulting data, and include these aspects in the agreement.

Intellectual Property Infringement

The license agreement should include a warranty of non-infringement and a clause indemnifying (providing compensation for a particular loss) the HCO and its users of the software against claims that the software or its licensed use infringes or misappropriates any patent, copyright, trade secret, or other intellectual property. Often, the vendor will not offer a warranty of non-infringement, saying instead that it only offers an indemnification clause. These clauses can be complex and include exceptions that need to be carefully considered. The clause might indemnify against monetary judgments payable to the owner of the intellectual property, but often not against the HCO's own losses or damages if it must suddenly cease use of the software because of an infringement claim. The HCO will want broader indemnification protection.

Indemnification by the Healthcare Organization and Disclaimers by the Vendor of Responsibility

The vendor may seek to have the HCO indemnify the vendor against claims by others arising from the HCO's use of or reliance on the software or its use, results, and output. It is not uncommon to see vendors disclaim responsibility for the results and output of the software and to require HCOs to examine and verify those results and output, such as accuracy of medication calculations. The best approach is to delete these types of provisions, especially indemnification by the HCO, and simply make each party responsible for its own fault in the event of any claims by a third party.

Restrictive Covenants and Feedback Clauses

The HCO should take careful note of restrictive covenants and feedback clauses and should only agree to them if they are reasonable and understood by the HCO. Restrictive covenants include non-compete clauses and other restrictions on doing business or conducting certain activities with others, as well as clauses that prohibit the hiring or solicitation of the other party's personnel.

Feedback clauses may require the HCO to assign ownership of feedback and its intellectual property to the vendor. Feedback is typically defined as suggestions, ideas, recommendations, improvements, and enhancements relating to the software or a service of the vendor. This can become a serious problem if the HCO wants to use or commercialize the feedback independent of the vendor or to share the feedback with other vendors. At most, a feedback clause should only grant to the vendor a nonexclusive license to use the feedback in the vendor's software and services. This license should be granted on an "as is" basis without any warranty. Any feedback clause requires careful consideration and possible exceptions (e.g., for copyrights and patents).

Governing Law and Forum Clauses

These clauses indicate which jurisdiction's law will govern the agreement. The forum clause indicates the jurisdiction and venue for any litigation between the parties (i.e., where a lawsuit will take place). It may seem odd, but a court in one state may apply the law of another state to the agreement and dispute. With respect to jurisdiction and venue, one compromise is to say that a party may only bring an action in the state (or more specific venue) of the other party. This may discourage litigation.

Right to Assign the Agreement and License

License agreements generally prohibit an assignment (of license and other rights and delegation or transfer of duties and obligations) or transfer of the agreement to a third party. Given the possibility that the HCO may merge with or be acquired by another entity in the future, it is a good idea to at least allow the HCO to assign or transfer the agreement if the HCO or its assets or business is acquired by sale, merger, or otherwise. A change of HCO control should not be deemed as a prohibited assignment or transfer.

Use of the Healthcare Organization's Name, Marks, and Logos

The license agreement should prohibit the vendor from using the HCO's name, trademark, service mark, or logo in any marketing, sales, or promotional materials; on a website; or in any other public communication without the written consent of the HCO in each case, including the right of prior review. Use of the HCO's name in a list of customers or a press release may be permitted by the agreement without that consent. Vendors should not be allowed to use these materials to imply any HCO affiliation, endorsement, or sponsorship of the vendor or its software, product, or service. Sometimes, HCOs may want to allow certain types of endorsement, for example, as a reference customer or by participating in a published case study, but these tend to be the exception for strategic relationships with vendors. In addition to HCO brand protections, similar restrictions should be considered

for the name of any officer, researcher, developer, clinical informatician, physician, or other healthcare professional employed by the HCO.

CONCLUSION AND FUTURE DIRECTIONS

License agreements are an essential part of an HCO's software procurement process. An understanding of those agreements and a willingness to negotiate for reasonable terms and conditions can reduce risk, save money, and protect the HCO against unpleasant surprises. An agreement, no matter how favorable to the HCO, is never an acceptable substitute for due diligence prior to the signing of the agreement or for a careful and systematic vendor selection process. After the agreement is signed, the HCO should have a process for ensuring and monitoring compliance with the agreement and for using the protections and advantages successfully negotiated into the agreement. Although it may seem obvious, the HCO should have an organized archive of agreements and an index and summary of the important agreements that can be consulted when needed. Finally, never underestimate the leverage that an HCO may have to contractually protect itself. The future of license agreements will only grow more complex as technology and data become more distributed over time. As data are merged from different sources, data ownership and security breaches will continue to be issues in the future.

ACKNOWLEDGMENT

The authors wish to acknowledge the contribution of Jon C. Christiansen to the previous edition of this chapter.

DISCUSSION QUESTIONS

1. Thinking about your own organization, outline the composition of a team to assist with generating a licensing agreement to integrate all imaging services in your facility across ultrasound, radiology, and cardiology. Give the rationale for each team member.
2. Discuss what steps organizations might take for due diligence. How might these protect the organization beyond having a good contract in place?
3. In this chapter, the author recommends numerous sections to a licensing agreement. Which ones surprised you?
4. Your electronic health record (EHR) vendor was sold to another company. What provisions in the agreement will be the ones you will look for to ensure patient care is not compromised as a transition occurs?

CASE STUDY

Best Bet Hospital is a tertiary care medical center with 500 acute care beds, 35 ambulatory clinics, a Level-1 emergency department, a 75-bed skilled nursing facility, and telehealth services for both stroke and dermatology services. The leadership decided to change its EHR after a 10-year life cycle and shift to a SaaS agreement. You are the long-term care representative on the selection committee. Due to your expertise in healthcare, leadership has asked you to assist with the licensing agreement for this purchase.

Discussion Questions

1. Give an overview of the particular needs (functional aspects) of long-term care that should be included in a licensing agreement.
2. Glancing over the sections in this chapter, create an outline of the most important areas to consider in the licensing agreement.
3. Best Bet wants to reduce maintenance and support costs. What are some ways this might be accomplished? What areas should be included in the licensing agreement to support these?

REFERENCES

Agile Alliance. Agile 101. Retrieved from https://www.agilealliance.org/agile101.

Cornell University Law School. (n.d.). Uniform Trade Secrets Act. Retrieved from https://www.law.cornell.edu/wex/trade_secret.

EHR contracts untangled: Selecting wisely, negotiating terms, and understanding the fine print. The Office of the National Coordinator for Health Information Technology. September 30, 2016.

Section 101 of the U.S. Patent Laws (35 U.S.C. 101), 2016.

20

Implementing and Upgrading an Information System

Madeline Araya, Meera Subash, and Nathan Yung

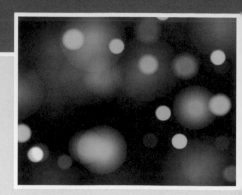

OBJECTIVES

At the completion of this chapter, the reader will be prepared to:

1. Summarize the genesis of electronic health record policy in the late 2000s in the United States.
2. Discuss how the phases of software development lifecycles influence the implementation or update of an EHR.
3. Describe the roles of superusers and informatics professionals in training and go-live activities.
4. Discuss factors to consider when planning for future system maintenance tasks.
5. Discuss potential future EHRs' technical requirements with increasing technology specifications.

KEY TERMS

big bang, 315	e-iatrogenesis, 310	scope creep, 311
change control, 312	information blocking, 308	superuser, 314
change freezes, 317	milestones, 312	user acceptance testing, 314
data abstraction, 317	phased go-live, 315	

ABSTRACT ❖

This chapter begins with a historical perspective of health information technology implementation and proceeds with process analyses for implementing a clinical health information system, centering on the electronic health record (EHR). The foci of clinical information system implementation and upgrading continue to focus on decision support, thereby (1) providing safe and up-to-date patient care, (2) promoting interoperability, and (3) leveraging advanced levels of clinical decision support (CDS). Implementing EHRs entails an effective internal and external communication process, multiple layers of decisions during each stage of the implementation, and a clear understanding of the project's complexity to ensure appropriate decision-making. Major decisions begin with a focus on what patient care needs are supported, usability, vendor and system selection, go-live options, workflows and processes redesign, and developing procedures and policies. The timeline and scope of the project is primarily dictated by expenses, staff, resources, and the drop-dead date for go-live. Success depends on a well-thought-out and detailed project plan with regular review and updating of the critical milestones, unwavering support from the organization's leadership, input from users during the design and build phases, thorough testing, end-user education, mitigation of identified risk factors, and control of scope creep. The implementation of an EHR is a continuous process requiring management and maintenance. Medication orders, nonmedication orders, and documentation screens or fields will continuously need to be added, modified, or inactivated; disruptions may require patch installation and tweaks to workflows and functionality. New virtual modes of care delivery are being integrated into pre-existing EHR builds to address the changing needs of patients and utilize new reimbursement structures.

INTRODUCTION

There are several reasons why a health organization (hospital organization, physician office, or clinic) may decide that a major change is needed. A careful review of the reasons for the change will start the process of deciding whether to install a new information system or upgrade the current system. Clinical information systems, specifically the electronic health record (EHR), are essential for the delivery of evidence-based care (EBC). EBC is patient-centered, relying on diagnostic information to provide cost effective and appropriate care. Information provided by EHRs facilitate effective patient-centered care through management of clinical activities resulting in reduction of medical errors and costs.

HISTORICAL REVIEW OF THE ELECTRONIC HEALTH RECORD

The American Recovery and Reinvestment Act (ARRA)

The American Recovery and Reinvestment Act (ARRA), enacted in 2009, spawned the Health Information Technology for Economic and Clinical Health (HITECH) Act. One of its primary goals was that each person in the United States would have a certified digital medical record by 2014, including the electronic exchange of health information across healthcare institutions, to improve quality of healthcare. As discussed in detail in Chapter 29, the HITECH Act created a $27 billion federally funded incentive program that provided Medicare and Medicaid payments over 5 to 10 years to three groups: (1) eligible providers (EPs), (2) eligible hospitals (EHs), and (3) critical access hospitals (CAHs). CAH were defined as rural hospitals certified to receive cost-based reimbursement from Medicare. Within the HITECH Act, two EHR incentive programs were developed, specifically the Medicare EHR Incentive Program administered by the Centers for Medicare and Medicaid Services (CMS) and the Medicaid EHR Incentive Program, which was governed by individual states and territories. It is important to note that these government incentive programs were not established to cover the total cost of implementing an EHR system but rather to encourage or "incentivize" healthcare organizations and healthcare providers to use an EHR in a meaningful way—called Meaningful Use (MU) (this term is now referred to as "promoting interoperability")—and to foster faster rates of adoption across the nation (One Hundred Eleventh Congress of the United States of America, 2009). Other terms often used for this incentive program were "stimulus funds," "stimulus package," or simply "ARRA funds" (Healthcare Information Technology Standards Panel [HITSP], n.d.).

CMS established the criteria for MU or promoting interoperability, including minimal thresholds for select objectives. There were three stages in the EHR Incentive Program. Stage 1 began in 2011 and emphasized capturing patient data that was expected to be shared with other healthcare professionals and the patient. Stage 2 began in 2014 and focused on advanced clinical practices and providing patient portals where patients could access their medical records. Stage 3 began in 2017 and accentuated data interoperability and patient outcomes while increasing the thresholds for the objectives and clinical measures (Centers for Medicare & Medicare Services [CMS], 2015). Additional requirements included the submission of detailed and timely reports demonstrating interoperability adoption to CMS and the appropriate state offices.

CMS requirements for promoting interoperability mandate that the EHR be a "certified complete EHR" or have individual modules that are "certified EHR modules." This means that they are certified by the Office of the National Coordinator for Health Information Technology (ONC). Complete EHR certification means that the system was required to prove it was functional with the appropriate data elements and logic to support all facility departments. EHR module certification means that the ancillary application met one or more requirements. Most hospitals and physician offices purchased commercial systems that incorporated all essential capabilities. A list of certified products can be found at CHPL (https://chpl.healthit.gov/#/search).

The Certification Commission for Health Information Technology (CCHIT) began testing and certifying new software applications in 2006. In 2014, it ceased testing and certifying EHRs for financial reasons and changed its role to advising healthcare providers on how to comply with the government's regulations and providing guidance to health IT developers on how to meet the government's requirements for a certified EHR. The CCHIT worked with the Health Information and Management Systems Society (HIMSS) to advance programs and policies that strongly promote interoperability and to advocate using IT between patients and providers as another tool to transform healthcare (Terry, 2014). CCHIT ceased all operations in 2014.

The ONC now manages the EHR certification program—which first began in 2010—using the process shown in Fig. 20.1. The ONC has increased the use of this program to other CMS and non-CMS programs. There are multiple editions of the program, each more robust than the last, to improve interoperability standards, increase transparency, and moderate costs for the programs and systems it supports. Modifications to this system have been instituted and documented in the Final Rule by the 21st Century Cures Act: Interoperability, Information Blocking, and the ONC Health IT Certification Program.

However, the MU criteria did not require purchasing a commercial, certified product. A few hospitals and EPs had developed their own "homegrown" EHRs that may or may not have included commercial components. CMS welcomed organizations to certify their systems using the EHR Alternative Certification for Healthcare Providers (EACH) program. The EACH program was a three-step program to certify homegrown systems or existing EHR technology not already covered by a vendor certification. The program provided a mechanism to obtain certification by demonstrating that the system met the U.S. Department of Health & Human Services (HHS) MU requirements (US DHHS Office of the National Coordinator [ONC], 2015). For example, the Regenstrief Medical Record System (RMRS) in Indiana is an EMR system that began in 1972 and expanded to several additional major hospitals (Duke, et al. 2014). Other medical centers that successfully opted for this alternative include Geisinger Health System, Marshfield Clinic Health System, Landmark Hospitals (Chartpad), and Brigham and Women's Hospital (Braunstein, 2015; Mace, 2016).

U.S. hospitals, while initially slow to adopt an EHR system, found that the HITECH could be clearly implemented. A 2011 survey conducted by the American Hospital Association found that EHR use doubled from 16% to 35% between 2009 and 2011. By 2014 the ONC reported that 76% of hospitals implemented at least a basic EHR system, and almost 97% of those implemented a certified EHR technology (Charles

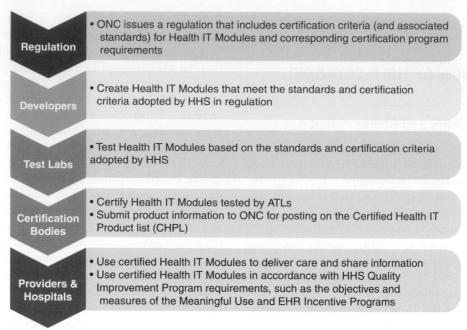

Fig. 20.1 The certification process at a glance. (Source: US DHHS Office of the National Coordinator. ONC. [2016, September 20]. About the ONC Health IT Certification Program. https://www.healthit.gov/policy-researchers-implementers/about-onc-health-it-certification-program)

et al., 2015). The American Hospital Association in a 2019 report noted that 9 of 10 hospitals used the EHR to inform their practice (https://www.aha.org/news/headline/2019-04-17-onc-nearly-all-hospitals-use-ehr-data-inform-clinical-practice).

The 21st Century CURES Act

On December 13, 2016, the 21st Century Cures Act ("Cures Act" for short) was signed into law with the goal of improving electronic access, exchange, and utilization of health information for patients and providers (ONC Cures Act). Specifically, the ONC enacted the Cures Act Final Rule to implement the interoperability and health information transparency terms of the Cures Act. The ultimate goal of the Final Rule was to facilitate patient control and engagement of their own health information. In addition to providing patients and their healthcare providers with access to health information, the Final Rule also aimed to increase incentives towards developing a health application ecosystem, such as a call to use more standardized application programming interfaces (APIs) to access structured healthcare data on smartphone applications. Furthermore, the rule required that patients have the ability to securely access their electronic health information (EHI) at no cost to them and in a timely fashion. Section 4004 of the Cures Act identified the role of information blocking and eight activities (Table 20.1) that do not qualify as information blocking according to this piece of legislation. Information blocking is a practice conducted usually by a health IT developer of certified health IT, health information network or exchange, or healthcare provider that is likely to interfere with the access, exchange, or use of EHI.

Federal rules implemented under the bipartisan Cures Act also specified eight types of clinical notes (as outlined in the United States Core Data for Interoperability) required to be available to patients free of charge. The eight note types included (1) consultation notes, (2) discharge summary notes, (3) history and physical, (4) imaging narratives, (5) lab reports, (6) pathology reports, (7) procedure notes, and (8) progress notes. Additional note type exceptions apply to protect patient confidentiality and sensitive matters (i.e. psychotherapy notes, those notes used in court proceedings).

The Cures 2.0 Act draft was released as follow-up legislation in June 2021. The Act aimed to galvanize medical product innovation, institute appropriate regulations for safety and quality, and modernize FDA and CMS processes. Additional aspects of the Act included bolstering future pandemic preparedness, supporting digital health technologies, and streamlining Medicare coverage processes (Locke et al., 2021).

TABLE 20.1 **Eight Exceptions to the Information Blocking Provision of Section 4004 of the Cures Act**	
Exceptions Involving Not Fulfilling Requests to Access, Exchange, or Use EHI	**Exceptions Involving Procedures for Fulfilling Requests to Access, Exchange, or Use EHI**
Preventing Harm	Licensing
Privacy	Fees
Security	Content and Manner
Infeasibility	
Health IT Performance	

Best Practices: Incorporating Evidence-Based Content and Clinical Decision Support Systems

With each new release, information systems become more complex and robust, enabling them to incorporate evidence-based content (called evidence-based practice [EBP]) and to use clinical decision support (CDS) features in the system. Detailed information on EBP and CDS is included in Chapters 11 and 12, respectively; however, one of the most frequently quoted definitions for EBP is one proposed by Sackett et al.—EBP is "the conscientious, explicit, and judicious use of current best evidence in making decisions about the care of individual patients. The practice of evidence-based medicine means integrating individual clinical expertise with the best available external clinical evidence from systematic research" (Sackett et al., 1996). EBP involves making decisions for clinical care based on the most current recommended treatments for specific diagnoses. These recommendations are derived from an ongoing review and analysis of high-caliber, peer-reviewed scientific studies in the literature. While entering orders from an EBP order set, the practitioner may override any of the recommended diagnostic or treatment options based on the individual needs of the patient. Some healthcare providers strongly object to a preconfigured EBP order set, referring to it as "cookbook medicine," and resist incorporating it into practice. Berner offers an analogy of CDS, including EBP similar to the nursing process of the traditional "five rights" for medication administration: "The clinical delivery system should provide the *Right* information to the *Right* person in the *Right* format through the *Right* channel at the *Right* time" (Berner, 2009).

A major challenge to EBP is remaining current due to the continuous discovery of new knowledge and the resulting changes to recommended best practices guidelines that are embedded in EHRs. Commercial products can assist organizations in updating protocols by providing current EBP clinical solutions, such as order sets and care plans. Most major EHRs have been upgraded with common CDS features that help meet some of the specific MU mandates, such as alerts for critical lab results or a history of methicillin-resistant *Staphylococcus aureus* (MRSA) on new admissions, pregnancy warnings on select medications and diagnostic tests, drug allergies, drug–drug interactions, drug–diagnosis warnings, dosage range limits, the capture of specific data such as smoking status and advance directives, and immunization reminders.

The advantages of using a system that incorporates evidence-based content and CDS include the following: Defines standardized, appropriate care and reduces variability of care for common diagnoses.

1. Defines local or facility-owned orderables (elements that can be ordered using computerized provider order entry [CPOE] available at that facility.
2. Triggers alerts and other CDS features based on locally built logic (rules). For instance, an alert may be triggered if (1) blood products are ordered on patients who request no blood products be administered, (2) pregnancy category teratogenic medications are ordered on patients of childbearing age with an unknown pregnancy status, or (3) the potassium level is below a preset level on patients receiving digitalis medications.
3. Collects detailed metrics for specific reports required to meet MU criteria. These reports address a variety of MU requirements, such as patient education, smoking status assessment, native language, discharge instructions, deep vein thrombosis prophylaxis in select patient populations, and the use of thrombolytic and antithrombotic medications in stroke patients.
4. Enables a more timely update of treatment plans based on best practices. The study Translating Research Into Practice (TRIP), conducted by researchers sponsored by the Agency for Healthcare Research and Quality (AHRQ) in 1999, concluded that it took an average of 10 to 20 years to incorporate new clinical findings into general clinical practice (Agency for Healthcare Research and Quality [AHRQ], 2001). This time lag between the discovery of new treatment options and the use of this new knowledge at the point of care is sometimes called the "lethal lag" or "fatal lag." CDS and EBP are likely to accelerate the incorporation of new findings into clinical practice.

Patient Safety and Improved Quality of Care

Before MU rules were initiated, most healthcare leadership and professionals cited patient safety as the primary reason for implementing an EHR; however, with the rapid adoption of EHRs it may appear to some healthcare professionals that the sole reason for implementing an EHR is to qualify for the incentive package. In response to this concern, leadership needs to communicate to staff that the primary deciding factors for implementing or upgrading an EHR include patient safety, improved quality of patient care, and efficiency.

EHRs help decrease medication errors, especially if closed-loop bedside barcoding medication administration is an integral piece of the system (Poon et al., 2010). Quality of care and outcomes improve when decision-support mechanisms, standardized order sets, and care plans based on best practices are incorporated in the EHR. Besides being aware of all the positive functionalities and advantages of the EHR, staff also need to be well informed on what the EHR cannot do.

Major implementations can elicit strong pushbacks from hospital staff for a variety of reasons. A primary reason is that a major implementation often involves changes in well-established workflows and processes, resulting in a temporary decrease in productivity, particularly in the early stages when clinicians are still learning the system. In addition, while the new system may offer significant advantages to the institution (e.g., a decrease in medication errors, reduced time between order entry and delivery of services, or a dramatic decrease in telephone calls from nursing and pharmacy to physicians about illegible or questionable orders), individual practitioners may focus on the disadvantages that personally affect them, such as an increase in time to enter admission orders or immediate post-op orders.

In a previously paper-based-records world, some healthcare providers created their own personal order sets for their practice and titled them using their name, such as Dr. Smith's

Routine Admission Orders for Surgery. Once records became electronic, personalized order sets were discouraged or even less likely to be made available in production. Each specialty benefits from creating a standardized order set for each of its common procedures, diagnoses, surgeries, and admissions, incorporating EBP. This approach minimizes wide variances in care and avoids an IT maintenance challenge to keep individual physicians' order sets up to date. One of the most important success factors in the implementation of an electronic health system is to involve as many users as possible in the design and planning of that system and discuss the inevitable changes to workflows, processes, policies, and procedures (Menachemi & Collum, 2011).

Using the EHR to perform a task for which it is not designed or using a poorly designed system may produce poor results or outcomes. Published studies report a variety of unintended consequences for EHRs. Ash et al. identified nine types of unintended consequences and corresponding interventions to minimize each of these risks (Ash et al., 2009). A few of the unintended consequences are associated with human error, such as selecting the wrong patient or the wrong medication from a list. They refer to this type of error as a juxtaposition error. Recommended strategies to decrease unintended consequences are very similar to the best practices for a successful implementation discussed later in this chapter (Ash et al., 2003). Weiner et al. coined a new term, e-iatrogenesis, to describe the most critical of the new type of errors seen in EHRs (Weiner et al., 2007). Other types of errors include users who fail to validate or read the list of all orders entered during a session before final acceptance or who accept the defaults for select orders without review.

The EHR may use **Tall Man lettering** (i.e., the use of mixed-case lettering) for look-alike names of medications recommended by the Institute for Safe Medication Practices (ISMP). Studies indicate that using mixed-case lettering in similar drug names helps decrease medication errors during order entry, medication dispensing, and medication administration by highlighting the differences in the drug names. A few examples of medication names using Tall Man lettering are NiFEDipine versus niCARDipine, DOBUTamine versus DOPamine, and CISplatin versus CARBOplatin (Institute for Safe Medication Practices [ISMP], 2011).

Another safety benefit associated with the implementation of an EHR is that it can enforce the use of CMS-approved abbreviations. In addition, EHRs can incorporate real-time updates or revisions to the order item master (a master list of orderable items) and electronic order sets. For example, Darvon and Darvocet were recalled in 2010 because of serious cardiac arrhythmias. Institutions with EHRs were able to quickly remove these medications from the pharmacy formulary, automatically inactivating Darvon and Darvon equivalents on all electronic order sets.

HIPAA legislation that was originally drafted in 1996 mandated unique national patient identifiers (NPIs) to ensure patient safety and promote interoperability. However, privacy advocates voiced strong opposition, and Congress passed laws preventing the development of unique NPIs. HIMSS has recently reintroduced a strong argument for an NPI and patient matching strategy using demographic attributes that are considered relatively stable and unlikely to change. Many proponents believe that we cannot achieve true interoperability until it is in place (Ritz 2013). Examples of attributes include first name, middle name, last name, maiden name, date of birth, gender, driver's license number, street address, city, state, ZIP Code, and phone number (Terry, 2015). Both proponents and opponents can cite scenarios in which data attributes may prove unstable, and the algorithms that are used do not address enough data elements. An ONC report found that patient matching accuracy oftentimes depended on whether it was matching patients internally or externally across organizations. The error rate varied widely from 10% in IT sophisticated organizations to an alarming 40% to 50% rate when matching across enterprises (Office of the National Coordinator for Health Information Technology, 2014).

Advances in EHR infrastructure have impacted the patient's experience with the healthcare system. The development of EMR-tethered patient portals for viewing lab results, messages from healthcare providers, and other notes has been associated with several reports of positive patient experiences, lower no-show rates, and self-reported decreases in healthcare system use (Graham et al., 2020). With the advent of the COVID-19 pandemic, telemedicine also came to the forefront as a necessary tool to continue providing healthcare to the masses. Systematic reviews and meta-analyses prior to the pandemic also identified that patients participating in telehealth visits described improved healthcare outcomes, increased ease of use, lower costs, and improved communication with healthcare providers (Kruse et al., 2017). E-visits have also been implemented in certain settings where patients can receive detailed diagnostic or treatment recommendations in an asynchronous messaging format with their healthcare provider team. Literature is pending on the effects of these visit types on long-term cost effectiveness and utility.

PLANNING AN EHR IMPLEMENTATION OR HEALTH INFORMATION SYSTEM UPGRADE PROJECT

Project Planning

While this section is going to be a brief overview of a structured planning process, it is our view that dedicated time by project management professionals who focus on coordinating the different phases within a project will be an invaluable resource. Although the typical training for project managers is designed to address a broad set of project types, a manager familiar with health care systems will have a combination of project management skills with the basics of software development lifecycles (SDLCs) which provides a more tailored outline for the vast number and types of health information systems and technologies that one may try to implement. This section hopes to shed light on the similarities between project management and SDLCs and to provide a framework to plan a system upgrade or new implementation.

Fundamentals of Project Management and Software Development Life Cycles

The PMBOK guide (Houston, 2017), which is a resource by the Project Management Institute for such professionals, divides the process of managing projects into five parts called process groups. The first two are the Initiating Process and the Planning Process (Houston, 2017). Briefly, the initiation process will ask important questions that weigh what the needs of the organization are; how the project will impact the organization; and risks, benefits, constraints, limitations, and contingencies at a broad level. This starting outline will require the assembly of a variety of stakeholders. During the planning process group, the outline from the initiation process is further defined with objectives and a basic course of action to complete the project. The outcome is of these process groups is a project charter that recruits organizational resources to complete the project.

Similarly, SDLCs are also grouped into overlapping phases. Table 20.2 highlights the main roles of the phases of project management and SDLC to illustrate the similarities (Gechman, 2019). While there are many ways to conceptualize and plan around software development and the software development life cycle, older conceptual approaches required more upfront knowledge, like in the traditional Waterfall Model. There have been gradual shifts towards more iterative approaches that allow for more flexibility, given that many of the facts are not yet known at the start of the development cycle. Some of the newer conceptual models include Spiral, Rapid prototype, Incremental, and Agile (Houston, 2017).

Regardless of which SDLC you are using to conceptualize the process, the major components addressed will always include system integration, testing, and verification processes. If your organization has decided to create a custom software, then the coders and developers will work closely with you to complete each phase of the SDLC.

Scope, Project Planning, and Change Control

This initiation process group is supposed to design a project charter that will ultimately create the list of objectives, the deliverables, a rough duration, a forecast of the resources necessary, and most importantly, the delegation of organizational resources for the completion of the project. Not all projects will require a charter, but it is likely that any new EHR or networked information system such as a laboratory information system (LIS) or picture archiving and communication system (PACS) will be complex enough to require formal project management and charter creation. A project charter will not only define the scope of the project but will also aid in the prevention of scope creep. Scope creep is the uncontrolled expansion to product or project scope without adjustments to time, cost, and resources (Healthcare Information and Management Systems Society, 2017). Scope creep can also be mitigated through tight change-control processes. It is in the group's best interest to mitigate scope creep because it commonly leads to burnout by team members or a project becoming delayed or over-budget.

Since the federal government introduced certification of EHRs, it has become more common for large health systems to implement a commercial-off-the-shelf (COTS) system. The

TABLE 20.2 **The Left Column Describes the Five Phases or Process Groups of Program Management, While the Right Column Describes the Stages of Software Development Also Known as the Software Development Lifecycle (SDLC)**	
Project Management	**Software Development Lifecycle**
Initiating: Comprised of all the activities leading up to formal authorization of the new project through a project charter, which has outlined the response to a problem and opportunity or a new business requirement	Planning or Exploratory: Focuses on research, analysis, and exploration which help determine the need for new software along with any existing software
Planning: The development of a project management plan after further discussions with stakeholders to gather detailed requirements and outline a course of actions.	Requirements Gathering: Determines who the intended users are and what the software must do to achieve the intended outcomes
Executing: The completion of the activities that have been formally defined in the project management plan.	Design Software: Creating specifications that outline all components of the software
Monitoring and Controlling: Typically concurrent to the executing process group. Fees activities monitor the execution of the project management plan to identify potential problems, deviations from the plan, changes in the plan, and corrective actions. Prevention of "Scope Creep"	Coding Phase: Physical programming also known as writing code
Closing: Completion of the project deliverables there have been accepted by the project sponsor. For ongoing activities, responsibility is transferred to the operations group to make use of the project's final deliverable	Testing: Occurs during various stages of development. The code is tested thoroughly, using a test plan and various testing methods. The tests well document the results of the code that satisfy the outlined requirements
	Deployment and Maintenance: How the different stages of development will occur and how the prototypes are used depending on the particular methodology. The methodology will guide the team through the development stages until the product is delivered.

21st Century Cures Act outlined changes to the testing and certification requirements of EHRs. While many organizations may use a commercial system, there are still information systems that are home-grown. For the purposes of this section, we will mostly assume that the implementation will be a single COTS system but will comment on more custom system design and implementation. If multiple systems are being implemented simultaneously or in success, it may be less common to select a single COTS system.

When starting to plan these projects, the correct stakeholders should be gathered for a variety of views and to define the boundaries of the project. This is also called creating a scope for the project. Defining what is included and excluded from the plan will aid in keeping the project from experiencing delays by trying to address too many issues. The planning process will require multiple different types of stakeholders, depending on what system is being implementing and how the organization's governance is structured. Table 20.3 is a list of potential stakeholders and some typical roles the stakeholders may play.

It is not uncommon for multiple problems to drive the need for changes or adjustments during and after the initial planning stage. Change control is a tool that should be agreed upon and implemented very early on to aid in the prevention of scope creep. Multiple stakeholders will identify different needs that are important to each one of them. Additionally, as work is done, new information not previously known during the planning will come to light. This continual problem of incomplete information during initial planning stages is one of the drivers of iterative SDLCs, such as Agile methodologies.

Milestones

In addition to defining the boundaries of the project, the charter or software master plans will also include milestones with approximate deadlines to ensure that progress is being made throughout the life of the project. Box 20.1 notes some examples of different milestones common to healthcare information system projects, but it is important to note that each project and the theoretical method used to plan it will determine the order

BOX 20.1	Example Milestones to Consider for Your Project

Request receipt and review
Governance review and approval decision
Architecture review in design
Hardware purchase
Project team training
Workflow in application design
Hardware and software installation
Application and reports configuration
Testing an issue resolution
User-acceptance testing
Development of training and support materials
Deployment

or parallel completion of these tasks. The unique requirements of each project will determine the issues and work breakdown structure (WBS)—which is a common phrase both in PM and SDLC, but it has slightly different meanings and interpretations depending on the individual background. To software developers, the WBS breaks down all the project tasks into smaller, more manageable, and controllable components and displays them in a hierarchical structure (Gechman, 2019). In project management, the various team members detail the activities or tasks needed to complete the objectives and the necessary resources and time. It is a listing of all deliverables and project work divided into manageable components with deadlines to maintain timely project deliverables.

If your organization is implementing a COTS system, much of the initial developments have already been decided and finalized into a finished product. The COTS system will fit a general need in the marketplace but will need local tailoring to your organization. The organization that identifies a new regulatory requirement or a new reason to change systems will need to evaluate if a COTS system's base functionality satisfies its needs. If so, the start of the project is focused on planning the local customization, upgrades, and tailoring to fulfill those strategic needs. Additional features may cost the organization additional licensing fees to obtain more prebuilt functionality. Once the selected features of the COTS have been decided upon, the local customization and integration starts. Most vendors will provide resources to guide and assist with planning the implementation, local customization, training, and rollout.

Analysis, Design, and Build
Analysts and Workflow Assessment

The analyst is going to be key in the development of the WBS, and their role in process design has been emphasized and outlined by the ONC. Carrying the ONC title of Practice Workflow and Information Management Redesign Specialist, they will be critical in designing the workflow that takes the most advantage of the features of the system. The successful analyst will understand the current clinical workflow, the data system, and the individual processes that need to be completed.

TABLE 20.3	List Common Stakeholders to Be Involved During the Life of the Project
Executive leadership	Defining how the project will meet the strategic mission of the organization and its goals within a particular budget
Project sponsors	The person or group authorizing the project, scope, and changes, and accepting the end deliverable
End-users	Commonly nurses, providers, and health care staff that will use the deliverable in regular operations
Vendors	Outside organizations involved in the project. Examples include the original COTS developer, a contacted company to develop a custom application, or consulting service
Project manager	The professional who oversees the planning, monitoring, controlling, closing, and timely delivery of the whole project
Project team	These people are typically the analysts who have a stake in the project's outcome and will influence the success of the final deliverable
Department managers	As a representative of the end-users or an actual end-user of the deliverable project, they will be influential in implementing the workflow changes and collecting feedback on the usability for the members of the department

Processes have several important key characteristics. Each process contains steps, inputs, and outputs, has a particular sequence or order, and is repeated multiple times for routine operation. Performing a process analysis can be part of the needs assessment prior to final selection of the new information system. Process analysis is the study of a current process to develop a report of the major observations, a list of the necessary functions, and suggestions describing how current processes can be improved. Process mapping documents the process analysis and commonly creates a visual diagram to illustrate the current process and workflow to allow for a redesign, considering the new information system. (Amatayakul, 2012). The act of process mapping can be divided into the type of task that underlies the process: physical, informational, and mental. The type of task and the process map will overlap with the current workflow for processes to be completed (Healthcare Information and Management Systems Society, 2015).

Informatics is a healthcare discipline that continues to grow while blending information science, computer science, and health care. Informaticists can be from any medical specialty or from any health care roll. There are nursing, pharmacist, physician, and PhD informaticists who may all play a role in these projects. Informaticists are typically early adopters and are very aware of the processes that analysts are trying to understand and redesign for the new system. They can serve as stakeholders outlining the needs requirements, change-management champions, and communication liaisons between analysts and end-users.

Components of System Configuration

There are multiple aspects that must be considered during this planning stage. Ideally, the architecture, security, and privacy teams are going to be involved early-on to address some design infrastructure and to ensure that there is good access, reliability, backup options, redundancies, and recovery times. Each system is unique, just like the HIT enterprise of the organization utilizing the new system. The following is a list of things that deserve some consideration for a generic system: the workstation, client technology, server, storage area network, disaster recovery, planned availability, network connectivity, interface with other components, and multiple sandbox, development, or testing environments (Houston, 2017). Tailoring describes the process of going through the unique requirements to match applicability of a broad checklist of tools and methods for the specific project. Depending on the size of the project and the role the new system will play in the day-to-day operations, the installation is relatively straightforward.

For systems that are very large and have a long list of requirements that it must meet for different end-users, such as an EHR, the maintenance of the system needs to be considered. Typically, an EHR will have development environments, testing environments, redundancies, and backups that will all need their own maintenance at regular cadence. It will take a significant amount of time and resources to maintain the operations of each environment, so forethought about aligning the skills of the analysts and IT personnel will pay off later.

Legacy Systems

The complex arrangement of health information systems and the interconnected nature of these systems make the legacy IT systems a unique challenge. Any system decommissioning or sun-setting process will also take careful planning. It is not uncommon that the integration of a new system replaces the now-inadequate functions of the old system. Understanding the usage of the old system and the workflows that depend on that system is vital to providing a potentially smooth transition. While complex, the disposition of these systems should ideally have a repeatable process in place at your organization. Typically, the team will include members representing the network, architecture, security, privacy, system and database administration, business analysts, application owners, vendors, application portfolio office, and IT leadership (Houston & Kennedy, 2020).

It may be the case that only parts are deactivated or removed as some specific pieces may be retained for a temporary time frame to allow smooth transitions from one system to another. Hopefully, any revisions or changes to the system over time will be documented to support the identification of the existing workflows in preparation for the sun-setting. The existing data with retained value needs to be identified and a plan to retain, store, or migrate the data should be developed by the architecture team, application owners, and possibly vendors depending on the individual architecture and destruction requirements. In addition to addressing the data, plans for the existing hardware should also be created.

Much of the planning around the legacy system will depend on the approach chosen for implementation or go-live.

Testing

Testing is integral to having a functional health information system, from small code updates to installation of a replacement system, to even full EHR implementations. The type of tests performed are determined by the functions that the system will do and how the system is addressing the identified business need. Regardless of the individual type of test, testing should be deployed heavily during the local customization of a COTS system or the development of a custom in-house system. Which type of system will also determine which kinds of tests will be necessary to ensure as much functionality in anticipation of the implementation step.

Table 20.4 details many different types of testing and what the role each type of test plays. Regardless of the system being implemented (custom versus COTS), some testing will be common to both scenarios. Internal testing techniques are commonly done before release to the customer including unit testing, function testing, and regression testing. A COTS developer will do this in isolation, but similar testing is done when the organization is planning for the implementation.

Prior to implementation or go-live, having a testing plan or phase ensures that the project will perform to the predetermined specifications for the project to be a success. Test plans will also commonly have phases and checks to ensure timely delivery of a functional system. As the project continues through the

TABLE 20.4   Descriptions of Different Software and Systems Testing That May Be Relevant During the Project Life

Alpha and Beta testing	Typically performed by COTS developers before formal release of a product to identify defects. Alpha testing is usually in-house testing by the developer while Beta testing is usually performed by external users
Back-to-Back testing	Type of testing strategy where multiple versions of the software are tested together, and the outputs are compared for consistency
Bottom-up testing	Testing that starts with the basic components and works towards the more complex
Configuration testing	Analyzes the software under various conditions to perform for different kinds of users
Installation testing	Verification that software is performing in a target environment
Performance testing	Verification that the developed software fulfills the specified requirements
Recovery testing	Forces the software to fail in multiple ways to assess the software's ability to recover
Regression testing	Testing after there has been modification to the software to screen for unintended consequences or effects
Security testing	Tests the built-in protection mechanisms that impede or prevent improper access
Stress test	Tests that exceed the designed loads and limits to assess for performance in overload situations
Thread test	Testing that verifies the key functional capabilities while performing a single or multiple tasks (threads)
Top-down testing	Testing that starts with the most abstract or complex components and works downwards
Unit testing	Testing of individual software components to ensure they function as designed without generating unexpected errors prior to integration weather components
Functional testing	Uses defined test scripts to verify specific requirements or groups of requirements are satisfied
System integration testing	Testing the system in the environment where it will run along with other software yet leads to user-acceptance testing. Individual software modules aren't combined and then tested and verified as a group
User acceptance testing	The final stage of testing performed and typically involves using the software product prior to software rollout.

timeline, it is important to perform integration testing throughout system development to ensure that necessary interfaces between software systems are functioning appropriately. This can apply to both unit integration and system integration.

One of the major components to the testing plan before go-live is **user acceptance testing** (UAT). This is the final stage of testing prior to go-live where the software manufacturer slash vendor and health care organization can further debug the software to ensure final functionality of the system. It is the closest testing to the end-user to identify any remaining problems. UAT is not one particular test, but it is considered the last step of tests

before the general roll-out. Three important features in UAT are the strategy, scenarios, and scripts (Healthcare Information and Management Systems Society, 2015). The strategy is the details of who will be involved, what equipment or software is needed, which procedures will be followed, and what support is necessary for a successful test. The scenarios should be a representative number of events to simulate the requirements of the software. The test scripts are the step-by-step instructions that will be used for each test and the associated expected results.

IMPLEMENTATION/GO-LIVE

Informatics Training Plan

Education of all end-users is a mini project and is best assigned to an education department to coordinate and oversee all components. A training plan must address the development of teaching plans, training manuals, and any training materials, like tip sheets, to provide instructions on common tasks to be used during training and on the job. Training falls into three major categories:

- **Superuser** training—Staff from the organization who take additional training and not only learn the EHR but understand the new workflows.
- Role-based training—Training focused on the roles of the user, such as a physician, nurse, therapist, unit clerk, or medical assistant.
- Process-based training—Workflow or a process, like an admission to a hospital (HealthIT.gov, 2019).

Training should be a requirement for any staff using the system, and policy and procedures should be developed for dealing with those who do not complete and/or pass the training. Considerations in planning training and education should include time for training, methodology of training, content, training rooms, and hardware needs (Table 20.5).

Trainers and the Role of Superusers/Informaticists

Depending on the organization's structure, the trainers might be in-house staff, vendor educators, temporary consultants, superusers, or a mix of these. In-house trainers are very familiar with the organization's policies and procedures and usually have experience and background in adult education. Sometimes organizations may need to bring in temporary trainers to get all users trained and then revert to in-house educators or superusers following go-live for new hires, system upgrades, and remediation training. Vendor educators and consultants frequently know the application very well but are not familiar with the organization's workflows and policies. Organizations may choose to leverage informatics professionals, such as nursing or provider informaticists, and use these informaticists as superusers. Superusers take additional training in addition to project team responsibilities and are typically present at go-live and can be assigned as "at-the-elbow" support with staff who are having difficulties during the first few days of implementation. They have been trained in advance on the basics as well as complex workflows introduced by the system. They can be valuable assets not just in training classes but also during the go-live

TABLE 20.5 Considerations for a Successful Training Plan

Hours of training	Enough time for users to become proficient in the system • Dependent on user role • Number of staff to be educated • Length of instruction may vary by user role • Schedule protected time away from regular responsibilities and shifts.
Methodology	May use a combination of methods • Classroom training, also known as instructor-led training • Web-based training, interactive video lessons • Competency testing of key learning objectives
Content	• Address common and standard workflows, including who is responsible for specific quality initiative documentation (i.e., smoking status, travel history, fall risk, etc.) • Highlight policy and standards for practice for each role as well as privacy and security policies and consequences for violation of said policies • Complex and important workflows should have dedicated training content (i.e., Blood administration)
Physical space and hardware	• Training rooms with enough computers and peripherals, like barcode scanners, printers, and even mobile devices for specific workflows • Training environment to simulate real-life scenarios and ideally a post-class environment to practice newly learned concepts should be made available

and beyond. Typically, the role of the superusers does not end at go-live but will continue with future projects, and they may also be used as new staff is hired and needs training. Training is an ongoing process which will continue post the go-live phase for any EHR project.

End-User Training

Most organizations use a combination of training methods. Using a variety of methods allows your training team to reach a broader audience for many purposes all at once. A drawback to using a variety of approaches is the constant need to update all the training materials with the introduction of new functionalities or upgrades. No matter the approach, the use of competency tests to assess proficiency is recommended. Education should be conducted as close to the go-live date as possible to facilitate retention of the new knowledge and skills, with a goal of no more than 4 to 6 weeks pre-go-live. Additionally, after class a practice environment should be made available where users can perform competency exercises; this ensures they are able to practice what they've learned. A learning management system (LMS) can be used to track how much training has occurred and by whom prior to go-live.

Training Modalities
Online Education Materials

Online materials or video-based learning are used by some institutions to teach EHR basics before attending an instructor-led class, or they can be used for more complicated or niche workflows after an instructor-led class which might be too generic or broad for a specialized group. For example, a phlebotomist would learn the basics of how to collect a specimen and complete a lab order (something a nurse, phlebotomist, and a respiratory therapist would also need to learn—role-based learning). But a more niche subject like how to process the lab specimen within the lab system would be a good candidate for an online module only available to those who perform this task. Or vice versa, the more generic workflow could be a great online module made available to a broad group of people, and in-person learning would be more specific. Online education materials like "FYI," "How Tos," and "Tip Sheets" may also be used as mini-refreshers or primers for later upgrades.

In-Person Training

One of the most popular methods is an instructor-led class in a classroom that contains all the equipment needed to demonstrate essential functionalities, including printers, barcode scanners, identification bands, medication labels, etc. The advantages of instructor-led training include the ability for end-users to ask questions, quick clarification of complex concepts, and easy identification of users who may need additional help. The primary disadvantages are the expense and resources needed to have multiple instructor-led classes. In addition, the number of students per session is limited. If users must attend class during their off-duty time, organizations will have to consider paying overtime. Alternately, if user education is incorporated into the 40-hour workweek, replacement staff may be required.

Preparing for Go-Live

Preparing for go-live involves deciding on the go-live approach, developing the go-live plan and support schedule, and preparing the end-users.

Deciding on the Go-Live Approach

There are two approaches to a go-live: big bang or incremental (also called a phased or a staged approach). The **big bang** approach occurs when all applications or modules are implemented at once. The advantages of the big bang approach are that it is usually less expensive and implementation time is shorter, allowing staff to return to a new normal and see early improvements in the project metrics more quickly. The negatives associated with the big bang approach are the significant reductions in productivity seen immediately at go-live and for a short time afterwards due to users' unfamiliarity with the new system and a large influx of requests to tweak the system (Box 20.2). With a **phased go-live** approach, both the old and new processes exist at the same time within the healthcare institution; the existence of both forces the clinician to use different workflows in patient units that have implemented the new system than in units that have not, potentially creating safety concerns. The incremental approach is usually selected when a facility has limited resources that cannot support a house-wide implementation or when the facility has a low tolerance for or ability to respond to institutional changes. Advantages of the incremental approach are that it allows time to make changes to

BOX 20.2   Advantages and Disadvantages of the Big Bang Approach

Advantages	Disadvantages
• Eliminates staff having to use two systems or processes in different departments, which decreases number of errors • Total cost of entire implementation is lower • Project is less likely to stall and is more likely to fully implement the new system • Shorter implementation cycle and shorter implementation pain • Quicker improvements in EHR-related metrics • On-site and remote consultants and vendor support are available for the duration of the go-live	• Significant decrease in productivity in the initial days and immediately after go-live, with gradual return to baseline • Less time to make changes to the build or workflows • Changes in workflows and processes are turned on house-wide with everyone on same learning curve, making implementation pain and anxiety greater • Must plan for large number of support personnel and roaming superusers to all departments.

BOX 20.3   Advantages and Disadvantages of the Incremental Approach

Advantages	Disadvantages
• Allows time to make changes to build and workflows with each new batch of users • Early reports of success breed enthusiasm and support to the upcoming departments • Less impact on productivity • Restricts implementation pain to a smaller number of select users or departments	• Staff who work in multiple departments in the organization must use two workflows, which can increase the number of errors • Project may stall due to users' dislike of using different processes or workflows in different departments • Total cost of entire implementation is higher due to extended support and training • Longer implementation time may leave staff with the feeling the system is not ready for prime time • Most vendors transition customers to their support division within 2 to 4 weeks post go-live and may not be available for further go-live phases • Early report of dissatisfaction may dissuade others from embracing the new system

the build or the workflows and does not decrease productivity house-wide while creating constant change for end-users. The disadvantages include the potential for errors due to multiple systems and the possibility that the project can be protracted and workflow disruptions will occur over a longer period, although on a smaller scale (Box 20.3).

Go-Live Plan

A detailed go-live plan includes each planned activity as a line item assigned to a specific individual or team with a completion date and time for each task. The go-live plan should include critical tasks that are scheduled to be completed a few days to a few weeks before the go-live date. Some project managers may break down the immediate days before go-live to the number of hours before go-live, marking tasks that must precede other tasks. Some of these may include cross-checking the patient census between the new and old systems, build migration, and data abstracting. Often the timing of tasks discovered during the practice migration events are accounted for in this plan. Avoid a go-live date that falls on a weekend, a Monday or Friday, or close to a major holiday when vendor support personnel may be less available. Two exceptions to this guideline are the implementation of a new financial system, which must start at midnight on the first day of the month for billing purposes, and a big bang implementation, which is typically scheduled to start on a weekend to minimally affect surgery and procedural services. When a go-live date is determined, it should be communicated to the organization and end-users

as soon as possible, especially within the last 2 to 3 months of the project.

Practicing Build Migration

In large-scale projects much of the development and testing is done in a test environment by many teams and people. Prior to the go-live it is wise to have a build migration practice event. These events give all persons from the project team a chance to move and migrate the build into a production-like environment. The purpose is to ensure all build is migrated appropriately, expose issues the teams may run into the night of go-live, and provide the project leadership timing of how long this portion of the go-live event will take. Often this means interfaces will need to be shut down and paper processes will need to be activated during the time it takes to migrate the new content or turn on the new system. For example, in a large-scale project like replacing a lab system, an admission order set (grouping of commonly placed orders on admission) would not be able to be migrated until all single lab orders are migrated first and exist in the target environment. For smaller projects like code upgrades or updates to an already existing system, the practicing of build migration may be scaled down; there could be content that can be moved into the live system "silently." This means the content can be made available by "activating" a newer version active during the go-live; this may be an automated process, or it may require manual updates. This should also be practiced prior to the go-live date to ensure no hiccups occur during the "activation" of the silent build.

Data Abstraction

Data abstraction is "the process of entering or 'populating' the electronic chart with clinical data from the traditional paper record or other sources" (Kushinka, 2017). Abstraction provides practice for end-users in entering critical data needed for a smooth transition, such as scheduling known surgical cases or future appointments for patients to be seen in clinic during the first days or weeks of the go-live date. Lab results and prescribed medications may be added into the new EHR, including any standing and future orders for patients in the new EHR. For inpatient locations like hospital units, data abstracting may need to be done in the hours before the go-live. Many EHRs require height, weight, and allergies to be entered on a patient before placing orders via CPOE. Having these data points for currently admitted patients in the new system will expedite the ordering process for providers when managing orders in the hours after go-live.

Change Freeze/Moratoriums

"Also known as 'Change Freezes,' moratoriums are often used to protect the core business from breaking changes during low staff resourcing times (public holidays etc.), major data migrations, facilities upgrades/maintenance and other disruptive situations (like office relocations, external infrastructure changes etc.)" ("Change moratorium" vs. organisational needs, 2018). Moratoriums ensure no unexpected consequences occur while making large changes for end-users. Working within the institutions' change management practices is critical. Placing the moratorium a week or two prior to data migration through the go-live date and even for a week or so after go-live ensures no other factors negatively affect the implementation and the go-live success. It's imperative that project managers engage with change management entities of the institution, as there may need to be negotiations between project managers and change management groups to justify any and all changes during go-live.

Marketing and Communication

Ensure people know the date and time of when the switch will happen and what to expect. Change moratoriums should also be communicated and expectations managed for all institutional projects. If users won't have access to electronic charting for 4 to 6 hours on the go-live date, it's important for all affected users to know and understand how they will manage and care for their patients during this time. Plans for how to continue with business as usual are imperative. Will they be charting on paper during that time? What will they be expected to chart in the new system once the system is up? A highly publicized helpdesk number or web conference (Zoom, Teams) for assistance should also be included in the communication for users to know whom to call if help is needed. Use of posters or banners in main lobbies, atriums, and waiting rooms as well as electronic messaging on the institutions' intranet and email distribution lists are common ways to advertise the go-live date.

Go-Live

This is the phase of the project when the system is made live and the older system is retired. This can extend to process or workflow; an old process is retired in favor of the newly developed process or workflow.

Command Center

Traditionally this is the physical space—a central location with adequate desk space, phones, computer screens, printers, wi-fi, and network access for the project team to be able to work during the go-live and the days or weeks after. Superusers, trainers, at-the-elbow (ATE) support, project teams, subject matter experts, analysts, vendor-supplied staff, contracted staff, and sometimes even stakeholders make up the personnel in the command center during the go-live activities. This is the project hub; it is typically staffed 24/7 for the first week or two after go-live. The purpose is to provide users and staff a central place to access project team members and knowledge experts as they get accustomed to the new system and workflows. The job of the command center staff is to gather, troubleshoot, and fix issues as they arise. Typically, during the go-live, many requests will be documented, and the project team will take the list and review with the organizational leaders each day to determine if a change will be required immediately or if the change can wait after the go-live phase. The command center may host daily or twice-daily meetings to review issues, fixes, and workarounds and provide quick tips/training if needed to all users and staff. A 100% virtual command center is possible. With the pressures of the 2020 worldwide pandemic, it became evident some institutions would need to proceed with implementation of projects without the ability to meet and support their staff in person in the traditional way. Innovation and technology made this possible. Valley Children's Hospital continued with their go-live activities via virtual support rooms, webinars, and one-on-one virtual sessions (Leventhal, 2020). The company ReMedi Health Solutions devised a successful virtual command center model for supporting clients and providing ATE support to staff via tablets, webcams, calls through Microsoft Teams, and remote screen access (Remedi Health Solutions, 2020). A hybrid approach would entail staffing a command center in person at a specific central location with minimal key staff (project manager, key stakeholders, superusers, and ATE support) who have a direct line to staff working remotely. The staff who is remote would need to be able to gain full access to the command center and end-users to timely work through any issues; this can easily be done via video conferencing tools like Teams and Zoom. Good candidates of roles to work remotely are IT analysts and vendor support who easily have access to remote tools.

At-the-Elbow (ATE) support

During the initial weeks of the go-live, organizations must plan to provide close support ("elbow-to-elbow" support) for end-users. Many institutions will provide 24/7 support for a week or two. Issues, questions, and misunderstandings should be reported to the project team, which then catalogs, prioritizes, and tracks them for resolution and future reference. This is a group of superusers, trainers, or even consultants who are familiar with the organization's workflows and software. They are key for an EHR implementation's success. They can resolve questions and frustrating issues quickly, which in turn allows your clinical staff to return to their other duties. They are typically roaming in clinical areas, or they can be available to staff via phone call to guide them through the more intricate workflows or the items forgotten since training. This group should be engaged early; they should be trained on the new system, and they should be supported during the go-live. They should have a direct line of communication with the command center or project team in case they do need to clarify a workflow or system issue (Jaimes, 2017).

Issue Tracking

A system for reporting, cataloging, assigning critical issues, and assigning skilled resources to identify issues and problems is critical to the success of the go-live phase. It is important to have a way to track what issues users are reporting. Most institutions have a helpdesk system for tracking the reporting of problems and issue resolution. Leverage the use of the tools already in place. You should be able to at minimum review the issue and what the resolution was (fix to system or training). It is important to report known issues and unresolved problems to project team leadership, stakeholders, and superusers. Immediate changes may be necessary if fixes are required; a mechanism for approving and updating build is needed. In addition, sending staff updated information via tip sheets of these fixes and changes is imperative. Emails with tip sheets should be distributed in a timely manner and discussed in debriefing meetings. If the resolution is deemed to be an enhancement, care needs to be taken to determine if the problem is due to an intentional change made by the new system or if the system is lacking in functionality. These "unresolved" issues should be reported, prioritized, and included in the future maintenance phase of the project.

POST-GO-LIVE AND SYSTEM MAINTENANCE

Post-Go-Live Maintenance

Maintenance is an ongoing process that involves a variety of tasks such as code updates, patches for identified defects, and a continuous revision of the system in response to users' requests, as well as new regulatory requirements and initiatives. The maintenance phase is an iterative process and will be ongoing. As a retrospective study reviewing changes made over a 6-year period of the Kaiser Permanente Institution points out, significant resources, expertise, and interdisciplinary collaboration are key. Over this time frame the number of changes tracked was significant and affected many users within the organization (Liu, 2019).

Change Control and Enhancements

Governance established during the build phase of the project should continue to oversee changes and be involved in changes to the system post-go-live. Users' requests captured

during the go-live and the days post-go-live plus any items cut from scope should be considered as part of future enhancements. Engage users and their ideas for system improvement. Informatics staff often round and engage with end-users to learn what needs improvement in the system. Continue to leverage end-users' experience to improve the EHR usability. Review the success criteria set out during the planning phase; review reports and data after the stabilization phase of the project to measure success. Define opportunities for improvement and include these in future projects or in future system enhancements.

FUTURE DIRECTIONS

Impact of COVID-19

The role of the CIO expanded greatly during the COVID-19 pandemic to include a rapid pivot to remote work, increased virtual care, and public health data management. A recent review of "10 Emerging Trends in Health IT for 2020" in *Becker's Hospital Review* suggests that the CIO's role will also include more operational and strategy components as the modern digital workforce continues to grow. IT teams serving with CIOs also have changed significantly in recent years to include more diverse members, including clinicians, data scientists, and cybersecurity professionals.

Integration Challenges
Voice Assistants

Health care systems had to react to the global pandemic of 2020, and many did by expanding telehealth functionality and integrating it with EHRs. The use of voice assistants (Google Assistant, Apple, Siri, and Amazon Alexa) tools could help improve healthcare by allowing users to dictate notes, manage and place orders, and assist providers in navigating the EHR hands-free (Sezgin et al., 2020). EHRs of the future will need to be able to meet the demand of ever-changing popular technologies like voice assistants to provide efficiencies to end-users while keeping patients' data safe and secure.

Standardized Application Programming Interfaces and Cybersecurity

The 2015 Edition Cures Update also introduced new technical certification criteria necessary for implementation of the 21st Century Cures Act. The goal is to advance interoperability between certified health IT systems and promote easy access to personal EHI. The technical criteria focus on the ability to export EHI to support patient access and requires the use of HL7 FHIR Release 4 Standard. In addition to these changes that promote a patient's access to their EHI, there were two cybersecurity criterion as well. These cybersecurity criteria focused on encryption and multi-factor authentication.

Conclusion and Future Directions

As of this writing, the number of Ransomware attacks targeting health systems has been increasing due to the recognized value of information stored in the EHRs. Health information systems will need upfront planning around keeping health information both secure from malicious actors but also broadly available to health care providers and patients to make the most informed decisions possible.

ACKNOWLEDGMENT

The authors wish to acknowledge the contribution of Christine D. Meyer to the previous edition of this chapter.

DISCUSSION QUESTIONS

1. Discuss the reasons why some institutions experience significantly more satisfaction or dissatisfaction during an implementation than do others.
2. What are some of the approaches that can be used to coordinate care during an incremental go-live as patients are transferred from units that have gone live to units still waiting to go live?
3. When developing new workflow processes using a systems approach, the work of patient care or specific tasks often shift from one department to another. While the new workflows can make the care provided to patients more efficient and effective for the institution as a whole, certain departments may experience more rather than less work. What are some approaches that can help users accept the new workflow?
4. Should insurers offer incentives to patients to select healthcare providers who are using EHRs to engage patients in managing their own care?
5. What are the advantages and disadvantages of a Healthcare Information Technology Standards Panel (HITSP)-certified health IT system versus a homegrown IT system that meets certification standards?
6. Should employees who have repeatedly failed to attend go-live classes be subjected to disciplinary measures?
7. Identify creative strategies to encourage physicians and other clinicians to participate in the implementation of a new health IT system.
8. Discuss ramifications and causes regarding interoperability issues among electronic health systems and applications.
9. Discuss the advantages and disadvantages of "information un-blocking" of clinical notes from both the patient and provider perspective. What would be important training considerations for physicians since the Cures Act Final Rule implementation?

CASE STUDY

You are a clinical informaticist and have been asked to work with your hospital to implement the clinical notes transparency element of the ONC Cures Act Final Rule. All clinical notes (as qualified under USCDI) written by attending providers for inpatients will be shared with the patient at discharge. This feature will be implemented in 2 months, and your team will be collaborating with the IT staff for patient portal modifications, HIM group, nursing informatics, risk management, provider leadership, and project managers to make this EHI available to patients.

Discussion Questions

1. How will you prepare adult, adolescent, and pediatric patients to understand and access the information newly available through their patient portal?
2. Develop a training plan for staff/providers taking into account the anticipated low acceptance rate of the new regulatory requirements.
3. How are you going to modify the patient-facing components of the EHR portal to ensure that patients maintain access to their information but are able to maintain a relationship with the providers?

REFERENCES

Agency for Healthcare Research and Quality (AHRQ). (2001). Translating Research into Practice (TRIP)-II: Fact Sheet. http://www.ahrq.gov/research/trip2fac.htm.

Amatayakul, M. K. (2012). *Process improvement with electronic health records: a stepwise approach to workflow and process management.* Productivity Press.

Ash, J. A., Sittig, D. F., Dykstra, R., Campbell, E., & Guappone, K. (2009). The unintended consequences of computerized provider order entry: findings from a mixed methods exploration. *International Journal of Medical Informatics, 78,* S69–S76. https://doi.org/10.1016/j.ijminf2008.07.15.

Ash, J. A., Stavri, Z., & Kuperman, G. J. (2003). A consensus statement on considerations for a successful CPOE implementation. *Journal of the American Medical Informatics Association, 10,* 229–234. https://doi.org/10.1197/jamia.M1204.

Berner, E.S. Clinical Decision Support Systems: State of the Art.; Agency for Healthcare Research and Quality; 2009.2009. http://healthit.ahrq.gov/images/jun09cdsreview/090069ef.html.

Braunstein, M. (2015). How a Healthcare Clinic Plans to Become a Software Company. InformationWeek. http://www.informationweek.com/software/enterprise-applications/how-a-healthcare-clinic-plans-to-become-a-software-company/a/d-id/1320339?.

Centers for Medicare & Medicare Services (CMS). (2015). CMS fact sheet: EHR incentive programs in 2015 and beyond. https://www.cms.gov/Newsroom/MediaReleaseDatabase/Fact-sheets/2015-Fact-sheets-items/2015-10-06-2.html.

"Change moratorium" vs. organisational needs. (2018, December 21). Thesumof.it. https://thesumof.it/blog/2018-12-21-change-moratorium-vs-organisational-needs

Charles, D., Gabriel, M., & Searcy, T. (2015, April). Adoption of Electronic Health Record Systems among U.S. Nonfederal Acute

Care Hospitals: 2008–2014. ONC Data Brief No. 23. https://www.healthit.gov/sites/default/files/data-brief/2014HospitalAdoptionDataBrief.pdf.

Duke, J. D., Morea, J., Mamlin, B., et al. (2014). Regenstrief Institute's Medical Gopher: A next-generation homegrown electronic medical record system. *International Journal of Medical Informatics*, 83(3), 170–179.

Gechman, M. (2019). *Project management of large software-intensive systems: controlling the software development process*. Boca Raton: CRC Press.

Graham, T. A. D., Ali, S., Avdagovska, M., & Ballermann, M. (2020, May 19). Effects of a web-based patient portal on patient satisfaction and missed appointment rates: Survey study. *Journal of Medical Internet Research*, 22(5), e17955. https://doi.org/10.2196/17955.

Healthcare Information And Management Systems Society. (2015). Preparing for success in healthcare information and management systems: the CAHIMS review guide. HIMSS.

Healthcare Information And Management Systems Society. (2017). *CPHIMS review guide: preparing for success in healthcare information and management systems*. Taylor & Francis: CRC Press.

Healthcare Information Technology Standards Panel (HITSP). (n.d.). HITSP Quality Measures Technical Note ED, VTE, and Stroke Examples for Implementation of the HITSP Quality Interoperability Specification: HITSP/TN906.

HealthIT.gov. (2019). *How should I train my staff?* https://www.healthit.gov/faq/how-should-i-train-my-staff

Houston, S. M. (2017). *The project manager's guide to health information technology implementation* (2nd Edition). Productivity Press.

Houston, S. M., & Kennedy, R. D. (2020). *Effective lifecycle management of healthcare applications: Achieving best practices by using a portfolio framework*. Productivity Press.

Institute for Safe Medication Practices (ISMP). (2011). FDA and ISMP lists of look-alike drug names with recommended tall man letters. http://www.ismp.org/tools/tallmanletters.pdf.

Jaimes, J. (2017, August 16). *Assembling the right stuff: The keys to gathering and supporting a successful EHR go-live support team*. Healthcare IT Today. https://www.healthcareittoday.com/2017/08/16/assembling-the-right-stuff-the-keys-to-gathering-and-supporting-a-successful-ehr-go-live-support-team/

Kruse, C. S., Krowski, N., Rodriguez, B., Tran, L., Vela, J., & Brooks, M. (2017, August 3). Telehealth and patient satisfaction: a systematic review and narrative analysis. *BMJ Open*, 7(8), e016242. https://doi.org/10.1136/bmjopen-2017-016242.

Leventhal, R. (2020, May 26). *StackPath*. www.hcinnovationgroup.com. https://www.hcinnovationgroup.com/clinical-it/electronic-health-record-electronic-medical-record-ehr-emr/news/21139682/valley-childrens-healthcare-completes-epic-golive-100-virtually

Locke, T., Ray, R., Hendricks-Sturrup, R., Lopez, M.H., Romine, M., McClellan, M. (2021). *Building a modern health data infrastructure: Cures 2.0 Act provisions on real-world evidence and federal agency communication*, https://healthpolicy.duke.edu/sites/default/files/2021-10/Cures%202.0%20Shared%20Evidence%20Data%20Infrastructure_0.pdf.

Mace, S. (2016). Tech Tactics for the Long-Term. HealthLeaders Media. http://www.healthleadersmedia.com/technology/tech-tactics-long-term?page=0%2C1.

Menachemi, N., & Collum, T. (2011). Benefits and drawbacks of electronic health record systems. Risk Manag Healthc Pol, 4, 47–55. https://doi.org/10.2147/RMHP.S12985.

Office of the National Coordinator for Health Information Technology. (2014). Patient identification and matching final report. https://www.healthit.gov/sites/default/files/patient_identification_matching_final_report.pdf.

ONC Cures Act: https://www.healthit.gov/curesrule/.

One Hundred Eleventh Congress of the United States of America. (2009). The American Recovery and Reinvestment Act of 2009, Title XIII. Heath Information Technology. http://www.gpo.gov/fdsys/pkg/BILLS-111hr1enr/pdf/BILLS-111hr1enr.pdf.

Poon, E. G., Keohane, C. A., Yoon, C. S., et al. (2010, May 6). Effect of bar-code technology on the safety of medication administration. *New England Journal of Medicine*, 362(18), 1698–1707. https://doi.org/10.1056/NEJMsa0907115. PMID: 20445181.

Ritz, D. (2013). Opinion: It's time for a national patient identifier. http://www.himss.org/News/NewsDetail.aspx?ItemNumber=21464.

S.A. Kushinka, M.B.A., Full Circle Projects, Inc. (2017). *California Health Care Foundation*. Retrieved from www.chcf.org: https://www.chcf.org/wp-content/uploads/2017/12/PDF-ChartAbstractionEHRDeploymentTechniques.pdf

Sackett, D. L., Rosenberg, W. M., Gray, J. A., Haynes, R. B., & Richardson, W. S. (1996). Evidence based medicine: What it is and what it isn't. *British Medical Journal*, 312(7023), 71–72.

Sezgin, E., Huang, Y., Ramtekkar, U., & Lin, S. (2020). Readiness for voice assistants to support healthcare delivery during a health crisis and pandemic. *npj Digital Medicine*, 3(1), 1–4. https://doi.org/10.1038/s41746-020-00332-0.

Terry, K. (2014). CCHIT exits EHR certification business. Information Week. http://www.informationweek.com/healthcare/policy-and-regulation/cchit-exits-ehr-certification-business/d/d-id/ 1113632.

Terry, K. (2015). National patient identifier struggles for life; CIO. http://www.cio.com/article/2972266/healthcare/national-patient-identifier-struggles-for-life.html.

US DHHS Office of the National Coordinator ONC. (2015, November 3). about the ONC health it certification program. https://www.healthit.gov/policy-researchers-implementers/about-onc-health-it-certification-program.

Vincent, X., & Liu, M. M. (2019, January 17). Inpatient electronic health record maintenance from 2010 to 2015. *The American Journal of Managed Care*, 18-21. https://www.ajmc.com/view/inpatient-electronic-health-record-maintenance-from-2010-to-2015

Weiner, J. P., Kfuri, T., Chan, K., & Fowles, J. B. (2007). e-Iatrogenesis: The most critical unintended consequence of CPOE and other HIT. *Journal of the American Medical Informatics Association*, 14, 387–388. https://doi.org/10.1197/jamia.M2338.

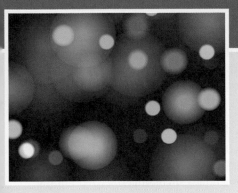

21

Downtime and Disaster Recovery for Health Information Systems

Nancy C. Brazelton and Ann M. Lyons

> *The primary objectives for downtime and disaster planning are to protect the organization and the patients served by minimizing operational disruptions.*

OBJECTIVES

At the completion of this chapter, the reader will be prepared to:
1. Discuss key factors to completing a downtime risk assessment.
2. Choose appropriate system downtime response plans.
3. Determine appropriate IT downtime response plans.
4. Summarize appropriate clinical and business downtime response plans.
5. Discuss the role of communication plans during an IT downtime.

KEY TERMS

business continuity, 331
clinical application, 324
cold site, 329
configuration management database (CMDB), 324
data center, 323
disaster recovery, 331
downtime, 322

electronic data interchange (EDI), 324
electronic health record (EHR), 323
enterprise resource planning (ERP), 324
high availability, 336
hot site, 329
human-made disaster, 323
incident response team (IRT), 331

Information Technology Infrastructure Library (ITIL), 324
Internet of Things (IoT), 323
natural disaster, 323
ransomware, 322
revenue cycle, 332
service level agreement (SLA), 329

ABSTRACT ❖

Healthcare entities are complex operations increasingly dependent on technology. This chapter identifies tactics related to planning for and responding to computer downtime events and disasters where systems are unavailable to users. Focus areas include the clinical impact, the information technology (IT) impact, business continuity, and communications. A model for assessing the level of downtime response is provided.

INTRODUCTION

Healthcare entities, no matter how small or large, are extremely complex businesses and are increasingly dependent on technology in their quest to provide exceptional healthcare. The employees of these healthcare organizations move through a unique labyrinth of systems, machines, workflows, regulatory requirements, business rules, and tools to provide the best care for patients and their families and to keep the business intact.

Healthcare organizations select from a variety of vendors, adopt information systems at different rates, and implement systems in the order that works best for them.

Given the importance of information systems within any healthcare entity, institutions and their employees must be prepared for the many variations of downtime, including those caused by human errors, software and hardware failures, severed power cables, intentionally placed malware with the intent to collect ransomware, and disruptions caused by Mother Nature (Acronis, n.d.). Even in 2021, much of the literature around the topic of downtime continues to be discussed in white papers, blogs, and industry group publications found via internet searches, a surprising trend given the number of academic institutions that rely on EHRs (Monica, 2018; Gecomo, Klopp, & Rouse 2020). When an article is presented in a peer-reviewed journal, the impetus to publish is usually spurred by a downtime event experienced by the authors, who want to encourage readers to create downtime plans (Polaneczky, 2007; Getz, 2009; Capital One, 2011).

The cost of downtimes in healthcare is staggering. A 2016 Ponemon Institute study found an average cost of $740,357 per incident (Ponemon Institute, 2016). Depending on the complexity and length of the downtime, this translates to roughly $8800/min. Because of the dramatic rise in incidents and media attention, ransomware attacks and their costs are being reported with much greater frequency both by the federal government and industry blogs and white papers (Coveware, 2021; Federal Trade Commission, n.d.; Bischoff, 2021). A Comparitech.com blog reported, "In 2020, 92 individual ransomware attacks affected over 600 separate clinics, hospitals, and organizations and more than 18 million patient records. We estimate the cost of these attacks to be almost $21 billion" (Bischoff, 2021). It is critical to understand the impact and cost of downtimes to your organization and you might even choose to calculate the true cost for your specific circumstance (Data Foundry, n.d.).

This chapter focuses on practical, tactical ways to put plans in place for managing health system downtime and disaster recovery. Tips and tools for downtime risk assessments, downtime and disaster response planning, clinical and information technology (IT) system recovery, and business continuity are provided. The chapter also provides information on developing a communication strategy and ideas for keeping patients safe and the business functioning, because downtime does happen.

ASSESSING RISK FOR DOWNTIMES

Planning for downtime can and should occur from project inception through system support and maintenance and must include all existing systems and infrastructure. The complexity and criticality of the organization will determine how extensive an exercise this must be. Potential types of downtime and their impacts on the systems should be anticipated, and mitigation plans must be put in place.

Downtimes can be classified by the root cause and the degree of impact. A general network-related incident or outage is different from a power outage or a planned software upgrade. A single noncritical software application may be unavailable, which will have a much lower impact than a total outage of the admission, discharge, and transfer (ADT) system. It is also important to consider the users or processes that are impacted.

Failure Points

Determining the root cause of a downtime is not always straightforward (Kill, 2018). The first step is to determine what is functioning and what is not. However, this first determination may not be the final answer. For example, a network downtime

may be diagnosed easily by asking the following questions: Can you access the internet *and* the intranet? How about the computer next to you? What about the computer on the unit downstairs? If the answer to these questions is "no," consider an entire network downtime. However, networks in many healthcare enterprises are now segmented for security purposes and include a series of switches, firewalls with coded rules, as well as the actual fiber network, cable pulls, and other components. This makes diagnosis of the specific network problem or the location of the problem more complex, potentially increasing the length of the network downtime. External factors may also exist, including telecommunication fiber vendors that may be having problems, as well as the millions of miles of fiber infrastructures vulnerable to physical damage, commonly referred to as a "backhoe outage."

Thus the first step in preventing or managing a downtime is to determine what might cause a downtime and then to perform a risk assessment of the impact for each potential downtime. This step can and should be iterative and involves compiling an inventory of existing applications and systems. Classifying all potential downtimes and putting them into mutually exclusive categories can be difficult. It is usually best to start by identifying the most common technology source of downtimes and documenting them. A systematic approach starting with infrastructure is more likely to ensure a comprehensive list. Begin by dividing the infrastructure into IT infrastructure and physical infrastructure.

IT infrastructure includes network and application delivery systems, such as those listed in Box 21.1. Examples of physical structures include those listed in Box 21.2. Some overlap exists

---

BOX 21.1 Sample Elements of Information Technology Infrastructure

- EHR software
- Clinical and ancillary system software (e.g., physiologic monitoring, endoscopy, registry databases)
- Picture archiving and communication system (PACS)
- Laboratory applications
- Cardiology applications
- Radiology applications
- Anesthesia and surgical services systems
- Surgical processing systems
- Revenue cycle software
- Interfaces or the interface engine
- Enterprise data warehouse
- General Ledger, Payroll, and Accounting systems

BOX 21.2 Examples of Information Technology Physical Structure

- Hardware related to the chillers that keep the data center cool
- Servers
- Storage (physical hardware that stores the EHR, e-mail, and other third-party systems)
- Electrical power
- Network switches and hubs, firewalls, and wireless access points
- Biomedical devices
- End user workstations and printers, bar code scanners
- Any component of the buildings themselves

BOX 21.3 Information Technology and Physical Infrastructure

Information Technology Infrastructure	Physical Infrastructure
• Application delivery system (e.g., Citrix)	• Batteries
• Asset management	• Biomedical devices
• Biomedical devices with software components and network requirements	• Buildings and facilities (list most likely maintained by an environment of care committee per requirements of accreditation and regulatory agencies)
• Bots	• Cabling
• Databases, E-mail, other communications	• Chillers for data center
• Enterprise data warehouse	• Electrical power
• Service/Help desk and computer support	• Emergency power outlets (red plugs)
• Identity management (e.g., active directory)	• Generators and fuel supply
• Interface engine	• Service/Help desk and computer support
• Interfaces	• Inventory (think broadly; replacement computer hardware to patient care supplies and paper forms)
• Internet of Things (IoT) patient monitoring devices	• Medical record (paper) storage
• Keyless entry systems or other security software	• Medical gasses
• Middleware servers	• Network cables and other physical components
• NetworkScanning software	• Operator switchboard
• Security systems	• Pneumatic tube systems
• Software applications list with interdependencies identified (will be unique to each organization)	• Physical security of buildings
• Telecommunication systems (hospital operators, paging, cellphone, analog, Voice Over Internet Protocol)	• Printers (include printers for patient ID labels/wristbands)
• Web services	• Reports
	• Storage area network; other storage
	• Scanners
	• Servers
	• Switches and hubs
	• UPS (uninterruptible power supply)
	• Utilities: power, heating, cooling, water

---

between the IT infrastructure and the physical infrastructure, and partial versus complete downtimes must be considered. Box 21.3 includes examples of both IT infrastructure and physical infrastructure. The order of the elements does not reflect their priority. Networks include both hardware and software components and therefore need to be examined from both aspects.

Common Causes of Downtime

The second step is to identify the most common potential causes of a downtime in the facility, areas of vulnerability, and the most likely scenarios of natural disasters or human-made disasters in the geographic area. Is the facility or data center on an old or outdated power grid? Is the building only rated to withstand a 6.5 magnitude earthquake in an area where experts predict one much stronger? Is the facility's generator located in an area that is vulnerable to flooding? Common disasters are noted in Table 21.1; these lists are not mutually exclusive but instead provide a starting point for planning at a specific organization.

System Inventory

The third step is to complete an inventory of all systems and document them. All systems in use at the organization should be inventoried because each is important to some aspect of the business. A sample inventory is located in Table 21.2.

An inventory list can be surprisingly difficult to compile and may involve walking through departments and units to observe systems and devices that clinicians use in their day-to-day workflow. This is especially critical if the institution has hybrid systems (i.e., a system using multiple vendors for specific

functionality). Ancillary systems within a hospital often have a limited but highly specific number of data requirements. For example, the pharmacy may have homegrown applications to assist with adjudicating pharmaceutical costs in addition to major modules in an electronic health record (EHR). These unique systems are added on to the main EHR because of the need for specific functionality or perhaps because the ancillary application was built and implemented prior to the EHR. Table 21.3 lists areas that may have special considerations within an acute care setting. In addition, readers should bear in mind the outpatient and ambulatory, as well as specialty populations such as pediatric or geriatric, settings will have unique requirements (Durry, 2015; MGH Center for Disaster Medicine, 2018; Larsen, Fong, Wernz, & Ratawani, 2018; Harrison et al., 2019).

To locate systems, applications or "apps," consider functional operations, type of personnel, data and information being processed or consumed, how and where vital records are housed, and policies and procedures that guide the business or practice (Larsen et al., 2019). This compilation will involve persistently reaching out to all members of the IT and business/operations members who host applications or provide some component of infrastructure for input. The more specific and complete the inventory, the more useful and helpful it will be in the event of an actual, planned, or unplanned downtime. Due to the difficulty of generating a complete inventory, it is best to start with the most critical applications and work on less critical ones later. Minimally, the inventory should include the items listed in Box 21.4.

TABLE 21.1   Downtime Vulnerabilities and Common Human-Made and Natural Disasters

Most Significant Downtime Vulnerabilities	Human-Made Disasters	Natural Disasters
Buildings or data center not up to current code or are vulnerable to natural or human-made disasters	Biologic: Intentional	Biologic
Cyber security attack	Cyber security attack	Dam failure
Lack of recovery site	Explosion: Intentional (bomb)	Drought
Lack of disaster planning or business continuity planning	Explosion: Unintentional (natural gas line rupture)	Earthquake
Lack of backups or inability to recover from backups	Fire	Fires, wildfires, (MGH Center for Disaster Medicine, 2018) wildfire smoke
Lack of high availability or failover for critical systems or applications	Hazmat incident	Flood, heatwave
Lack of downtime planning	Nuclear incident	Hurricane
Outdated or aging physical infrastructure	Pandemic	Landslide, mudslide, debris flow
Outdated or aging technology (i.e., not on current or supported level of code or servers that are no longer supported)	Terrorist attack	Pandemic
Power grid and supply	Workforce violence, shootings, loss of life of key personnel	Snowstorm, blizzard
System resources at or near capacity (disk space, database, storage, etc.)		Space weather, geomagnetic storm, tornado, tsunami

TABLE 21.2   System Inventory Considerations

Type of System	Examples
Core clinical applications	Patient registration and admitting, EHR computerized provider order entry (CPOE), clinical documentation, medication administration record (MAR), surgical services, and anesthesia information system
Ancillary service and procedure area information services	Pharmacy, radiology and imaging, laboratory, arterial blood gas, cardiology, endoscopy, respiratory, neurology, nutrition care, dictation, health information management, biomedical devices (physiologic monitors, vital sign machines, intravenous pumps, ventilators, pneumatic tube systems, etc.)
Online reference databases	Drug information references; patient education; policies and procedures; disease, diagnosis, and interventional protocol databases; formulas or health-related calculators
Revenue cycle	Admission, discharge, and transfer; enterprise scheduling; preauthorization; facility and technical billing; health information (HIM), document management (scanning), coding; professional and physician billing; claim scrubbers; print vendors; address verification; electronic data interchange (EDI) transactions; benefit checking
Business, finance, and personnel	E-mail, office software, cash collections, credit card transactions, banking, business intelligence, reports and reporting, supply chain and enterprise resource planning (ERP), budgeting, human resources, payroll, staff scheduling, keyless entry, facilities and engineering, telephone systems and wiring, telephone operators, paging systems, wireless communication devices
Miscellaneous	Printers, Bluetooth devices (scanners, label printers), reports, data warehouse, barcode scanning, print vendor, internet-based public web pages, intranet and related internal web sites, wikis, clinical health information exchanges, retail outlets (retail pharmacies, gift shops, food service)

Note: This is not a complete list.

System dependencies, configuration diagrams, and interface data should be documented and stored in a place that is easily accessible and backed up on a routine basis as the final step. Best practices for maintaining this inventory and documentation from an Information Technology Infrastructure Library (ITIL) (Information Technology Infrastructure Library ITIL 2021) perspective is a configuration management database (CMDB) that has configuration items unique to the organization. However, many tools or combinations of tools are available for this purpose, such as shared drives and folders, spreadsheets, databases, vendor-supplied tools, wiki sites, collaboration software, document management systems repositories, or even simple paper notebooks.

Emergency Preparedness

With the appropriate data collected, IT should work very closely with the organization's emergency preparedness and disaster planning groups in planning for disasters. Having some component of IT downtime as a part of disaster drills is an efficient and effective way for IT and staff to practice disaster response and hone plans. The federal government has published many helpful articles and websites to assist in institutional and personal planning. These include Ready.Gov, (Ready.Gov, n.d.) which partners with many of the following: Federal Emergency Management Agency (FEMA), the US Department of Education, the US Department of the Interior,

TABLE 21.3 Special Considerations by Area for Acute Care Setting

Area	Specialty Requirements
Anesthesia	Ventilators, anesthetic gases, frequent vital signs
Automated charge capture	Can be from many systems
Cardiac catheterization lab	Hemodynamic monitors, image capture, documentation for registries
Emergency department	Tracking patients in the waiting room and through the department
Endoscopy	Image capture and specific discreet documentation for registries or billing
Health information	Coding, release of information, maintenance of the legal medical record, legal cases, insurance queries, scanning solutions
Physicians, advanced practice clinicians	CPOE, clinical decision support systems, diagnostic test results, dictation
Newborn intensive care	Bedside monitoring and extracorporeal membrane oxygenation devices, ventilators, intravenous pumps
Nursing	Care planning, CPOE, Bar Code Medication Administration or electronic medication administration record, telemetry, patient communication systems with nurses, clinical decision support reminders, nursing databases (e.g., patient education resources)
Nutrition care	Assessments, nutrition care system, consultation notes, CPOE
Obstetrics	Fetal monitoring, mother and baby monitoring and documentation during the labor period, preterm wave forms, information from mother's record that needs to be available on newborn's record for continuity of care
Outpatient procedure areas	Point of care systems, registration and scheduling, medication-dispensing machines (i.e., Pyxis and Omnicell)
Pharmacy	Medication dispensing machines (Pyxis and Omnicell), robots, inpatient versus retail pharmacy ordering systems, intravenous pumps that contain drug-specific information (Alaris, etc.), and pharmacy ordering system often interfaces with the medication supplier
Physical, occupational, and speech therapies	Therapy systems have specific patient education content
Physiologic monitoring	Often supported by biomedical engineering and has vendor-specific content
Radiology, imaging, and picture archiving and communication system	Image and procedure capture, multiple modalities, questionnaires
Respiratory therapy	Contains respiratory measures like ventilator settings, ventilator weaning parameters, respiratory treatments and measurements

CPOE, Computerized provider order entry.

BOX 21.4 Inventory Items

- Vendor name
  - If developed in-house, where is the source code and other documentation?
  - Date of contract and its current location
- Application or module name
  - Date of original go-live
- Current version
  - Date of upgrade
- Categorization (site defined): major/minor, Tier I/II/III, other
- Host model (where the application or service is located): in-house or remote
- If remote, supported by whom?
- Interfaces, both inbound and outbound
- Third-party bolt-on systems
- Other key dependencies
- Primary use
- Primary users and number of users
- Business owners
- Information technology contacts
- Notes and comments

Health Resources and Services Administration (HRSA), and the Veterans Administration (FEMA, 2021; US Department of Education, n.d.; US Department of the Interior, n.d.; US Health and Human Services, n.d.; US Veteran's Administration, n.d.).

SYSTEM AND IT RESPONSE PLANS

Downtime Types

Once the system documentation is developed and the risks are understood, the healthcare institution is ready to define the different types of potential downtimes. These can be depicted on a continuum, indicating the degree of significance. The significance of the different downtimes will depend on the level of complexity and the suite of applications installed at your institution/organization. For example, a cloud-hosted system at a single physician's office is much less complex than the multitude of systems/applications installed at an academic medical center or large integrated delivery network (IDN) spread across multiple states or geographic regions. Context makes a difference.

Downtime Impact

Consider both planned and unplanned downtimes. If a downtime is scheduled, there should be ample time to plan. However, if the downtime is unexpected, no contingency plans may be in place. A worst-case scenario of an unplanned downtime is a total loss of the network function occurring midweek at the start of the business day when the hospital and clinic schedules are full, all operating rooms are in use, and the emergency department is busy and expecting two traumas (one via flight service) on a snowy winter day when 20% of staff are late due to road conditions.

Table 21.4 identifies a number of elements that will influence the impact of an individual downtime and is not intended to be followed linearly. Different scenarios or error messages will lead you down different paths, just as different symptoms might lead to different diagnoses in patient care. In direct patient care, readers would take different actions if a patient's temperature increased by a half-degree Celsius and the heart rate increased by 10 beats/min over the last 45 minutes, as opposed to if a patient had a sudden decrease in heart rate to 30 beats/min. Some events allow for a measured response, whereas others require immediate attention. The same process occurs when managing EHRs or other systems. Being able to quickly translate error messages and recognize patterns are keys to reducing the length of the downtime and restoring clinician and staff workflow.

Once the organization has clear definitions for downtimes and has methods of assessing the significance of potential events, (Morse, 2015) the emergency preparedness and disaster planning team can develop the response, communication, and recovery plans. A comprehensive and accurate assessment will provide a reliable starting point for the team responding to the downtime, thereby decreasing chaos and saving critical time at the start of an event.

System Level Method for Calculating Downtime Impact

The downtime plan will include different levels of interventions for various events. For example, a downtime event with a simple application may be managed with a decision tool. An example of a simple decision tree is shown in Fig. 21.1. However, using this same approach may become too cumbersome when dealing with multiple systems. In these cases, an organization may use a "level" system such as the one shown in Table 21.5.

Downtime Determinator

With a downtime event involving multiple systems, the use of a tool to quickly assess the significance of the downtime event will help the IT team and clinical users determine which of the predefined responses should be invoked. One example of such a tool is the Downtime Determinator depicted in Fig. 21.2, a tool developed by the authors. The x-axis is the length of downtime (or time to recovery), and the y-axis represents impact and risk. Each of the seven risk components is plotted on the Downtime Determinator tool in one of the four quadrants, and a pattern or cluster of numbers will begin to emerge. The pattern of numbers becomes the basis for evaluating the event. Quadrant response needs to be defined by the institution/organization.

When the majority of numbers cluster in the lower left quadrant, this should invoke a quadrant 1 response; numbers clustered in the upper right quadrant should invoke a quadrant 4 response. The lower left quadrant represents the least critical events, and the upper right quadrant represents the most critical events. The Downtime Determinator displays the numbers 2/3 and 3/2 in the upper left and lower right quadrants, respectively. Each organization will need to assign quadrants 2 and 3 based on its assessment of each individual downtime event, after considering the impact and risk versus time. There may be times when the length of the downtime is so long that the event warrants a quadrant 3 (more intense) response. There may be other times when the event scope is so massive that even though the downtime is scheduled for 30 minutes, it warrants a quadrant 3 response.

TABLE 21.4 Impact Considerations	
Attribute	**Continuum**
Expected or actual duration	≤1 h to >4 h; should also plan for catastrophic events in which network or systems may take weeks to months to rebuild
Time of day	The slowest night of the week to about the busiest day of the week (think OR scheduling pattern)
Number of users affected and scope of outage	Single user or department to the entire facility; partial to full; single system or infrastructure component to complete loss of application, network, or building
IT infrastructure	Intact to completely damaged and replacement parts need to be ordered
Impact on workflow	Users are able to carry on activities with minimal disruption to complete change in workflow reverting to paper/manual systems
Complexity of IT installs and criticality of applications	Single system with review-only functionality to an organization that is >90% electronic and paperless with multiple systems for all business and healthcare requirements
Planned or unplanned	Downtime scheduled during agreed-upon service level agreement and system comes back up as promised to an unexpected system-wide downtime with no estimated time to recovery
Complexity of health system or complexity and criticality of unit or department affected	Single office to multistate integrated delivery network; office that still keeps paper records to a fully electronic ICU with patients on multiple assistive devices
Communication methods and mechanisms	Communicate in person or via two-way radios or satellite phones until communications systems are back online (analog phones, VOIP phones, paging, cellphones, internet, intranet, faxing)
Redundancy of infrastructure and the ability to recover	No redundant systems or infrastructure to fully redundant, highly available system in a co-located data center
Maturity of downtime plans, policies, and procedures and availability of backup supplies	No plans or supplies to mature and tested policy, procedure, and plans with stocked supplies and staff aware of them

ICU, Intensive care unit; *IT*, information technology; *VOIP*, Voice Over Internet Protocol.

The Downtime Determinator is similar to the "level" system in Table 21.5. However, the Downtime Determinator allows for more specificity and nuances in responses because each of the attributes can be considered separately and responded to in relation to other attributes. When using a tool such as the Downtime Determinator, each organization should customize the tool by defining each attribute/component and delineating time along the *x*-axis. Four scenarios are outlined below using the Downtime Determinator, ranging from least to most impact:

Scenario 1: Level I trauma center and teaching hospital. Planned EHR downtime from 02:00 to 05:00 on a Wednesday night. IT infrastructure and communications intact (Fig. 21.3).

Scenario 2: Community hospital and associated outpatient clinics. Unplanned downtime of the scheduling and billing systems at 15:30 on a Monday. Multiple staff unable to do work, but clinical care is not affected. Recovery expected in 3 hours. System requires replacement of a hard drive; the hard drive is available locally, and it should be delivered to the data center by the vendor shortly. Communications intact (Fig. 21.4).

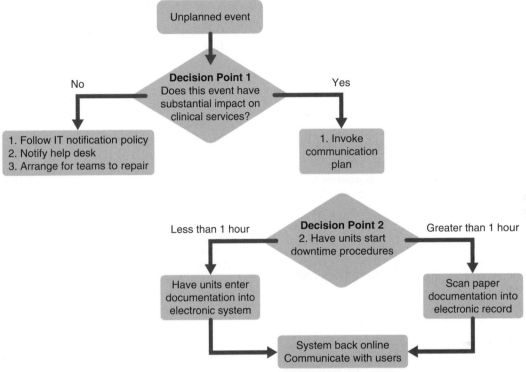

Fig. 21.1 Simple downtime decision tree.

	TABLE 21.5 **Downtime Levels**	
	Definition	**Response Examples**
Level 1	Part of a system down or unavailable but minimal impact and no loss of content or data integrity. Expected time to recovery less than 1 h.	IT team and targeted users only are involved per standard SLA. Service desk agent communicates with user.
Level 2	Complete system unavailable, data may be unavailable, and data will have to be entered into the system to maintain integrity. Expected time to recovery up to 4 h.	IT team and targeted users are involved per standard SLA. Unit-based downtime plans invoked. May require additional communication to stakeholders and plans for reentry of data.
Level 3	Multiple systems unavailable, big impact on workflow and content may be unavailable and will have to be entered into the system to maintain integrity. Expected time to recovery greater than 4 h.	IT incident response team involved along with multiple teams. Downtime plans invoked. Broad communication to the organization. Notification to key stakeholders and administration. Plan for reentry of data.
Level 4	All systems and network unavailable but root cause is known and recovery is possible. Users must complete downtime plans. Estimated time to recovery greater than 4 h.	IT incident response team involved, along with multiple teams. Downtime plans invoked. Broad communication to the organization. Notification to key stakeholders and administration. Plan for reentry of data. May involve emergency response team and opening of command center.
Level 5	All systems and network unavailable. Ransomware attack or major catastrophic event and facility structure may be compromised. Systems and infrastructure need to be rebuilt. System-wide emergency plans and response invoked.	All hands on deck and event directed per emergency response team or administration. May require communication to the wider community.

IT, Information technology; *SLA*, service level agreement.

Scenario 3: Acute care hospital with multiple intensive care units (ICUs) with a physiologic monitoring system interfaced to the EHR via bedside medical device integration (BMDI). The vendor-specific server is damaged due to a water spill in the communication closet, and the BMDI unexpectedly quits working at 08:00 on a Saturday morning. The vendor indicates a 2-week lag until a replacement server will be available (Fig. 21.5).

Scenario 4: An F-16 military airplane crashes, during training exercises, into the data center of an academic medical center at 19:00 on a Friday night. The data center is destroyed physically, a large fuel spill covers the area, and there is complete

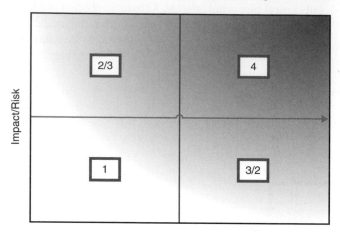

Plot each component in one of the four quadrants to determine where the items cluster

1. Time of day/number of users
2. IT infrastructure affected
3. System criticality
4. Planned versus unplanned
5. Health system complexity
6. Communication: Amount required and are methods affected?
7. Ability to recover

Fig. 21.2 Downtime Determinator Model.

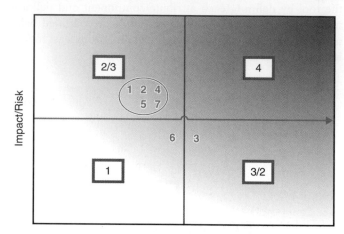

Plot each component in one of the four quadrants to determine where the items cluster

1. Time of day/number of users
2. IT infrastructure affected
3. System criticality
4. Planned versus unplanned
5. Health system complexity
6. Communication: Amount required and are methods affected?
7. Ability to recover

Fig. 21.4 Downtime Determinator quadrant 2 example.

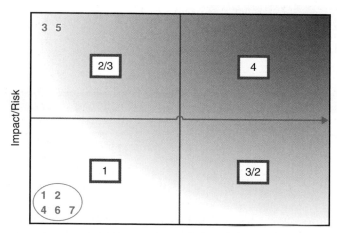

Plot each component in one of the four quadrants to determine where the items cluster

1. Time of day/number of users
2. IT infrastructure affected
3. System criticality
4. Planned versus unplanned
5. Health system complexity
6. Communication: Amount required and are methods affected?
7. Ability to recover

Fig. 21.3 Downtime Determinator quadrant 1 example.

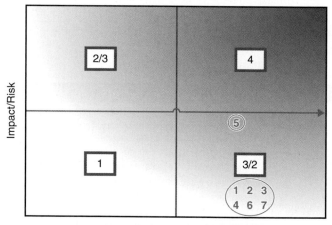

Plot each component in one of the four quadrants to determine where the items cluster

1. Time of day/number of users
2. IT infrastructure affected
3. System criticality
4. Planned versus unplanned
5. Health system complexity
6. Communication: Amount required and are methods affected?
7. Ability to recover

Fig. 21.5 Downtime Determinator quadrant 3 example.

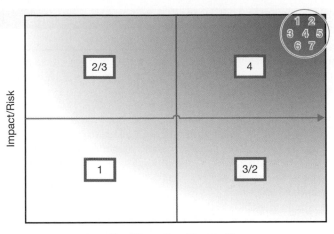

Plot each component in one of the four quadrants to
determine where the items cluster

1. Time of day/number of users
2. IT infrastructure affected
3. System criticality
4. Planned versus unplanned
5. Health system complexity
6. Communication: Amount required and are methods affected?
7. Ability to recover

Fig. 21.6 Downtime Determinator quadrant 4 example.

IT system downtime. The hospital and campus are otherwise intact. The academic medical center has a **hot site** that can host approximately 30% of critical systems and a **cold site** that has the capacity to host the remainder of the systems. The critical hot site applications can be available in 24 hours, but the remaining 70% of applications to be built on the cold site will take 30 days for complete recovery (Fig. 21.6).

As seen with these scenarios, the clustering of numbers helps guide the response of the organization in managing the event or disaster. A quadrant 1 event (scenario 1) should be a routine event that is managed with standard downtime processes, communications, and **service level agreements (SLAs)** that are already in place. With a quadrant 4 major disaster (scenario 4), the response should be all inclusive. Such a disaster would have a significant impact on the ability to continue providing all clinical and business operations. Recently, there has been a spate of major ransomware attacks where the EHR has been unavailable for multiple days and qualifies as a quadrant 4 disaster. Taking time to plan and put realistic processes into place before the event will determine whether the organization will continue to care for patients safely and have the business remain intact.

IT RESPONSE PLANS

Organizations are obligated to maintain contingency and disaster plans in order to be compliant with the HIPAA security rule of 1996, the U.S. Department of Health and Human Services, and accreditation bodies. A separate set of IT policies should exist to supplement the organization's overall disaster plan and include security and privacy components. Senior leadership of the IT department, the security and privacy office, the emergency preparedness group, and senior leadership from the broader organization should review and approve the plans (Monica, 2018). These plans should be frequently reviewed, tested, and revised as needed. Staff need to be updated on a consistent basis so they are prepared to implement contingency and disaster plans with minimum effort. Considerations for the IT components of an IT disaster plan are listed in Table 21.6.

At the point when the institution is converting back to its standard systems, the organization needs to be prepared to test the clinical system rapidly to ensure that all aspects of the system are functioning as planned. Having up-to-date test plans for all systems is an integral part of quickly resuming clinical and business operations. Software upgrades can and do occur frequently. If the test plans are not current, the testing process may not be reliable and valid. A benefit of keeping test plans up to date is the ability to enlist the help of non-IT staff during the recovery phase.

Redundant Systems

Redundant systems, also known as backup systems, provide clinicians the ability to access critical data during an electronic downtime. If clinicians can recover just enough information to carry on with patient care from the point at which the downtime begins, care can proceed safely (Larsen et al., 2019). Therefore, a subset of critical data must always be available, even during downtime. Each individual organization should define the required subset of data according to applications and services. Suggestions are basic demographics, orders, medication administration records (MARs), most recent vitals, laboratory values, imaging reports, and physician and provider progress notes.

Vendors are increasingly responding to the need for improved downtime solutions. As an example, a vendor might install one or more stand-alone machines in each patient care area, depending on the average patient census and geographic layout of the unit. Each machine can be designed to store a subset of historical patient data for up to 30 days. During a downtime, staff access these machines to retrieve patient-related data. Obviously, once the downtime begins, these systems will no longer be updated, and new patient data that are generated must be maintained manually. These data must be entered back into the EHR by keying them into the system or scanning them in after the system is up again. Because healthcare providers may need printed data during the downtime event, each machine should be directly connected by cable to a printer so it is not dependent on the down network connection for printing services. Another benefit of these machines is that they can be portable. In the event of a hospital evacuation, these machines can be removed from the premises and data from these machines can be used until a recovery plan is in place.

However, this particular redundant downtime solution has limitations. One concept that is difficult for clinical and IT staff to understand is that once the network becomes unavailable, these downtime machines are no longer updated with patient information. This requires the healthcare providers to check the new manually recorded data as well as the historical data maintained in the temporary system when providing care. Another

TABLE 21.6 Information Technology Contingency and Disaster Recovery Plan Considerations

Element	Activities
Staff competencies	• Identify and agree on roles and responsibilities. • Create comprehensive system documentation and make it widely available. • Demand "knowledge transfers"; all members to avoid SPOFs. • Develop stakeholder relationships. • Update emergency contacts for vendors and IT staff.
Data backups	• Preserve all critical data associated with the patient, the business, finances, payroll, and personnel. • Be knowledgeable about the retention policies of medical records and business documents for the organization and state. • Schedule backups on duplicate data on tapes, disks, and optical disks. • Store data in one of the clouds and/or across multiple servers.
Off-site storage of removable media	• Include a secure plan for transporting the media to an offsite location. • Encrypt data.
Adequate storage	• Evaluate storage capacity and procedures proactively.
Development and test domains for all systems	• Test all changes to production prior to promoting the code to production using a formal process.
System monitoring and notifications	• Keep a spreadsheet of common errors to help speed up diagnostics. • Introduce various types of downtimes to a test (nonproduction) system and evaluate the error messages or system issues. For example, in the nonproduction system, turn off the interfaces to see what types of errors or alerts you receive in the monitoring. • Work with the database team to mimic at-capacity database tables and carefully monitor system errors that are displayed.
Continuity plans	• Design systems that are highly available and redundant. • Archive source code with a reputable third-party company. • Complete negotiations up front for replacement hardware with commitments on days to ship and configure. • Arrange colocation sites with adequate network bandwidth and dual network pathways. • Develop reciprocal agreements or consortium arrangements. • Consider hot sites, warm sites, and cold sites. • If Cloud hosted, pay particular attention to their disaster recovery and business continuity plans, including things such as at least two separate internet pathways to and from their site.
Postevent review and revision	• Have formal process for the review that is inclusive of stakeholders. • Complete and document the event review as near to the event as possible.

IT, Information technology; *SPOF,* single point of failure.
Data from Federal Emergency Management Agency (FEMA), 2021. Ready.gov, 2021.

limitation is that the data may be organized differently than in the EHR, and as a result, information may be displayed or printed in a different format. This can cause confusion and even errors in patient care. Also, data entry for the downtime may not be complete, resulting in a fragmented or incomplete record.

The downtime solution using temporary machines must meet Health Insurance Portability and Accountability Act (HIPAA) requirements for security, privacy, and confidentiality. As a result, these machines require an extra layer of encryption to prevent information theft in the event that the machine is removed from the hospital.

Other terms used to describe redundant systems are *shadow, mirror,* or *read-only systems* (Bailey, 2020*)*. The downtime system described previously is a shadow or mirror system that is only able to be read by clinicians. Clinicians cannot add any patient data to this type of system. Some shadow or mirror systems duplicate the EHR. In the event that the primary system crashes, the secondary system automatically, and hopefully seamlessly, transitions the clinician to the secondary system. The clinician continues to document orders, medications, or care. Generally, these systems reside on separate hardware that "mirrors" the configuration of the primary system. These

systems are generally more robust than the redundant downtime solution described previously, encompassing a similar look and feel and often with read and write capability. These systems are beneficial because clinicians use their current log-in and password to access the system; the look and feel of the system are almost identical to the EHR; and printing can be available.

Redundant systems that resemble the configuration of the existing EHR will require a substantial financial investment from both infrastructure and software vendors. The financial investment can be an obstacle. Therefore a business case should be made with and for the clinicians on behalf of patients. The more mature the EHR, the more dependent the clinicians are on the system to retrieve information to provide patient care. Investing in a backup system of this caliber is arguably a necessity after institutions have reached a certain level of EHR maturity and may protect against the emerging threats of malware and ransomware attacks. Encourage your organization to frequently assess this requirement and, if one is already in place, encourage the optimization and maturation of these solutions (Gymarthy, 2019).

In addition to the previously discussed solutions, homegrown, web-based solutions may be available for use by clinicians prior to a planned downtime. For example, a web-based solution may be configured so that clinicians can print an MAR or all current patient orders. These have proven helpful during planned upgrades because they provide clinicians with enough information to weather the upgrade as well as provide a place to begin manual documentation of patient care during the downtime.

Downtime Policies and Procedures

The IT impact and downtime risk can be reduced by following a systematic process when changes are applied to the "production" or "live" system. One approach is to organize a service management program to organize a risk assessment and downtime planning document. Service management is a discipline for managing IT systems that focuses on the customer and the business and its operations as opposed to simply being technology-centric. The service life cycle includes strategy, design, transition, operation, and continual improvement (Invensis, n.d.). Interestingly, this life cycle is similar to both the system development life cycle used to implement computer systems and the nursing process (Wilson & Morrisroe, 2005; Toney-Butler & Thayer, 2021). Various process-based systems exist to assist the IT team in instituting a service management program, including ITIL (ITIL, 2021), Six Sigma, and total quality management (TQM). These systems require the use of standardized terminology, problem identification and management, change control measures, and communication patterns. The benefits of using these systems are agreed-upon realistic service levels, predictable and consistent processes, metrics, and alignment with business needs.

Implementing a service management program requires financial and time commitments from the organization, IT executives, and all members of the IT team, but is well worth the investment. Commitments are needed from the IT staff to fill roles on committees such as the change advisory board, incident response team (IRT), and IT service management. A major benefit of a service management program includes having a framework with clear rules and processes to structure IT activities so fewer unplanned events occur. One of the disadvantages of a service management program is that the program will invariably increase the time to implement new code or new functionality. This additional time might turn into an advantage, as waiting may reduce knee-jerk reactions from users. It also gives the IT team more time to test the new functionality and discover any dependencies. Waiting also benefits clinicians because they can negotiate a standard change time and reduce unnecessary downtimes.

Disaster Planning Manuals

The IT department should have a full set of written manuals that are available in multiple media formats, including something that does not require network connectivity. When stress is high, having a written reminder of steps is invaluable and will reduce the time to recovery (EMA, 2021). A downtime or disaster is not the time to soley rely on memory, a specific person, or knowledge known yet undocumented. This document and plan should have copies of relevant policies, specific procedures, and team responsibilities outlining steps to diagnose, recover, and validate systems. The plan should be evaluated and updated frequently, at least annually, and drilled or tested.

Creation of the plan should be completed by an interdisciplinary group. It often starts with the inventory that has been completed and assigns recovery point objectives and recovery time objectives to each system and service. This is a way to establish the recovery priority and identify dependencies. Key systems such as the EHR will be priority zero. Security software, such as key entry systems for perimeter doors and security cameras, should also be considered priority zero. The priority of the plan should be to facilitate the safest and most expedient recovery possible and reduce risk. Even if a site has great redundancy of systems or high availabilty, a formal written plan will facilitate recovery. Vendors and consultants are often used in this space as they have experience and templates that can guide the process (Kaur, 2021).

Business Continuity

Preparedness and planning are the keys to disaster recovery (Gecomo et al., 2020) following either a simple incident or a catastrophic event. In fact, the process of planning can be as beneficial to an organization as the final written plan. Recovery (Pipkin, 2020) should include all components identified as crucial: network, servers, storage, data, connectivity, telecommunications, hardware, software, desktops, security, and wireless to name a few.

The goal of disaster recovery is to reinstate business operations quickly and completely. Can the system/organization pay its employees? How do you determine how many people are currently taking family medical leave (FMLA)? Has the supply chain been reestablished? Can you send claims to the payors?

Depending on the severity of the event or disaster, it may be necessary to implement an incremental recovery. Key administrative leaders, with input from the staff, should be involved in the decisions about the recovery sequence for systems and applications. Including staff in the planning will likely facilitate the recovery process. It is important to consider expanded roles during events that require all hands on deck. One example occurred in our institution when our clinical analysts were asked to help reboot servers in the data center during a malware attack that lasted 72 hours. The steps to actual recovery will be different for each event and for each organization. Because of this complexity and the time involved in developing comprehensive plans, an organization may choose to hire outside consultants instead of using internal resources (Gartner Peer Insights, n.d.).

Business continuity management is a complementary process to disaster recovery. Business continuity has a larger scope than recovering only IT systems. It also includes determining which administrative and healthcare services must be available using a defined timeline and identifying which systems can be excluded from initial recovery. Business continuity management outlines the functions, processes, and systems needed to allow the core business of providing health services to continue.

A tier system works well for this purpose, and each organization will have unique requirements. For example, Tier I applications would be identified as critical and recovered first. The organization defines the expected time to recovery based on the requirement for service and available resources. As a general rule, the faster the recovery must occur, the more expensive the recovery process will be. The cost should also be evaluated in comparison with the cost of the downtime. For a Tier I application to be recovered in 24 hours or less, it is likely that a hot site would be required with hardware standing by. Tier II applications would come next and may be identified as needing to be available within 72 hours. Finally, Tier III and Tier IV may be identified as requiring recovery within 1 week and 1 month, respectively. For healthcare, business continuity includes providing care for both patients and the revenue cycle. Defining business continuity should be a formal process that includes the following:

- A business impact analysis that takes into consideration the institution's business needs and the needs of the community for healthcare services
- Definition of recovery strategies
- Development of a formal plan
- Exercises to test the plan

As with other elements discussed previously, this process will need resources (both human and financial) from the organization's senior leadership (Ready.Gov, n.d.b.).

The IT group should assure and consult with every business unit (including themselves) to make sure business continuity plans are in place and that they have a downtime box that includes items such as registration forms, charge sheets, fax forms, and other commonly used forms for that business area. Consider keeping paper instructions about how to fill out and use paper forms in a downtime box. In addition, it is a good idea to have these documents stored on a portable media device to be kept in the downtime box. In the event of a disaster, these forms can be stored on a second portable device and kept in a secure location. Organizations should make specific assignments to ensure that these are kept up to date and staff review the downtime box procedures periodically.

CLINICAL AND BUSINESS OPERATIONS RESPONSE PLANS

With the increased use of technology healthcare organizations must now precisely determine their response when technology is unavailable. How do clinicians find historical data, including recent vital signs, the first of three troponin results, the history and physical prior to surgery, and the last time the PRN (as needed) pain medication was given, with the patient's response to it? How do healthcare providers document new events, medications, orders, and treatments? How does the pharmacy dispense a medication and keep track it? How do ancillary systems such as radiology and pharmacy receive handwritten orders? Do the computerized supply cabinets have programming that permits overriding the system and, if so, how are charges captured after the fact? How will you register a patient in the clinic? Can the gift shop sell items to family members? How will the cafeteria provide food to patients, staff, and family members? These are a few of the potential problems that may arise at institutions in the event of system unavailability.

Data useful for general system support and downtime planning should be carefully documented as well. These items may be part of the application inventory, or they may be housed in a separate document, including those listed in Box 21.5. Each addition to the technology in use can produce unintended consequences and in turn affect the initial assessment and resulting plan. A landmark, 4-year analysis of the unintended consequences of computerized provider order entry (CPOE) identified nine types of unintended consequences (Ash et al., 2007). A list of these unintended consequences is included in Box 21.6. Additional studies show EHR adoption introduces failed expectations, innovation, and burnout, as well as impacts on patient care (Colicchio et al., 2019; Lyons et al., 2017).

BOX 21.5   Elements for General Systems Support

- A checklist for the IT team to follow when a planned or unplanned downtime occurs
- Checklists and role definition cards for the clinicians, caregivers, and registration staff
- Known system vulnerabilities
- Documentation of frequent error messages
- Patterns of error messages indicating known problems or pending system failure
- Knowledge objects used in supporting or maintaining system
- Contact information with phone numbers for vendors and the teams supporting the application
- Service level agreements with key users of the application
- Preferred user communication plan for planned and unplanned downtimes
- Plan to deploy nonclinical staff to support clinicians or perform duties assigned by the command center
- Unit- or department-based workflow diagrams
- Unit or department blueprints that document all electronic devices connected to the wired or wireless network
- Agreed-upon time for planned changes and maintenance work, also known as a change window
- Policies, procedures, rules, or standards from information technology or the broader organization that apply to the particular application

---

BOX 21.6   Unintended Consequences of the Impact of Computerized Provider Order Entry

- More/new work issues
- Workflow issues with mismatch of order entry and related activities
- Never-ending demands
- Paper persistence
- Communication issues with changes in communication patterns
- Emotions
- New types of errors introduced by use of a computer
- Changes in the power structure
- Overdependence on technology

Modified from the classic article Ash, J. S., Sittig, D. F., Poon, E. G., Guappone, K., Campbell, E., & Dykstra, R. H. (2007). The extent and importance of unintended consequences related to computerized provider order entry. *Journal of the American Medical Informatics Association. 14*(4), 415–s423.

Logically, the more electronic components in the organization, the more complex troubleshooting becomes. The elements that need to be considered include inpatient and outpatient venues, networks, intranets, printers, databases, interfaces, storage hardware, published applications, and layering software used to manage the myriad devices in an organization. Failure at any of these points may result in some sort of downtime for clinicians. Reducing the risk of a downtime can be accomplished by using the approaches outlined in the following sections.

Reviewing Clinical Downtime Plans

Approved downtime policies and procedures are needed to guide the clinical team. It is imperative that the clinical teams be involved with the development of the policies, and it is best if clinicians and business owners lead this effort. These policies should be prescriptive, include roles and responsibilities, and define workarounds or manual procedures that allow for the continuity of critical functions. They should include specific instructions about required data entry to the legal and permanent EHR record at the conclusion of the downtime. Examples of downtime policies are available in literature and on the internet (Larsen et al., 2018; Harrison et al., 2019).

The organization will have an overreaching disaster plan to guide you through the variety of downtimes. However, every clinical and business unit needs to have their specific policies and procedures in place. Begin by taking an inventory of current policies and procedures for your unit. Hopefully, some have been started and you can use them to expedite this process. If none are in place, assign one person in your unit to this task. Informaticists are subject matter experts, uniquely qualified and perfectly positioned to initiate the inventory process for their unit and the entire organization. Informaticists often lead interdisciplinary committees from inventory, through development of plans, through on-going maintenance and annual testing of the plans (Larsen et al., 2018).

Downtime in the Acute Care Setting

In order to make a response to a downtime on a clinical unit as stress-free as possible, make sure the checklists, key telephone numbers, reference materials, and instructions are easily accessible in a central place on the unit. Visual cues such as a specific color box or binder and bold labeling are helpful. Some facilities have downtime carts that are symbolically similar to a "crash cart." Each unit will be unique based on the services that are provided. For example, OR case cards should be available in printed format or in a media that can be printed on a local (non-networked) printer. In acute settings, printed medical reference materials are helpful for drug dosing, drug interactions, and treatment protocols.

The plan should account for all aspects of patient care, including documentation, ordering, order sets, results reporting, discharge, communication protocols, as well as patient tracking and bed planning. In addition to patient care, there should be documentation about key infrastructure such as electricity, "red plugs," entrance security, policies and processes to access supplies and medications, telephones, and emergency communication such as radios and "runners." Likewise, managing

the time-card system will impact the ability to generate payroll for staff. The hospital disaster plan will inform the unit-specific plans, including interaction with the hospital command center.

Policies regarding back-entry of data into the EHR, especially noting the need to take special care with inpatient admissions and transfers, medication reconciliation (MGH Center for Disaster Medicine, 2018). The organization will need to determine the cost/benefit of back-entering data into the EHR. The longer the downtime, the more time it takes to re-enter data.

A component of the logistics of planning for disasters and downtimes is considering the staff needs. They will experience increased anxiety and stress as well as an increased work load. Consider and plan for the human needs of nutrition, rest, and stress relief if possible. Also consider the staff's personal needs, such as childcare, transportation needs, and their health care needs. When there is a planned prolonged downtime, it is wise to staff (Larsen et al., 2018) up if possible so that patient care can proceed without interruption while tasks such as medication administration, supply acquisition, and documentation take much longer due to manual workflows. In today's world of remote work, there may be new and innovative ways that remote staff can assist with tasks to reduce the burden on the direct care givers.

Downtime in the Ambulatory Care Setting

Ambulatory care relies on many of the same systems as an inpatient care unit but has some unique needs, such as more real-time chart closure so that medical coding can occur. However, it has processes and patient flow that are decidedly different than those found in inpatient units. Knowing who is on the current schedule and creating future appointments are instrumental in running a clinic in the ambulatory setting. Likewise, imminently canceling patients during an unplanned downtime may need to occur. How will you contact patients to cancel their appointments if the EHR is unavailable? A brief hand-written progress note will likely suffice for an ambulatory visit, but how will you communicate discharge instructions, referral telephone numbers, and new prescriptions to the patient? Will they be hand-written? Can the medication prescription be called into the patient's pharmacy? How will you find the pharmacy's phone number? The ambulatory care area should also have a downtime resources that are highly visible, updated, and well known to the staff.

Downtime Box

A best practice is for all patient units and business areas to have up-to-date, physical "downtime" boxes (Gecomo et al., 2020). Each box contains documentation forms specific to the patient care area, instructions for paper form completion, and a plan for managing the paper documents on the unit. For example, ICUs may revert to traditional six-panel paper flow sheets. Other patient care areas have screenshots of the electronic "patient admission" form or other forms directly from the EHR. When no preprinted forms are available, blank or lined pieces of paper are used and work as long as healthcare providers are aware of documentation requirements. Each downtime box should be stocked to last at least 24 hours and have instructions for restocking the forms. Each patient care area is expected to maintain and customize the contents of its "downtime" box. Informaticians can partner closely with clinicians to create downtime policies and procedures to ensure that clinical requirements are matched with available IT solutions.

Business Continuity Plan

Business continuity focuses less on patient care and patient care systems and more on promoting the business's health and viability (Ready.Gov, n.d.b.). These plans also focus on areas of greatest risk to the organization. For example, if your IT systems are unavailable and charting is on paper, what will the process be for creating claims and getting them sent to the payers so that revenue can come back to the organization? How will payroll work if your timekeeping system is suddenly on paper? How will you obtain supplies from all of the vendors in your supply chain? How will you contact staff if you need additional resources? How will you manage Release of Information? Business continuity plans will be unique for each aspect of the business and must be approached methodically across the organization (Roush, Opsahl, Parker, & Davis, 2021).

Many organizations use consultants or vendors who have experience in this area to get the project started or get it updated. They have a plethora of tools available to make the process more efficient and timely and often start with a questionnaire for each specific area. Someone from outside the organization will often be able to bring a fresh set of eyes to processes and help think through key outcome indicators and forecasting. Business continuity plans require ongoing review and updating, and having a person in your organization accountable for overseeing this activity is critical. Remember to include your broader community in this plan.

Downtime Simulation

Disaster and downtime planning exercises are very beneficial (Hout, 2019). Exercises may also be required by regulatory or accreditation agencies (The Joint Commission, n.d.). Training should be done for all new employees at orientation and updated at least annually as a component of employee competency. Disaster simulations and exercises can help (Sano, 2020):
- Test staff readiness and response to an event
- Provide helpful information on additional staff training needs
- Identify holes and weak areas in the plan
- Improve workflows and processes during the event and for recovery
- Support the impetus to keep the plan updated and current

Exercises should be well planned ahead of time, sponsored by senior leaders of the organization and the emergency response plan, well communicated, well staffed, and inclusive of all staff. Both announced and unannounced exercises are beneficial. For an acute hospital, practicing both intake and evacuation of patients are critical.

Lessons learned from each exercise should be applied to improving the plan for the next time. The debrief of the planners and staff can also be useful in updating training materials, disaster references and boxes, and team building.

DOWNTIME COMMUNICATION PLANS

Plan Components

Communication is an integral part of any downtime, as the events can be very stressful. In addition to being your customer, they also have customers or patients that need information. Accurate, clear, and timely information can help reduce the stress and build confidence that the situation is under control (Patterson, n.d.). Five components of communication plans are needed to determine the following:
- Who needs to know the details?
- What details are needed?
- What media or modes of communication will be used?
- Who will communicate what information?
- What systems or workflow processes are affected?

Of course, the more complex the downtime is, the more people need to be notified and the more information needs to be communicated. For example, if the bedside monitoring device is not transmitting data to the EHR, only the ICU staff needs to be notified. If the EHR database becomes corrupt, then all clinicians who use the system will need to be notified, as well as all IT teams, and possibly hospital administration, and the risk management department.

Planned Downtime Communication Template

We have provided examples below, and other templated resources are available (Larsen et al., 2018). Having consistent templates helps the organization and end-users pivot to downtime procedures and gives them confidence in the procedural changes. Some general guidelines are listed here:
- When will the downtime begin?
- How long will the system be unavailable?
- Why will the system be down?
- What changes are being made to the system?
- Who will be affected and what can the end user expect?
- What procedures should be followed during the downtime?

These guidelines and templates can be adapted for use during both planned and unexpected downtimes.

Unplanned Downtime Communication Template

A good start to communicating an unplanned downtime is to acknowledge the issue as soon as possible and be clear on the scope of the outage with a focus on user impact. Give direction on using downtime procedures if appropriate, and let the users know about the estimated time to recovery (ETR) if known. Make a commitment to follow-up regularly during the incident and then also let them know when the incident is resolved. Consider having templates for your service desk site, an email message, a paged or text message, and any other social media in use by your organization (Patterson, n.d.).

For paging or text: Users are experiencing [problem]. ETR [time]. [Action]

Examples for paging or texting:
- Users are unable to log into EHR. No known ETR. Use business continuity application.
- Users continue to be unable to log into EHR. Root cause identified. ETR 4 hours. Go to downtime procedures.

- EHR is now available. Clinical documents will be scanned into EHR.

Postings on the service desk/incident site or sending email messages can contain more details. Some customers are seeing [problem]. We are aware of the issue, teams and the vendor are engaged. [List of workarounds or other instructions]. We do not have a current ETR but will update you at [time].

Example for service desk posting:

- Users are unable to order supplies through our ERP system. We are aware of the issue and have engaged the ERP team and the vendor. Please fax your requests to Central Supply. We do not have a current ETR but will update you hourly.

Example for email:

To: All Users distribution list

Subject: Network downtime December 2, 00:30 to 04:00

There will be a Network downtime on December 2, 00:30 to 04:00. This downtime will allow important IT Infrastructure updates, creating greater stability within the environment. During this downtime EHR, network access, internet access, VPN, and other network connected devices will be unavailable.

Please prepare for the IT downtime per your department's guidelines. During the maintenance, place lab orders via the pneumatic tube. Critical results will be telephoned to the unit. All normal lab results will be sent to the EHR when maintenance is complete.

Please contact the ITS Service Desk at [number] with any questions.

Thank You,

ITS Service Desk

Help or Service Desk Training

If your organization uses a tool for IT service management such as ITIL, the procedures discussed here will be used. If your facility does not use one of these systems, they might use other sources (ITIL, 2021; Atlassian, n.d.) to develop policies and procedures to ensure that communication is managed properly. Communication occurs most predictably and reliably when the responsibility belongs to one consistent team or group of people. A service management or an equivalent team works well to manage the communications. Whoever is designated as the primary communication team must work very closely with the IRT and the help desk. The help desk is critical to communication, as in most cases, staff experiencing technical problems have been instructed to contact the help desk first. Plus, in most healthcare organizations, the help desk staff are on-site and have on-call agents available 24 hours a day. Training the help desk staff to manage these communications allows the infrastructure and other IT teams to work on resolving the problems. Clearly stating the message and quickly informing the help desk will facilitate distribution of the intended message.

Other tools that can be used in addition to the trouble ticket queue include: continuous or intermittent conference calls, individual and group paging for the IT department, individual and group instant messaging, webcasts, updated web pages, group e-mail updates, recorded phone messages, social media

sites, sanctioned organizational applications, and coordination with hospital operators. Multiple means of communication need to be considered when planning for an event. The technical problems causing the downtime or the disaster event may also eliminate certain communication modes. For example, if the network is down, an e-mail cannot be sent with information about managing the event to the clinical units, and Voice Over Internet Protocol (VOIP) phones will not work.

The hospital telecommunications operators can manage many aspects of the communication plan, including individual and group pagers, cellphones, tablets, and other communication devices for clinicians and the operational areas. Sending information to these communication devices may help manage information distribution during sudden or extended downtimes. A best practice in the age of internet-based phone systems is to have some analog phones available in key hospital areas because they function during network and electrical downtimes. These phones can be identified by using a different color of phone, such as red. Hospital telecommunications operators can also use the overhead paging system in the hospital to distribute information. The point is to be sure to include these hospital operators in the downtime communication plans.

In the event of a major disaster, satellite radios and phones can be used. Satellite phones and radios are network independent but require electricity to recharge their batteries. The local emergency management office in the organization will have more information about these capabilities.

Coordinating Between IT and Response Teams

The IT staff is responsible for communicating the necessary information to the help desk agents. In addition, some electronic systems contain notification alert capability. For example, planned downtimes can be communicated using the notification system in the organization's EHR. Obviously, this method would not be available during an EHR downtime, but it can be used to announce a planned downtime or when any of the ancillary systems are offline.

IT leaders are responsible for communicating with the organization's senior leadership and the public relations department so they can manage media relations with the community. Social media applications can also be used to manage information with the media and to distribute information to staff in the event of a downtime (assuming that staff members have subscribed to the service and that the service provides the appropriate level of security and privacy).

Other mechanisms may be in place depending on the institution and the setting. For example, if the organization is affiliated with a university, a "campus alert" system may be available. Using this system, notifications can be sent via e-mail, cellphone, work phone, home phone, or a combination of these. This communication strategy can be very helpful during disaster drills as well as other types of unexpected events. Numerous ways exist to communicate with hospital employees and leadership, IT staff, the news media, and the public. Finding the right combination for the facility's budget and staff and formalizing the ownership of specific communication will facilitate the workflow transitions during EHR downtimes at the facility.

CONCLUSION AND FUTURE DIRECTIONS

This chapter identifies tactics for health system downtime planning and disaster recovery. It challenges clinicians and informaticians to assess, plan for, respond to, recover from, communicate about, continue business during, and prevent downtimes and disasters when possible. Trained informaticists can step into many of these roles and play an integral role in designing, planning, maintaining, and evaluating downtime and disaster recovery planning.

The primary objective for downtime and disaster planning is to protect the organization and the patients who are served by minimizing disruption to operations. This includes minimizing economic loss; ensuring stability; protecting critical assets; ensuring safety for personnel, patients, and other customers; and reducing variability in decision making during a disaster. In healthcare and health IT, the single most important reason to carry out the activities described in the chapter carefully and methodically is the ability to provide uninterrupted, exceptional service and safe care to all patients.

The reliance on technology and the impact of downtimes, disasters, security events, and ransomware attacks has increased. This should drive administrators to invest additional human and material resources in assessing and planning to minimize the impact of potential threats. Advances in technology can be expected, which means you'll need to reevaluate on at least a yearly basis. These solutions may be less costly as new and improved technology eventually reduces the potential for downtimes. Additional research is very much needed to help clinicians and health systems understand the experience of downtime workflow interruptions, the patient safety implications, and the operational impacts. In addition, research should be initiated to drive a standard approach to downtime planning for health systems, disaster recovery, and business continuity efforts. Many focus areas might be addressed along the continuum of disaster planning to business continuity, where research could have a very positive impact on the health system and its clients.

DISCUSSION QUESTIONS

1. Explain the importance of an organization-specific downtime risk assessment.
2. Describe the pros and cons of different assessment tools for evaluating downtime events and discuss scenarios in which they might be used to their greatest advantage.
3. Compare and contrast the roles of the informatician, the clinician, and IT personnel in system downtime planning.
4. Describe key components of a business continuity plan and (a) how they might differ for different types of organizations and (b) how the clinical and business units differ.
5. Contrast different communication methods for system downtime events and summarize the pros and cons of each.
6. How has your organization prepared for a ransomware attack or major security breach?

CASE STUDY

At your Level 2 trauma center, an unplanned EHR downtime occurs at 17:00 on a Tuesday. After 1 hour of troubleshooting and working with the vendor's help desk, the IT team attempts a system reboot, which is unsuccessful. The vendor is in a different time zone, so specialists have to be called in from home to respond to this incident. The initial assessment is that the downtime is due to database corruption and that the system will have to be recovered from backup systems. Unfortunately, the system is not configured with high availability techniques nor is it redundant. The IT department estimates that it will take 8 hours to recover the system, for a total downtime of 10 hours.

DISCUSSION QUESTIONS

1. Plot each component on the Downtime Determinator for both part 1 and part 2 of the scenario as it unfolds, and document your IT response, end user response, and communication plans.
2. Make changes to the assessment and plans to account for changes to the scenario.

REFERENCES

Acronis. (n.d.). What is a disaster recovery plan? Accessed August 26, 2020. https://www.acronis.com/en-us/articles/disaster-recovery-plan/?gclid=EAlalQobChMIw8GRzNis8gIVMGpcBB1VwwkeEAAYASAAEgJ6T_D_BwE

Ash, J. S., Sittig, D. F., Poon, E. G., Guappone, K., Campbell, E., & Dykstra, R. H. (2007). The extent and importance of unintended consequences related to computerized provider order entry. *Journal of the American Medical Informatics Association, 14*(4), 415–423.

Atlassian. (n.d.). The path to better incident management starts here. Accessed August 26, 2021. https://www.atlassian.com/incident-management/incident-communication.

Bailey, R. (2020). Overview of redundant systems. https://www.atlantic.net/dedicated-server-hosting/overview-of-redundant-systems/.

Bischoff, P. (2021). Ransomware attaches on US healthcare organizations cost $20.8 bn in 2020. Comparitech. https://www.comparitech.com/blog/information-security/ransomware-attacks-hospitals-data/

Capital One. (2011). Business continuity and disaster recovery checklist for small business owners. Continuity Central. http://www.continuitycentral.com/feature0501.htm.

Colicchio, T. K., Cimino, J. J., & Del Fiol, G. (2019 Jun 3). Unintended consequences of nationwide electronic health record adoption: challenges and opportunities in the post-meaningful use era. *Journal of Medical Internet Research, 21*(6), e13313. https://doi.org/10.2196/13313.

Coveware. (2021). What we can learn from ransomware actor "security reports." https://www.coveware.com/blog/2021/6/24/what-we-can-learn-from-ransomware-actor-security-reports

Data Foundry. (n.d.). How to calculate the true cost of downtime. Accessed August 26, 2020. https://www.datafoundry.com/blog/how-to-calculate-the-true-cost-of-downtime

Durry, A. (2015). Are we ready? Pediatric disaster planning. *Nursing Made Incredibly Easy, 13*(5), 30–37. https://doi.org/10.1097/01.NME.0000470082.48212.01.

EMA. (2021). National Incident Management System. https://www.fema.gov/emergency-managers/national-preparedness/plan.

Federal Trade Commission. (n.d.). Data security. Accessed August 26, 2021. https://www.ftc.gov/tips-advice/business-center/privacy-and-security/data-security

FEMA. (2021). National incident management system. https://www.fema.gov/national-incident-management-system.

Gartner Peer Insights. (n.d.). Business continuity management program solutions reviews and ratings. Accessed August 26, 2021. https://www.gartner.com/reviews/market/business-continuity-management-program-solutions.

Gecomo, J. G., Klopp, A., Rouse, M. Implementation of an evidence-based electronic health record (EHR) downtime readiness and recovery plan. HIMSS Core Technologies; 2020. https://www.himss.org/resources/implementation-evidence-based-electronic-health-record-ehr-downtime-readiness-and.

Getz, L. (2009). Dealing with downtime: How to survive if your EHR system fails. *For the Record, 21*(21), 16. http://www.fortherecordmag.com/archives/110909p16.shtml.

Gymarthy, K. (2019). 5 Reasons data centers are important to your backup strategy. https://www.vxchnge.com/blog/data-center-backup-strategy.

Harrison, A. M., Siwani, R., Pickering, B. W., & Herasevich, V. (2019 Oct 1). Clinical impact of intraoperative electronic health record downtime on surgical patients. *Journal of the American Medical*

Informatics Association, 26(10), 928–933. https://doi.org/10.1093/jamia/ocz029.

Hout, O. (2019). Six scenarios for business continuity plan testing. https://www.agilityrecovery.com/article/6-scenarios-business-continuity-plan-testing.

Information Technology Infrastructure Library (ITIL). (2021). ITIL Open Guide. https://www.itlibrary.org/.

Invensis. (n.d.). An overview of ITL service lifecycle modules. Accessed August 26, 2021. https://www.invensislearning.com/articles/itil/overview-of-itil-service-lifecycle-modules.

Kaur, G. (2021). Top 8 disaster recovery companies in 2021. https://www.toolbox.com/it-security/vulnerability-management/articles/disaster-recovery-software-companies/.

Kill, G. (2018). The 11 leading causes of downtime. https://integracon.com/11-leading-causes-downtime/.

Larsen, E., Fong, A., Wernz, C., & Ratawani, R. M. (2018). Implications of electronic health record downtime: an analysis of patient safety event reports. *Journal of the American Medical Informatics Association, 25*(2), 187–191.

Larsen, E., Hoffman, D., Rivera, C., Kleiner, B. M., Wernz, C., & Ratwani, R. M. (2019 May). Continuing patient care during electronic health record downtime. *Applied Clinical Informatics, 10*(3), 495–504.

Lyons, A. M., Sward, K. A., Deshmukh, V. G., Pett, M. A., Donaldson, G. W., & Turnbull, J. (2017). Impact of computerized provider order entry. *Journal of the American Medical Informatics Association, 24*(2), 303–309.

MGH Center for Disaster Medicine. (2018). Hospital Preparedness for unplanned information technology downtime events. https://www.massgeneral.org/assets/mgh/pdf/emergency-medicine/downtime-toolkit.pdf.

Monica, K. (2018). How to optimize EHR downtime preparedness, reduce slowdowns. https://ehrintelligence.com/news/how-to-optimize-ehr-downtime-preparedness-reduce-slowdowns.

Morse S. (2015). California hospitals prepared as wildfires rage, association says. http://www.healthcarefinancenews.com/news/california-hospitals-prepared-wildfires-rage-association-says.

Patterson M. (n.d.). Communicating with customers during a system outage. Accessed August 26, 2021. https://www.helpscout.com/helpu/outage-status-update/.

Pipkin C. (2020). Seven ways to build an effective disaster recovery & business plan. https://www.toolbox.com/collaboration/remote-support/guest-article/7-ways-to-build-an-effective-disaster-recovery-business-continuity-plan/.

Polaneczky M. (2007). When the electronic medical record goes down. The blog that ate manhattan. http://www.tbtam.com/2007/03/when-the-electronic-medical-record-goes-down.html.

Ponemon Institute. (2016). Cost of cyber crime study and the risk of business innovation. 2016 HPE CC Global Report Final 3. https://www.ponemon.org/local/upload/file/2016%20HPE%20CCC%20GLOBAL%20REPORT%20FINAL%203.pdf

Ready.Gov (n.d.a). Business continuity plan. Accessed August 26, 2021a. https://www.ready.gov/business-continuity-plan.

Ready.Gov (n.d.b). Home page. Accessed August 26, 2021. https://www.ready.gov.

Roush K. Opsahl A. Parker K. Davis J. (2021). Business continuity planning: An effective strategy during and electronic health record downtime. Nurse Leader. https://www.nurseleader.com/article/S1541-4612(21)00014-8/fulltext.

Sano, A. (2020 Jan). Using an evidence-based approach for EHR downtime education in nurse onboarding. *Computers,*

Informatics, Nursing, 38(1), 36–44. https://doi.org/10.1097/CIN.0000000000000582.

The Joint Commission. (n.d.). Emergency management. Accessed August 26, 2021. https://www.jointcommission.org/resources/patient-safety-topics/emergency-management/.

Toney-Butler T. J., & Thayer J. M. "Nursing process." Statpearls. Statpearls publishing 2021. https://www.ncbi.nlm.nih.gov/books/NBK499937/

US Department of Education. (n.d.). Natural disaster resources. Accessed August 26, 2021. https://www.ed.gov/hurricane-help.

US Department of the Interior. (n.d.). Natural disaster response and recovery. Accessed August 26, 2021. https://www.doi.gov/recovery.

US Health and Human Services. (n.d.). Emergency preparedness & continuity of operations. Accessed August 26, 2021. https://www.hrsa.gov/emergency/index.html.

US Veteran's Administration. (n.d.). VHA office of emergency management. Accessed August 26, 2021. https://www.va.gov/vhaemergencymanagement/.

Wilson, J. R., & Morrisroe, G. (2005 Apr 4). Systems analysis and design. *Evaluation of Human Work, 3*, 241–279.

22

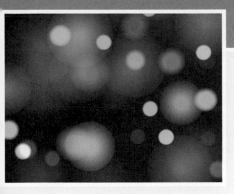

Improving the User Experience for Health Information Technology

Aaron Zachary Hettinger, Lynda R. Hardy, and Sadaf Kazi

Usability has a strong, often direct relationship with clinical productivity, error rates, user fatigue, and user satisfaction[1]

OBJECTIVES

At the completion of this chapter, the reader will be prepared to:
1. Discuss the role of human factors, ergonomics, human-computer interaction, usability, and user-centered design in improving health IT systems usability.
2. Describe the major aspects of the user-centered design process.
3. Describe frameworks related to the user experience, processes, and usability tests.
4. Distinguish between the methods of discount usability, traditional usability methods, and formal user testing.
5. Distinguish between multiple types of user testing.
6. Describe the steps involved in conducting a usability test.

KEY TERMS

contextual inquiry, 348
discount usability methods, 345
ergonomics, 342
focused ethnographies, 348
heuristic evaluations, 345

human-computer interaction (HCI), 342
human factors, 341
joint cognitive systems, 343
sociotechnical system, 340
task analysis, 348

think-aloud protocol, 346
usability, 340
user-centered design, 341

ABSTRACT ❖

The usability of health information technology (IT) products is a worldwide concern. U.S. federal agencies are responding to this challenge by developing regulations and reports to increase cognitive support for using health IT products, thereby reducing errors associated with health IT, and improving safety. Health professionals and informaticians require a suite of skills to understand and apply concepts in usability and translate them to improve healthcare safety. This chapter provides an introduction to the knowledge and skills required to meet those needs. First, the chapter outlines the need for attention to usability in health IT. Terms are defined, the concepts of usability goals are presented, and user-centered design precepts are discussed. Potential benefits for improved usability are outlined. Available human-computer interaction (HCI) frameworks are listed; one framework is explained in detail, and selected methods particular to usability evaluations are explained. Types of usability tests are discussed and linked to the systems life cycle. Examples of actual usability studies in health settings are provided. These techniques will provide assistance to readers to design and conduct usability tests to determine the effectiveness and efficiency of and satisfaction with health IT products.

INTRODUCTION TO IMPROVING USABILITY IN HEALTH IT SYSTEMS

Readers can easily describe their frustrations with poorly designed health information technology (IT) products. Solutions to these health IT issues involve the systematic study of health IT usability that incorporates a wide variety of available resources. This section of the chapter outlines users' current experiences with health IT. After terms are defined, potential benefits are discussed for improved usability to health IT product users and health organizations.

The Current Usability of Health Information Technology Products

Usability issues with health IT products are a worldwide concern. The expansion of mobile health (mHealth) and electronic health records (EHRs) have resulted in complex interactions among multiple users, IT products, and environments, all with varying characteristics. These complex interactions, known as a sociotechnical system, coupled with complex health systems, are magnified as users interact with health IT.

Convincing evidence exists that usability issues in health IT can result in patient safety problems and errors (Health Information Management and Systems Society [HIMSS], 2009; Beuscart-Zephir et al., 2013; Carayon et al., 2014). In the United States, The Joint Commission (TJC) issued an alert in mid-2015 concerning sentinel events related to health IT. TJC evaluated 3375 previous adverse event reports, identifying 120 health IT-related sentinel events (The Joint Commission [TJC], 2015). One-third of these stemmed from factors related to the human-computer interface, while 24% stemmed from workflow and communication issues. Lack of interoperability and difficulties in extracting relevant data from vast quantities of information can result in omissions and errors in care continuity mechanisms such as handoffs (Staggers et al., 2011; Pew Charitable Trust, 2015). Moreover, providers have difficulty finding critical information and developing the "big picture" of the patient (Stead and Lin, 2009; HIMSS, 2016). In the federal sector, an ambulatory EHR application serving more than nine million patients failed to support providers during patient encounters, did not allow them to obtain situational awareness of the patient (the "big picture" of the patient), promoted workarounds for the existing nonintegrated systems, and greatly increased frustrations because of required structured documentation (Staggers et al., 2010). Last, potential patient safety issues occurred with two different Electronic Medication Administration Records (eMARs) because nurses could not easily view patients' medications to determine those missed and those due (Staggers et al., 2015; Guo et al., 2011).

Physicians are currently very vocal about their dissatisfaction and productivity issues with EHRs. Their perceptions about EHR usability were increasingly negative between 2010 and 2013, according to a national survey (ACP, 2013). In a letter signed by 30 physician organizations in 2015, the American Medical Association (AMA) issued a call for solutions to poorly designed EHRs (AMA, 2014).

Other healthcare professions are similarly affected but less outspoken. However, a recent call to action was issued to improve nurses' user experiences (UXs), especially for EHRs (Staggers et al., 2015). Nurses are particularly affected by excessive documentation requirements. For example, admission assessments in acute care can take from 30 to 60 minutes and involve 532 clicks, structured documentation does not reflect the nuances of care (a pick list cannot capture how a patient feels about dying, for example), and nurses indicated that EHRs are a hindrance to care because they take time away from patients (HIMSS, 2016). These issues could be ameliorated by incorporating known usability principles and processes to improve the usability of health IT.

Usability

The term usability is often used interchangeably with HCI when the product is a computer, but usability also concerns products beyond computers. Usability is also more focused on interactions within a specific context or environment for a specific product. Formally, the ISO defines usability as the extent to which a product can be used by specific users in a specific context to achieve specific goals with effectiveness, efficiency, and satisfaction (ISO, 1998). A product with good usability allows users in a particular context to achieve their goals when interacting with a product (Rubin & Chisnell, 2008). Usability is, however, fundamentally concerned with human performance, and in the case of healthcare, interactions that promote safety rather than only subjective data. Usability can be measured by the following dimensions:

- Speed and errors in interactions with a health IT product
- Ease of learning and remembering interactions after time has elapsed
- User satisfaction or perceptions about the interactions with health IT
- Efficiency and accuracy of interactions
- Designs to promote error-free or error-forgiving products
- Seamless fit of an information system to the tasks and goals of users

The Goals of Usability

The overall goals of usability are established by the ISO. Fig. 22.1 depicts the ISO usability goals (HIMSS, 2011):

- *Effectiveness* is the accuracy and completeness with which specified users achieve specified goals in particular environments, including worker and consumer or patient safety.
- *Efficiency* includes the resources expended in relation to the accuracy and completeness of goals achieved.
- *Satisfaction* is the level of comfort and acceptability that users and other people associate with the product or work system and deals with users' perceptions (HIMSS, 2011).

Dimensions of usability correlate to potential benefits of usability depicted in Fig. 22.2, and (as discussed in detail in the next section) include improvements for individuals or groups of

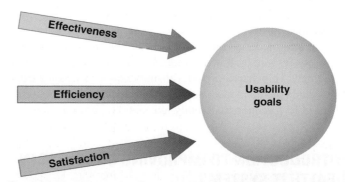

Fig. 22.1 Usability goals. (From HIMSS Usability Task Force. [2011]. Promoting usability in health organizations: Initial steps and progress toward a healthcare usability maturity model. Chicago, IL: Healthcare Information and Management Systems Society. Reprinted with permission from HIMSS.)

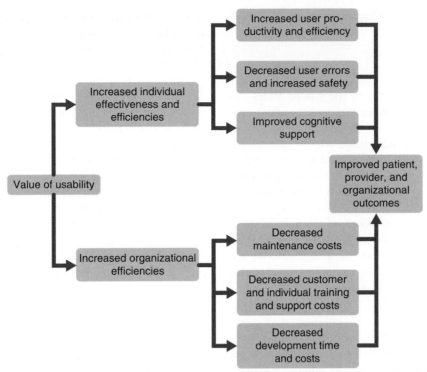

Fig. 22.2 The value of usability to health organizations. (From HIMSS Usability Task Force. [2011]. Promoting usability in health organizations: Initial steps and progress toward a healthcare usability maturity model. Chicago, IL. Copyright © Healthcare Information and Management Systems Society.)

individuals in the following areas: productivity and efficiency, effectiveness in product use, safety, and cognitive support (an aspect of effectiveness).

USER-CENTERED DESIGN

Usability experts employ a process of a **user-centered design (UCD)** composed of the following three axioms:
- An early and central focus on users in the design and development of products
- Iterative design
- Systematic measures of the interactions between users and products (Rubin & Chisnell, 2008; Dix et al., 2004)

These principles were derived nearly 30 years ago by Gould and Lewis and are more salient than ever because contemporary environments are filled with an array of complex tools. An early and central focus on users means understanding users in depth—that is, their characteristics, environment, and tasks (Rubin & Chisnell, 2008). Direct contact with actual users is needed early and often throughout a design or redesign process. *Iterative design* means having rounds of design expansions where key users evaluate product prototypes to determine their effectiveness and efficiency in the care process and health decisions. One design is never adequate, and typically at least three rounds are necessary. Once a design is available, even on paper or in PowerPoint, designers or informaticians work with users to determine any issues by having them systematically interact with and respond to the design. Specific methods to accomplish this are explained in subsequent sections. The goals are for major usability issues to be identified and corrected early in the process. Design and evaluation then occur in a cycle until

major usability issues are corrected. This dynamic, iterative process, which includes the three axioms listed above, is known as user-centered design. Structured and systematic observations, including identified measures, are necessary. Usability goals and axioms apply not only to developing products but also to the selection, purchase, customization, and redesign of products. This type of design allows us to integrate health data, information, and knowledge into health IT products. For example, a well-designed eMAR would filter medication routes to match the particular medication, eliminating inappropriate options (e.g., being able to chart an antacid as an intravenous medication or administer a tablet in the left arm). Although this sounds like common sense, current designs in major EHRs often do not accommodate this type of cognitive support and safe design.

Human Factors

According to the Human Factors and Ergonomics Society (HFES), **human factors** is "the scientific discipline concerned with the understanding of interactions among humans and other elements of a system, and the profession that applies theory, principles, data, and methods to design in order to optimize human well-being and overall system performance" (HFES, 2012). Simple examples include a design for opening a door efficiently, how to turn on the lighting for one area of a room from a bank of light switches, and how to safely and efficiently operate the controls to drive a car. In healthcare, human factors might concern the design of a new operating room to better support workflow, teamwork, and patient flow, or identifying obstacles to intensive care nurses in their task performance (Gurses & Carayon, 2007). Human factors engineering principles have been applied specifically to understand the needs of EHR users.

Productivity suffers when human factors are not well understood and managed.

Ergonomics

The term ergonomics is used interchangeably with human factors by the HFES in Europe, but in the United States and other countries, its focus is on human performance with physical characteristics of tools, systems, and machines (Dix et al., 2004). For example, ergonomics issues might address the design of a power drill to fit a human hand or the design of chairs to promote comfort and safety. In healthcare, ergonomics can be the number, types, and locations of computer workstations or the physical design of a mobile device to support care. Ergonomics also pertains to the design of a surgical instrument to fit the human hand to perform desired functions effectively and efficiently. Some practitioners would describe the distinction as between physical ergonomics (e.g. workstation and seating design) versus cognitive ergonomics (e.g. interface design) (Hollnagel, 1997).

Human-Computer Interaction

Human-computer interaction (HCI) is the study of how people design, implement, and evaluate interactive computer systems in the context of users' tasks and work (Rubin & Chisnell, 2008). HCI, as with human factors, draws on the disciplines of psychology and cognitive science, computer science, sociology, and information science and on the discipline of the user at hand. HCI can be addressed throughout the systems life cycle to include the design, development, purchase, implementation, and evaluation of applications. HCI topics can include the following:

- The design and use of devices such as an intravenous pump or a touchpad on a computer
- User satisfaction with computerized provider order entry (CPOE)
- Patient usage rates of mHealth apps or personal health records
- Users' perceptions of eMARs
- The standardization (or not) and meaning of icons on a patient portal
- Principles of effective screen design, including mobile application design
- Analysis of the capabilities and limitations of users and matching these to mHealth designs

Cognitive Informatics

The field of cognitive informatics is relatively new and often not well understood. It includes both the development of human artificial cognition (artificial intelligence) as well as seeking to better describe human behavior and cognition through the application of informatics (Wang, 2003; Wang, 2007). Cognitive informatics combines cognitive and information sciences to increase the understanding, description, and prediction of healthcare products and outcomes to improve healthcare decision-making (Patel & Kannampallil, 2015). There can be significant overlap with human factors engineering principles, however where usability studies may utilize 5 to 15 users per iterative process, cognitive informatics can utilize thousands or millions of recorded interactions to understand real world behaviors in complex systems like healthcare (Hettinger et al., 2017).

Potential Benefits of Improving Usability

A white paper from HIMSS describes how to incorporate usability in health organizations (HIMSS, 2011). This publicly available white paper includes a section on the benefits of usability to healthcare summarized here.

Usability can add value to organizations across a range of areas. Usability return on investment (ROI) material is available from (1) non-healthcare projects such as Bias and Mayhew (Bias & Mayhew, 2005) and Nielsen, (Nielsen & Gilutz, 2003) (2) the User Experience Professionals Association website, and (3) Dey Alexander Consulting (Dey Consulting, 2009). To the author's knowledge, no research is yet available about large-scale ROI or cost savings for usability efforts in healthcare projects. Thus material is cited from non-healthcare applications. However, findings from non-healthcare IT projects are likely to extend to healthcare because of the often dramatic changes that usability can create. Fig. 22.2 outlines potential areas of value when usability is improved in health organizations. In addition, the Office of the National Coordinator (ONC) sponsored the development of the ONC Change Package for Improving EHR Usability to help healthcare systems incorporate basic concepts and publicly available tools (Office of the National Coordinator for Health Information Technology, 2018).

Increased Individual Effectiveness

Usability can positively affect at least three areas of particular interest in health IT:

1. Increased user productivity and efficiency
2. Decreased user errors and increased safety
3. Improved cognitive support

Increased User Productivity and Efficiency

One of the most prevalent complaints about health IT in general and EHRs specifically is that the technology impedes users' productivity. For example, outpatient visits were reduced from four to three per hour after an ambulatory EHR was fielded (Philpott, 2009). A cognitive work analysis of the same system in a laboratory setting showed a large number of average steps to complete common tasks, a high average execution time, and a large percentage of required mental operators (Saitwal et al., 2010).

Employing usability processes helps improve productivity and efficiency. The Nielsen Norman Group estimated that "productivity gains from redesigning an intranet to improve usability are eight times larger than costs for a company with 1000 employees; 20 times larger for a company with 10,000 employees; and 50 times larger for a company with 100,000 employees" (Nielsen & Gilutz, 2003). Website redesign statistics for the 42 cases collected by Nielsen Norman yielded an average increase in user productivity of 161%. After testing intranets for low and high usability, these authors projected a savings of 48 hours per employee if intranets were redesigned for high usability. Souza et al. cited usability research showing that two-thirds of buyers failed in shopping attempts on well-known sites (Souza et al., 2001). Thus poor usability on intranets can mean poor employee productivity.

Decreased User Errors and Increased Safety

One major reason why health IT is installed is to reduce healthcare errors (Institute of Medicine, 2011). While some classes of errors such as medication prescribing errors can be reduced with health IT, technology itself can create unintended consequences and new errors due to poor usability (Ash et al., 2007, 2009). For example, Kushniruk et al. identified how certain types of usability problems were related to errors as physicians entered prescriptions into handheld devices (Kushniruk et al., 2004). Nielsen and Levy collected case studies and found a decrease in user error rates in 46 redesign projects measuring user error (Nielsen & Levy, 1994). Another study showed a 25% decrease in user errors after screen redesign (Dray & Karat, 1994). Users found needed information only 42% of the time on 15 large commercial websites, even when they were directed to the correct home page; 62% gave up looking for desired items on websites (Nielsen & Gilutz, 2003). Redesigns could prevent errors in these types of interactions; thus incorporating usability can potentially decrease errors in health IT products. A study by Ratwani and colleagues (2021) showed a tremendous difference across two EHRs in four health systems in terms of the time on task and error rates in a simulated setting (Ratwani et al., 2018). One CPOE task (prescribing a steroid taper) demonstrated error rates of more than 50%.

Improved Cognitive Support

Stead and Lin concluded that the premier EHRs in the United States in 2009 did not provide the required cognitive support for clinicians (i.e., tools for thinking about and solving health problems) (Stead & Lin, 2009). This is still true today. Cognitive support may include designs to provide an overview or summary of the patient, information "at a glance," intuitive designs, and tailored support for clinicians in specific contexts. An example of how usability can provide cognitive support is the work on novel physiologic monitoring designs. Researchers employed user-centered design and usability testing techniques to create novel designs integrating physiologic data in a graphic object (Drews & Westenskow, 2006; Syroid et al., 2002; Wachter et al., 2006). The new design provided integrated, "at a glance" pictorial data to show changes to clinicians. These graphic objects are now being incorporated in vendors' products as an adjunct to numeric data displays. Another example is the design and testing of new displays for ICU nurses after researchers performed a comprehensive study of their tasks and cognitive requirements (Koch et al., 2012). Unintended consequences can occur with the introduction of new technology, including one study that showed increased task switching with the implementation of new health IT systems (Benda et al., 2016).

Increased Organizational Efficiencies

Well-designed user interfaces and systems translate into organizational efficiencies, including the following:

- Decreased maintenance costs
- Decreased customer and individual training and support costs
- Decreased development time and costs

HUMAN-COMPUTER INTERACTION FRAMEWORKS FOR HEALTH INFORMATICS

Frameworks provide guidance for understanding essential components that improve the usability of the system. They are helpful in completing UCD processes, usability tests, IT adoption evaluations, and usability research. This section of the chapter provides an overview of existing frameworks and describes in detail the Health Human–Computer Interaction Framework (HHCI).

Human Factors and Human–Computer Interaction Frameworks (Benda et al., 2016; Carayon et al., 2020)

Various HCI frameworks and models with different foci are available:

- Fit Between Individuals, Task, and Technology (FITT) (Ammenwerth et al., 2006)
- User, Function, Representation, and Task Analyses (UFuRT, or TURF) (Zhang & Butler; Zhang & Walji, 2011)
- A framework for employing usability methods to redesign a fielded system (Johnson et al., 2005)
- A framework for technology-induced error (Borycki et al., 2012)
- A combined health IT adoption and HCI model (Despont-Gros et al., 2005)
- Joint cognitive systems (Hollnagel & Woods, 2005)
- Systems Engineering Initiative for Patient Safety (SEIPS) (Carayon et al., 2020; Holden et al., 2013)
  The last two models bear more discussion.

Joint Cognitive Systems

Hollnagel and Woods coined the term *cognitive systems engineering*, acknowledging that sociotechnical systems, or complex technologies embedded within social systems, are increasingly prevalent yet have frequent system failures (Hollnagel & Woods, 2005). The authors devised a cyclic model called contextual control model, or CoCom, with the following elements: event, modifies, constructs, determines, acts, and produces. Users and context are major components of the model. Importantly, joint cognitive systems imply that information is shared or distributed among humans and technology. This framework is useful for examining teamwork in healthcare, such as those for patient care.

Systems Engineering Initiative for Patient Safety

SEIPS 3.0, shown in Fig. 22.3, is a model centered on work systems and patient centeredness. Work performance results in a sociotechnical system with people as one component. People (or a person) are central to work systems, and support for the

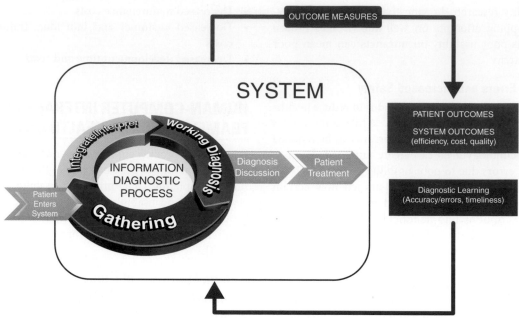

Fig. 22.3 SEIPS Model 3.0. (National Academies of Sciences, Engineering, and Medicine. 2015. Improving Diagnosis in Health Care. https://doi.org/10.17226/21794. Adapted and reproduced with permission from the National Academy of Sciences, Courtesy of the National Academies Press, Washington, D.C.)

design of work is necessary. Support includes the design of work structures and processes using human factors science. Often work systems include technology, but SEIPS may also be used to examine work without technology (Holden et al., 2013). The most recent SEIPS iteration, 3.0 includes an expanded focus on the patient journey and that episodes of care can be distributed across time and location and a more complex framework is required for improved context (Carayon et al., 2020).

An analysis of the existing frameworks found each helpful but inadequate for health usability studies. Missing elements across frameworks included (1) interactions among disparate users, including patients, although SEIPS acknowledges groups of people and CoCom and TURF mention information distribution, (2) characteristics and actions of products and users, (3) a focus on context, and (4) a developmental timeline. Context is critical in particular because it defines the kinds of users, tasks, and work design (Zhang & Butler; Zhang & Walji, 2011). A developmental time element is also necessary because it accounts for users changing (maturing) in their interactions over time (Despont-Gros et al., 2005; Staggers, 2001). Therefore a new framework was created.

The Health Human–Computer Interaction Framework

The current HHCI framework builds on early work by Staggers and Parks describing nurse-computer interaction (Staggers & Parks, 1992). It was expanded to include groups of healthcare providers and interactions with patients (Staggers, 2001). The framework is adapted further here to acknowledge that IT may be only one example of an available health IT product (e.g., others might be physiologic monitors or intravenous pumps).

The elements of the framework are outlined in Fig. 22.4. Information (e.g., patient care, administrative, or educational information) is the exchange mechanism. Interactions occur in a system of mutual influences where elements (e.g., individuals, health IT) act and respond based on specific characteristics. Context is paramount with all interactions embedded within a context. This means that any outcomes of interactions are distinct, as they are defined by a context. The developmental timeline indicates that interactions change over time. Thus the outcomes of interactions are different based on when an interaction occurs in time.

Humans or products can initiate interactions. The information is processed through either the product or the humans, according to characteristics. The recipient then reacts to the information; for example, a healthcare provider could read and respond to an e-mail from a patient, or a product might process interactions after the Enter key is pressed. Iterative cycles continue as humans behave and products act according to defined characteristics. Goals and planning are implicit within the tasks displayed in the framework.

Essential Components for Improving Usability

The important point in this section is that using a framework or model can greatly assist readers to think comprehensively about usability for health IT and the conduct of usability studies. Readers may choose a framework to match the need at hand. Methods can then be applied as appropriate, while ensuring that critical elements are under consideration. This idea is expanded in later sections to illustrate how the framework assists usability testing. In summary, product interactions are a complex part of a sociotechnical system. Critical elements to consider are as follows:

- Users and their characteristics
- Interactions
- Tasks (goals of tasks)

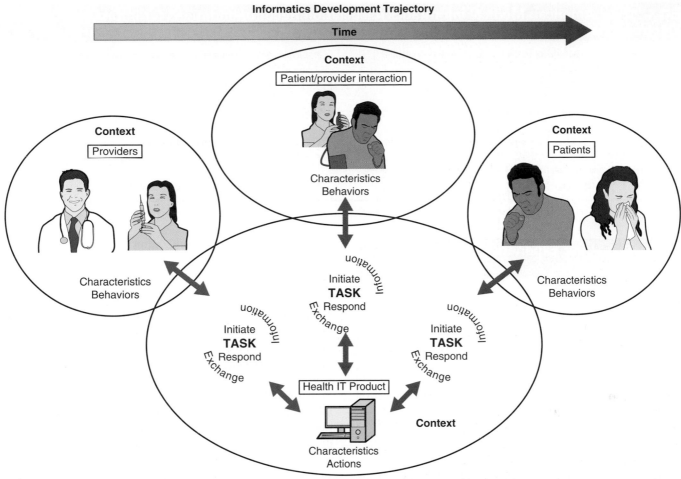

Fig. 22.4 Health human–computer interaction framework. (Copyright Nancy Staggers. Reprinted with permission.)

- Information
- Products and their characteristics
- Context
- Interactions mature over time (developmental timeline)

SELECTING METHODS TO IMPROVE USABILITY

Usability methods can be at a more strategic level or project-based. For instance, strategic UX methods were outlined by the American Medical Informatics Association (AMIA) in 10 recommendations to improve patient safety and quality of care by improving the usability of EHRs (Box 22.1) (Middleton et al., 2013).

Readers should be aware of some specific methods for analyzing usability in health IT systems to effect recommendations and apply concepts to health IT in local projects. Techniques to improve the usability can be informal or formal, simple or complex, and employ a few individuals or a wide range of users. Readers or researchers can design small projects or sophisticated studies by combining usability precepts with usability-specific or traditional research designs and methods such as quantitative, qualitative, or mixed methods. The type of usability study is dependent on the purpose of the project; when the assessment is targeted within the systems life cycle; the desired

outcome of the project; and available resources, including time, people, and money. However, any study can use the elements from the HHCI framework as a guide (Box 22.2).

Usability methods were developed over decades and are robust. This section of the chapter concentrates on unique, proven methods to choose and apply. These include discount usability methods and other usability methods described later.

Discount Usability Methods

Nielsen developed techniques he called discount usability methods to reduce the number of required users in usability projects and to use early design prototypes. Meant for usability experts, this method has proven useful for others involved in designing projects (Nielsen, 1993, 1994). A discount usability method offers economies of time, effort, and cost and can be completed at any point in the systems life cycle. The most common technique is heuristic evaluation.

Heuristic Evaluation

The definition of a heuristic is a "rule of thumb" or guideline. Heuristic evaluations (HEs) compare products against accepted usability guidelines to reveal issues. Nielsen recommends that three to five experts complete independent evaluations and then combine issues into a master list after discussion and

---

BOX 22.1   American Medical Informatics Association Recommendations for Improving Electronic Health Records Usability

- Accelerate a research agenda for usability a human factors in health IT.
  - Prioritize standard use cases.
  - Develop a core set of measures for adverse events related to health IT use.
  - Research and promote best practice for safe implementations of EHRs.
- Create new policies.
  - Include usability concerns as a part of the standardization and interoperability across EHRs.
  - Establish an adverse event reporting system for health IT and voluntary health IT event reporting.

- Develop and disseminate an education campaign on the safe and effective use of EHRs.
- Develop industry guidelines.
  - Develop a common user interface style guide for select EHR functionalities.
  - Perform actual usability assessment on patient-safety sensitive EHR functionalities.
- Create clinical end-user recommendations.
  - Adopt best practices for EHR system implementations and ongoing management.
  - Monitor how IT systems are used and report IT-related adverse events.

AMIA, American Medical Informatics Association; *EHR*, electronic health records; *IT*, information technology.

BOX 22.2   User Experience Methods and Techniques

An excellent resource for usability methods and techniques is the Usability. gov website. This resource includes content such as the basics about usability, project management, and visual design. For our purposes here, the most relevant content is the section on "how to and tools."

Usability projects can be done at any point in the systems life cycle from initial work (to identify usability issues; clarify requirements; and assess initial designs, technical prototypes, or simple computerized applications) to iterative development of solutions, product selection, product customization, or evaluation of a system after installation (Thompson et al., 1999).

UX, User experience.

---

consolidation. HE violations of guidelines are made and severity scores are then assigned to the identified issues (Nielsen, 1994). Importantly, dual domain experts (experts in both usability and the field to which the application is geared) can find 81% to 90% of existing usability problems and increased numbers of major issues with the application (Nielsen, 1992). HE is a commonly employed technique, and readers can complete an HE after only a modest amount of training.

- A number of usability heuristics are available to evaluate applications: Nielsen's 10 heuristics (Nielsen, 1995)
- Zhang et al.'s 14 heuristics (Zhang et al., 2003)
- Dix et al.'s 10 heuristics (Dix et al., 2004)
- Shneiderman's 8 golden rules (Shneiderman & Plaisant, 2005)
- HIMSS's 9 usability principles (Health Information Management and Systems Society HIMSS, 2009)

Zhang et al.'s guidelines have been used extensively in health applications and devices. These authors combined Nielsen's and Shneiderman's heuristics and applied them to a project evaluating two infusion pumps, finding 192 and 121 heuristic violations, respectively, categorized into 89 and 52 usability problems. Using this technique, they concluded that the pump with the higher violations might contribute to more medical errors than the other one (Zhang et al., 2003). Zhang et al.'s 14 adapted heuristics and definitions are outlined in Table 22.1. Once readers develop a basic understanding of the meaning of each heuristic, they can evaluate a health IT product against the heuristics as in the following examples.

Examples of a Heuristic Evaluation Project

Guo et al. used Zhang's heuristics to evaluate a vendor's eMAR installed at a tertiary care center (Guo et al., 2011). The authors received training on the eMAR, defined typical tasks that nurses complete using the product, and also modified Zhang's heuristics to include concepts about patient safety. The authors independently completed the defined tasks and compared their interactions to the heuristics, synthesized results, and found 233 violations for 60 usability problems. Problems included having to manually update the screen by clicking an "as of" button to refresh the screen and ensure that the most current medication orders were being viewed. Nurses had great difficulty in determining medications given "at a glance." These results have implications across all three usability goals of effectiveness, efficiency, and satisfaction, and also raise potential patient safety issues.

Researchers evaluated the Veterans' Administration's eMAR using a similar process to the one listed above; however, they also validated usability findings with the site barcode medication administration nurse coordinators (Staggers et al., 2015). Findings included 90 usability problems and 440 heuristic evaluation violations. Fifteen issues were rated as catastrophic, with nurses particularly impaired in situation awareness or having the ability to develop a "big picture" of what was happening with patients and their medications. An example was medication preparation for a group of patients. The application allowed nurses to access only one patient's medication list at a time even though they cared for groups of patients, so they developed workarounds such as using paper 4 × 6 index cards to organize medications for times throughout a shift. HE provided insights about how this application needed to be improved to support nurses' cognitive processes and medication activities.

Traditional Usability Methods

A large suite of methods is available to conduct usability examinations of health products and processes. Three of these methods—think-aloud protocol, task analysis, and contextual inquiry/focused ethnographies—are presented here.

Think-Aloud Protocol

Think-aloud protocol involves a small number of actual application users (vs. experts). Even as few as five users can offer rich

TABLE 22.1 Zhang Heuristics and Nielsen Severity Rating Scheme

Heuristic Category	Definition
Consistency and standards	Consistency across all aspects of the product: methods of navigation, messages and actions, meaning of buttons, and terms and icons. Congruence with known screen design principles for color and screen layout. Consistency with ISO (International Organization for Standardization) usability guidelines.
Visibility of system state	Users understand what the system is doing and what they can do with the product from the system messages, information, and displays.
Match between system and world	The technology matches the way users think and do work, uses appropriate information flow, has typical options that users need, and includes expected actions by the system.
Minimalist	No superfluous information. System and screen design targeted to primary information users' needs. Use of progressive disclosure to display details of a category of information only when needed. The exception can be designs for expert users where screen density is preferred.
Minimize memory load	Minimizing the amount of information and tasks users have to memorize to adequately use the technology. Product makes use of sample formats for data input, such as a calendar for date format.
Informative feedback	The technology provides prompt and useful feedback about users' interactions and actions (e.g., feedback that orders were placed).
Flexibility and efficiency	The ability to tailor and customize to suit individuals' needs. Includes novice and expert capabilities (e.g., string searches).
Good error messages	Tell users what error occurred and how users can recover from the error. Not abstract or general such as "Forbidden!" Need to be precise and polite and not blame the user.
Prevent errors	Catastrophic errors must be prevented (e.g., mixing pediatric medication order dosing between kilograms and pounds or delivering a radiation dose with the device left wide open instead of being tailored to tumor size).
Clear closure	Users should know when a task is completed and all information is accepted. Displays should include progress toward 100% completion versus using a series of bars.
Reversible actions	Whenever possible, actions and interactions should be able to be undone within legal limits in electronic health records. If actions cannot be reversed, there is a consistent procedure for documenting the correction of any misinformation in the system.
Use the users' language	The technology uses language and terms the targeted users can comprehend and expect. Health terms are used appropriately.
Users in control	Users initiate actions versus having the perception that the technology is in control. Avoid surprising actions, ending up in unexpected places, and loud sounds with errors.
Help and documentation	Provide help for users within the context the actions occur (context sensitive). Embed help functions throughout the application.
Severity Scale Rating Element	Definition
0—No usability problem	No need to correct the issue.
1—Cosmetic problem	Correct the issue only if extra time and fiscal resources allow. Lowest priority.
2—Minor problem	Annoying issue with minor impact. Low priority to fix.
3—Major usability problem	Issue with major impact to use or training or both. Important to fix. Considerations are the numbers and kinds of users affected by a persistent problem.
4—Usability catastrophe	Severe issue that must be corrected before product release, especially those related to patient safety.

Data from Zhang, J., Johnson, T. R., Patel, V. L., Paige, D. L., & Kubose, T. (2003). Using usability heuristics to evaluate patient safety of medical devices. *Journal of Biomedical Informatics. 36*(1,2), 23–30; Nielsen, J. (1993). Severity ratings for usability problems. http://www.useit.com/papers/heursitic/severityrating.html/.

data about usability issues. Users talk aloud while they interact with a product and observers record their experienced usability problems. As users voice what they are trying to do, they indicate where interactions are confusing and provide other thoughts about the product. This allows a detailed examination of the specified tasks, in particular to uncover major effectiveness issues. This method may be used in the design, redesign, development, or evaluation of applications at any time in the systems life cycle. Think-aloud methods are often used in conjunction with other techniques.

With this technique, researchers first determine a specific set of tasks for users to complete, such as tasks to operate an infusion pump or use an mHealth app. Defining tasks ahead of time provides structure and consistency across participants and guides users through the procedure. Participants are asked to complete the tasks and talk aloud during the session. Methods to capture the session can include observing and taking notes, audio- or video-recording using software such as Morae or even a smartphone, and handwritten diaries or issue logs (Dix et al., 2004). The resulting material is then analyzed by grouping issues or using a schema such as HE categories to label findings. The analysis portion of this method can be time consuming, depending on the complexity of the product, the number of users tested, and the number of tasks. However, the information gained by using this method is robust and helpful in pinpointing areas needing redesign.

Task Analysis

Task analysis is a generic term for a set of more than 100 techniques that range from a focus on cognitive tasks and processes (called cognitive task analysis) to observable user interactions with an application (e.g., a systematic mapping of team interactions during a patient code). Task analyses are systematic methods used to understand what users are doing or required to do with a health IT product. They focus on tasks and behavioral actions of the users interacting with products. These methods provide a process for learning about and documenting how ordinary users complete actions in a specific context (Ash et al., 2007; Hackos & Redish, 1998; Courage et al., 2008). Task analyses are helpful to identify task completeness, the correct or incorrect sequencing of tasks (especially their fit to cognitive tasks), accuracy of actions, error recovery, and task allocation between humans and products. Task analysis is typically used early in the systems life cycle to determine user requirements for design or to determine redesign when rich data are needed. This technique may be used to analyze areas for redesign. One type of analysis, cognitive task analysis, is particularly useful for understanding users' goals while interacting with products (Crandall et al., 2006). A task analysis can be used, for example, to determine who is attending to patients' preventive health alerts in a clinic because alerts are seen by a variety of healthcare providers.

Sample methods of task analysis include the following:

- Interviews
- Observations
- Shadowing users at their actual work sites
- Observing users doing tasks
- Conducting ethnographic studies or interviews (Courage et al., 2008)

A critique of cognitive task techniques is available for readers who want to find the right method for their project (Wei & Salvendy, 2004). References on the specifics of performing task analyses are available (Hackos & Redish, 1998; Courage et al., 2008; Crandall et al., 2006).

Sample output from a task analysis is listed in Table 22.2. After observations and interviews, evaluators record user actions (e.g., a flow chart with task descriptions). Evaluators might video-record users as they interact with an mHealth application, asking users to perform specific tasks and use a think-aloud protocol to uncover tasks (especially cognitive tasks) and requirements.

Example of a Task Analysis

Researchers video-recorded nurses as they interacted with an existing eMAR in an inpatient application (Staggers et al., 2007). They also observed nurses' medication management tasks in the actual setting in a variety of acute care units. The researchers created a task flow diagram of medication tasks that included cognitive tasks and delineated deficiencies with the current application. By using task analysis to define requirements, the researchers could then develop a novel and more effective eMAR.

Contextual Inquiry or Focused Ethnographies

Ethnography methods are borrowed from anthropology and sociology, where fieldwork and analyses of people in cultural and social settings are completed. Focused ethnographies and contextual inquiry involve interacting with users in their actual sites or "field settings." They concentrate on individuals' points of view and their experiences and interactions in social settings, rather than on just the actions of those individuals (Hammersley & Atkinson, 2007; Viitanen, 2011). However, researchers are observers rather than a part of the society. During observations, detailed descriptions are generated with an emphasis on social relationships, interactions with IT, and their impact on work. Ethnographies have become important in understanding the usability and describing the impact of complex products.

Example of a Focused Ethnography or Contextual Inquiry

Ash et al. used this method to research the impact of CPOE on users in acute care facilities in the United States (Ash et al., 2009, 2007, 2004) They completed interviews, focus groups, and observations and outlined unintended consequences for CPOE: new and more work, workflow issues, unusual system demands, disruptions in routine communications, extreme user emotions, and overdependence on the technology. Their studies are considered seminal works in informatics.

FORMAL USER TESTING

Usability Measures

"Usability measurements are to user interface design what physical exams are to patient care" (Staggers, 2011).

User tests may be done at any point in the systems life cycle, but they are often completed as summative tests—that is, after

TABLE 22.2 Sample Output From Task Analyses

Type of Task Analysis Output	Description
Profiles of users or personas	Short narrative, visual descriptions, and/or summaries about the characteristics of users
Workflow diagrams	A flow diagram of tasks or cognitive processes performed by users
Task sequences or hierarchies	Lists of tasks order by sequence or arranged to show interrelationships
Task scenarios	Detailed descriptions of events or incidents, including how users handle situations
Usability issues	A list and classification of usability problems with a product
Affinity diagrams	Bottom-up groupings of facts and issues about users, tasks, and environments to generate design ideas
Video and audiotape highlights	Clips that illustrate particular observations about users and tasks in a context

Adapted from Staggers, N. (2001). Human-computer interaction. In: S. Englebardt and R. Nelson (Eds.), *Information technology in health care: An interdisciplinary approach* (pp. 321–345). Philadelphia, PA: Harcourt Health Science Company.

a product is nearly or completely developed and/or fielded. At that point, more objective methods are employed. A critical aspect of conducting a usability test is measuring human performance and having a larger sample of users. To assist readers, a taxonomy of usability measures is presented in Table 22.3. This table is adapted from Sweeney et al. and from Staggers and expanded here (Staggers, 2001, 2013; Sweeney et al., 1993). The taxonomy includes measures from three perspectives: users, experts, and organizations. Researchers recommend at least 15 users for summative testing (Virzi, 1992). The important points are that usability is measurable and that a suite of measures is available. In addition to the objective measures in the table, questionnaires are available to measure users' perceptions of or satisfaction with their product interactions.

TABLE 22.3 Sample Usability Measures

Usability Focus	Usability Measures
User behaviors (performance)	Task times (speed, reaction times)
	Percentage of tasks completed
	Number, kinds of errors
	Percentage of tasks completed accurately
	Time, frequency spent on any one option
	Number of hits and/or amount of time spent on a website
	Training time
	Eye tracking
	Facial expressions
	Breadth and depth of application usage in actual settings
	Quality of completed tasks (e.g., quality of decisions)
	Users' comments (think-aloud) as they interact with technology
	System setup or installation time, complexity of setup
	Model of tasks and user behaviors
	Description of problems when interacting with an application
User behaviors (cognitive)	Description of or systems fit with cognitive information processing
	Retention of application knowledge over time
	Comprehension of system
	Fit with workflow
User behaviors (perceptions)	Usability ratings of products
	Perceptions about any aspect of technology (speed, effectiveness)
	Comments during interviews
	Questionnaires and rating responses (workload, satisfaction)
User behaviors (physiologic)	Heart rate
	EEG
	Galvanic skin response
	Brain-evoked potentials
User behaviors (perceptions about physiologic reactions)	Perceptions about anxiety, stress
User behaviors (motivation)	Willingness to use system
	Enthusiasm
Expert evaluations (performance)	Model predictions for task performance times, learning, ease of understanding
	Observations of users as they use applications in a setting to determine fit with work
Expert evaluations (conformance to guidelines)	Level of adherence to guidelines, design criteria, usability principles (heuristic evaluation)
Expert evaluations (perception)	Ratings of technology, informal or formal comments
Context (organization)	Economic costs (increased FTEs for the help desk for a new application)
	Number of support staff, time needed to support product
	Number of training staff, time needed to support product
	Costs (for support, training, loss of productivity)
	Observations about the fit with work design and workflow in departments, organizations, networks of institutions
Combined	Videotaping and audiotaping users as they interact with an application and capturing keystrokes. Can capture any combination of the above.

EEG, Electroencephalography; *FTE*, full-time equivalent.
Adapted from Staggers N. (2001). Human-computer interaction. In: S. Englebardt and R. Nelson (Eds.), *Information technology in health care: An interdisciplinary approach* (pp. 321–345). Philadelphia, PA: Harcourt Health Science Company; Staggers, N. (2012). Improving the usability of health informatics applications. In: T. Hebda and P. Czar (Eds.), *Handbook of informatics for nurses and health professionals* (170–193). Upper Saddle River, NJ: Pearson Education.

Usability Questionnaires

There are multiple types of usability questionnaires. This section describes four questionnaires available to measure user interaction or user interface satisfaction:

- System Usability Scale (SUS) (Bangor et al., 2008; Sauro, 2011)
- Questionnaire for User Interaction Satisfaction (QUIS) (Norman et al., 1998)
- Purdue Usability Testing Questionnaire (Lin et al., 1997)
- Software Usability Measurement Inventory (SUMI) (Kirakowski & Corbett, 1993)

The SUS is considered an industry standard among UX professionals and has been used widely on a variety of products outside of and internal to healthcare (Bangor et al., 2008; Sauro, 2011). The SUS is a publicly available, 10-item scale developed in 1986 by John Brooke at Digital Equipment Corporation (Bangor et al., 2008).

Developed in the late 1990s, QUIS addresses users' overall perceptions of a product, including overall reaction, terminology, screen layout, learning, system capabilities, and other subscales such as multimedia applications (Norman et al., 1998). QUIS subscales can be mixed and matched to fit the application at hand. Participants can complete the QUIS in about 5 to 10 minutes. Reliability and validity assessments are available for this tool.

The Purdue Usability Testing Questionnaire has 100 open-ended questions about how features adhere to accepted guidelines. Students would need to be familiar with design guidelines before using this questionnaire (Lin et al., 1997). However, reliability and validity assessments of the questionnaire are not reported.

Less information is available about the SUMI, including its assessed reliability and validity. The instrument has three components: an overall assessment, a usability profile, and an item consensus analysis (Kirakowski & Corbett, 1993). The usability profile examines areas such as efficiency, helpfulness, control, and learnability. The consensus component addresses adherence to well-known design alternatives such as categorical ordering of data in a simple search task.

SELECTING A TYPE OF USABILITY TEST

A key decision before beginning a UX assessment is determining the type of study to conduct in a specific case. This section expands on work by Rubin and Chisnell and uses the system's life cycle to organize the types of tests available (Rubin & Chisnell, 2008).

Determining User Needs and Requirements

Informaticians determine user needs and requirements during the initial design or redesign process, at the beginning of the systems life cycle, using the following:

- Users' characteristics
- Tasks (including cognitive tasks)
- Work design
- Interactions among workers and tasks and products
- Requirements about the specific environments and particular needs related to the context of interactions

Studies can be conducted with limited resources if the scope of the investigation is focused. As the complexity increases, resource consumption increases concomitantly. Assessments early in the systems life cycle seek to answer the following questions:

- Who are the users and what are their characteristics?
- What are basic activities and tasks in this context?
- How do users cognitively process information?
- What information processing can be supported by products?
- What special considerations should be made for users in this environment?
- What attributes need to be in place for an initial design?

Observations using think-aloud protocol and task analysis can be used to determine users' needs and requirements and answer the questions listed previously.

Example of a Requirements Determination Usability Study

Researchers completed a series of studies focused on nurses' acute care handoffs or change of shift reports to determine the current state of the activity and to develop requirements to support handoff tasks (Staggers et al., 2011; Staggers & Jennings, 2009; Staggers et al., 2012). Handoffs are highly complex and cognitively intensive periods where nurses going off shift synthesize information about patients and communicate it to nurses coming on shift. Methods that would generate rich details about the process, such as observation, field notes, and interviews, were selected. The HHCI framework guided the thinking about requirements analysis for different aspects of the handoff process. For example, researchers considered nurses (expertise levels, regular vs. travel nurses), types of units (critical care, emergency department, medical, and surgical), and types of product support in place (EHRs, CPOE, eMAR). Handoff tasks can be completed in a variety of ways, including audio recordings, face-to-face interactions, and bedside reports. The researchers completed a focused ethnography across available medical and surgical units in different facilities. They observed change of shift reports, audiotaped nurses, photographed nurses' tools, and took field notes about nurses' interactions with the existing EHRs in the facilities. From the findings, the researchers were able to derive detailed information about requirements for computerized support for change of shift activities (Staggers et al., 2012).

Formative Tests

Formative tests are conducted earlier in the systems life cycle after requirements are determined. These tests are conducted on preliminary designs/redesigns when fewer resources have been committed to programming the product. Methods are often more informal and involve extensive interactions between the evaluator and user. Results often produce rich data (e.g., from think-alouds). The objective of a very early formative test is to assess the effectiveness of emerging design concepts by asking the following:

- Is the basic functionality of value to users?
- Is basic navigation and information flow intuitive?
- Is fundamental content missing?

- How much computer experience does a user need to use this module (Rubin & Chisnell, 2008)?

The usability focus is on the effectiveness goal. Users are asked to perform common tasks with the prototype or step through paper mockups of the application using the think-aloud method. At this assessment, researchers strive to understand *why* users are behaving as they do with the application rather than how quickly they perform (Staggers et al., 2011). To assess effectiveness, the researcher is interested in finding cognitive disconnects with basic functions, missing information or steps, and assessing how easily users understand the task at hand.

Nielsen recommends having at least five users perform think-aloud protocols as an observer watches them and records any issues. This number of users can detect as much as 60% to 80% of design errors (Nielsen, 1993, 2000). Later research confirmed that as few as five to eight users are sufficient for most early usability tests (Shneiderman & Plaisant, 2010; Dumas & Fox, 2008).

Examples of Formative Tests

A public health researcher wanted to develop an application to display reportable patient conditions across jurisdictions. After researching available applications and completing requirements, she developed a prototype using PowerPoint to meet initial requirements and to assess usability for the following sample tasks: (1) find out whether chlamydia is a reportable condition in Utah, Colorado, or Washington; (2) determine the time frame for reporting the condition; and (3) ascertain whether a specimen must be submitted and the location for the submission. She selected key public health, clinical, and laboratory users as participants in the test. These users were asked to think aloud as they completed common tasks. The researcher took notes to record the data related to their responses. Using these data, several iterations of the prototype were designed to improve the usability in completing the tasks (Rajeev, 2012).

A second example of a formative test is one conducted midway through the development of a product application (Rubin & Chisnell, 2008). After the organization and general design were determined, this type of test assessed lower-level operations of the application, stressing the efficiency goals of the product (vs. effectiveness in the above example) and how well the task is presented to users. The researcher assessed a subsequent version of the public health application described previously. She asked the same key users to use the same tasks, but now participants commented on operations, icons, and the arrangement of the radio buttons.

Questions during this test might include the following:
- How quickly and accurately can users perform selected tasks?
- Are the terms in the system consistent across modules?
- Are operations displayed in a manner that allows quick detection of critical information?

Users performed common tasks with a product that was partially developed. Usability measures (see Table 22.3) such as performance time and errors are often selected. Users can perform tasks silently or researchers can use think-aloud methods to elicit issues. Again, designers use the results to craft a redesigned prototype to correct issues.

Validation Test

A validation test is completed later in the systems life cycle using a more mature product. This type of test assesses how this particular product compares to a predetermined standard, benchmark, or performance measure. A second purpose might be to assess how all modules in a technology application work as an integrated whole. For instance, a validation test can be useful in a system selection process to decide how a new vendor supports critical tasks such as medication barcoding or medication reconciliation. Questions for a validation test might include the following:
- Can 80% of users retrieve the correct complete blood count (CBC) test results within 10 seconds of interacting with the system?
- How many heuristic violations are identified for this product?
- Can users complete admission orders for a trauma patient with no errors?

This type of test is more structured, so it precludes interactions between testers and users. Performance measures mentioned earlier are employed as users interact to complete the benchmark testing. The methods are carefully structured. Accurate testing with representative end users is critical to successful formative and validation testing. The use of publicly available use case for testing can help identify known hazards across health IT systems to allow for mitigation and safe design (Ways to Improve Electronic Health Record Safety, 2018).

Example of a Validation Test

A nurse researcher wanted to ensure that a new mobile device for rural care in Tanzania mirrored the established algorithms on paper. The goal was to assess whether the algorithms used with the mobile device were 100% accurate. She enlisted key users and informaticians to interact with each pathway in the device. Deviations from the established algorithms were documented and corrected (Perri, 2012).

Comparison Test

Readers can conduct comparison tests at any point in the systems life cycle, but they are more commonly done to compare an existing design with a redesign or to compare two different design solutions for the same application. The major objective of this usability test is to determine which application, design, or product is more effective, efficient, and satisfying (Rubin & Chisnell, 2008). The study design can range from an informal side-by-side comparison with structured tasks or use of a classic experimental study design. Results are more dramatic if the designs are substantially different.

Examples of a Comparison Study

The purpose of this study was to determine whether a new user interface for orders management was different than an older interface in terms of performance times, errors, and user satisfaction (Staggers et al., 2007). The tasks and interactions were planned to minimize the amount of time that nurses would be away from patient care. The informaticians used an HCI framework to guide elements in the study. Users interacted on identical computers to test both interfaces. Tasks were "real-world" orders and identical for the two designs. The environment was a computer training room away from patient care units and distractions. The developmental trajectory was considered in this study to ensure that results were not affected by practice time. Therefore 40 tasks for each interface allowed nurses to become practiced at each user interface. (The threshold of task numbers was determined in pilot work.) Tasks, keystrokes, and errors were captured automatically by the computer. The QUIS was administered after each interface to assess user satisfaction. Each nurse interacted with both interfaces, but the order in which they were presented was randomized. The results showed the new interface was significantly faster, had fewer errors, and produced high user satisfaction.

A nurse researcher, in a second study, wanted to compare the traditional design of physiologic monitors and other products to a new design that integrated data across physiologic parameters, medication management, and communication (Koch et al., 2013). His target population was intensive care unit (ICU) nurses. The tasks were designed so that the study could be completed in about 20 to 30 minutes in each of two sessions. Paper prototypes were used to assess effectiveness, efficiency, and satisfaction before resources were expended to code bidirectional interfaces to the devices. Tasks were defined, and nurses interacted with the prototypes. Findings were that the new, integrated monitor view resulted in faster task times, higher detection of potential medication interactions, lower perceived mental workload, and higher satisfaction.

Identifying Usability Issues With Fielded Health IT Products

As organizations begin to understand the importance of the UX, leaders may be unsure where to begin identifying usability issues in their current environments. The following list includes symptoms of potential strategic usability issues and provides a framework for determining where initial energy and resources could be focused (HIMSS, 2011):

- Products or applications requiring long training times
- Support calls categorized by product or application
- Adverse events related to product interactions
- Lists of requested system change requests typically tracked in a database of system change requests across users and products
- User group requests for updates or changes
- Users' descriptions of their most vexing applications and interactions
- Users' identified delays or errors when they interact with complex applications, especially any requiring information synthesis such as eMARs, clinical summaries, and handoffs

Once a usability problem is suspected, researchers or students begin assessing the issue more systematically using the techniques described previously.

Steps for Conducting User Experience Tests

Readers, at some point in their careers, will likely want to conduct a usability project. Step-by-step guides are available (Health Information Management and Systems Society [HIMSS], 2009; Rubin & Chisnell, 2008; Lowry et al., 2012).

The texts by Crandell, Klein, and Hoffman; (Crandall et al., 2006) Rubin and Chisnell; (Rubin & Chisnell, 2008) and Tullis and Albert (Tullis & Albert, 2008) can act as specific guides. HIMSS (Health Information Management and Systems Society [HIMSS], 2009) and the National Institute of Standards and Technology (NIST) (Lowry et al., 2012) have published guides for conducting usability tests on EHRs. For instance, the NIST suggests using both HE and summative testing to evaluate products, especially EHRs.

1. The basic steps for conducting usability tests can be summarized as follows: *Define a clear purpose.* The specific purpose guides testers to determine the type of study, methods, and users required. For example, if the purpose relates to assessment of a redesign of a CPOE module for an intraoperative surgical team, an exploratory test may be indicated.

2. *Assess constraints.* Testers are always mindful of study constraints: time; resources; availability of the software to be evaluated; and availability of other equipment such as video cameras, testing labs, or users, especially if the users are specialists. These constraints may drive the type of usability test. For example, if the tester's goal is to evaluate an application to support anesthesiologists, these time-constrained physicians may not be willing to spend more than 15 to 20 minutes participating in a usability test. Tasks, methods, and products are defined to work within this constraint.

3. *Use an HCI framework to define pertinent components.* Use a framework to assess each component against the planned study. Who are the key users? What are typical tasks? What information needs to be exchanged? What product characteristics and which actions are needed? What is the setting or context? Will it be a naturalistic setting to determine exactly how an application will be used or a laboratory setting to control interruptions? What is a representative time in the developmental trajectory? How much practice time needs to be considered, especially if the design is new? Be sure to examine the latter component carefully to ensure a valid comparison between users' interactions with a new product and a current one by including practice time in the study.

4. *Match methods to the purpose, constraints, and framework assessment.* Methods that produce rich results such as a think-aloud protocol will match a purpose of understanding key user requirements, while a more structured method will allow a comparison of new and old designs. Long training and practice times for complex devices may constrain the number of tasks testers can offer. Other basic methodological steps are as follows:

- Select representative end users.
- Select a usability test appropriate to the purpose and point in the systems life cycle.
- Define and validate tasks.
- Measure key elements and control for others (e.g., measure performance time but control interruptions unless the effect of interruptions is the focus).
- Define the context to be used.
- Consider training and practice for new products.

- Pilot test methods before running the main study to smooth out procedures and bugs.

Once the methods are defined, all of these pieces can be put into action and the evaluation can be conducted.

CONCLUSION AND FUTURE DIRECTIONS

Usability issues have clear impacts on health IT users. In the United States, agencies are engaging in activities to improve the usability for health IT products (e.g., NIST, the Office of the National Coordinator for Health Information Technology, Agency for Healthcare Research & Quality). The Food and Drug Administration has required usability testing on medical devices for over 20 years, but other health IT vendors and health organizations are only beginning to employ the principles and processes for improving usability. The most immediate future direction concerns usability education and understanding action steps to be taken. Organizations need to increase their knowledge and skills related to improving usability. One way is to use the material outlined by the HIMSS Usability Task Force in 2011 on a Health Usability Maturity Model (HIMSS, 2011). The ONC Change Package for Improving EHR Usability also contains resources to help health systems identify and improve EHR usability in coordination with health IT vendors, usability professionals, and front-line healthcare providers (Office of the National Coordinator for Health Information Technology, 2018). These materials can guide organizations in assessing their current level of usability, employing methods to market usability to the organization, and increasing the usability to reach a strategic level.

Future usability directions will require multiple routes for improvement. Strategic directions might include the development of a national clearinghouse or organization to track usability issues and solutions. In particular, tracking for issues related to patient safety and health IT use is needed. A 2019 study demonstrated potential safety issues the recently implemented ONC EHR surveillance program (Pacheco et al., 2019).

Continued reporting and distribution of hazards will help all vendors and health systems improve the usability of the technology by improving safety and efficiency in implemented tools. Usability recommendations from AMIA and other organizations should be implemented to include an expanded research agenda for health IT and usability. Identified usability issues should also have a "home" within respective professional organizations (e.g., nurses might collaborate with HIMSS or the American Nurses Association on a repository for usability solutions). The future might include the use of automated methods to ensure that designs conform to known standards, especially basic screen designs. Best practices in usability and implementations should be employed. The future must include a focus on health IT products that support the way users think and work in health settings. There is evidence that health IT vendors have also significantly improved their usability practices over time (Ratwani et al., 2015; Hettinger et al., 2021).

This chapter described current issues with technology, definitions, or terms and the potential benefits of improving the usability in health organizations. Axioms of usability were defined: an early and central focus on users in the design and development of systems, iterative design of applications, and systematic usability measures. Across HCI frameworks, these major elements exist: users, products, contexts, tasks, information, interactions, and a developmental trajectory. Common usability methods and tests were discussed, and examples were provided. Readers are now prepared to conduct discount usability tests and several types of formative, summative, validation, and comparison usability tests. Readers have examples of performance and benchmark measures and four steps outlining the planning and conducting of usability tests.

ACKNOWLEDGMENT

The authors wish to acknowledge the contribution of Nancy Staggers to the previous edition of this chapter.

▮ DISCUSSION QUESTIONS

1. Complex interactions of users, information technology, and the environment make up the sociotechnical system. Why is the consideration of this system important to patient care and safety?
2. Usability can be defined as the ability of an individual to interact with a product. Usability can affect any work environment and impact work outcomes. Explain how computer usability effects your work effectiveness, efficiency, and satisfaction.
3. Ergonomics, or the ability to interface with the physical characteristics of a tool, system, or machine, is essential for safety and comfort. Identify a tool in your work environment and describe how ergonomics impacts tool use and outcomes.
4. What are considerations that go into selecting different types of formative vs. summative usability tests?
5. Identify key human-computer interaction (HCI) issues and considerations about HCI and cognitive informatics that affect the use of a computer in a healthcare environment.

CASE STUDY

Midcity Hospital System, the largest hospital system in a metropolitan area, was slow to adopt an electronic health record (EHR). Midcity was comprised of six smaller facilities and urgent care centers and needed a better method of communicating for patient care. Senior leadership decided to install a new EHR.

DISCUSSION QUESTIONS

1. What factors should leadership consider when deciding whether to install a new EHR or modify the current EHR? Include team membership, task characteristics, and considerations about human-computer interaction.

2. What key issues related to hospital personnel and other stakeholders are important to consider when determining what hardware components should be used and where they should be located?

3. What factors and users should be considered when addressing the EHR's usability?

4. What types of usability testing should the leadership team consider before a 'go live' with the new system? What types of usability testing should be considered to determine the success of adoption?

REFERENCES

ACP. (2013). Survey of clinicians: user satisfaction with electronic health records has decreased since 2010. http://www.acponline.org/pressroom/ehrs_survey.htm/.

AMA. (2014). AMA calls for design overhaul of electronic health records to improve usability. http://www.ama-assn.org/ama/pub/news/news/2014/2014-09-16-solutions-to-ehr-systems.page/.

Ammenwerth, E., Iller, C., & Mahler, C. (2006). IT-adoption and the interaction of task, technology and individuals: A fit framework and a case study. *BMC Medical Informatics and Decision Making,* 6(3), 1–13.

Ash, J. S., Berg, M., & Coiera, E. (2004). Some unintended consequences of information technology in health care: the nature of patient care information system-related errors. *Journal of the American Medical Informatics Association,* 11(2), 104–112.

Ash, J. S., Sittig, D. F., Dykstra, R., Campbell, E., & Guappone, K. (2007). Exploring the unintended consequences of computerized physician order entry. *Studies in Health Technology and Informatics,* 129(Pt 1), 198–202.

Ash, J. S., Sittig, D. F., Dykstra, R., Campbell, E., & Guappone, K. (2009). The unintended consequences of computerized provider order entry: findings from a mixed methods exploration. *International Journal of Medical Informatics,* 78(Suppl 1), S69–S76.

Ash, J. S., Sittig, D. F., Poon, E. G., Guappone, K., Campbell, E., & Dykstra, R. H. (2007). The extent and importance of unintended consequences related to computerized provider order entry. *Journal of the American Medical Informatics Association,* 14(4), 415–423.

Bangor, A., Kortum, P., & Miller, J. T. (2008). An empirical evaluation of the system usability scale. *International Journal of Human–Computer Interaction,* 24(6), 574–594.

Benda, N. C., Meadors, M. L., Hettinger, A. Z., & Ratwani, R. M. (2016 Jun 1). Emergency physician task switching increases with the introduction of a commercial electronic health record. *Annals of Emergency Medicine,* 67(6), 741–746.

Benda, N. C., Meadors, M. L., Hettinger, A. Z., & Ratwani, R. M. (2016 Jun 1). Emergency physician task switching increases with the introduction of a commercial electronic health record. *Annals of Emergency Medicine,* 67(6), 741–746.

Beuscart-Zephir, M. C., Borycki, E., Carayon, P., Jaspers, M. W., & Pelayo, S. (2013). Evolution of human factors research and studies of health information technologies: the role of patient safety. *Yearbook of Medical Informatics,* 8(1), 67–77.

Bias, R. G., & Mayhew, D. J. (2005). *Cost-justifying usability: An update for the internet age.* San Francisco, CA: Morgan Kaufman.

Borycki, E. M., Kushniruk, A. W., Bellwood, P., & Brender, J. (2012). Technology-induced errors. The current use of frameworks and models from the biomedical and life sciences literatures. *Methods of Information in Medicine,* 51(2), 95–103.

Carayon P., Wooldridge A., Hoonakker P., Hundt A.S., Kelly M. M. (2020). SEIPS 3.0: Human-centered design of the patient journey for patient safety. *Applied Ergonomics,* 84: 103033. doi: 10.1016/j.apergo.2019.103033.

Carayon, P., Xie, A., & Kianfar, S. (2014). Human factors and ergonomics as a patient safety practice. *BMJ Quality & Safety,* 23(3), 196–205.

Courage, C., Redish, J., & Wixon, D. (2008). Task analysis. In A. Sears & J. Jacko (Eds.), *The human-computer interaction handbook* (pp. 928–937). New York: Lawrence Erlbaum Associates.

Crandall, B., Klein, G., & Hoffman, R. (2006). Incident-based CTA: helping practitioners "tell stories." In B. Crandall, G. Klein, & R. R. Hoffman (Eds.), *Working minds: A practitioner's guide to cognitive task analysis* (pp. 69–90). Cambridge, MA: The MIT Press.

Despont-Gros, C., Mueller, H., & Lovis, C. (2005). Evaluating user interactions with clinical information systems: a model based on human- computer interaction models. *Journal of Biomedical Informatics,* 38(3), 244–255.

Dey Consulting. (2009). Return on investment discussion articles. http://www.deyalexander.com.au/resources/uxd/roi.html/.

Dix, A., Finlay, J. E., Abowd, G. D., & Beale, R. (2004). *Human-computer interaction* (3rd ed.). Essex, England: Prentice-Hall.

Dray, S. M., & Karat, C. (1994). Human factors cost justification for an internal development project. In R. G. Bias & D. J. Mayhew (Eds.), *Cost-justifying usability* (pp. 111–122). San Francisco: Morgan Kauffman Publishers.

Drews, F. A., & Westenskow, D. R. (2006). The right picture is worth a thousand numbers: Data displays in anesthesia. *Human Factors,* 48(1), 59–71.

Dumas, J. S., & Fox, J. E. (2008). Usability testing: current practice and future directions. In A. Sears & J. Jacko (Eds.), *The human-computer interaction handbook: fundamentals, evolving* technologies and emerging applications (2nd ed.). New York: Lawrence Erlbaum.

Guo, J., Iribarren, S., Kapsandoy, S., Perri, S., & Staggers, N. (2011). eMAR user interfaces: A call for ubiquitous usability evaluations and product redesign. *Applied Clinical Informatics, 2*(2), 202–224.

Gurses, A. P., & Carayon, P. (2007). Performance obstacles of intensive care nurses. *Nursing Research, 56*(3), 185–194.

Hackos, J. T., & Redish, J. C. (1998). *User and task analysis for interface design.* New York: John Wiley & Sons.

Hammersley, M., & Atkinson, P. (2007). *Ethnography: Principles in practice* (3rd ed.). London: Routledge.

Healthcare Information and Management Systems Society (HIMSS). User Experience Committee. (2009). Defining and testing EMR usability: principles and proposed methods of EMR usability evaluation and rating. http://www.himss.org/ResourceLibrary/ContentTabsDetail.aspx?ItemNumber=41050/.

Healthcare Information and Management Systems Society (HIMSS). (2011). *Promoting usability in health organizations: Initial steps and progress toward a healthcare usability maturity model.* Chicago, IL: Health Information Management Systems Society.

Healthcare Information and Management Systems Society (HIMSS). (2016). Issues and solutions to nurses' user experiences with health IT; 2016. http://www.himss.org/library/user-experience-healthcare-it/.

Hettinger, A. Z., Melnick, E. R., & Ratwani, R. M. (2021 May). Advancing electronic health record vendor usability maturity: Progress and next steps. *Journal of the American Medical Informatics Association, 28*(5), 1029–1031.

Hettinger, A. Z., Roth, E. M., & Bisantz, A. M. (2017 Mar 1). Cognitive engineering and health informatics: applications and intersections. *Journal of Biomedical Informatics, 67*, 21–33.

HFES. (2012). Definitions of human factors and ergonomics. http://www.hfes.org/Web/EducationalResources/HFEdefinitionsmain.html#govagencies/.

Holden, R. J., Carayon, P., Gurses, A. P., Hoonakker, Peter, Schoofs Hundt, Ann, Ant Ozok, A., et al. (2013). SEIPS 2.0: A human factors framework for studying and improving the work of healthcare professionals and patients. *Ergonomics, 56*(11), 1669–1686.

Hollnagel, E., & Woods, D. (2005). *Joint cognitive systems: Foundations of cognitive systems engineering.* Boca Raton, FL: Taylor & Francis Group.

Hollnagel, E. (1997 Oct 1). Cognitive ergonomics: It's all in the mind. *Ergonomics, 40*(10), 1170–1182.

IOM. (2011). *Health IT and patient safety: Building safer systems for better care.* Washington, DC: The National Academies Press.

ISO. (1998). International Organization of Standards 9241-11. http://www.usabilitynet.org/tools/r_international.htm#9241-11/.

Johnson, C. M., Johnson, T. R., & Zhang, J. (2005). A user-centered framework for redesigning health care interfaces. *Journal of Biomedical Informatics, 38*(1), 75–87.

Kirakowski, J., & Corbett, M. (1993). SUMI: The software measurement inventory. *British Journal of Educational Technology, 24*, 210–212.

Koch S., Westenskow D., Weir C., James Agutter, Maral Haar, Matthias Görges, et al. ICU nurses' evaluations of integrated information integration in displays for ICU nurses on user satisfaction and perceived mental workload. Paper presented at the Medical Informatics Europe. Pisa, Italy.

Koch, S. H., Weir, C., Haar, M., et al. (2012). Intensive care unit nurses' information needs and recommendations for integrated displays to improve nurses' situation awareness. *Journal of the American Medical Informatics Association, 19*(4), 583–590.

Koch, S. H., Weir, C., Westenskow, D., et al. (2013). Evaluation of the effect of information integration in displays for ICU nurses on situation awareness and task completion time: A prospective randomized controlled study. *International Journal of Medical Informatics, 82*(8), 665–675.

Kushniruk, A., Triola, M., Stein, B., Borycki, E., & Kannry, J. (2004). The relationship of usability to medical error: An evaluation of errors associated with usability problems in the use of a handheld application for prescribing medications. *Studies in Health Technology and Informatics, 107*(Pt 2), 1073–1076.

Lin, H., Choong, Y., & Salvendy, G. (1997). A proposed index of usability: A method for comparing the relative usability of different software systems. *Behaviour & Information Technology, 16*(4-5), 267–278.

Lowry, S. Z., Quinn, M. T., Ramaiah, M., Schumacher, Robert M., Patterson, Emily S., North, Robert, et al. (2012). Technical evaluation, testing and validation of the usability of electronic health records. Rockville, MD: National Institute of Standards and Technology.

Middleton, B., Bloomrosen, M., Dente, M. A., Hashmat, Bill, Koppel, Ross, Marc Overhage, J., et al. (2013). Enhancing patient safety and quality of care by improving the usability of electronic health record systems: recommendations from AMIA. *Journal of the American Medical Informatics Association, 20*(e1), e2–e8.

Nielsen, J., & Gilutz, S. (2003). *Usability return on investment.* Fremont, CA: Nielsen Norman Group.

Nielsen, J., & Levy, J. (1994). Measuring usability-preference vs performance. *Communications of the ACM, 37*(4), 66–75.

Nielsen J. (1995). 10 Usability heuristics for interface design. http://www.nngroup.com/articles/ten-usability-heuristics/.

Nielsen J. (1992). Finding usability problems through heuristic evaluation. In: Paper presented at Proceedings of the SIGCHI Conference on Human Factors in Computing Systems. Monterey, CA.

Nielsen, J. (1994). Heuristic evaluation. In J. Nielsen & R. L. Mack (Eds.), *Usability inspection methods* (pp. 25–62). New York: John Wiley & Sons Inc.

Nielsen, J. (1993). *Usability engineering.* Cambridge, MA: AP Professional.

Nielsen, J. (2000). Why you only need to test with five users. http://www.nngroup.com/articles/why-you-only-need-to-test-with-5-users/.

Norman K., Shneiderman B., Harper B., Slaughter L. (1998). Questionnaire for user interaction satisfaction, version 7.0.1. http://lap.umd.edu/quis/.

Office of the National Coordinator for Health Information Technology. (2018). ONC change package for improving EHR usability. https://www.healthit.gov/sites/default/files/playbook/pdf/usability-change-plan.pdf Accessed September 20, 2021.

Pacheco, T. B., Hettinger, A. Z., & Ratwani, R. M. (2019 Dec 17). Identifying potential patient safety issues from the federal electronic health record surveillance program. *Journal of the American Medical Association, 322*(23), 2339–2340.

Patel, V. L., & Kannampallil, T. G. (2015). Cognitive informatics in biomedicine and healthcare. *Journal of Biomedical Informatics, 53*(3-14).

Perri, S. (2012). *Using electronic decision support to enhance provider-caretaker communication for treatment of children under five in Tanzania.* Salt Lake City, UT: University of Utah.

Pew Charitable Trust, (2015). *Conference on issues and solutions to electronic health record usability.* Washington DC: Pew Charitable Trust.

Philpott T. (2009). Doctors See bigger role in Electronic Health Record Reform. Stars and Stripes. http://www.stripes.com/.

Rajeev, D. (2012). *Development and evaluation of new strategies to enhance public health reporting.* Salt Lake City, UT: University of Utah.

Ratwani, R. M., Fairbanks, R. J., Hettinger, A. Z., & Benda, N. C. (2015 Nov 1). Electronic health record usability: analysis of the user-centered design processes of eleven electronic health record vendors. *Journal of the American Medical Informatics Association,* 22(6), 1179–1182.

Ratwani, R. M., Savage, E., Will, A., Arnold, R., Khairat, S., Miller, K., Fairbanks, R. J., Hodgkins, M., & Hettinger, A. Z. (2018 Sep). A usability and safety analysis of electronic health records: A multi-center study. *Journal of the American Medical Informatics Association,* 25(9), 1197–1201.

Rubin, J., & Chisnell, D. (2008). *Handbook of usability testing: How to plan, design and conduct effective tests.* New York: John Wiley & Sons.

Saitwal, H., Feng, X., Walji, M., Patel, V., & Zhang, J. (2010). Assessing performance of an electronic health record (EHR) using cognitive task analysis. *International Journal of Medical Informatics,* 79(7), 501–506.

Sauro J. (2011). Measuring usability with the system usability scale (SUS). http://www.measuringusability.com/sus.php/.

Shneiderman, B., & Plaisant, C. (2010). *Designing the user interface: Strategies for effective human-computer interaction* (5th ed.). Boston: Addison-Wesley.

Shneiderman, B., & Plaisant, K. (2005). Designing the user interface: Strategies for effective human-computer interaction (4th ed.). Boston, MA: Pearson/Addison-Wesley.

Souza, R., Sonderegger, P., Roshan, S., & Dorsey, M. (2001). *Get ROI from design.* Cambridge, MA: Forrester Research;.

Staggers, N., Clark, L., Blaz, J. W., & Kapsandoy, S. (2012). Nurses' information management and use of electronic tools during acute care handoffs. *Western Journal of Nursing Research,* 34(2), 153–173.

Staggers, N., Clark, L., Blaz, J. W., & Kapsandoy, S. (2011). Why patient summaries in electronic health records do not provide the cognitive support necessary for nurses' handoffs on medical and surgical units: insights from interviews and observations. *Health Informatics Journal,* 17(3), 209–223.

Staggers, N., Elias, B. L., Hunt, J. R., Makar, E., & Alexander, G. L. (2015). Nursing-centric technology and usability a call to action. *Computers, Informatics, Nursing: CIN,* 33(8), 325–332.

Staggers, N., Iribarren, S., Guo, J. W., & Weir, C. (2015). Evaluation of a BCMA's Electronic Medication Administration Record. *Western Journal of Nursing Research,* 37(7), 899–921.

Staggers, N., Jennings, B. M., & Lasome, C. E. (2010). A usability assessment of AHLTA in ambulatory clinics at a military medical center. *Military Medicine,* 175(7), 518–524.

Staggers, N., & Jennings, B. M. (2009). The content and context of change of shift report on medical and surgical units. *Journal of Nursing Administration,* 39(9), 393–398.

Staggers, N., Kobus, D., & Brown, C. (2007). Nurses' evaluations of a novel design for an electronic medication administration record. *Computers, informatics, nursing: CIN* 25(2), 67–75.

Staggers, N., & Parks, P. L. (1992). Collaboration between unlikely disciplines in the creation of a conceptual framework for nurse-computer interactions. *Proceedings of the Annual Symposium on Computer Applications in Medical Care,* 661–665.

Staggers, N. (2001). Human-computer interaction. In S. Englebardt & R. Nelson (Eds.), *Information technology in health care: An interdisciplinary approach* (pp. 321–345). Orlando, FL: Harcourt Health Science Company.

Staggers, N. (2013). Improving the usability of health informatics applications. In T. Hebda & P. Czar (Eds.), *Handbook of informatics for nurses and health professionals* (pp. 170–193). Upper Saddle River, NJ: Pearson.

Staggers, N. (2011). The April 2011 hearing on EHR usability. Column on crucial conversations about optimal design column. *Online Journal of Nursing Informatics (OJNI),* 15(2).

Stead, W., & Lin, H. (2009). *Computational technology for effective healthcare: Immediate steps and strategic directions.* Washington, DC: National Academies Press.

Sweeney, M., Maguire, M., & Shackel, B. (1993). Evaluating user-computer interaction: a framework. *International Journal of Man-Machine Studies,* 38, 689–711.

Syroid, N. D., Agutter, J., Drews, F. A., et al. (2002). Development and evaluation of a graphical anesthesia drug display. *Anesthesiology,* 96(3), 565–575.

The Joint Commission (TJC). (2015). Safe Use of Health Information Technology; www.jointcommission.org/.

Thompson, C. B., Snyder-Halpern, R., & Staggers, N. (1999). Analysis, processes, and techniques. Case study. *Computers in Nursing,* 17(5), 203–206.

Tullis, T., & Albert, B. (2008). *Measuring the user experience: Collecting, analyzing and presenting usability metrics.* New York: Elsevier.

Viitanen, J. (2011). Contextual inquiry method for user-centred clinical IT system design. *Studies in Health Technology and Informatics,* 169, 965–969.

Virzi, R. A. (1992). Refining the test phase of usability evaluation: how many subjects is enough? *Human Factors,* 34(4), 457–468.

Wachter, S. B., Johnson, K., Albert, R., Syroid, N., Drews, F., & Westenskow, D. (2006). The evaluation of a pulmonary display to detect adverse respiratory events using high resolution human simulator. *Journal of the American Medical Informatics Association,* 13(6), 635–642.

Wang, Y. (2003 Aug). On cognitive informatics. *Brain and Mind,* 4(2), 151–167.

Wang, Y. (2007 Jan 1). The theoretical framework of cognitive informatics. *International Journal of Cognitive Informatics and Natural Intelligence (IJCINI),* 1(1), 1–27.

Ways to Improve Electronic Health Record Safety. A report from The Pew Charitable Trusts, American Medical Association, & Medstar Health, Aug 2018. https://www.pewtrusts.org/-/media/assets/2018/08/healthit_safe_use_of_ehrs_report.pdf. Accessed 9/21/21.

Wei, J., & Salvendy, G. (2004). The cognitive task analysis methods for job and task design: Review and reappraisal. *Behavior & Information Technology,* 23(4), 273–299.

Zhang J., Butler K.A. UFuRT: A work-centered framework and process for design and evaluation of information systems. Paper presented at Proceedings of HCI International; July 22–27. Beijing, China.

Zhang, J., Johnson, T. R., Patel, V. L., Paige, D. L., & Kubose, T. (2003). Using usability heuristics to evaluate patient safety of medical devices. *Journal of Biomedical Informatics,* 36(1–2), 23–30.

Zhang, J., & Walji, M. F. (2011). TURF: Toward a unified framework of EHR usability. *Journal of Biomedical Informatics,* 44(6), 1056–1067.

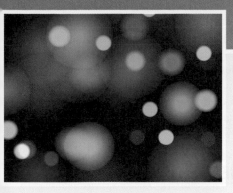

23

Data Science and Analytics in Healthcare

Louis Luangkesorn

OBJECTIVES

At the completion of this chapter, the reader will be prepared to:
1. Describe terms and concepts related to data science in healthcare.
2. Describe how the 3 Vs encapsulate the innate characteristics of complex data.
3. Discuss the fundamentals of data science.
4. Discuss the 3 types of data analytics.
5. Describe components of the data science life cycle.
6. Describe key factors in preprocessing data.
7. Describe the overarching premise of predictive analytics.
8. Discuss basic organizational considerations within data science.

KEY TERMS

data analytics, 360
data governance, 371
data science, 359
ethics, 372

exploratory data analysis, 361
learning health system, 358
machine learning, 358
model evaluation, 365

predictive analytics, 361
prescriptive analytics, 361

ABSTRACT ❖

On December 15, 2019, the National Center for Advancing Translational Sciences (NCATS), one of the National Institutes of Health (NIH), set up an Open Data Portal to share data on rare tropical diseases. Less than a month later the first COVID-19 diagnosis was added to the database. This fast-track response and sharing of critical information enabled the prioritization of drugs, development of protocols, and clinical trials to move faster than ever in a coordinated fashion. Christopher Austin of the NIH stated, "what's different is that inefficiency, duplication, time lags, and lack of sharing was wrung out of the system," leading to the speed of development (National Academies of Science, Engineering, and Medicine, 2021). This rapid discovery and dissemination of clinical data and the resulting rapid development of therapeutics illustrates the promise of data science in healthcare, using a large volume of data from disparate sources and types to lead to a rapid advance in patient care. The President's Council of Advisors on Science and Technology (PCAST) routinely reviews the status of the United States (US) abilities to manage the health and welfare of the population through technology and data science. More recent reports address three main pillars supporting their decisions, (1) enhancing a multicenter engagement in research and innovation,

(2) creating a new institute structure integrating Industries of the Future in discovery research to product development, and (3) creating new modalities for ensuring the availability of a qualitative diverse IoTF workforce. Within these pillars, PCAST makes special note of the discovery of new therapies and acceleration of their translation to novel healthcare treatments, diagnoses, care delivery, and cost lowering; all performed using informatics (President's Council of Advisors on Science and Technology, 2020). However, in its 2010 report, *Realizing the Full Potential of Health Information Technology to Improve Healthcare for Americans: The Path Forward*, the PCAST (President's Council of Advisors on Science and Technology, 2010) noted that information technology has the potential to transform healthcare as it has transformed many other aspects of society. It can give clinicians access to complete patient data and provide them with support to make decisions, help patients become more involved in their care, enable population level public health monitoring, and streamline processes to improve healthcare delivery. However, it does not happen automatically. Oracle defines data science as combining multiple quantitative fields, including statistics, artificial intelligence, and data analysis, as extracting value from data (Oracle, 2021). This includes preparing data for

analysis, applying quantitative methods, and reviewing the results to uncover and interpret patterns and enable leaders to draw insights that inform decisions. Achieving the promise of healthcare analytics requires infrastructure and analysts who can integrate the information available and synthesize it to inform medical decision-making and healthcare organizations' activity. This chapter introduces approaches to data science, analytics, and knowledge building from health data. It then explores the application of data analytic processes in healthcare and describes organizational needs for data science, such as personnel and data governance. The chapter concludes with discussions on data governance, privacy, and ethical considerations in the application of data science in healthcare.

INTRODUCTION

Data science and data analytics have the potential to transform healthcare in many dimensions. Individual patient-doctor relationships can be extended from only occasional in-person visits by medical devices that can monitor body measurements over time and add the measurements to the patient record. Physician experience and intuition may be informed by decision support systems that draw on information from a wide range of patients with a range of characteristics, providing more variety than just "typical" patients. Ongoing care may be customized for an individual's genetic and physical characteristics (Ginsburg et al., 2018). Clinic or hospital operations can be evaluated to ensure the availability of healthcare providers when they are needed.

However, there are obstacles to achieving this. Organizations must develop strategies for data governance, to include data storage and analytics, ensuring the organization achieves to protect and respect the privacy and rights of patients and personnel. These strategies are supported through multidisciplinary leadership that uses a learning health system culture for healthcare improvement. This culture builds a team science approach combining subject matter experts, database and computational programmers, and data science specialists collaborating with all levels of stakeholders to design, develop, and deploy these solutions.

DATA SCIENCE IN HEALTHCARE

Defining Data Science

Defining *data science* is like defining *health informatics*; there is no single definition, and it depends on whom you are asking. Data science is the knowledge, organization, testing, organizing, and understanding of scientific methods and processes associated with structured or unstructured data. Fig. 23.1 provides a visual understanding of the components required within the data science ecosystem, using systems that include data, computing, programming, statistics and analytics, machine learning (ML), and mathematics.

Data science in healthcare is multifocal. Physician *data scientists* may consider the diagnostic abilities of machine learning (ML) to identify an illness or the use of an algorithm to determine a medical action. A nurse *informaticist* may consider the use of hospital data to determine overall resource use or the use of public health statistics to determine the incidence or prevalence of illness in their geographical area. A pharmacist may consider the use of medication distribution to determine overall drug expenses or collecting adverse events to determine medication adverse events. A computational data scientist may consider the aggregation of large data sets for predictive or preventive measures within a healthcare setting. Everyone loves data and the power it has to improve healthcare.

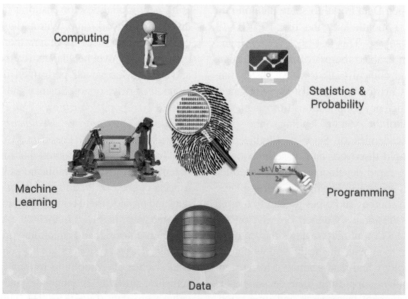

Fig. 23.1 Components of Data Science. (Copyrighted by Lynda R. Hardy.)

TABLE 23.1 Data Categories and Examples of Datasets in healthcare (Institute for Health Technology Transformation, 2013)

Data Category	Examples of Collected Data
Web and social media	Anything found on the internet
Transaction records	Claims data and billing records
Biometric	Vital signs, medical imaging, fingerprints, genetics, retinal scans, data from home use medical devices, robotics, handwriting
Machine generated	Uploads and readings from sensors and other devices
Human generated	Electronic health records, e-mail, paper documents

Data from Institute for Health Technology Transformation. (2013). *Transforming health care through big data: Strategies for leveraging big data in the health care industry.* Institute for Health Technology Transformation. http://c4fd63cb482ce6861463-bc6183f1c18e748a49b 87a25911a0555.r93.cf2.rackcdn.com/iHT2_BigData_2013.pdf.

Data science is the general process of converting raw data into actionable insights, meaning it offers a systematic approach to answering analytical questions to improve decision-making. Examples of applications areas within healthcare are listed in Table 23.1 (Institute for Health Technology Transformation, 2013).

Data sources in healthcare are a mixture of structured (e.g., laboratory values) and unstructured information (e.g., clinical notes). Using analytical techniques, data science has the potential to provide powerful insights across and within patients, institutions, regions, and nations. These data sources constitute an incredible resource that is currently underused for scientific research in healthcare.

- Analysis can be conducted to support the decision-making process at the individual patient or population level.
- Analyses can be used to develop policies and systems for population-level care.
- Analyses can be used to design healthcare delivery systems.
- Specific questions useful to analyze the population health management across millions of patients might include:
- Which treatments are associated with better outcomes for patients with kidney disease or specific carcinomas?
- How does obesity affect the need for joint replacement surgery at younger ages, and at what costs?
- How do patients' physiologic parameters compare to newer and previous cardiac medications?
- What algorithms are available to assist in patient care decision-making, such as atherosclerotic cardiovascular disease (ASCVD)?

Unlike traditional business reporting, these analyses require information across multiple sources such as patients' problem lists, histories, medications, lab and imaging results, and claims data (Peters & Buntrock, 2014). Some may include data aggregated from multiple sites or institutions.

Data science analyses for individual patients allow for more personalized care (precision medicine). For instance, a patient with diabetes might have metabolic rates, biochemical reactions, and responses to the insulin that could be analyzed against norms to pinpoint specific, individualized medication delivery doses and times, along with tailored nutritional guidance (Peters & Buntrock, 2014). Another example is the IBM Watson project that combines information from the entire corpus of published medical journals along with individuals' health records from healthcare organizations to suggest treatment pathways tailored to the individual, a method of personalized medicine (IBM, 2014). Similar individualized questions could be completed for genetic test results (O'Reilly et al., 2012). Data science also allows for rapid response on a population level. The same data used for personalized medicine can then be analyzed to identify population health trends, enabling a healthcare organization to monitor emerging health trends and issues among its patient population.

Part of the U.S. response to COVID-19 included actions by the National Center for Advancing Translational Sciences (NCATS) in accelerating translational research for developing treatment and informing responses to COVID-19. The Open Data Portal was used to share information on cases in a secure and privacy protecting manner. Healthcare workers were able to easily and safely share case data to contribute to the nationwide knowledge base and learn from others. This was especially important in the early days when the geographic region affected by COVID-19 was changing rapidly, and no one location had enough experience in working with it. The Center for Data to Health has enabled the linking of data on a million patients, 100 s of millions of lab results, and a billion rows of data. This has enabled faster development of therapies and vaccines than what had been historically the case. Christopher Austin of the National Institutes of Health (NIH) stated, "what's different is that inefficiency, duplication, time lags, and lack of sharing was wrung out of the system," leading to the speed of development (National Academies of Science, Engineering, and Medicine, 2021). Another source of near real-time data aggregation during the COVID-19 pandemic is the Johns Hopkins University Center for Systems Science and Engineering (CSSE) COVID-19 Dashboard (Dong et al., 2020). Fig. 23.2 shows real-time data representing the global incidence of COVID-19 from a public website by the JHU CSSE.

Other data science applications are quality improvement initiatives and learning health system projects. The potential for knowledge development is seemingly unlimited.

Informatics and US Healthcare Expenditures

Health informatics provides essential information related to the health of our nation. U.S. healthcare expenditures were 17.7% of the U.S. gross domestic product in 2019, an increase of 4.6% from the previous year (Centers for Medicare and Medicaid, 2020) and are expected to increase over time based on CMS National Health Expenditure Data (Keehan et al., 2020).

Health information technology (IT) can help leverage those monies by reducing costs and improving outcomes. However, routine use of IT, in and of itself, does not automatically lead to these benefits. Instead, these benefits are tied to specific uses of health IT within and across healthcare organizations, including the application of data science to improve healthcare delivery and patient care.

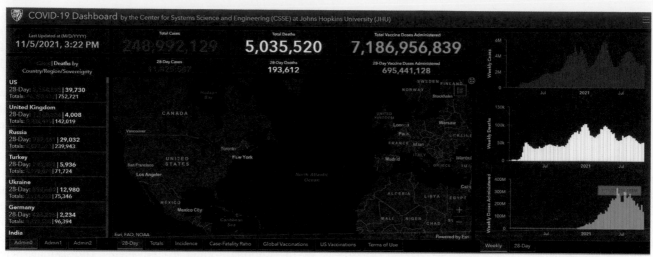

Fig. 23.2 Johns Hopkins COVID-19 Dashboard. (Johns Hopkins University https://coronavirus.jhu.edu/map.html.)

CHARACTERISTICS OF COMPLEX DATA

Volume, Velocity, Variety

Data science techniques are needed in settings where the data sets have complex characteristics. Five data characteristics are important in understanding the complex available data in healthcare, as seen in Box 23.1 (Eaton et al., 2012).

Volume refers to the sheer quantity of data generated and analyzed. In practical terms, data are often stored in distributed locations, and their size overwhelms the capability of individual workstations to process and analyze. Therefore, techniques for working with distributed data storage, such as cloud computing or computing clusters, need to be employed.

Velocity refers to the speed that data are generated and change over time. One important implication is that decisions need to be made rapidly in an evolving environment. Any analysis must be completed quickly enough to support decisions relevant to that data. Otherwise, decisions may not be useful or timely. Alternatively, we need the right information at the right time!

Variety means that the data come from many different sources simultaneously and in many different formats, as seen in Table 23.1. These include varied forms of storing or sharing data, different types of media (e.g., visual, audio, text, molecular), different rules surrounding data (e.g., security for HIPAA protected data), and alternate levels and sources of granularity (e.g., census data, billing, public health, electronic health records [EHRs], or social media). For example, payment data provided by the Centers for Medicare and Medicaid Services, hospital patient data, and hospital billing data are all from different sources and have different rules for use.

Veracity, Value

Veracity and *value* are two aspects that need to be addressed to make data useful to a healthcare organization. Veracity refers to the accuracy and completeness (the "truth") of the data or its opposite, the messiness of the data. The quality of individual data elements can vary greatly, especially when they are from multiple sources. The meaning of data elements must also be verified to confirm what a particular source assigns to a given data element that corresponds to the analyst's understanding of the same data element and its intended use.

Value recognizes that the purposes of collecting, processing, and analyzing data are to fill a need. For example, an acute care staffing mix that emphasizes more highly educated nurses can result in fewer patient complications; however, there is a point beyond which increased labor costs do not produce fewer complications (or produce value). In the context of value, a key component of any data project is the question the data are expected to answer and how a healthcare organization will respond to the results of the analysis.

A data scientist or analyst needs to manage data with mindful consideration of the five Vs of big data. An analyst or analytic team member should have computer programming skills to manage the data and have subject matter expertise to recognize how to test for the veracity of the data. The mathematical and statistical knowledge to perform correct analyses and present the results in a meaningful format to provide value to the organization.

BENEFITS OF DATA SCIENCE

Data Analytics Tools

Data science benefits are generated from using data aggregated from a wide range of resources that are beyond the ability of an individual person to aggregate and synthesize. Various forms of **data analytics** and tools are used to analyze healthcare operations across healthcare areas, including financial, operational, and clinical data. They can be used to coordinate care and/or business decisions over time and venues. The benefits can be

---

BOX 23.1	**The 5 Vs of Big Data**

- Volume
- Velocity
- Variety
- Veracity
- Value

seen in a better quality of care for the individual and the population as a whole and increased understanding while potentially lowering costs.

Deriving Benefits of Analytics

However, insights from data are not realized automatically through the installation of an analytics IT infrastructure and/or an EHR system. Deriving benefits of analytics requires a healthcare organization to (1) identify the required analytic capabilities at all levels of the organization, (2) ensure that the system has the required capabilities, and (3) commission appropriately educated personnel to plan and implement the analytic process from data to deployment, thereby ensuring ultimate translation (Trotter & Uhlman, 2013).

Regardless of whether data analytics are used for research or decision making, the approaches to analyses are similar. In the next section, these sample approaches are outlined.

APPROACHES TO APPLYING ANALYSES

There are three general categories of analytics: descriptive, predictive, and prescriptive (Lustig et al., 2010).

Descriptive Analytics

Descriptive analytics prepares and analyzes retrospective data to understand and analyze business performance or population demographics. The process of exploratory data analysis (EDA) includes the use of descriptive statistics (including summaries and data visualizations) and statistical analysis. The goal of EDA is to understand the state of a system, such as the distribution of inpatient stays among current patients in a hospital or the outcome of population-related data and information over time. Information and knowledge gained by revealing patterns and trends through EDA support more effective administrative or clinical decision-making. EDA can also be used to generate hypotheses that can be answered by analyzing available system data (e.g., the frequency of lab tests and their costs over the past year). The information discovered using EDA produces data reports or information dashboards using spreadsheets or web-based applications to view and interpret specific information to aid decision-makers.

Summary statistics are associated with two categories of measures: measures of centrality and measures of variability. Measures of centrality include the mean, median, or mode. These measures are what is meant when asked to quantify some characteristic often. The mean suggests a central value or the sum of values divided by the number of values. The median is the value that separates the higher numbers of a data set from the lower numbers. The mode is simply the number that appears most frequently in a given data set. These numbers may have little meaning in isolation. There must be a comparison of the observation. Observations are often compared to a standard but could be compared to other local observations or even the same subject over time. In this comparison, the next question is if any difference is meaningful. Healthcare professionals often ask this question—the difference may be statistically significant—but is it *clinically* significant? This requires a measure of variation. Some measures include the standard deviation, variance, interquartile range, or the range. Statistical methods use these measures to calculate specific statistics that can quantify the concepts of meaningful differences.

For graphical methods of EDA, there are a number of different types of charts that can be used that are available through various software packages and plotting programming libraries. The choice of chart types depends on the information being communicated and often the types of comparisons that will help the viewer provide context for the data. Fig. 23.3 provides a range of different chart types and the purposes they are used (Abela, 2020).

Another class of descriptive analytics is statistical inference. These include hypothesis testing such as t-tests and analysis of variance. These statistical tests are often used in combination with designed experiments to test a hypothesis about the source of the data to create insights into past observations. Bayesian statistics, which determine the probability of a hypothesis, can be applied where the goal is a probability model, and there is both observed data and additional information that can be used to form a prior belief about the underlying system (Gelman et al., 2013). For example, Bayesian methods can be used to estimate a probability distribution for the duration of surgical procedures, even in the case where a procedure has not been performed before (Luangkesorn & Eren-Doğu, 2015).

Predictive Analytics

Predictive analytics is the use of data and mathematical techniques to develop models of business performance that represent the relationship between data inputs and outputs/outcomes. Predictive analytics is a component of artificial intelligence (AI) or imitating intelligence or patterns. Within AI is ML, or how a computer can "learn" from data. Deeper into AI is deep learning that is inspired by how the human brain works or neural networks. This chapter will focus on the ML component of analytics. Predictive analytics methods, including machine and statistical learning (ML) methods, are commonly used in predictive analytics. Types of problems addressed in predictive analytics include:

Regression. Predicting an outcome or a new observation (e.g., predicting the effect of a treatment).

Classification. Predicting the category for a new outcome (e.g., predicting which patients will respond to a specific medication or treatment protocol).

Clustering. Grouping observations into similar groups (e.g., seeing that women who smoke have a higher rate of premature infants).

Association rules. Determining a new characteristic based on known characteristics of an observation (e.g., noting that people in a lower socioeconomic group have a higher rate of health literacy problems).

Predictive analytics will be described in more detail in the section on Predictive analytics.

Prescriptive Analytics

Prescriptive analytics refers to the use of models that determine a set of high-value alternative actions or decisions given a set of objectives, requirements, and constraints. These work

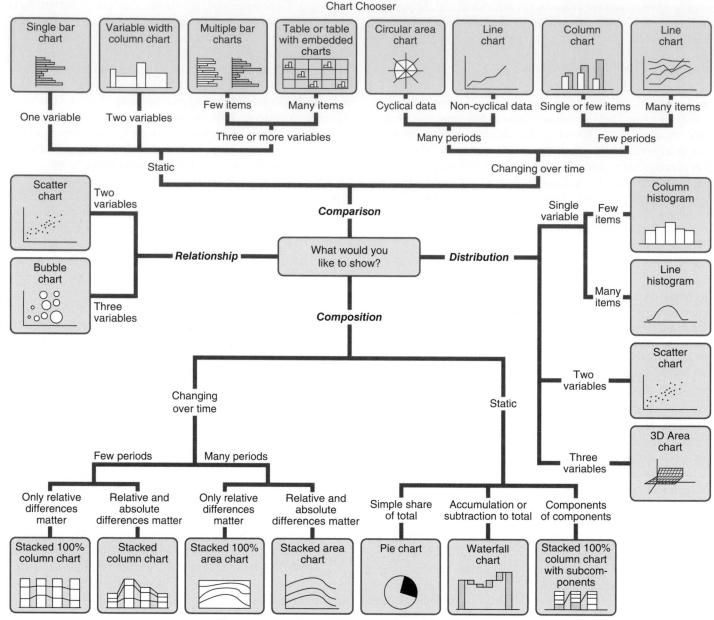

Fig. 23.3 Chart Chooser. (© 2020 Andrew, V. and Abela, A.)

through modeling the system and potential alternatives, considering requirements and constraints, and choosing between alternatives to improve system performance. Methods used in prescriptive analytics include decision models, including decision trees, queuing models, mathematical programming methods for optimization, and simulation. These methods have the advantage of being able to predict system output under a range of system configurations, allowing decision makers to choose the best of potential alternatives. This includes modeling systems that do not yet exist or will have major changes so that the historical experience may have little to do with the future. For example, simulation can be used to simulate a clinic under forecasted demands to test new design concepts and staffing plans (Luangkesorn et al., 2012). A range of these types of models,

including simulation, linear, decision trees, compartmental models, Markov models, and optimization models, have been used for evaluating policies for infectious disease control while looking at the decisions for individuals and institutions as well as population level policies. These models can evaluate options on a number of criteria, including health, economics, and equity (Long & Brandeau, 2009). During the COVID-19 pandemic, models were used to predict the spread of COVID-19 under a range of interventions in different settings, identified populations at high risk of infection and mortality based on individual characteristics, and informed government and healthcare providers in making decisions on meeting the demand for equipment and personnel (Bertsimas et al., 2021; Parker et al., 2021).

DATA SCIENCE LIFE CYCLE

Data science is an interactive process where that data scientists work with stakeholders (a team approach) to understand the problem, data experts to identify and understand the data available, then convert the data into forms suitable for the analytic methods that will be used. With every round of results presented to stakeholders, stakeholders typically respond to the insights with new questions and directions. This iterative nature of development, with the messiness of real-world data that is complex and ever changing, makes it different from most software environments that computer programming and software development experts are used to working in (Tuulos & Bowne-Anderson, 2021).

Data Science Applications

Developing data science applications is a mix of software engineering and experimental science. Compared to most software development projects, data science applications have exposure to constantly changing real-world conditions through the data and the real-world operations that collect that data. The need for empirical observation to learn the behavior of data science models, the behavior of people who interact with the models, and the relative importance of working with data and experimentation instead of computer code that is the focus of traditional software engineering creates additional complications in managing data science projects.

CRISP-DM Data Science Model

One framework used to organize the data science life cycle is the cross-industry standard process for data mining (CRISP-DM) (Fig. 23.4) (Chapman et al., 2000).

The CRISP-DM model provides an overview of the life cycle of a data science project. It covers the phases of a project, key relationships between phases, and highlights the cyclical nature of data science projects.

The first phase of the data science project is business understanding. This phase focuses on understanding the project objectives and requirements from a business perspective. This greater context allows developing a problem definition and a plan that can achieve the data science problem.

Data understanding starts with the initial data collection, then understanding the data through (EDA) and discussions with subject matter experts and stakeholders. Data dictionaries can provide some definitions of what available data fields are intended to represent. However, having an operational understanding of a data element requires a discussion with SMEs who are familiar with how the data element was collected and what was intended by the data collector. During this phase, initial insights gained during EDA and initial discussions lead to updating the business understanding.

The data preparation phase involves creating the datasets that will be used in analytic models. This starts with working with database administrators and data owners on accessing datasets. Database administrators refer to this process as Extract,

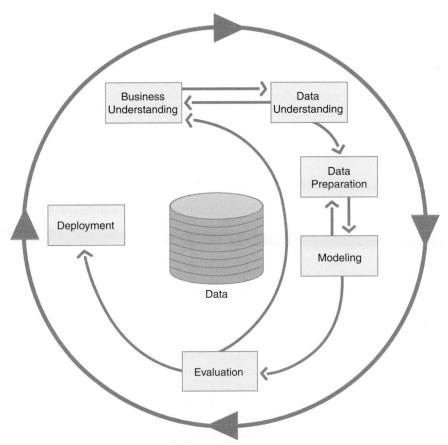

Fig. 23.4 CRISP-DM Life Cycle Phases.

Transform, Load (ETL). Almost all data analysis environments have included capabilities to extract data from data sources such as relational databases or formatted data files. More capable data analysis environments will include the capability to manipulate data using data manipulation language that implements the grammar of data manipulation: select, filter, mutate, arrange, group by and summarize, and join.

SQL is a common language used within relational databases. The grammar of data manipulation is also implemented in programming languages focused on data analysis using data frames such as R, Python, Scala, and Julia. Often SQL is used in extracting data from databases to take advantage of the database server capability then further transformation will be done within the data analysis environment. This stage will include data cleaning and data munging, where the data are transformed from the elements that are stored into elements that will be used within analytical methods.

Modeling is implementing the analytical method that will be applied. While CRISP-DM was originally developed in the context of data mining and ML, this also includes EDA and other analytical methods such as statistics or operations research.

After a model is developed, the output of the model must be reviewed with stakeholders in the evaluation phase. Here, the model and the steps to create it must be reviewed to be certain that the model can be used to achieve the business objectives. In early rounds, this evaluation will often reveal that important business issues have not been properly considered. The evaluation will lead to a decision on the goals for the next round of the CRISP-DM cycle or how the model will be implemented for use by decision makers or stakeholders.

The end goal for data science is deployment. In some cases, this would be a model that can be applied using up-to-date data by decision makers or stakeholders as part of the organization's decision-making process. In other cases, it will be a report that outlines the model, the insights, and how these insights can be used to inform ongoing decisions. In either case, the task of the analyst is to present that the model results in a form that is useful to the customer in the business context and leads to a course of action.

The outer circle in the CRISP-DM diagram emphasizes the cyclical nature of the CRISP-DM process. In contrast to waterfall development models, where known inputs are taken to create a previously specified product, data science follows a life cycle more familiar to experimental scientists. The first cycle through CRISP-DM is often an EDA, and the models are often statistical or graphical. The insights in the first cycle very frequently lead to large changes in the direction of the project compared to the initial idea, as disparate stakeholders are presented with a picture of the business context. The next cycles are often rough prototype models intended to provide stakeholders an understanding of what is possible and provoke reaction and feedback into what will be a final model that is usable for decision making. While it may be tempting to develop a project plan upfront and deliver features along a set timeline, using CRISP-DM in an agile manner and organizing the project into cycles has been shown to create value for stakeholders sooner. It allows for timely and meaningful stakeholder feedback, leads to earlier assessments of model performance, and allows for adjusting plans based on stakeholder feedback (Hotz, 2020).

PREPROCESSING DATA

Preprocessing Clinical Data

To illustrate preprocessing, this section uses EHR data as an example. The process can be extrapolated to other datasets. EHRs include both coded (structured) data and unstructured text data that must be cleaned and processed prior to analysis. EHRs collect and store data according to a coding system consisting of one or more terminologies. While standard terminologies exist, many systems make use of local terminology, a distinct set of variables, and a distinct coding system for those variables that are not necessarily shared across systems. Different sites, clinics, or hospitals within a healthcare organization could use different terminologies, coding data in different ways. Within a single site, changes in information systems and terminologies over time can also result in variations in data coding. When data are aggregated across time and across sites, the variations in terminology result in a dataset that represents similar concepts in multiple ways. Unlike data collected using a prospective approach, such as for use in randomized control trials, clinical data often require extensive cleaning and preprocessing. See Box 23.2 for information concerning tools that can be used in this process.

Preprocessing Text Data

In clinical records, the richest and most descriptive data are often unstructured, captured only in the text notes entered by clinicians. Text data can be analyzed in a large number of clinical records using a specialized approach known as natural language processing (NLP) or, more specifically, information extraction (Meystre et al., 2008). Methods of information extraction identify pieces of meaningful information in sequences of text, pieces of information that represent concepts and can be coded as such for further analysis. Machine interpretation of text written in the form of natural language is not straightforward because natural language is rife with spelling errors, acronyms, and abbreviations, among other issues (Nadkarni et al., 2011). Consequently, information extraction is usually a computationally expensive, multistep process in which text data are passed through a pipeline of sequential NLP procedures. These procedures deal with common NLP challenges such as word disambiguation and negation and may involve the use of ML methods. However, each pipeline may differ according to the NLP task at hand (Nadkarni et al., 2011).

BOX 23.2 **Tools for Processing Clinical Data**

The U.S. National Library of Medicine maintains a repository of the many available informatics tools called the Online Registry of Biomedical Informatics Tools (ORBIT) Project at http://orbit.nlm.nih.gov. However, given the complexities of processing clinical data with these tools, investigators should consider collaboration or consultation with an informatics specialist versed in the use of these techniques.

Preprocessing Coded (Structured) Data

In a set of consistently coded clinical data, the data should be analyzed using descriptive statistics and visualization with respect to the following:

Distribution. Normally distributed data are most amenable to modeling. If the data distribution is not normally distributed, the data can be transformed using a function or analyzed using nonparametric statistical methods.

Frequency. The frequency of specific values for categorical variables may reveal a need for additional preprocessing. It is not uncommon for identical concepts to be represented using multiple outcome values. Some values represent events that are so rare they should be considered outliers and excluded.

Missing data. Missing data can be meaningful. For example, a missing hemoglobin A1c (HgA1c) laboratory test may indicate that a patient does not have diabetes. In that case, a binary variable indicating whether HgA1c values are truly missing can be added to the dataset. In other circumstances, the values are simply missing at random. If values are missing at random, they can be replaced using a number of statistical imputation approaches.

Sparsity. Sparse data are data for which binary values are mostly zero. Categorical variables with a large number of possible values contribute to sparsity. For example, a field called "primary diagnosis" has a set of possible values equal to the number of diagnoses found in the International Classification of Diseases (ICD)-10 coding system. Some diagnoses will be more common than others will. For uncommon diagnoses, the value of "uncommon diagnosis" will almost always equal zero. The value of "1" will be found in only a small percentage of records.

Outliers. Outliers, data points that fall far outside the distribution of data, should be considered for elimination or further analysis prior to modeling.

Identifiers. Codes or other values that uniquely identify patients should be excluded from the modeling process.

Erroneous data. Absurd, impossible data values are routinely found in clinical data. These can be treated as randomly missing values and replaced.

The considerations in preprocessing the data at this stage are numerous and beyond the scope of this chapter. Preprocessing is always best accomplished through a joint effort by the analyst and one or more domain experts, such as clinicians who are familiar with the concepts the data represent. The domain experts can lend valuable insight to the analyst, who must develop an optimal representation of each variable. Review of the data at this point may reveal conceptual gaps, the absence of data, or the lack of quality data that represents important concepts. For example, age and functional status (e.g., activities of daily living) might be important data to include in a project related to predicting patient falls in the hospital. By mapping concepts to variables, or vice versa, teams can communicate about gaps and weaknesses in the data as well as potential solutions.

PREDICTIVE ANALYTICS

Predictive analytics is the use of quantitative methods to make predictions on future observations from the same source. The methods used to accomplish this are varied and include both statistical approaches and ML.

Statistical Approaches

Statistical approaches fit a model to the data. A common approach is a logistic or linear regression, representing the observed relationship between input variables and a classification or a dependent variable.

Bayesian networks, a class of models based on the Bayes theorem, constitute another popular approach. Bayesian models are robust, tolerate missing data, and can be computed quickly over a set of data.

Machine Learning

ML methods are computer algorithms that learn to perform a task based on examples. In data mining, the task is typically prediction or regression (predict a real number) or classification (predict class membership). ML algorithms vary in the way they learn to perform tasks. Many algorithms begin with an initial working theory of how a set of input data predict an output (a.k.a. target), a future event, or an unknown value. The algorithm then makes incremental adjustments to the working theory based on examples of both the input and the target. The examples are contained in a set of training data. A complete discussion of ML and specific ML algorithms is beyond the scope of this chapter. However, key methods and characteristics are summarized in Table 23.2. All methods listed in this table are commonly implemented in general-purpose data mining software and programming language ML libraries.

Multiple variant algorithms can be used to implement each approach, and specialized method-specific software is available to support more flexible configurations. Data mining software allows users to implement versions of these algorithms via point-and-click graphic user interfaces. However, these algorithms can also be written and executed using analytical environments as part of a larger system. It is important that users understand how to apply each unique method properly in order to produce optimal models and avoid spurious results. For clients of data analytics, it is important to understand the considerations for choosing and evaluating models in order to productively discuss these with the analysts in the problem setting.

Sampling and Partitioning

Once the data have been fully cleaned and preprocessed, they must be sampled and partitioned to enable model evaluation. Sampling is the step in which a smaller subset of the data is chosen for analysis. Sampling is important because excessive amounts of data slow computer processing time during analysis without significantly improving the quality of the results. Sampling for classification tasks is typically random or stratified on class membership.

Partitioning refers to the assignment of individual records or rows in a dataset for a specific purpose: model development (training, incremental testing of models during development) or model validation (data held out from the development process for the purpose of unbiased performance estimation). There are multiple approaches to sampling and partitioning, and the suitability of the approach depends on the nature of the project

TABLE 23.2   Examples of Machine Learning Methods

Method	Description
Decision trees	• Recursive partitioning of data is based on an information criterion (entropy, information gain, etc.) • Common algorithms: C4.5, Classification and Regression Trees (CART), recursive partitioning • Easily interpreted • Require pruning based on coverage to avoid overfitting • More difficult to calibrate to new populations and settings
Decision rules	• Classification rules in the form of if-then-else rule sets • Easily interpreted • Require pruning based on coverage to avoid overfitting • Closely related to decision trees; decision trees can be easily converted to decision rules
Artificial neural networks	• Networks of processing units • Output a probability of class membership • Computationally expensive • Effective for modeling complex, nonlinear solutions • Not easily interpreted
Support vector machines	• Linear functions implemented in a transformed feature space • Computationally efficient • Effective for modeling complex, nonlinear solutions • Not easily interpreted
Ensemble methods	• Combines the output of multiple decision trees • Common algorithms: Random forests, Boosting, Bagging • Scalable (computationally feasible even with very large amounts of data) • Not easily interpreted
Bayesian networks	• Probabilistic models based on the Bayes theorem • Models are easily calibrated for use with new settings and populations • Models may assume conditional independence among variables • Not as scalable as other methods; it may not work well with very large amounts of data due to the way in which Bayesian networks are computed

and the quantity of available data. If very large amounts of data are available, large sets can be sampled for model development and validation. If more limited amounts of data are available, it will be necessary to optimize the use of that data through resampling approaches. Two common resampling approaches are termed *bootstrapping* and *cross-validation* (Sahiner et al., 2007).

Model Evaluation

The most critical step in the evaluation, the partitioning of data, begins before ML methods are applied (Fig. 23.5). Performance estimates are calculated by comparing a model's predictions to actual values on a set of data for which the actual values are known. If this comparison is made using the training data—the same data used to parameterize the model—the performance estimates will be optimistically biased. It is critical that a sizable sample of the original data is set aside and not used in any way to train or calibrate models. This holdout sample of

data is often termed the validation set or testing set. Used solely for performance estimation, testing using the held-out data will yield unbiased estimates of the error in the predictions.

For regression problems, the model evaluation is generally done on the based on the error when comparing the observed test data and the prediction made by the candidate model applied to the test data. Measures include:

- Mean absolute error (MAE) $= \frac{1}{n}\sum_{i=1}^{n}|y_i - \breve{y}_i|$,

- Mean squared error (MSE) $= \frac{1}{n}\sum_{i=1}^{n}(y_i - \breve{y}_i)^2$, and

- Root mean squared error (RMSE) $= \frac{1}{n}\sqrt{\sum_{i=1}^{n}(y_i - \breve{y}_i)^2}$.

While the coefficient of determination is familiar from traditional statistics, in ML the goal is typically accuracy in the predictions, so error-based metrics are more common. In particular, RMSE is commonly used; it has the same units as the error being measured.

In classification, comparing predictions and actual observations in test data yields a confusion matrix that can be used to derive performance measures, similar to the performance measures used in evaluating clinical diagnostic tests, such as accuracy, true-positive rate, false-positive rate, true-negative rate, false-negative rate, sensitivity, and specificity. The specific performance measures used should be selected based on the goals of the project.

Accuracy (TP + TN)/(TP + FP + FN + TN) is perhaps the most intuitive measure; however, there is no distinction between the type of error made, and it is very dependent on the composition of that particular sample. In some cases, the cost of a false positive can be much higher than the cost of a false negative or vice versa. In addition, the accuracy (or its converse, the error rate) is highly dependent on the natural frequency of a class. Where one class overwhelmingly dominates, very high accuracy can be obtained by always choosing the dominant class. However, if the goal of the analysis is to identify minority class members, this is not useful.

Specificity and Sensitivity

Another set of measures is sensitivity and specificity. This dual measure separately addresses both false positives and false negatives. Sensitivity is calculated as the number of true positives (predicted to be true and actually is true) over the number of sample that are true. (TP/(TP + FN)) This represents the model's ability to identify cases that are true. Specificity is calculated as the number of samples that are false and that the model predicted to be false over the number of samples that are false. (TN/(TN + FP)) This represents the ability of the model to correctly identify that the sample was false. What may be a more intuitive way of thinking of specificity is the false positive rate, which is [1 −Specificity]. This would represent the rate that the model incorrectly identifies a sample as true when in fact, it was false. Sensitivity and specificity can be combined into the Receiver Operating Characteristic (ROC) curve, which will be discussed later.

If there is an observation where a prediction as well as the overall prevalence are known (common in a medical diagnostic test), the measures of positive predicted value (PPV) and

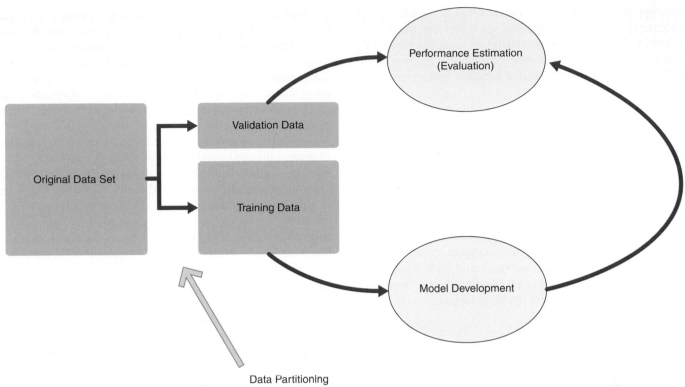

Data Partitioning

Fig. 23.5 The relationship of data partitioning to both model development and evaluation.

negative predictive value (NPV) may be useful. PPV is TP/(TP + FP) NPV is TN/(TN + FN). Therefore, these are conditional based on the results of the test (compared to sensitivity and specificity that are conditional on the actual value of observations). PPV can also be calculated as Sensitivity/(Sensitivity * [1 − Specificity]).

Receiver Operating Characteristic

Sensitivity and specificity can then be used to develop the Receiver Operating Characteristic (ROC) curve. Classification models will calculate a value that is used to determine if an observation is in a class or not. By changing the threshold where the model makes a prediction that an observation is a member of a class, the model can increase or decrease the number of positive predictions and the number of false positives that are included among the positive predictions.

To evaluate and compare overall model performance, the ROC curve and the area under the ROC curve (AUC) are important measures of performance. The ROC curve, depicted in Fig. 23.6, is obtained by plotting the false-positive fraction and true-positive fraction based on cumulative comparison of predicted and actual values at increasing values of probability. The resulting curve shows the trade-off between sensitivity and specificity exhibited by a classifier at any given threshold. AUC is the probability that a randomly chosen positive case will be selected as more likely to be positive than a randomly selected negative case (Hanley & McNeil, 1982). As such, it serves as an overall measure of model performance. An area under the ROC curve of $A_z = 0.5$ is equivalent to random chance. Better performance is indicated by higher

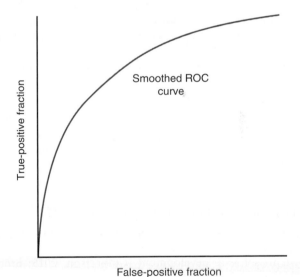

Fig. 23.6 Smoothed receiver operating characteristic *(ROC)* curve.

values of A_z. Interpretation of the area under the ROC curve, especially in relation to other models or classifiers, requires the calculation of confidence intervals.

The first step in out of sample testing is to divide the data into training and testing data sets. This is usually done by random selection, which can be adjusted to ensure demographic balance. A certain fraction (often 0.2) of the data is set aside for scoring (testing) the model that is developed and the remainder is used to train the model.

Within the training data, the data can be again divided into training and test data. When done repeatedly, this is cross validation. The purpose of repeatedly dividing the model into training and test data is to develop a measure of an error on the results of the model, which includes both a mean error and a standard deviation of the error.

There are several forms of cross-validation. The most common and often desired form is k-fold cross validation. In this setting, the data is divided into several parts (commonly $k = 10$). For each fold, the remaining parts are used to develop a model that predicts the first part. This yields 10 estimates of error that can be used to calculate a mean estimate and a standard deviation. Other variations are stratified (where each fold is created to have a balanced distribution of some predictor). Leave one out (where all other data is used to predict each observation one at a time), or Monte Carlo or random cross-validation (where a holdout set is selected randomly with replacement each time, with the possibility of selections of the same data point in different holdout sets) (Kuhn & Johnson, 2013).

Model Deployment

Deployment refers to the actual use of analytic models or tools. In this step, analysts determine how the models or tools are optimally delivered to a decision maker—that is, they translate the models or tools to the problem at hand. In the simplest sense, deployment could consist of merely reporting analyses. Another model involves routine prospective use of analytic models to offer predictions or decision support based upon real-time data. The latter entails either configuring the system, such as an EHR, or adding a module that functions to provide analyses within the live information system.

A key aspect of deployment is the ability of an analyst to adapt models to changes in the nature of the data and to calibrate models for different settings and patient populations. Sometimes, the analyst and the developer are the same. In other cases, the developer works in response to analyst needs and feedback. Often, analysts will request changes to the model to address a specific need or issue. These types of changes are best developed and tested in conjunction with a source code version of the model. Once the changes are well tested in the source code environment, these changes can be examined for potential inclusion into the main model functioning in a live system. The concept of "make one to throw it away" is well known in software development (Culbertson, 2015; Brooks, 1995), but in analytics, it is common to have many iterations to allow institutional knowledge to grow as initial results are shared with decision-makers, allowing them to react to the initial results and shape the ongoing direction of the analysis and its use.

Another method of deployment is the direct delivery of results to a decision maker without explicit analyst intervention. One way to accomplish this is through delivery of spreadsheets such as Microsoft Excel, with graphical user interfaces (GUIs) that can be used by the decision maker to select the data and generate pre-developed summaries and charts. For example, a display may show registered nurse (RN) staffing patterns and projected infection rates occurring within the next few days. The user may drill down into the data by looking at education level of the staff or into the type or location of specific infections.

A third deployment method is the intranet delivery of reports, where decision-makers access a site that allows them to tailor a report request or details. Their requested details are run using a data analysis environment hosted on a remote server and delivered through an internet browser, such as with Tableau or Power BI.

A fourth method is automated report generation. Programming can be embedded into statistical software such as Sweave or knitr, platforms such as Jupyter notebooks, or other reproducible research tools (Stodden et al., 2014). These can be used to specify the subject of the analysis, directed to run the analysis in the hosted data analysis software, and produce a report in Adobe PDF or word processor formats with tables, charts, and other results embedded. A descriptive narrative can be included so that the analysis can be reproduced with the same or new datasets as needed. For instance, one neurological practice uses a combination of R and Sweave to analyze the data and deliver a customized, comprehensive report immediately after the completion of a series of neuropsychological tests (Garbade & Burgard, 2006). Another example is shown in Fig. 23.7, which displays intensive care unit (ICU) and step-down unit usage over time (Luangkesorn et al., 2012).

Modern software development methodologies such as the spiral development model incorporate multiple rounds of feedback. Once deployed, this model is in continual use in a live environment with constant feedback within its cycle. That is, as decision makers' stated requirements change and the organization builds experience using this approach, new information is incorporated into the analysis used in making decisions. This process can improve business and data understanding, which changes the way that analysis products are used, as well as decision makers' future requirements.

ORGANIZATIONAL CONSIDERATIONS FOR DATA SCIENCE

Organizations can mature over time in their use of data science and analytics. A model showing this progression is in Fig. 23.8. Organizations begin with retrospective analysis (exploratory data analyses discussed earlier in the chapter) and gradually move up the scale of difficulty and value toward prescriptive analytics. As organizations gain maturity, several elements are important in this growth: data science personnel, tools and platforms, data standardization, and data governance.

Data Science Personnel

An analytics group needs to be established and grown over time. Analytics has a superficial overlap with traditional data analysis and/or software engineering, but requirements for modern analytics cannot be satisfied by a traditional data analyst or a pure programmer. Traditional data analysts are normally asked to perform descriptive analysis or to run standard summary or review procedures on standard datasets (e.g., to produce a chart for a report or to produce summary statistics using statistical

```
In [13]:  pyl.figure(figsize=(5.5,4))
          pyl.plot(hospNonstatEmp.icu.actMon.tseries(),hospNonstatEmp.icu.actMon.yseries())
          pyl.plot(hospNonstatEmp.icu.actMon.tseries(),
                  [G.icubeds for xi in hospNonstatEmp.icu.actMon.tseries()])
          pyl.title("ICU Utilization over time",
                  fontsize=12,fontweight="bold")
          pyl.xlabel("time",fontsize=9,fontweight="bold")
          pyl.ylabel("Beds",fontsize=9,fontweight="bold")
          pyl.grid(True)
          pyl.savefig(r".\icuutilization.png")
          pyl.show()
          pyl.clf()
```

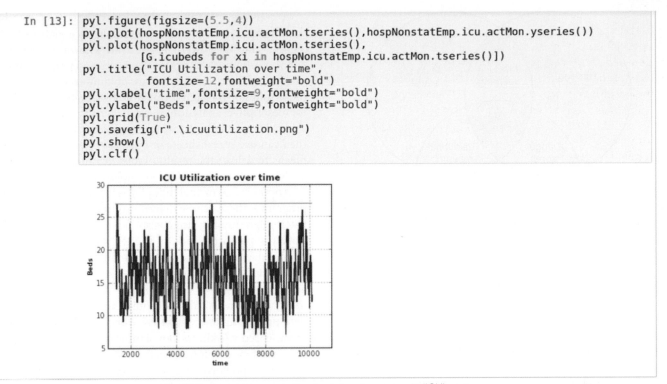

Fig. 23.7 A sample report showing intensive care unit *(ICU)* usage.

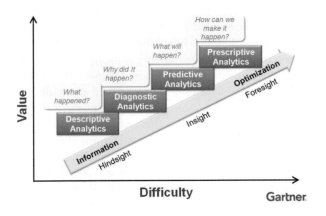

Fig. 23.8 Gartner Analytics Maturity Model. (Reprinted with permission of Gartner, Inc.)

software). Data science groups, on the other hand, are generally asked to be creative in developing analytics procedures across a range of datasets to meet the specific needs of decision makers and to present the results in ways that enhance decision makers' understanding of problems as they make decisions.

An example of this kind of project would be predicting the impact of adding another operating room to the current suite of rooms. Subject matter experts could explain workflows and identify reasonable alternatives. Analysts could then develop models that implement the alternative interventions and the case mix, estimate the downtime of rooms, the number and kinds of staff required, and projected revenue or loss as number of cases changes. Software engineers and programmers may

then be asked to implement the models into a dashboard or an application that decision makers could use to have the model run in different scenarios. A data scientist must have sufficient understanding of the subject matter and computer programming techniques to work with all of these professionals to create value for the organization.

Recommended Skills for a Data Science/Health Analytics Professional

To be of the most benefit to a healthcare system a data scientist is required to be multifaceted in the skills of computer information systems and in healthcare operations (Meer, 2016). Drew Conway describes the requirements of analytics professionals as a three-part Venn diagram (Fig. 23.9) (Conway, 2013). The three areas of knowledge required by analytics professionals are computer hacking (programming and databases), mathematics and statistics, and subject matter expertise.

Computer hacking skills are required because of the way the data used in analytics is electronically stored and because of potential errors in the collection and recording of data. Without the ability to manipulate electronic data, including various types of numerical and text data, and to think algorithmically, this data is essentially unavailable. This means that the analytics professional needs a fair proficiency in programming data, although a formal degree in programming may not be necessary. In addition, the data scientist needs enough understanding of IT infrastructure to discuss issues with the computer and IT engineers who manage the IT infrastructure and databases.

To develop true insight from data, the data scientist requires mathematical and statistical understanding. Although the computational work of mathematical and statistical methods may

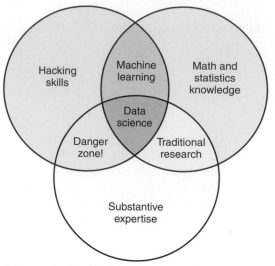

Fig. 23.9 Data scientist skills Venn diagram. (Copyright © 2015 Drew Conway Data Consulting, LLC.)

be performed through the use of computer packages, an understanding of mathematical and statistical concepts is necessary to identify what methods are valid for a given situation, how decision makers should interpret the results, and how to determine if the results are of practical significance.

The need for subject matter expertise is the biggest divergence of data science from the practice of most analytical fields. This expertise is required for examining the healthcare business process to identify important values, translate the business requirements to mathematical and statistical models, and interpret the results in terms that make sense in the business setting. This separates data science from academic fields such as ML, which are typically developed separately from the subject matter of potential applications (Conway, 2013).

One issue is the difficulty in finding someone with the combination of all these skills. Each of the three knowledge areas could be a career in its own right, so finding a person who embodies strength in all three of these knowledge areas is often compared to looking for a mythical unicorn (Bartolucci, 2013). But what is often truly needed is a team of people whom each are deep in one area while having a level of skills and understanding in all other aspects that facilitates collaboration and teamwork, sometimes known as a t-shaped analyst. Then, the organization assembles a team that collectively have strength and depth in every aspect of the analytics role from working with databases such as EHR, computational programming skills, quantitative analysis techniques such as statistics or ML, and working with the clinicians and subject matter experts who deliver care, provide services, build models, and make decisions for designing the systems that assist and inform those who provide healthcare services.

Tools and Platforms

A second decision the organization needs to make in conjunction with the analytics group is the choice of computer platform. While many of the platforms are made to interact well with others a basic understanding of choices is helpful.

A common platform for analytics is spreadsheet software such as MS Excel and business intelligence platforms such as Tableau and MS Power BI. These are known for being able to connect or import data from databases and perform basic summaries and charting. As they are ubiquitous as part of software office suites or through intranet interfaces, these are often used for descriptive analytics or as a delivery platform for more sophisticated methods, which can create databases as output then can use spreadsheets or business intelligence platforms as means to deliver the results. Table 23.3 illustrates categories of analytics tools and provides examples.

Another class of analytics platforms is stand-alone analytical programs. These can be driven through GUI menus or custom batch programming languages. These include many traditional statistical platforms such as SAS, SPSS, and Minitab, as well as graphical ML platforms such as Rapidminer, KNIME, or Weka. These packages are specialized for statistics and data analysis and include ways of connecting to common databases. Often they include graphical model building capabilities to specify the data processing and analytical workflow. These graphical and menu-based workflows can significantly ease the initial development of models for use in the analysis.

A third platform class is data analysis environments based on programming languages with special facilities for data analysis. Two characteristics are common to these languages: a data frame data structure that stores information about entities and allows for SQL-like data manipulation and libraries that implement numerical and statistical methods. These languages include R, Python, Julia, and Scala. One advantage of the programming language–based platforms is that they are often extensible, meaning that capabilities not originally considered by the initial developer can be created and added to the platform.

Applications written using these languages can be connected to or embedded in other applications. For example, the big data platform Apache Hadoop can embed the ML capabilities of Apache Spark, (Meng et al., 2016) which can be scripted (programmed) using Java, R, Python, or Scala. Similarly, the cloud data platform MS Azure (Microsoft, 2016) can include the Azure ML extension, which can be scripted using Python or R. These allow for easy embedding of analytical models that use these analytical environments into a larger IT platform.

In the end, the choice of platform is dependent on the type of expected deployment for analytical products and the people available to the analytics group.

TABLE 23.3	**Examples of Analytics Tools**
Class	**Examples**
Spreadsheets and data visualization tools	MS Excel, Pentaho, Tableau, Power BI
Statistical analysis programs	SAS, SPSS, Stata, Weka, KNIME, Rapidminer
Programming languages	R, Python, Matlab, Scala, Julia

Data Governance

Organizations need to make myriad decisions around managing and obtaining value from data, such as minimizing cost and complexity, managing risk, and ensuring adherence to regulations and legal requirements. As organizations mature in their data science analyses, they need formal mechanisms, called data governance, to oversee these analytic processes. **Data governance** means decision-making and authority over data-related matters. The concept can have many nuances, such as organizational structures for managing data, rules and policies, data decision rights, methods for accountability, and methods of enforcement for data-related processes (The DGI, 2016).

Thus, organizations need a structure for enterprise-wide data management. This is the first step in transforming an organization's adoption of data science.

Data governance typically addresses these types of vendor-agnostic topics:
- Tools
- Techniques
- Models
- Best practices

The Data Governance Institute (DGI) provides a data governance framework seen in Fig. 23.10 that includes 10 components every data governance program should employ (The DGI, 2016).

Ethical considerations

Two ethical considerations with data science in healthcare are related to privacy and the application of analytics in the context of human society.

In healthcare, data scientists deal with personal data, such as patients or clients of healthcare services. This data is often covered by the *Standards for Privacy of Individually Identifiable Health Information* (Privacy Rule) of the Health Insurance Portability and Accountability Act of 1996 (HIPAA). The Privacy Rule standards address the use and disclosure of individuals' health information, also known as protected health information (PHI) as well as standards for individual's privacy rights to understand how their personal information will be used. In particular, it protects all "individually identifiable health information" (U.S. Department of Health & Human Services). In a broader context, this is known as Personal Identifiable Information (PII). The goal of the Privacy Rule within HIPAA is to assure that PHI is protected while still allowing for the flow of information needed to provide and promote quality healthcare and promote public health.

PHI includes information such as:
- individuals physical or mental health or condition,
- provision of healthcare to an individual,
- provisions of payment for healthcare, and
- demographic data.

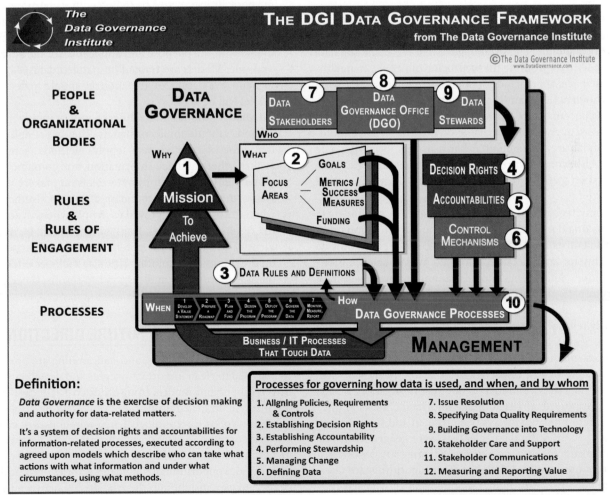

Fig. 23.10 Data governance framework. (Reprinted with permission of The Data Governance Institute.)

For data scientists more interested in populations rather than individual patients, one way of working with healthcare data while respecting the individual's privacy is to de-identify PHI. The goal of de-identification is to remove data elements that can identify individuals by themselves, in combination with other data elements, or through statistical methods (U.S. National Institutes of Health, 2021). De-identification can include removing names, address, contact information, medical record numbers, account numbers, license number, biometric data, dates, age, and geographic data. In addition, various groups of people may be in a protected class (e.g., race/ethnicity or veterans), If the specific research aim requires some of these elements, care must be taken to reduce the specificity of the data used so that individuals privacy is protected and the interests of protected classes are respected (U.S. Department of Health & Human Services Office for Civil Rights, 2015).

In addition to regulatory issues such as HIPAA and the Privacy Rule, there are ethical considerations that data scientist dealing with applications with societal impacts should be applying in their work. While there is not an authoritative set of considerations in data science, one applicable set comes from bioethics. Floridi and Cowls (Floridi & Cowls, 2019) suggest five core principles for ethical AI:

- beneficence,
- non-maleficence,
- autonomy,
- justice, and
- explicability.

The principle of beneficence suggests that AI (including data science) be used to promote the well-being of people. In healthcare data science, this includes patients, providers, and associated stakeholders (e.g., family and communities).

Non-maleficence asks that data scientists guard against the negative consequences of overusing or misusing AI technologies. Particular areas of potential harm include privacy, using results of AI beyond secure constraints, and guarding against societal risks (such as reinforcing existing harmful societal structures).

Autonomy recognizes that while data science methods can assist in making decisions, in the end, people are decision makers. Data scientists may not allow decision makers to abdicate responsibility for actions taken informed by data science models. In addition, data science models cannot remove freedom of choice from patients or providers. Therefore, the autonomy of machines (e.g., data science models) should be restricted and intrinsically reversible. People should retain the ability to make the final decisions, including the ability to delegate decisions to a data science model for the sake of efficacy or efficiency.

The principle of justice recognizes that the healthcare system and the data science model do not exist in isolation. Access to healthcare and the ability to make informed choices in one's own best interest has not always been true. In addition, the historical data sets used by data scientists were generated in this world. For example, Buolamwini and Gebru (2018) observed that datasets used to train facial analysis algorithms are overwhelmingly composed of lighter-skinned subjects. When they created a test dataset that was balanced by gender and skin type

and evaluated three commercial gender classification systems, they found the error rate for black females was up to 34.7% compared to an error rate for white males of 0.8%. O'Neill (2016) describes how insurance companies have indirectly included race through the use of proxies that are affected by historical racial discrimination, setting rates to the extent that race becomes more important than actual customer history or behavior. Therefore, attention must be made so that data science models do not merely repeat or encode past wrongs such as discrimination and threats to diversity due to the composition of the datasets used to train the models.

Explicability asks that the decision-making process of data science and AI is understandable. While many ML algorithms used in data science are not interpretable, analysts and decision makers should understand the source and composition of the data that is used by data science methods, what the goals of the ML algorithm were, and agree that these are appropriate to the decision or action that is being made based on the model.

These ethical considerations need to be accounted for at all stages of the data science project, not only at the end. The Stanford Center for Research on Foundation Models points out how **ethics** can be applied to various aspects of data science projects (Bommasani et al., 2021).

- Data creation: Data are created by people and is at least implicitly about people. It is also created and collected for a purpose, its use should be in line with its purpose.
- Data curation: Data are selected into datasets. The analyst needs to ensure that the data is relevant and the selection is in line with the purpose and application of the analysis.
- Training: Models are trained on curated datasets. The training and evaluation of the models should reflect how the model will be used.
- Adaptation: Models in healthcare are not purely mathematical and computational constructs. They are added to systems that process curated data, apply methods, screen results against other validated information, and combine the results with other indicators for use by decision makers.
- Deployment: The impact of data science in healthcare occurs when the model is deployed to people who will act based on the results of the model. Deployment should be managed to identify and correct for potential issues that arise in acting on the results of the model. This also includes understanding on how to interpret and respond to results, especially problematic results.

CONCLUSIONS AND FUTURE DIRECTIONS

Data science, data analytics, and data mining are processes that can be used to glean important insights and develop useful, data-driven output and models from collected healthcare data. With each patient and each healthcare event, data describing numerous aspects of care accumulate. Large warehouses of clinical data are now commonplace, and as time passes, the data will become increasingly longitudinal in nature. This future direction presents an enormous opportunity, as large repositories of clinical data can be used to gain insight into the relationship between the characteristics of patient, diagnoses, interventions, outcomes, and other elements such as costs and operational processes. Data can also be used to identify prospective patient cohorts for scientific research. They can be used to assist healthcare providers with clinical decisions and avoid a medical error. However, the sheer size and complexity of the data necessitate specialized approaches to data management and analysis. The methods of data science enable us to analyze the data efficiently and effectively and develop clinical knowledge models for decision support.

Using data science and data analytics, informaticians and health professionals can leverage the vast amounts of data generated in the course of providing healthcare in order to improve healthcare. However, analysts and health professionals should always be aware that in the end, healthcare is delivered to individuals, and the capabilities afforded by data science assist but do not take over from individual judgment on individual cases.

ACKNOWLEDGMENTS

The author wishes to acknowledge the contributions of Mollie R. Cummins and Nancy Staggers to the previous edition of this chapter.

DISCUSSION QUESTIONS

1. Write a statement outlining the three top big data or data analytics questions you would want to consider in your work setting.
2. Compare and contrast the types and methods that are available for EDA, predictive, and prescriptive analytics. Give examples of each.
3. Why is it necessary to process coded and text data before using data mining methods?
4. Fig. 23.10 includes 10 components every data governance program should employ. For each component, provide one implication of that component within a healthcare setting.

CASE STUDY

1. You are a new hire in a regional office that oversees 35 long-term care facilities. One of your goals is to build a regional knowledge development program. You have support from your supervisor in developing this new program. Your supervisor went to a recent conference and now understands the potential of using data across facilities for improved decision-making. However, your supervisor does not understand how to even begin such a program and is looking to you to provide some guidance. Using the information in this chapter, answer the following questions: Thinking about the Gartner model that outlines how analytics mature in organizations, what would be your initial goals for a knowledge development program? Discuss initial characteristics of output for a beginning program.

2. One of your first steps would be to assess the health IT capabilities in each of your facilities and at the regional level. Think about what you would want to know about each of these. Consider available local functions, interoperability (information transfer) of systems, repositories at the local or regional level, and support personnel.
3. Thinking about the skills needed for data science analysts, outline an initial team of people you would need to begin the program.
4. Discuss marketing efforts for this program targeted at the executive staff of the long-term care facilities. Create a list of the kinds of questions that might be answered by using data science.

REFERENCES

Abela, A. (2006, September 6). "Choosing a good chart." Available: https://extremepresentation.typepad.com/blog/2006/09/choosing_a_good.html. Accessed February 2020.

Bartolucci, J. (2013, November 21). "Are you recruiting a data scientist, or unicorn?" *Information Week*

Bertsimas, D., Boussioux, L., Cory-Wright, R., Delarue, A., Digalakis, V., Jacquillat, A., Kitane, D. L., Lukin, G., Li, M., Mingardi, L., Nohadani, O., Orfanoudaki, A., Papalexopoulos, T., Paskov, I., & Pau, J. (2021). "From predictions to prescriptions: A data-driven response to COVID-19." *Healthcare Management Science*, 24, 253–272.

Bommasani, R., Hudson, D. A., Adeli, E., Altman, R., Arora, S., Arx, S. v., Bernstein, M. S., Bohg, J., Bosselut, A., Brunskill, E., Brynjolfsson, E., Buch, S., Card, D., Castellon, R., Chatterji, N., & Chen, A. (2021). "On the opportunities and risks of foundation models." *Arxiv*

Brooks, F. (1995). *The mythical man month: Essays on software engineering*. Boston: Addison-Wesley Pub. Co.

Buolamwini, J., & Gebru, T. (2018). "Gender shades: intersectional accuracy disparities in commercial gender classification." *Proceedings of Machine Learning Research*, 81, 77–91.

Centers for Medicare and Medicaid, "National Health Expenditure Data—Historical," December 16, 2020. [Online]. Available: https://www.cms.gov/Research-Statistics-Data-and-Systems/Statistics-Trends-and-Reports/NationalHealthExpendData/NationalHealthAccountsHistorical.

Chapman, P., Clinton, J., Kerber, R., Khabaza, T., Reinartz, T., Shearer, C., & Wirth, R. (2000). "CRISP-DM 1.0," CRISP-DM consortium.

Conway, D. (2013). "The Data Science Venn Diagram," (2013, March 26). [Online]. Available: http://drewconway.com/zia/2013/3/26/the-data-science-venn-diagram.

Culbertson, R. (2015). "The ethics of big data. There's a fine line between patient privacy and identifying better forms of treatment." *Healthcare Executive, 30*(6), 44. 46-47.

Dong, E., Du, H., & Gardner, L. (2020). "An interactive web-based dashboard to track COVID-19 in real time." *The Lancet: Infectious Diseases, 20*(5). P533-534.

Eaton, C., Deroos, D., Deutsch, T., Lapis, G., & Zikopoulos, P. (2012). *Understanding big data: Analytics for enterprise class hadoop and streaming data.* New York: McGraw-Hill.

Floridi, L., & Cowls, J. (2019). "A unified framework of five principles for AI in society." *Harvard Data Science Review, 7*(1).

Garbade, S., & Burgard, P. (2006). "Using {R}/{Sweave} in everyday clinical practice." *R News, 6*(2).

Gelman, A., Carlin, J., Stern, H., Dunson, D., Vehtari, A., & Rubin, D. (2013). *Bayesian data analysis* (3rd ed.). New York: Chapman and Hall/CRC,.

Ginsburg, P. B., Loera-Brust, A. d, Brandt, C., & Durak, A. (2018). *The opportunities and challenges of data analytics in health care.* Washington, DC: Brookings Institution.

Hanley, J. A., & McNeil, B. J. (1982). "The meaning and use of the area under a receiver operating characteristic (ROC) curve." *Radiology, 143*(1), 29–36.

Hotz, N. (2020). "What is CRISP DM?" [Online]. Available: https://www.datascience-pm.com/crisp-dm-2/.

IBM. (2014). "IBM Watson Health." [Online]. Available: https://www.ibm.com/smarterplanet/us/en/ibmwatson/health/. [Accessed April 13, 2014].

Institute for Health Technology Transformation. (2013). *"Transforming health care through big data: Strategies for leveraging big data in the health care industry."* Institute for Health Technology Transformation.

Keehan, S. P., Cuckler, G. A., Poisal, J. A., Sisko, A. M., Smith, S. D., Madison, A. J., Rennie, K. E., Fiore, J. A., & Hardesty, J. C. (2020). "National Health Expenditure Projections, 2019–28: Expected rebound in prices drives rising spending growth." *Health Affairs, 39*(4), 704–714.

Kuhn, M., & Johnson, K. (2013). *Applied predictive modeling.* New York: Springer.

Long, E., & Brandeau, M. (2009). "OR's next top model: Decision models for infectious disease control." *Tutorials in Operations Research,* 123–138.

Luangkesorn, K. L., Bountourelis, T., Schaefer, A., Nabors, S., & Clermont, G. (2012b). "The case against utilization: deceptive performance measures in inpatient care capacity models," *Proceedings of the 2012 Winter Simulation Conference (WSC),* Berlin.

Lustig, I., Dietrich, B., Johnson, C., & Dziekan, C. (2010, December 5). "The analytics journey." Analytics. Available at: https://pubsonline.informs.org/do/10.1287/LYTX.2010.06.01/full/.

Luangkesorn, K., & Eren-Doğu, Z. (2015). "Markov Chain Monte Carlo methods for estimating surgery duration." *Journal of Statistical Computation and Simulation, 86*(2), 1–17.

Luangkesorn, K., Norman, B., Zhuang, Y., Falbo, M., & Sysko, J. (2012a). "Practice summaries: designing disease prevention and screening centers in Abu Dhabi." *Interfaces, 42*(4), 406–409.

Meer, D. (2016). "Educating the next analytics 'bilinguals.'" *Strategy+Business.*

Meng, X., Bradley, J., Yavuz, B., Sparks, E., Venkataraman, S., Liu, D., Freeman, J., Tsai, D., Amde, M., Owen, S., Xin, D., Xin, R., Franklin, M. J., Zadeh, R., Zaharia, M., & Tal, A. (2016). "MLlib: machine learning in apache spark." *Journal of Machine Learning Research, 17,* 1–7.

Meystre, S. M., Savova, G. K., Kipper-Schuler, K. C., & Hurdle, J. F. (2008). "Extracting information from textual documents in the electronic health record: a review of recent research." *Yearbook of Medical Informatics, 17*(1), 128–144.

Microsoft. (2016). "Microsoft Azure machine learning." [Online]. Available: https://azure.microsoft.com/en-us/services/machine-learning.

National Academies of Science, Engineering, and Medicine. (2021). *Learning from rapid response, innovation, and adaptation to the COVID-19 crisis: Proceedings of a workshop—in brief.* Washington, DC: The National Acadamies Press.

Nadkarni, P. M., Ohno-Machado, L., & Chapman, W. W. (2011). "Natural language processing: an introduction." *Journal of the American Medical Informatics Association, 18*(5), 544–551.

O'Reilly, T., Steele, J., Loukides, M., & Hill, C. (2012). *How data science is transforming health care: Solving the wanamaker dilemma.* Sebastopol, CA: O'Reilly Media.

O'Neil, C. (2016). *Weapons of math destruction,* New York: Crown.

Oracle. (2021). "What is Data Science?" [Online]. Available: https://www.oracle.com/data-science/what-is-data-science/. Accessed October 5, 2021.

Parker, F., Sawczu, H., Ganjkhanlo, F., Ahmad, F., & Ghobadi, K. (2021). "Optimal resource and demand redistribution for healthcare systems under stress from COVID-19." *arXiv.*

President's Council of Advisors on Science and Technology. (2010). *Realizing the full potential of health information technology to Improve healthcare for Americans: The path forward.* Washington, DC: Executive Office of the President.

President's Council of Advisors on Science and Technology. (2020). *Recommendations for strengthening American leadership in industries of the future.* Washington, DC: Office of Science and Technology Policy.

Peters, S. G., & Buntrock, J. D. (2014, July). "Big data and the electronic health record." *The Journal of Ambulatory Care, 37*(3), 206–210.

Sahiner, B., Chan, H. -P., & Hadjiiski, L. (2007). "Classifier performance estimation under the constraint of a finite sample size: Resampling schemes applied to neural network classifiers." *Neural Networks, 21*(2-3), 476–483.

Stodden, V., Leisch, F., & Peng, R. D. (2014). *Implementing reproducible research.* New York: Chapman and Hall/CRC.

The DGI. (2016). "The Data Governance Institute." [Online]. Available: http://www.datagovernance.com/. [Accessed April 26, 2016].

Trotter, F., & Uhlman, D. (2013). *Hacking healthcare.* Stebatopol, CA: O'Reilly Media.

U.S. Department of Health & Human Services Office for Civil Rights. (2015). "Guidance regarding methods for de-identification of protected health information in accordance with the Health Insurance Portability and Accountability Act (HIPAA) Privacy Rule," published November 6, 2015. [Online]. Available: https://www.hhs.gov/hipaa/for-professionals/privacy/special-topics/de-identification/index.html. [Accessed August 21, 2021].

U.S. Department of Health & Human Services. (2003). "Summary of the HIPAA privacy rule." [Online]. Available: https://www.hhs.gov/hipaa/for-professionals/privacy/laws-regulations/index.html. [Accessed June 28, 2021].

U.S. National Institutes of Health. (2004). "Protecting personal health information in research: understanding the HIPAA Privacy Rule." [Online]. Available: https://privacyruleandresearch.nih.gov/pdf/HIPAA_Booklet_4-14-2003.pdf. [Accessed August 21 2021].

V. Tuulos and H. Bowne-Anderson (2021). "MLOps and DevOps: Why data makes it different." [Online]. Available: https://www.oreilly.com/radar/mlops-and-devops-why-data-makes-it-different/. [Accessed October 24 2021].

24

Safety and Quality Initiatives in Health Informatics

Juliana J. Brixey, Lynda R. Hardy, and Zach Burningham

Due to the complexity of the errors in healthcare, multifaceted strategies, including health information technology tools, are needed to realize improvement in clinical processes and patient outcomes when striving to improve safety and quality.

OBJECTIVES

At the completion of this chapter, the reader will be prepared to:
1. Describe key concepts of patient safety and quality care.
2. Describe federal efforts to improve patient safety and quality.
3. Discuss the theoretical underpinnings and needs for patient safety and quality.

KEY TERMS

adverse event, 377

American Recovery and Reinvestment Act, 376

Bar Code Medication Administration (BCMA), 382

Complex Adaptive System (CAS), 382

Electronic Medication Administration Record (eMAR), 382

health information technology (HIT), 376

patient safety, 377

pay for performance, 384

quality of care, 376

workarounds, 383

ABSTRACT ❖

This chapter focuses on patient safety and quality of care through the perspective of health informatics. It begins with a concept definition and discusses key regulatory initiatives for improving patient safety and care quality in the United States. The chapter reviews the Patient Safety and Quality Research Design (PSQRD) framework and classifies and evaluates adverse patient safety and quality events. It will continue with discussions related to Singh and Sittig's Sociotechnical Work System that integrates health information technology within the context of patient safety and quality. The chapter culminates with a discussion related to the integrations of the two frameworks noting successes, lessons learned, and future directions to guide health practitioners and informaticists to improve patient outcomes, practice, and research.

INTRODUCTION

This chapter examines the use of health information technology (health IT) to improve patient safety and care quality. The concepts *quality of care* and *patient safety* are defined, and selected key regulatory initiatives that are driving a focus on the quality of care and patient safety in the United States are discussed. Two frameworks are reviewed indicating the association between the Patient Safety and Quality Research Design (PSQRD) framework (Brown et al., 2008) and the Sociotechnological Work System framework (Singh & Sittig, 2016). The frameworks are introduced and used to classify adverse patient safety and quality events, identify health information technology (HIT) patient safety and quality measures, discuss key success factors, lessons learned, and challenges, and then make recommendations for implementation and future research.

A series of Institute of Medicine (IOM)[a,b] reports on the quality of healthcare have led to widespread recognition that preventable medical errors occur far too often and that the quality of patient care has been inconsistent across the U.S. healthcare system for more than a decade (Adams &

[a]Effective July 1, 2015, the National Academy of Science, Engineering, and Medicine voted to change the name of the IOM to the National Academy of Medicine. In March 2016, the National Academy of Sciences announced that the division of the National Academies of Sciences, Engineering, and Medicine (the Academies) that focuses on health and medicine was renamed the Health and Medicine Division (HMD) in place of the name IOM. In this textbook, you may see any of these three names used, depending on the date of the publication or report.

[b]The term "meaningful use" references the association with Centers for Medicare & Medicaid Services (CMS) rules for the electronic medical record incentive program. This term has been retired and CMS now refers to as *promoting interoperability* (https://www.cms.gov/Regulations-and-Guidance/Legislation/EHRIncentivePrograms).

Corrigan, 2003; Institute of Medicine, 2001; Kohn et al., 1999; Lohr, 1990; Page, 2004; National Academies of Sciences and Engineering, and Medicine, 2015). Research generated evidence (Bates & Gawande, 2003; Kaushal et al., 2003; The Joint Commission, 2016) demonstrates that health information technology (HIT) can improve communication and reduce errors (Bates & Gawande, 2003; Kaushal et al., 2003) and indicates positive public attitudes towards HIT use and healthcare quality, costs, and privacy (Gaylin et al., 2011). The IOM recommended the widespread adoption of health IT to facilitate effective, high-quality, and safe patient care (The Joint Commission, 2016).

The American Recovery and Reinvestment Act (ARRA) of 2009 was expected to improve the quality of care by promoting and incentivizing the adoption of electronic health records (EHRs) as well as supporting the Meaningful Use of EHRs (Centers for Medicare and Medicaid Services, 2009) to achieve widespread improvement in the ability to detect and reduce clinical errors (Bradley et al., 2012). Examples of specific ARRA requirements directed at improving the quality of care are included in Box 24.1.

Early data indicate that Meaningful Use was effective in promoting the use of certified EHRs. Early adoption of EHRs was slow, but the Center for Medicare and Medicaid Services (CMS) incentive program provided the financial impetus for clinical settings to implement a system. A 2017 report noted that 96% of acute care facilities used a certified EHR, and 99% of large hospitals (those with more than 300 beds) had effective health information systems (ONC, https://www.healthit.gov/data/quick-stats/percent-hospitals-type-possess-certified-health-it). The Centers for Disease Control and Prevention (CDC) currently reports that 72.3% of office-based healthcare providers use certified EHRs or electronic medical records (EMRs). Furthermore, nearly 90% are using some type of system (https://www.cdc.gov/nchs/fastats/electronic-medical-records.htm). Improved care coordination, exchange of electronic health information or interoperability, and automated submission of quality data continue to be monitored and used. The Medicare Access and CHIP Reauthorization Act of 2015 (MACRA) details are discussed in Chapter 29. The Act includes several provisions related to patient safety (Better, Smarter, Healthier, 2015; Medicare Access and CHIP, 2015).

DEFINITIONS

Inconsistent use of language and variations in definitions are barriers to understanding the concepts of patient safety and quality, as well as to benchmarking beyond the organizational level (Runciman et al., 2009). The definitions of *patient safety and quality of care* put forth by the Academies and the World Health Organization (WHO) provide a solid foundation for the consistent use of these terms.

Quality of Care

In its 1990 report titled *Medicare: A Strategy for Quality Assurance*, the IOM defined quality of care as "the degree to which health services for individuals and populations increase the likelihood of desired health outcomes and are consistent with current professional knowledge." (p. 21) In 2001, in its report titled *Crossing the Quality Chasm*, the IOM proposed six aims as a means to narrow the quality chasm that exists in the U.S. healthcare system (Adams & Corrigan, 2003). It proposed that healthcare should be:

Safe. Prevents injury or other adverse outcomes.

Effective. Ensures that evidence-based interventions are used, with patients consistently receiving the treatments most likely to be beneficial.

Patient-centered. Ensures that patient preferences, needs, and values are front and center in the process of clinical decision-making.

Timely. Delivered when needed and without harmful delays.

Efficient. Prevents the waste of valuable human and material resources.

Equitable. Provided to all individuals without regard for ethnic, racial, socioeconomic, or other personal characteristics.

The WHO identifies key facts related to patient safety that are consistent with the IOM report. They further suggest that patient safety is fundamental to quality of care and should be patient-centered (https://www.who.int/news-room/fact-sheets/detail/patient-safety).

Patient Safety

"Patient safety is a fundamental principle of health care" (Patient safety, 2017). Global research indicates that significant medical errors occur injuring patients and extending the

---

BOX 24.1   Examples of Specific ARRA Requirements for Improving the Quality of Care

Meaningful Use Requirement	Rationale
Use of a certified EHR	Ensures that EHRs in practice have the capability of achieving the goals of Meaningful Use (e.g., they are not simply used as "word processors")
Facilitation of care coordination and quality by participating in the exchange of electronic health information	Ensures that the correct data is available to support evidence-based care at each encounter across the healthcare continuum
Submission of data for quality reporting	To improve the quality of care in the United States, consistent data are needed to support measurement and quality improvement

ARRA, American Recovery and Reinvestment Act; *EHR,* electronic health record.

length of care or resulting in death. All income-level countries indicate the importance of providing the safest form of health care possible, given available resources (Patient safety, 2017). The complexity of health care continues to rise as we face global health provider shortages, increased health care needs, and global pandemics.

The IOM defines patient safety as "freedom from accidental injury due to medical care, or medical errors," where error is defined as "the failure of a planned action to be completed as intended or the use of a wrong plan to achieve an aim." (Institute of Medicine, 2001 p. 4).

The International Classification for Patient Safety (ICPS) defines safety as "the reduction of risk and unnecessary harm to an acceptable minimum" and patient safety as "the reduction of risk of unnecessary harm associated with healthcare to an acceptable minimum." (Runciman et al., 2009 p. 21). The ICPS defines error as "failure to carry out a planned action as intended or application of an incorrect plan" and healthcare-associated harm as "harm arising from or associated with plans or actions taken during the provision of healthcare, rather than an underlying disease or injury." (Runciman et al., 2009 pp. 19,21).

These definitions highlight the multifaceted nature of safety and quality and the notion that failures of both omission (e.g., failure to provide evidence-based care) and commission (e.g., providing care incorrectly) can compromise the quality and safety of healthcare.

National Initiatives Driving Adoption and Use of Health IT

A key lesson learned from the IOM's *Quality Chasm Series* is that achieving higher quality and safer care in the United States requires a systemic redesign of established clinical processes and that health IT is needed to support and maintain the transition to best practices.[c] Several initiatives on the national level have maintained a steady focus on patient safety and care quality. Recent U.S. policy aligns incentives with the goal of adoption and widespread use of health IT to ensure a healthcare system characterized by uniform high quality and safe patient care (Centers for Medicare et al., 2010).

The Office of the National Coordinator for Health Information Technology (ONC) published a report titled *Federal Health Information Technology Strategic Plan: 2011–2015* (Office of the National Coordinator for Health Information Technology, 2011). This report defined the ONC's plan for working with the private and public sectors to achieve the nation's health IT agenda. Specific examples of accreditation and policy efforts designed to achieve the six quality aims defined by the IOM through a focus on the redesign of clinical processes and adoption and Meaningful Use of health IT are included in Table 24.1. The ONC and the CDC began tracking the adoption of certified EHRs by office-based physicians in 2014. Since 2008, office-based physician adoption of any EHRs has more than doubled, from 42% to 86%. Provider and hospital adoption of EHRs continued to grow, but as of 2015,

not all Meaningful Use aims were achieved due to a lack of interoperability (Bradley et al., 2012). As of 2017, office-based physician adoption of EHRs doubled since 2008 where nearly 9 in 10 (86%) of office-based physicians had adopted any EHR, (Adams & Corrigan, 2003) and nearly 4 in 5 (80%) had adopted a certified EHR (Brown et al., 2008; Healthit, 2015; Agency for Healthcare Research and Quality, 2014; Office of the National Coordinator for Health Information Technology, 2019). Without interoperability, the larger vision of achieving a learning healthcare system (LHS) is in peril. In response, the ONC has released its first version of its shared nationwide interoperability roadmap, *Connecting Health and Care for the Nation*, which lays out a plan to achieve interoperability of health IT and to support a functional learning health system by 2024 (Office of the National Coordinator for Health Information Technology, 2014).

The ONC also released an updated *Federal Health Information Technology Strategic Plan: 2015–2020*, (Agency for Healthcare Research and Quality, 2014) highlighting both the achievements of Meaningful Use (e.g., widespread adoption of health IT) and those areas where the U.S. IT infrastructure is lacking (e.g., interoperability, patient-centeredness). In this report, the ONC calls on public, private, consumer, and industry stakeholders to align to achieve the federal health IT vision of high-quality care, lower costs, a healthy population, and engaged people (Agency for Healthcare Research and Quality, 2014).

FEDERAL INITIATIVES

Federal Health Information Technology Strategic Plan: 2015–2020

The Federal Health Information Technology Strategic Plan: 2015–2020 links safety-related initiatives to the Health Information Technology Patient Safety Action and Surveillance Plan: June 2013 (Office of the National Coordinator for Health Information Technology, 2013). This plan addresses health IT through two objectives: (1) to use health IT to make care safer and (2) to improve the safety of health IT. In September 2014, ONC issued an update on the progress achieved by implementing the plan. "The report explains that we now have a better understanding of the types of safety events related to health IT and, more importantly, the interventions available to prevent unintended consequences of the use of health IT tools" (Office of the National Coordinator for Health Information Technology, 2014). Information about this plan and continuing progress can be found at http://www.healthit.gov/policy-researchers-implementers/health-it-and-patient-safety.

Key afocal areas for ongoing accreditation and policy efforts include improving the quality of care and preventing adverse events. An adverse event (U.S. Food & Drug Administration [FDA], 2021). is any undesirable experience associated with the use of a medical product in a patient. Evidence suggests that the United States may be making progress in the quest for higher quality and safer care, but

---

[c]References 1, 3, 4, 6, 19, 20.

TABLE 24.1 Accreditation and Policy Initiatives Focusing on Improving Quality of Care and Patient Safety Through Health Information Technology

Initiative	Description
The Joint Commission National Patient Safety Goals (NSPG) (Medicare Access and CHIP, 2015)	Program established in 2002 by The Joint Commission to assist accredited organizations in addressing patient safety concerns (The Joint Commission, 2015). Examples of 2012 NPSG facilitated by health IT include the following: • Reduce the likelihood of patient harm associated with the use of anticoagulant therapy (NPSG.03.05.01). (1) EMR-based clinical decision support to alert and manage potential food and drug interactions, (2) use of "smart pumps" to provide consistent and accurate dosing, and (3) use of MedlinePlus to educate patients about the importance of follow-up monitoring, compliance, drug–food interactions, and the potential for adverse drug reactions and interactions. • Maintain and communicate accurate patient medication information (NPSG.03.06.01). (1) Use of an electronic medication reconciliation system to obtain information on the medications the patient is currently taking at all care transitions and (2) use of MedlinePlus to provide the patient (or family) with written information about the medications prescribed.
The Leapfrog Group (The Leapfrog Group, 2015)	Initiative led by healthcare purchasers designed to improve the quality, safety, and affordability of healthcare by reducing preventable medical mistakes (Office of the National Coordinator for Health Information Technology, 2015). Examples of 2015 Leapfrog goals facilitated by health IT include the following: • Prevent medication errors: Use of CPOE. • Avoid harm: Use of clinical decision support in EMR decision support to prevent medical mistakes. • Reduce pressure ulcers: Electronic assessment and plan of care application to link areas of risk with tailored interventions to prevent pressure ulcers from occurring. • Reduce in-hospital injuries: Electronic assessment and plan of care application to link areas of risk with tailored interventions to prevent falls and related injuries.
CMS Hospital-Acquired Conditions (Kaushal et al., 2003)	In response to the Deficit Reduction Act of 2006, CMS identified a list of preventable hospital-acquired conditions for which hospitals would no longer receive additional payment (The Joint Commission, 2016). Examples of hospital-acquired conditions that could be prevented using health IT include the following: • Pressure ulcers: Electronic assessment and plan of care application to link areas of risk with tailored interventions to prevent pressure ulcers from occurring. • Patient falls with injury: Electronic assessment and plan of care application to link areas of risk with tailored interventions to prevent falls and related injury. • Manifestations of poor glycemic control: Use of clinical decision support in EMR for postoperative insulin dosing.
Pay for Performance (P4P) (Aspden et al., 2007)	Medicare initiative designed to improve quality of care in all healthcare settings through collaboration with providers and other stakeholders to ensure that valid, reliable measures of quality and determine levels of reimbursement for care provided (Office of the National Coordinator for Health Information Technology, 2011). Examples of P4P measures facilitated by health IT include the following: • Cholesterol management–LDL control <100: Patient use of self-management tools through a patient portal. • HbA1c control <7.0%: Patient use of self-management tools through a patient portal. • Implement drug-drug and drug-allergy interaction checks: Use of clinical decision support in EMR for automated interaction checking.
Meaningful Use (The Joint Commission, 2015)	American Recovery and Reinvestment Act (ARRA) of 2009 initiative was designed to provide incentives for providers and healthcare organizations to improve quality of care through meaningful use of EHRs. Examples of meaningful use of health IT performance measures include the following: • Use CPOE. • Use Emar. • Provide online access to health information to patients (Office of the National Coordinator for Health Information Technology, 2015).
National Committee for Quality Assurance (NCQA)	A nonprofit organization established in 1990 by the Robert Wood Johnson Foundation to improve the consumer's ability to evaluate health plans through voluntary public reporting (Cohen et al., 2016). The Healthcare Effectiveness Data and Information Set (HEDIS) was developed and is maintained by NCQA.
Utilization Review Accreditation Commission (URAC)	An independent, nonprofit organization that aims to promote continuous improvement in the quality and efficiency of healthcare management through processes of accreditation and education (Downey et al., 2012).

CMS, Centers for Medicare and Medicaid Services; *CPOE*, computerized provider order entry; *EHR*, electronic health record; *eMAR*, Electronic Medication Administration Record; *EMR*, electronic medical record; *Health IT*, health information technology; *LDL*, low-density lipoprotein; *NPSG*, National Patient Safety Goals.

there is much room for improvement. Cohen et al. (2015) (Cohen et al., 2016) examined national trends in surgical outcomes from 2006 to 2013. The team reported long-term improvement in surgical outcomes for hospitals participating in the American College of Surgery National Surgical Quality Improvement Program. Improved outcomes included mortality, morbidity, and surgical site infections (Downey et al., 2012). Downey et al. evaluated national trends in patient safety indicators (PSI) such as postoperative pulmonary embolism, deep vein thrombosis, and pressure ulcers. The researchers found significant PSI trends for the decade 1998 to 2007. PSIs with the greatest levels of improvement during that period included birth trauma injury to neonates, postoperative physiologic and metabolic derangements, and iatrogenic pneumothorax. The PSIs with the greatest increase in incidence included pressure ulcers, postoperative sepsis, and infections due to improper medical care. Downey et al. noted that health IT holds potential for decreasing PSIs through standard reporting requirements and by supporting evidence-based practices through decision support and the use of order sets (Downey et al., 2012).

National Efforts Related to Quality Data Standards

The purpose of the Meaningful Use initiative was to improve the quality of care in the United States through the routine exchange of electronic health information for care delivery and quality reporting purposes. However, substantial work was needed to build the informatics infrastructure required to support system interoperability and routine data exchange (Healthit, 2015; Agency for Healthcare Research and Quality, 2014; Office of the National Coordinator for Health Information Technology, 2014). One component of the informatics infrastructure was establishing and adopting multilevel standards to support semantic interoperability. Semantic interoperability means that data are exchanged without a loss of context or meaning and therefore can be reused without special effort on the part of the user (Office of the National Coordinator for Health Information Technology, 2014). Semantic interoperability is only possible when all organizations adopt the same standards for quality measurement and reporting and use those standards in their electronic systems. The goal was to capture data for quality reporting in the context of existing documentation workflows. This required the adoption and use of standard clinical content in electronic systems, standard taxonomies or vocabularies are used to encode the content, and messaging standards are used to transfer information from one healthcare organization to another.

Automatic tracking of quality of care requires standard quality measures to ensure that all organizations use consistent metrics for benchmarking and use similar data types to populate the quality metrics. The standard quality metrics must define standard value sets (allowed values), taxonomies (standard terminologies), concept codes (codes assigned by the terminology developer), attributes (characteristics that provide context), and data structures for data to be collected as a by-product of documentation. These standards must be used to encode the content in the electronic record.

The ongoing work that maps (i.e., links) specific quality concepts to recommended terminologies for CMS quality measures is published on the electronic Clinical Quality Improvement (eCQI) website. The eCQI website is coordinated by the CMS and ONC to provide the most up-to-date measures, tools, and resources for applying existing standards to specify measures electronically (Office of the National Coordinator for Health Information Technology, 2015; USA, 2021).

Defined standards supporting Meaningful Use are included in Table 24.2. Representation of the complete data element set (e.g., the entire question-answer pair) by standardized terminologies and codes within an EHR system is required to fully automate quality reporting. Adopting and using the same standards by all organizations are required for quality reporting and benchmarking beyond the organizational level. These standards were included in the Stage 2 Meaningful Use initiative that provided incentives for their use in EHR systems and subsequently to provide the informatics infrastructure needed across the United States to collect and report quality data as a by-product of documentation. Stage 3 Meaningful Use proposed a focus on outcomes and was scheduled to begin in 2017 (Centers for Medicare and Medicaid, 2015). However, in 2018, CMS renamed the EHR Incentive Program to the Promoting Interoperability Program (CMS, 2018).

EVALUATING PATIENT SAFETY AND QUALITY

The foundation for the approach used to evaluate patient safety and care quality in healthcare organizations in the United States is based on the work of Avedis Donabedian. Donabedian developed a framework for measuring quality based on organizational structure, processes, and their linkages to patient outcomes (Donabedian, 1988). Donabedian's model provides the underpinnings for the framework used to assess PSQRD. Box 24.2 provides definitions of the primary concepts of the Donabedian model in terms of healthcare. Fig. 24.1 demonstrated the links and interactions between the concepts (Medicare Access and CHIP, 2015). Donabedian's model assesses quality through three domains: structure, process, and outcomes. Introducing the Singh and Sittig model (Fig. 24.2) increases the use of HIT to understand fundamental principles of the use of data, the need to verify and validate the data, and use a continuous feedback loop with the EHR to provide rationale and importance for safety events.

Conceptual Framework for Patient Safety and Quality

The framework for PSQRD builds on Donabedian's structure-process-outcome model to support the evaluation of an intervention from the pre-implementation testing phase through implementation and evaluation (Medicare Access and CHIP, 2015). The expanded HIT framework should have the greatest organizational effect related to the causal chain of quality and safety events (see Fig. 24.1). The PSQRD framework provides a means to categorize interventions according to areas of the causal chain targeted (e.g., the structure, the management or clinical processes, and the patient outcomes or throughput

TABLE 24.2   A Sample of Categories and Types of Data Elements Common to High-Priority Measures and Adopted Terminologies[a]

Data Categories	Data Types		2016 Interoperability Standards Vocabulary Standards to Support Meaningful Use
Adverse drug event	Allergy	Intolerance	National Drug File - Reference Terminology (NDF-RT)
Communication	Provider-provider	Provider-patient	
Diagnostic study	Order	Result	CPT 4/ICD-10 CM, CPT 4
Diagnosis	Outpatient (billing)	Inpatient	SNOMED CT/ICD-10 CM, SNOMED CT
	Outpatient (problem list)		
History	Behavioral (smoking)	Language	SNOMED CT
	Birth	Payment source	
	Care classification	Primary care provider	
	Death	Sex	
	Enrollment trial	Symptoms	
	Ethnicity/race		
Laboratory	Order	Result	LOINC
Location	Source/current/target	Transfer type	HL7 2.x ADT message
Medication	Discontinue order	Outpatient duration	RxNorm
	Inpatient administered	Outpatient order	
	Inpatient ordered	Outpatient filled	
Opt out	Other reason		
Physical exam	Vitals		LOINC
Procedure	Inpatient end	Outpatient	ICD-10 CM, CPT 4
	Inpatient start	Past history	
	Order	Consult results	

[a]For a complete list of data elements and codes, see the 2016 Interoperability Standards Advisor at https://www.healthit.gov/standards-advisory/2016.

Adapted with permission from American Medical Informatics Association and based on Dykes, P. C., Caligtan, C., Novack, A., Thomas, D., Winfield, L., Zuccotti, G., et al. (2010). Development of automated quality reporting: Aligning local efforts with national standards. *AMIA Annual Symposium Proceedings.* 2010, 187–191.

CPT, Current procedural terminology; *ICD*, international classification of diseases; *LOINC*, logical observation identifier names and codes; *SNOMED*, systematized nomenclature of medicine.

BOX 24.2   Definitions of the Primary Concepts for the Donabedian Model in Terms of Healthcare

Structure	The healthcare setting and its attributes include buildings, staffing ratios, available equipment, and the care provision budget.
	Includes exogenous factors not under the local control of a hospital or healthcare organization. Examples include: The Joint Commission (TJC) accreditation standards Meaningful Use requirements accreditation, licensing, and payment directives
Process	The managerial and clinical processes are in place to support the provision of care. Includes both managerial and clinical processes.
	Managerial process interventions have a latent effect on outcomes, as they influence communication and care practices that aim to affect patient care delivery.
	Clinical process interventions may have an immediate effect on patient outcomes.
Outcomes	The result of the structures and processes in place. May include both clinical outcomes and throughput. The outcomes are often the aim of health information technology and other interventions implemented to improve patient status.

---

targeted by the intervention or that drive adoption and use of the intervention in clinical practice).

The PSQRD framework is pertinent for evaluating the effect of health IT interventions on quality and patient safety, explaining why a health IT intervention was successful (or not). There are many reasons why health IT interventions are not adopted in practice (Jha et al., 2009). Health IT tools not widely adopted and used will have a limited effect on patient outcomes. The PSQRD framework is used to evaluate health IT interventions

designed to improve patient safety and care quality and to make recommendations for improving the implementation and evaluation of health IT interventions aimed at enhancing patient safety and care quality.

The PSQRD framework suggests that safety and quality issues are not mutually exclusive entities but exist on a "vector of egregiousness." Quality is at one end of the vector, representing frequent events with lower levels of immediacy. Causality ("the confidence with which a bad outcome, if it occurs, can be

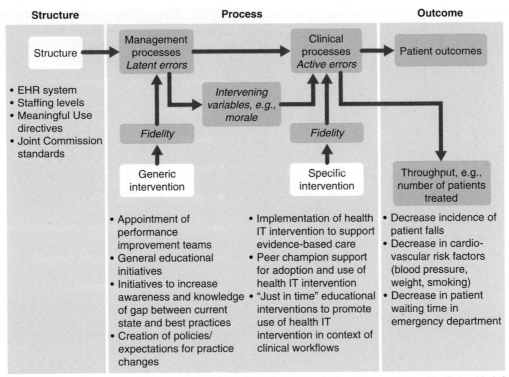

Fig. 24.1 A framework for patient safety and quality research design. *EHR*, Electronic health record; *Health IT*, health information technology. (Modified from Brown, C., Hofer, T., Johal, A., Thomson, R., Nicholl, J., Franklin, B. D., et al. An epistemology of patient safety research: A framework for study design and interpretation. Part 1. Conceptualising and developing interventions. *Quality & Safety in Health Care, 17*[3], 158–162.)

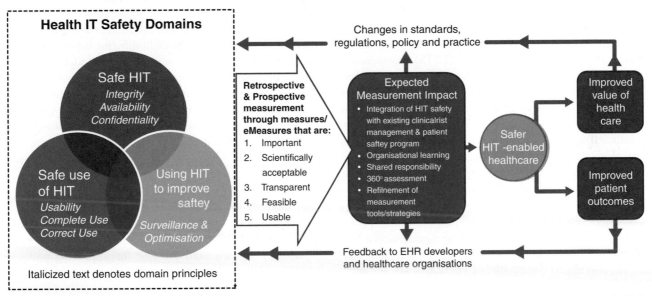

Fig. 24.2 he Sociotechnical Work System. *EHR*, Electronic health record; *Health IT*, health information technology. From Singh, H., & Sittig, D. F. [2016]. Measuring and improving patient safety through health information technology: The health IT safety framework. BMJ Quality & Safety, 25[4], 226–232.

attributed to an error") and patient safety are at opposing ends of the vector, encompassing more immediate events with high levels of causality. Errors or events that do not fall on or close to the vector are included within the safety-quality continuum and classified as having components of both (Medicare, 2015). For example, there is good evidence on the population level that screening mammography decreases breast cancer mortality in women (Moss et al., 2006, 2015). When an unscreened woman

develops end-stage breast cancer, the adverse outcome was preventable. However, the causal link is low, and the time over which breast cancer occurs is typically not immediate or rapid.

Using this model as a framework, a hospital-acquired infection from poor hand-washing practices has a high degree of causality and a low to moderate degree of immediacy. For example, there is sufficient evidence that poor hand-washing causes infections, though there is typically a time delay between exposure and onset of the infection. Patient falls and pressure ulcers are located midway up the vector of egregiousness, with the lack of tailored interventions to mitigate risk, placing patients at risk for injury with moderate degrees of causality and immediacy. Serious medication errors are higher on the vector, as they may occur due to inadequate adherence to the "five rights" for medication safety (right patient, right time, right drug, right dose, and right route). Medication errors are the most common adverse event (an unintended and unfavorable effect of medical care or treatment) in hospital settings. The errors are preventable using health IT systems with decision support at the bedside (i.e., closed-loop barcoding, medication administration, and smart pumps) (Garrouste-Orgeas et al., 2012). Medication errors are high on the vector of egregiousness toward safety because these types of errors are preventable through adherence to the "five rights" and, when they occur, have the potential to cause immediate and significant patient harm.

Conceptual Framework for Sociotechnical Work System

The implementation of health IT has been undertaken to reduce or eliminate preventable medical errors. Regrettably, health IT has introduced new errors. For example, many health IT solutions have led to provider burnout which can increase the risk of medical errors due to information overload, click fatigue, or inefficient user interfaces (Motluk, 2018; Collier, 2018; Dunn Lopez et al., 2021). It is essential to fix and learn from system problems to improve safety, ultimately creating a learning environment.

Fundamentally, the Health IT Safety (HITS) measurement framework proposes a foundation for health IT-related patient safety measurement, monitoring, and improvement within the context of a complex, adaptive, sociotechnical system. Furthermore, the sociotechnical work system considers the "many interacting technical (hardware, software, networking infrastructure) and non-technical (clinical workflow, internal organization policies, people, physical environment, and external policies) variables that affect health-IT related patient safety." The HITS measurement framework could be used by a LHS in the quest for improved measurement of underreported HITS events.

Conceptual frameworks have been used to increase the understanding of applying HIT to healthcare safety, efficacy, and quality. These frameworks include Roger's diffusion of innovation theory (Rogers, 2003), Venkateshe's user acceptance theory (Venkatesh et al., 2003), and Hutchins' theory of distributed cognition (Hutchins, 1995; Furniss et al., 2019). These frameworks fail to address in needs of today's fast-paced, complex adaptive healthcare systems. Sittig and Singh's sociotechnical model integrates eight interrelated dimensions to address the HIT needs in a complex adaptive healthcare system. These eight dimensions articulated in Box 24.3 are interdependent and interrelated concepts that represent a compilation of complex adaptive systems (CAS). The development of this framework emanated from design, implementation, and evaluation challenges that faced HIT within healthcare due to the advancement

---

BOX 24.3   Eight Concepts of Complex Adaptive Systems That Address Health Information Technology Needs

Hardware and Software Computing Infrastructure: Required to run applications

Clinical Content: Structured and unstructured data on the data-information-knowledge continuum

Human Computer Interface: Interaction of unrelated entities that users see, touch, and hear

People: All humans within the system (patients, clinicians, health information technology personnel, software developers)

Workflow and Communication: Steps required to ensure patients received quality care

Internal Organizational Polices, Procedures, and Culture: Organizational beliefs affect all other dimensions

External Rules, Regulations, and Pressures: Forces placing constraints on design, implementation, and use

System Measurement and Monitoring: Requirements for systematic measurement and monitoring

---

of healthcare needs, patient-related diagnostics, and rapidity of network interactions required to ensure the system's veracity and integrity. A CAS, by nature, is one where many interdependent elements occur at a fast pace requiring accurate and immediate intervention.

The Sociotechnical Model addresses the need for EHR system success by viewing the eight dimensions as interrelated and relational. Fig. 24.2, the Sociotechnical Model (Singh & Sittig, 2016) provides the relationship of the Sociotechnical Model to patient safety and care quality, noting the requirement interrelationship of integrity, availability, confidentiality, usability, surveillance, and optimization to meet improved patient outcomes. The eight dimensions, shown in Fig. 24.3, reflect the interrelationship of HIT related to a CAS and should not be considered independent nor hierarchical. The Socio-technical Framework addresses patient safety and quality care through the interactive and interrelation use of the EHR.

Medication Safety

Health IT systems hold promise for improving patient safety and improving care quality, particularly in medication safety. To date, computerized provider order entry (CPOE) and clinical decision support (CDS) systems have been used successfully in clinical practice to reduce errors during the process of ordering medications (National Academies of Sciences and Engineering, and Medicine, 2015; Bates & Gawande, 2003). In addition, Bar Code Medication Administration (BCMA) and Electronic Medication Administration Record (eMAR) systems have been adopted in many hospitals to improve patient safety and streamline clinical workflow, focusing on improving administration processes at the point of care (Paoletti et al., 2007; Sakowski et al., 2005; Yates, 2007). These systems leverage barcoding applications, with barcode labels placed on patient wristbands and medications. The systems can ensure adherence to the "five rights"

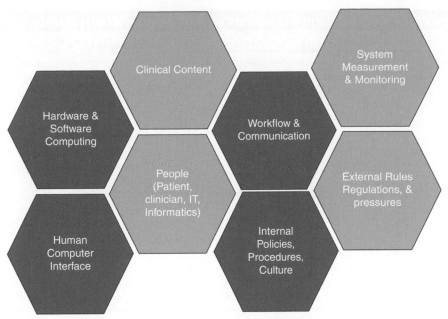

Fig. 24.3 Sociotechnical dimensions (Created by Lynda R. Hardy.)

to reduce medication errors and document drug administration in real-time. BCMA and eMAR systems are effective when implemented and used correctly (Mills et al., 2006; Patterson et al., 2002; van Onzenoort et al., 2008). For example, after BCMA system implementation, the scanning compliance rate is often suboptimal for scanning drugs and patient IDs (Franklin et al., 2007; Koppel et al., 2008). One study found that compliance with scanning medications was only 55.3% (Franklin et al., 2007). Another study revealed that nurses sometimes bypass scanning processes and create workarounds to reduce workloads or prevent the delay of medication administration (van Onzenoort et al., 2008). **Workarounds** are defined as any use of an operating system outside its designed protocol (van Onzenoort et al., 2008). This problem occurs most often in the system implementation stage and may create potential new paths to medical errors or other negative effects, such as inefficiency (Patterson et al., 2002, 2006).

Another important medication safety system that functions at the point of care is the smart infusion pump. Smart infusion pumps (also known as "smart pumps" or computerized patient infusion devices) include features designed to reduce administration errors and represent transformational clinical tools with the potential to decrease the number of IV medication errors in hospitals (Pedersen et al., 2012). This technology provides medication error reduction capabilities via a preprogrammed drug library with dose limit alerts and audio/visual feedback to users regarding entries programmed beyond predetermined dose, concentration, and duration thresholds. Smart pumps have been widely used in the United States. Notably, the adoption rate in the United States has doubled from 2005 to 2012 (Pedersen et al., 2012). A 2012 national survey by the American Society of Healthcare System Pharmacists found a 77% adoption rate of IV Smart pumps by US hospitals (Pederson et al., 2013). The growing adoption rate corresponds with the implementation of other technologies for safety and quality improvements, such as

EHRs, CPOE, and BCMA (Mills et al., 2006). One review paper found that smart pumps could reduce programming error rates. However, other types of errors may persist after implementing smart pumps (e.g., wrong drug errors, administration timing errors, and wrong patient errors) (Ohashi et al., 2014). A combination of smart pumps along with other clinical systems can prevent these errors. Furthermore, interoperability between currently implemented clinical systems and smart pumps is key to making meaningful improvements in IV medication safety. A lack of smart pump integration with other clinical systems in practice may limit the benefit of smart pumps (Harrington, 2018; Joseph et al., 2020).

The IOM reports, The Joint Commission Standards, and the National Patient Safety Goals (NPSG) represent structural incentives for the use of health IT to improve medication safety (Kaushal et al., 2003; The Joint Commission, 2015). The Joint Commission is an international nonprofit organization that accredits healthcare organizations that excel in providing safe and effective care of the highest quality and value. The NPSG and The Joint Commission Standards relevant to medication administrations (Table 24.3) are requirements for institutions in the United States and other countries that seek The Joint Commission accreditation.

Published studies suggest that successful implementation of BCMA and eMAR systems that improve patient safety depends on several factors, including the following (Paoletti et al., 2007; Sakowski et al., 2005; Yates, 2007):

A positive workplace culture (leadership, teamwork, and clinician ownership)

1. Training and support
2. Acceptance of the major impact of work practices by all team staff
3. A usable system with adequate decision support

Systems implemented using these principles can meet TJC Standards and NPSG and are hypothesized to improve patient safety.

TABLE 24.3	The Joint Commission Standards and National Patient Safety Goals	
	Requirements	**Elements of Performance**
National Patient Safety Goals (NPSG): NPSG.01.01.01	Use at least two patient identifiers when providing care, treatment, and services	Use at least two patient identifiers when administering medications, blood, or blood components, when collecting blood samples and other specimens for clinical testing, and when providing treatments or procedures. The patient's room number or physical location is not used as an identifier.
NPSG.03.04.01	Label all medications, medication containers, and other solutions on and off the sterile field in perioperative and other procedural settings[a]	In perioperative and other procedural settings, both on and off the sterile field, label medications, and solutions that are not immediately administered. This applies even if there is only one medication being used.
Medication Management: MM.06.01.01	The hospital safely administers medications	Before administration, the individual administering the medication does the following: Verifies that the medication selected matches the medication order and product label Verifies that the medication has not expired Verifies that no contraindications exist Verifies that the medication is being administered at the proper time, in the prescribed dose, and by the correct route

[a]Medication containers include syringes, medicine cups, and basins.
NPSG, National Patient Safety Goals.
Data from The Joint Commission. National Patient Safety Goals. Effective January 1, 2015. http://www.jointcommission.org/assets/1/6/2015_NPSG_HAP.pdf.

Chronic Illness Screening and Management

Health IT has demonstrated potential in improving the quality of care regarding chronic illness screening and management (Atlas et al., 2011; Cebul et al., 2011; Knaevelsrud & Maercker, 2010; Kwok et al., 2009; Park & Kim, 2012; Ruland et al., 2013; Simon et al., 2011; Saposnik et al., 2010). As noted in Fig. 24.2, health IT interventions that target chronic illness screening and management fall on the quality end of the vector of egregiousness, with lower levels of causality and immediacy.

Examples of structural incentives for using health IT to improve clinical processes include CDS based on practice guidelines such as the U.S. Preventive Services Task Force (USPSTF) recommendations on screening for breast cancer (U.S. Preventative Services Task Force, 2015) and depression, (U.S. Preventative Services Task Force, 2009) pay-for-performance measures, (Werner et al., 2011) and CMS core measures (Chassin et al., 2010). Analysis of these types of external programs on process improvement and patients' outcomes suggests that the long-term effect is limited and that tailoring quality improvement programs (e.g., the management and clinical processes) based on organization-specific situations is recommended (Werner et al., 2011).

One strategy that is successful in improving quality outcomes for those with chronic illness is the use of health IT interventions that target patients to improve access to treatment, (Knaevelsrud and Maercker, 2010) adherence to medication, diet, and exercise regimens, (Carson et al., 2012; Park & Kim, 2012) adherence to recommended screening guidelines, (Atlas et al., 2011) and engagement in symptom management (Ruland et al., 2013). Engagement of patients using health IT is a successful strategy for improving adherence to screening and best

practices management of chronic illness and improved quality outcomes (Shade et al., 2015; Bowles et al., 2015).

Nursing Sensitive Quality Outcomes: Patient Falls and Pressure Ulcers

Health IT interventions are also effective for improving patient safety and care quality related to fall and pressure ulcer prevention (Carson et al., 2012; Dowding et al., 2012; Dykes et al., 2010; Fossum et al., 2011, 2013; Garrett et al., 2009). The patient characteristics and factors related to risks for falls and pressure ulcers are multifaceted. For example, the patient's risks increase when skin surveillance is inadequate or fall prevention interventions are not ordered and taught to the patient and family. Fig. 24.2 illustrates that patient falls and pressure ulcers are located midway on the vector of egregiousness between safety and quality, with moderate levels of causality (failure to consistently implement tailored interventions) and immediacy (time to patient fall or development of pressure ulcer). An important structural component present for hospitals in the United States was the Deficit Reduction Act of 2006. CMS identified a list of preventable, hospital-acquired conditions for which hospitals would no longer receive additional payment (The Joint Commission, 2016). The regulations regarding nonpayment for hospital-acquired conditions included patient falls and pressure ulcers (The Joint Commission, 2016). The regulations provided an external directive (e.g., structure) that created a sense of urgency within organizations to eliminate preventable patient falls and pressure ulcers.

Management processes, including an administrative focus on fall and pressure ulcer prevention, are key factors in improving the quality of care. At the organizational level, interventions such as training, the use of health IT systems for decision support, and the involvement of peer champions in identifying and implementing interventions that are both feasible and effective provide an environment conducive to fall and pressure ulcer prevention (Dykes et al., 2010; Garrett et al., 2009). The use of clinical experts to improve the knowledge base of nurses and other healthcare providers (Carson et al., 2012) and the use of a peer champion model (Carson et al., 2012; Dykes et al., 2010; Garrett et al., 2009; Riggio et al., 2009; Schnipper et al., 2010) support fidelity of both management processes (e.g., communication, importance of behavior change, advocacy for fall and pressure ulcer prevention initiatives) and clinical processes (e.g., end-user training, support, modeling the intervention set on patient care units).

When implementing complex practice changes, as required for fall and pressure ulcer prevention, health IT is often a single component of a multifaceted performance improvement intervention. Moreover, leadership support for the practice change is essential. Health IT interventions are most effective when both clinical and management processes are addressed and where organizational leadership demonstrates strong support for improvement strategies (Carson et al., 2012; Dykes et al., 2010; Garrett et al., 2009).

Success Factors and Lessons Learned

The effects of health IT interventions aimed at improving patient safety and care quality using the key frameworks have been evaluated to identify key success factors and provide a foundation for making recommendations for continued use, design, and implementation for health IT research. The PSQRD framework, through the expansion of Donabedian's model, is useful for exploring the relationships between the organization's structural forces (e.g., setting attributes, exogenous factors) that support organizational change, including the adoption and use of health IT as a tool to improve clinical processes and patient outcomes. External accreditation or regulatory requirements provide structural incentives for the changes in clinical processes that are supported by health IT interventions. The PSQRD framework focuses on intervening variables that improve staff commitment to process changes, such as incentive payments and morale (Riggio et al., 2009). Additional examples of management strategies to improve fidelity with the intervention include peer champion support networks, (Carson et al., 2012; Day et al., 2011; Dykes & Carroll, 2009) and enduser education (Garrett et al., 2009; Riggio et al., 2009; Dykes & Carroll, 2009).

The PSQRD framework provides a means to plan for and evaluate health IT interventions designed to improve patient safety and care quality. Characteristics of successful health IT implementation projects are provided in Box 24.4. The PSQRD framework is a useful guide for developing a comprehensive implementation and evaluation plan that addresses these success factors. It provides an effective strategy for evaluating the effect of health IT on patient safety and care quality outcomes.

The Sociotechnical framework is key to understanding the application of HIT to CAS, where decisions are made based on the interrelationship of clinical information, alerts, usability,

---

BOX 24.4 Characteristics of Successful Health IT Implementation Projects Supporting Quality and Safety

Factor	Description
Leadership support	Leaders support the adoption and use of health IT to improve patient care and facilitate practice changes.
Comprehensive health IT implementation and adoption strategy	Attention to both management and clinical processes to promote fidelity with the intervention.
Health IT as a "tool"	Health IT applications are considered a tool or a single component of a multifaceted intervention to improve the underlying clinical processes and patient outcomes.
Patient engagement	Patients engaged in clinical process changes to deliver evidence-based care, to improve safe practices, and to improve patient outcomes. Health IT is one tool to support process changes.
End-user involvement	End-users involved in iterative development and implementation of health IT interventions to improve quality and safety.
Peer champion support	The use of peer support to facilitate the adoption and proper use of health IT applications within clinical workflows.

Health IT, Health information technology.

---

and continuous measurement and monitoring. The clinical and the informational domains coexist in a CAS environment where the safe and effective use of the EHR involves multiple factors that provide data, information, and knowledge for decision-making. This framework expands theories and frameworks that use technology but do not address the need to effectively dissect disruptions that affect the process. Ensuring that the appropriate health care decisions are made and the safety and quality of patient care provided may require a multiframework approach that integrates key components and continued measurement and monitoring of patient care flow, dynamics, and HIT.

Even well-designed health IT interventions require a comprehensive plan that includes a focus on structure, management, clinical processes, and intervening variables to address fidelity with the intervention. Failure to address these factors may prevent the adoption and use of health IT tools and serve as a barrier to patient safety and quality in clinical practice. For example, Schnipper et al. describe a Smartforms application, a clinical documentation tool designed to facilitate real-time, documentation-based decision support to capture structured, coded data in the context of documentation (Schnipper et al., 2008). A randomized controlled trial demonstrated a limited impact of the Smartforms on patient outcomes because only 5.6% of eligible healthcare providers used the application (Schnipper et al., 2010). Investigators summarized their lessons learned, stating that in addition to well-designed health IT tools, improvements in chronic disease management require a comprehensive approach that includes the following:

Financial incentives (structure)

Multifaceted quality improvement efforts (management processes including interventions to promote fidelity with the intervention)

Reorganization of patient care activities (clinical processes) across care team members (Schnipper et al., 2010)

While many frameworks exist, this chapter introduced two frameworks that have been successful in integrating patient care and HIT.

CONCLUSION AND FUTURE DIRECTIONS

Medical errors and poor-quality care continue to occur in healthcare organizations. Failure to understand the interrelationship of care and technology to maximize the EHR in decision-making suggests that the understanding of healthcare systems as CAS is missing. This chapter demonstrates that the progress continues in the United States to address inadequacies in patient care and quality recognized by sentinel publications (i.e., IOM reports) and the need for continuous quality reporting and promoting EHR interoperability. Health IT innovations continue to be associated with improved patient safety and quality medication errors.

Further improvements require that healthcare organizations use a learning health system approach to healthcare and health IT evaluation. The two frameworks provided indicate the emphasis placed on the intersection between clinical care and HIT, noting the strength of the combination. The PSQRD framework considers the supporting structures and processes (management and clinical) that drive healthcare outcomes. This approach can facilitate the adoption and interoperability of health IT tools that will systematically drive patient safety and quality in clinical practice and inform effective research. The Sociotechnical framework provides eight intersecting dimensions that consider how the HIT software and hardware, coupled with clinical content, workflow, and communication, can work towards patient safety and quality care.

Predicated on the complexity of the errors in healthcare, multifaceted strategies, including evaluation frameworks and innovative health IT tools, are needed to realize additional improvement in clinical processes and patient outcomes by improving the quality and safety of healthcare.[c] Prerequisites for health IT systems that will improve patient safety and quality include strong clinical leadership and a solid informatics infrastructure. Clinical leadership characterized by technical skill, experience with managing IT projects, and a vision for the value of technology for improving patient care are associated with successful IT adoption (Ingebrigtsen et al., 2014). Such attributes are needed to lead the clinical team from planning to implementation, where the optimal benefits of health IT can be realized. A solid informatics infrastructure across healthcare organizations, where standards are adopted and used by all, is vital to improving safety and quality. Continued work with standardized measures and benchmarks, standard clinical content used in electronic systems, standard taxonomies or vocabularies to encode that content, and messaging standards to transfer information from one healthcare organization to another are the foundational requirements for improved safety and quality of care.

New legislation continues to develop standards that will create an informatics infrastructure to support patient safety and care quality across the United States (Office of the National Coordinator for Health Information Technology, 2015). However, continued emphasis on standards is necessary to advance best practices in each setting. Standards are a place to ensure safety and care quality at a basic level, but patients often define (and expect) quality at a much higher level. Moving forward, all healthcare organizations and institutions must strive to meet and exceed patient expectations of safety and care quality through the adoption and use of health IT.

ACKNOWLEDGMENTS

The authors wish to acknowledge the contributions of Patricia C. Dykes and Kumiko O. Schnock to the previous edition of this chapter.

[c] References 49–51, 69, 70, 75, 79, 80, 85, 86

DISCUSSION QUESTIONS

1. The U.S. Department of Health and Human Services Agency for Healthcare Research and Quality has identified seven Portfolios of Research. The full list can be viewed at http://www.ahrq.gov/cpi/portfolios/index.html. Two of the Portfolios of Research that are of key importance to this chapter are (1) Health Information Technology and (2) Patient Safety. Describe how these two Portfolios of Research relate to the ONC's *Health Information Technology Patient Safety Action and Surveillance Plan: June 2013* (Washington, DC: Office of the National Coordinator for Health Information Technology, 2013).

2. What is the utility of Donabedian's structure-process-outcome model as the basis for evaluating quality of care and patient safety associated with a health IT application? Describe two limitations. Discuss how the framework for patient safety and research design can be used to overcome these limitations.

3. Use the framework for patient safety and quality research design to create a comprehensive plan to support the successful implementation of Bar Code Medication Administration.

4. The Office of the National Coordinator (ONC) is taking actions on health IT and patient safety as described in their *Health IT Patient Safety Action and Surveillance Plan* by *improving* the safe use of health IT, *learning* more about the impact of health IT on patient safety, and *leading* to

create a culture of shared responsibility among all users of health IT. A description of this initiative is located at https://www.healthit.gov/policy-researchers-implementers/health-it-and-safety. Describe the implications of this initiative from an interprofessional perspective for either your current work setting or that of the case study presented in the chapter.

CASE STUDY

Western Heights Hospital (WHH) is a 1125-bed, 5-hospital academic healthcare system servicing central and western Massachusetts. WHH is the only designated Level I Trauma Center for adults and children in the area. It is home to New England's first hospital-based air ambulance and the region's only Level III Neonatal Intensive Care Center. WHH launched a 5-year strategic plan with a fundamental goal of a system-wide move from a paper environment to an electronic one. Phase I included implementing an EHR system consisting of order entry for all laboratory, radiology, and patient care orders. Additionally, clinical documentation was implemented, including admission assessments and all nursing flow sheets. The nursing informatics counsel, a 25-member group of nurses representing all disciplines, developed the clinical content. The clinical content was custom built using both free text and structured data entry fields within the application.

Three months after go-live, hospital leadership is reporting that it is unable to report on various state and federally mandated quality measures. These measures track healthcare quality based on national standards, are compared to nationally accepted benchmarks, and are used to plan ways to improve quality. Leadership has communicated that the reports generated by the system are incomplete and are putting the hospital at financial risk due to lower reimbursement rates.

Clinicians are eager and excited to continue to develop content in the application. However, the project's program manager is proposing a stabilization and optimization approach and does not want to go forward with content development until the issue of reporting has been assessed and addressed.

Discussion Questions

1. Assuming that you are the clinical content manager and lead all reporting efforts, what approach would you take to address the reporting problem?
2. Preadmission testing data are currently collected on paper. The chief of surgery has identified an opportunity to collect these data in the new EHR system by the preadmission testing area in the outpatient setting. Many of the collected data elements are shared with the current admission assessment. Describe how this effort can be approached. What methods can be used to implement the process?
3. Using the PSQRD methodology, identify an area of quality improvement in the hospital setting, develop a process plan, and identify the expected outcomes.

REFERENCES

Adams, K., & Corrigan, J. (2003). *Priority areas for national action: Transforming health care quality*. Washington, DC: Institute of Medicine;.

Agency for Healthcare Research and Quality. (2014). A robust health data infrastructure. Rockville, MD. AHRQ Publication No. 14-0041-EF 14-0041-EF. https://www.healthit.gov/sites/default/files/ptp13-700hhs_white.pdf.

Aspden, P., Wolcott, J., Bootman, J., & Cronenwett, L. (2007). *Preventing medication errors: Quality chasm series* (pp. 463). Washington, DC: National Academies Press.

Atlas, S. J., Grant, R. W., Lester, W. T., Ashburner, J. M., Chang, Y., Barry, M. J., et al. (2011). A cluster-randomized trial of a primary care informatics-based system for breast cancer screening. *Journal of General Internal Medicine, 26*(2), 154–161.

Bates, D. W., & Gawande, A. A. (2003). Improving safety with information technology. *The New England Journal of Medicine, 348*(25), 2526–2534.

Better, Smarter, Healthier: In Historic Announcement, HHS Sets Clear Goals and Timeline for Shifting Medicare Reimbursements from Volume to Value. http://www.hhs.gov/news/press/2015pres/01/20150126a.html. Accessed January 26, 2015.

Bowles, K. H., Dykes, P., & Demiris, G. (2015). The use of health information technology to improve care and outcomes for older adults. *Research in Gerontological Nursing, 8*(1), 5–10.

Bradley R., Pratt R., Thrasher E., Byrd T., & Thomas C. (2012). An examination of the relationships among IT capability intentions, IT infrastructure integration and quality of care: A study in U.S. Hospitals. In: Paper presented at: 45th Hawaii International Conference on System Sciences. Hawaii.

Brown, C., Hofer, T., Johal, A., Thomson, R., Nicholl, J., Franklin, B. D., et al. (2008). An epistemology of patient safety research: A framework for study design and interpretation. Part 4. One size does not fit all. *Quality and Safety in Health Care, 17*(3), 178–181.

Carson, D., Emmons, K., Falone, W., & Preston, A. M. (2012). Development of pressure ulcer program across a university health system. *Journal of Nursing Care Quality, 27*(1), 20–27.

Cebul, R. D., Love, T. E., Jain, A. K., & Hebert, C. J. (2011). Electronic health records and quality of diabetes care. *The New England Journal of Medicine, 365*(9), 825–833.

Centers for Medicare, Medicaid Services (CMS), & HHS. (2010). Medicare and Medicaid programs; electronic health record incentive program; final rule. *Federal Register, 75*(144), 44313–44588.

Centers for Medicare and Medicaid Services. (2009). Hospital-Acquired Conditions (Present on Admission Indicator). http://www.cms.hhs.gov/HospitalAcqCond/01_Overview.asp#TopOfPage.

Centers for Medicare and Medicaid. (2015). Medicare and Medicaid Programs; Electronic Health Record Incentive Program—Stage 3. 2015 edition health information technology (health IT) certification criteria, 2015 edition base electronic health record (EHR) definition, and ONC health IT certification program modifications; final rules. *Federal Register, 80*(60), 62601–62759.

Chassin, M. R., Loeb, J. M., Schmaltz, S. P., & Wachter, R. M. (2010). Accountability measures—using measurement to promote quality improvement. *The New England Journal of Medicine, 363*(7), 683–688.

CMS. (2018). Stage 3 Program requirements for providers attesting to their state's Medicaid Promoting Interoperability (PI) programs. https://www.cms.gov/Regulations-and-Guidance/Legislation/EHRIncentivePrograms/Stage3Medicaid_Require.

Cohen, M. E., Liu, Y., Ko, C. Y., & Hall, B. L. (2016). Improved surgical outcomes for ACS NSQIP hospitals over time: Evaluation of hospital cohorts with up to 8 years of participation. *Annals of Surgery, 263*(2), 267–273.

Collier, R. (2018). Rethinking EHR interfaces to reduce click fatigue and physician burnout. *Canadian Medical Association Journal, 190*(33), E994–E995.

Day, R. O., Roffe, D. J., Richardson, K. L., Baysari, M. T., Brennan, N. J., Beveridge, S., et al. (2011). Implementing electronic medication management at an Australian teaching hospital. *The Medical Journal of Australia, 195*(9), 498–502.

Donabedian, A. (1988). The quality of care. How can it be assessed? *Journal of the American Medical Association, 260*(12), 1743–1748.

Dowding, D. W., Turley, M., & Garrido, T. (Jul-Aug 2012). The impact of an electronic health record on nurse sensitive patient outcomes: An interrupted time series analysis. *Journal of the American Medical Informatics Association: JAMIA, 19*(4), 615–620.

Downey, J. R., Hernandez-Boussard, T., Banka, G., & Morton, J. M. (Feb 2012). Is patient safety improving? National trends in patient safety indicators: 1998–2007. *Health Services Research, 47*(1 Pt 2), 414–430.

Dunn Lopez, K., Chin, C. -L., Leitão Azevedo, R. F., Kaushik, V., Roy, B., Schuh, W., et al. (2021). Electronic health record usability and workload changes over time for provider and nursing staff following transition to new EHR. *Applied Ergonomics, 93*, 103359.

Dykes, P., & Carroll, D. A. H. (2009). Fall TIPS: Strategies to promote adoption and use of a fall prevention toolkit. *AMIA Annual Symposium Proceedings, 2009*, 153–157.

Dykes, P. C., Carroll, D. L., Hurley, A., Lipsitz, S., Benoit, A., Chang, F., et al. (2010). Fall prevention in acute care hospitals: A randomized trial. *JAMA., 304*(17), 1912–1918.

Fossum, M., Alexander, G. L., Ehnfors, M., & Ehrenberg, A. (2011). Effects of a computerized decision support system on pressure ulcers and malnutrition in nursing homes for the elderly. *International Journal of Medical Informatics, 80*(9), 607–617.

Fossum, M., Ehnfors, M., Svensson, E., Hansen, L. M., & Ehrenberg, A. (2013). Effects of a computerized decision support system on care planning for pressure ulcers and malnutrition in nursing homes: An intervention study. *International Journal of Medical Informatics, 82*(10), 911–921.

Franklin, B. D., O'Grady, K., Donyai, P., Jacklin, A., & Barber, N. (2007). The impact of a closed-loop electronic prescribing and administration system on prescribing errors, administration errors and staff time: A before-and-after study. *Quality & Safety in Health Care, 16*(4), 279–284.

Furniss, D., Garfield, S., Husson, F., Blandford, A., & Franklin, B. D. (2019). Distributed cognition: understanding complex sociotechnical informatics. *Studies in Health Technology and Informatics, 263*, 75–86. https://doi.org/10.3233/SHTI190113.

Garrett, J., Wheeler, H., Goetz, K., Majewski, M., Langlois, P., & Payson, C. (2009). Implementing an "always practice" to redefine skin care management. *The Journal of Nursing Administration, 39*(9), 382–387.

Garrouste-Orgeas, M., Philippart, F., Bruel, C., Max, A., Lau, N., & Misset, B. (2012). Overview of medical errors and adverse events. *Annals of Intensive Care, 2*(1), 2.

Gaylin, D. S., Moiduddin, A., Mohamoud, S., Lundeen, K., & Kelly, J. A. (2011). Public attitudes about health information technology, and its relationship to health care quality, costs, and privacy. *Health Services Research, 46*(3), 920–938. https://doi.org/10.1111/j.1475-6773.2010.01233.x.

Harrington, L. (2018). Interoperability of infusion pumps with electronic health records. *AACN Advanced Critical Care, 29*(4), 377–381. https://doi.org/10.4037/aacnacc2018874.

Healthit.gov. (2015). Health IT quick stats. http://dashboard.healthit.gov/quickstats/quickstats.php.

Hutchins, E. (1995). *Cognition in the wild*. MIT Press.

Ingebrigtsen, T., Georgiou, A., Clay-Williams, R., Magrabi, F., Hordern, A., Prgomet, M., et al. (2014). The impact of clinical leadership on health information technology adoption: Systematic review. *International Journal of Medical Informatics, 83*(6), 393–405.

Institute of Medicine. (2001). *Crossing the quality chasm: A new health system for the 21st century*. Washington, DC: Institute of Medicine;.

Jha, A. K., Bates, D. W., Jenter, C., Orav, E. J., Zheng, J., Cleary, P., et al. (2009). Electronic health records: Use, barriers and satisfaction among physicians who care for black and Hispanic patients. *Journal of Evaluation in Clinical Practice, 15*(1), 158–163.

Jha, A. K., DesRoches, C. M., Campbell, E. G., Donelan, K., Rao, S. R., Ferris, T. G., et al. (2009). Use of electronic health records in U.S. hospitals. *The New England Journal of Medicine, 360*(16), 1628–1638.

Joseph, R., Lee, S. W., Anderson, S. V., & Morrisette, M. J. (2020). Impact of interoperability of smart infusion pumps and an electronic medical record in critical care. *American Journal of Health-System Pharmacy, 77*(15), 1231–1236.

Kaushal, R., Shojania, K. G., & Bates, D. W. (2003). Effects of computerized physician order entry and clinical decision support systems on medication safety: A systematic review. *Archives of Internal Medicine, 163*(12), 1409–1416.

Knaevelsrud, C., & Maercker, A. (2010). Long-term effects of an internet-based treatment for posttraumatic stress. *Cognitive Behaviour Therapy, 39*(1), 72–77.

Kohn, L., Corrigan, J., & Donaldson, M. (1999). *To err is human: Building a safer health system*. Washington, DC: IOM.

Koppel, R., Wetterneck, T., Telles, J. L., & Karsh, B. -T. (2008). Workarounds to barcode medication administration systems: Their occurrences, causes, and threats to patient safety. *Journal of the American Medical Informatics Association: JAMIA, 15*(4), 408–423.

Kwok, R., Dinh, M., Dinh, D., & Chu, M. (2009). Improving adherence to asthma clinical guidelines and discharge documentation from emergency departments: Implementation of a dynamic and integrated electronic decision support system. *Emergency Medicine Australasia, 21*(1), 31–37.

Lohr, K. (1990). *Medicare: A strategy for quality assurance* (Vol. 1). Washington, DC: Institute of Medicine.

Medicare Access and CHIP Reauthorization Act of 2015. H.R.2.EN. http://thomas.loc.gov/cgi-bin/query/D?c114:4:/temp/~c1144daAw2::&gt.

Mills, P. D., Neily, J., Mims, E., Burkhardt, M. E., & Bagian, J. (2006). Improving the bar-coded medication administration system at the Department of Veterans Affairs. *American Journal of Health-System Pharmacy, 63*(15), 1442–1447.

Moss, S. M., Cuckle, H., Evans, A., Johns, L., Waller, M., Bobrow, L., et al. (2006). Effect of mammographic screening from age 40 years on breast cancer mortality at 10 years' follow-up: A randomised controlled trial. *Lancet*, 368(9552), 2053–2060.

Moss, S. M., Wale, C., Smith, R., Evans, A., Cuckle, H., & Duffy, S. W. (2015). Effect of mammographic screening from age 40 years on breast cancer mortality in the UK Age trial at 17 years' follow-up: A randomised controlled trial. The. *Lancet Oncology*, 16(9), 1123–1132.

Motluk, A. (2018). Do doctors experiencing burnout make more errors. *Canadian Medical Association Journal*, 190(40), E1216–E1217. https://doi.org/10.1503/cmaj.109-5663.

National Academies of Sciences, & Engineering, and Medicine. (2015). *Improving diagnosis in health care*. Washington, DC: The National Academies Press.

Office of the National Coordinator for Health Information Technology. (2011). *Federal health information technology strategic plan 2011—2015*. Washington, DC: Office of the National Coordinator for Health Information Technology;.

Office of the National Coordinator for Health Information Technology. (2019). Office-based physician electronic health record adoption, health IT quick-stat #50. https://www.healthit.gov/data/quickstats/office-based-physician-electronic-health-record-adoption.

Office of the National Coordinator for Health Information Technology. (2014). *Connecting health and care for the nation: A 10-year vision to achieve an interoperable health IT infrastructure*. Washington, DC: Office of the National Coordinator for Health Information Technology. https://www.healthit.gov/sites/default/files/ONC10yearInteroperabilityConceptPaper.pdf.

Office of the National Coordinator for Health Information Technology. (2013). *Health information technology patient safety action & surveillance plan: June 2013*. Washington, DC: Office of the National Coordinator for Health Information Technology. https://www.healthit.gov/sites/default/files/safety_plan_master.pdf.

Office of the National Coordinator for Health Information Technology. (2014). *ONC Health IT Safety Program—Progress on health IT patient safety action and surveillance plan*. Washington, DC: Office of the National Coordinator for Health Information Technology. https://www.healthit.gov/sites/default/files/ONC_HIT_SafetyProgramReport_9-9-14_.pdf.

Office of the National Coordinator for Health Information Technology. (2015). The one-stop shop for the most current resources to support electronic clinical quality improvement. https://ecqi.healthit.gov/.

Office of the National Coordinator for Health Information Technology. (2015). Interoperability standards advisory, draft for comment. https://www.healthit.gov/standards-advisory/2016.

Ohashi, K., Dalleur, O., Dykes, P. C., & Bates, D. W. (2014). Benefits and risks of using smart pumps to reduce medication error rates: A systematic review. *Drug Safety*, 37(12), 1011–1020.

Page, A. (2004). *Keeping patients safe: Transforming the work environment of nurses*. Washington, DC: Institute of Medicine.

Paoletti, R. D., Suess, T. M., Lesko, M. G., Feroli, A. A., Kennel, J. A., Mahler, J. M., et al. (2007). Using bar-code technology and medication observation methodology for safer medication administration. *American Journal of Health-System Pharmacy*, 64(5), 536–543.

Park, M.-J., & Kim, H.-S. (2012). Evaluation of mobile phone and Internet intervention on waist circumference and blood pressure in post-menopausal women with abdominal obesity. *International Journal of Medical Informatics*, 81(6), 388–394.

Park, M.-J., & Kim, H.-S. (2012). Evaluation of mobile phone and Internet intervention on waist circumference and blood pressure in post-menopausal women with abdominal obesity. *International Journal of Medical Informatics*, 81(6), 388–394.

Patterson, E. S., Cook, R. I., & Render, M. L. (2002). Improving patient safety by identifying side effects from introducing bar coding in medication administration. *Journal of the American Medical Informatics Association: JAMIA*, 9(5), 540–553.

Patterson, E. S., Rogers, M. L., Chapman, R. J., & Render, M. L. (2006). Compliance with intended use of Bar Code Medication Administration in acute and long-term care: An observational study. *Human Factors*, 48(1), 15–22.

Pedersen, C. A., Schneider, P. J., & Scheckelhoff, D. J. (2012). ASHP national survey of pharmacy practice in hospital settings: Dispensing and administration—2011. *American Journal of Health-System Pharmacy*, 69(9), 768–785.

Pederson, C. A., Schneider, P. J., & Scheckelhoff, D. J. (2013). ASHP national survey of pharmacy practice in hospital settings: Monitoring and patient education—2012. *American Journal of Health-System Pharmacy*, 70, 787–803.

Riggio, J. M., Sorokin, R., Moxey, E. D., Mather, P., Gould, S., & Kane, G. C. (2009). Effectiveness of a clinical-decision-support system in improving compliance with cardiac-care quality measures and supporting resident training. *Academic Medicine*, 84(12), 1719–1726.

Rogers, E. M. (2003). *Diffusion of innovations* (5th ed.). New York, NY: Free Press.

Ruland, C. M., Andersen, T., Jeneson, A., Moore, S., Grimsbø, G. H., Børøsund, E., et al. (2013). Effects of an internet support system to assist cancer patients in reducing symptom distress: A randomized controlled trial. *Cancer Nursing*, 36(1), 6–17.

Runciman, W., Hibbert, P., Thomson, R., Van Der Schaaf, T., Sherman, H., & Lewalle, P. (2009). Towards an international classification for patient safety: Key concepts and terms. *International Journal for Quality in Health Care*, 21(1), 18–26.

Sakowski, J., Leonard, T., Colburn, S., Michaelsen, B., Schiro, T., Schneider, J., et al. (2005). Using a bar-coded medication administration system to prevent medication errors in a community hospital network. *American Journal of Health-System Pharmacy*, 62(24), 2619–2625.

Saposnik, G., Teasell, R., Mamdani, M., Hall, J., McIlroy, W., Cheung, D., et al. (2010). Effectiveness of virtual reality using Wii gaming technology in stroke rehabilitation: A pilot randomized clinical trial and proof of principle. *Stroke*, 41(7), 1477–1484.

Schnipper, J. L., Linder, J. A., Palchuk, M. B., Yu, D. T., McColgan, K. E., Volk, L. A., et al. (2010). Effects of documentation-based decision support on chronic disease management. *The American Journal of Managed Care*, 16(12 Suppl HIT), SP72–SP81.

Schnipper, J. L., McColgan, K. E., Linder, J. A., Yu, T., Fiskio, J., Tsurikova, R., et al. (2008). Improving management of chronic diseases with documentation-based clinical decision support: Results of a pilot study. *AMIA Annual Symposium Proceedings*, 1050.

Shade, S. B., Steward, W. T., Koester, K. A., Chakravarty, D., & Myers, J. J. (2015). Health information technology interventions enhance care completion, engagement in HIV care and treatment, and viral suppression among HIV-infected patients in publicly funded settings. *Journal of the American Medical Informatics Association: JAMIA*, 22(e1), e104–e111.

Simon, G. E., Ralston, J. D., Savarino, J., Pabiniak, C., Wentzel, C., & Operskalski, B. H. (2011). Randomized trial of depression follow-up care by online messaging. *Journal of General Internal Medicine, 26*(7), 698–704.

Singh, H., & Sittig, D. F. (2016 Apr). Measuring and improving patient safety through health information technology: The health IT safety framework. *BMJ Quality and Safety, 25*(4), 226–232. https://doi.org/10.1136/bmjqs-2015-004486.

The Joint Commission. (2016). National patient safety goals. http://www.jointcommission.org/standards_information/npsgs.aspx.

The Joint Commission. (2015). The joint commission e-dition. https://e-dition.jcrinc.com/MainContent.aspx.

The Leapfrog Group. (2015). http://www.leapfroggroup.org/home.

U.S. Food & Drug Administration (FDA). What is a Serious Adverse Event? Reporting Serious Problems to FDA. Available at: https://www.fda.gov/safety/reporting-serious-problems-fda/what-serious-adverse-event. Accessed December 14, 2021.

U.S. Preventative Services Task Force. 2015. Breast cancer screening draft recommendations. http://screeningforbreastcancer.org/.

U.S. Preventative Services Task Force. (2009). Depression in adults: Screening. http://www.uspreventiveservicestaskforce.org/Page/ Document/RecommendationStatementFinal/depression-in-adults-screening.

USA.gov. eCQI Resource Center. (2021). eCQM standards. Available at https://ecqi.healthit.gov/ecqm-standards?qt-standards=1. Accessed December 14, 2021.

van Onzenoort, H. A., van de Plas, A., Kessels, A. G., Veldhorst-Janssen, N. M., van der Kuy, P. H., & Neef, C. (2008). Factors influencing bar-code verification by nurses during medication administration in a Dutch hospital. *American Journal of Health-System Pharmacy, 65*(7), 644–648.

Venkatesh, V., Morris, M. G., Davis, G. B., & Davis, F. D. (2003). User acceptance of information technology: Toward a unified view. *MIS Quarterly, 27* 425e78.

Werner, R. M., Kolstad, J. T., Stuart, E. A., & Polsky, D. (2011). The effect of pay-for-performance in hospitals: Lessons for quality improvement. *Health Affairs, 30*(4), 690–698.

World Health Organization. (2017). Patient safety: Making health care safer. https://apps.who.int/iris/handle/10665/255507. Licence: CC BY-NC-SA 3.0 IGO.

Yates, C. (2007). Implementing a bar-coded bedside medication administration system. *Critical Care Nursing Quarterly, 30*(2), 189–195.

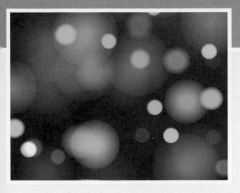

25

Informatics in the Curriculum

Marisa L. Wilson

OBJECTIVES

At the completion of this chapter, the reader will be prepared to:
1. Summarize key issues transforming healthcare into a digital environment.
2. Give examples of formal efforts to define expected informatics competencies produced by health profession organizations.
3. Discuss how supporting educators and ensuring education quality can close the informatics competency gap.
4. Summarize key challenges of technology-enhanced education.
5. Give examples of how teaching and learning processes adapt to support healthcare.
6. Describe frameworks and models that guide informatics curriculum.
7. Discuss the roles available to healthcare professionals with informatics training.

KEY TERMS

accreditation, 396	credentialing, 398	informatics competencies, 398
certification, 398	digital health, 392	

ABSTRACT ❖

This chapter focuses on the multiple complex forces pushing change to ensure a competent and capable healthcare workforce. While there are multiple topics to explore, this chapter will highlight: (1) drivers propelling the need for a competent and capable healthcare workforce; (2) response by healthcare provider educational associations and institutions to meet this demand; and (3) accreditation and certification agencies charged with ensuring educational quality and safe practitioners. These requirements are necessary to ensure the healthcare workforce is capable of practicing in an environment that is rapidly shifting to an all-digital system. This chapter also reviews key Institute of Medicine reports and the Health Information Technology for Economic and Clinical Health application to educational issues.

INTRODUCTION

Medical and health care and, a patient, consumer, or population's overall state of health and wellbeing are being radically transformed by advances in healthcare information and communication technology (health IT and ICT). The desire and need to use digital technology at the point of care—whether it be in an acute hospital, an ambulatory center, a long-term care facility, or a home—are being driven by need, increasing familiarity and comfort with using technology, and with the proliferative use of technology in other business sectors such as retail, communications, entertainment, banking, and education. Current public health crises, the rising cost of medical care, and consumer expectations, not only in the United States but around the globe, have created an urgency for accurate data and

information to form actionable knowledge to guide care. This requires efficient digital collection tools, a usable end user interface, analytics capability, and the ability for clinicians to easily consume information at an appropriate point in a cognitive workflow when transformation of care processes using the data and information generated using health information technology (health IT) can occur. In many countries, innovative technologies, and the reconceptualization of the fundamental nature of Medicine and healthcare are quickly reshaping the industry into an almost digital platform. Traditional face-to-face care with in-person interactions between the provider and patient, occurring within the confines of a physical space and at a specified time, are being converted into virtual interactions that remove the constraints of location, time, and in-person requirements. These interactions are now rapidly evolving into digital health modalities using technologies and processes which totally remove the time and location barriers from the interactions between the provider and patients or consumers. In its current state, digital health, uses telecare and telehealth tools, wearables and mobile applications, health analytics inclusive of genomics, precision medicine, data analytics, and digitized information systems such as the electronic health record (EHR) (Lundgren et al., 2021; Buchanan et al., 2021). The medical and healthcare industries are increasingly turning to digital information and the use of electronic communication to fundamentally change the services provided. In the United States, the 2009 American Recovery and Reinvestment Act included measures to provide financial incentives and other types of support to modernize the healthcare technology infrastructure of the United States. The Health Information Technology for Economic and Clinical Health (HITECH) Act of 2009 was one of the measures within the act (Centers for Medicare and Medicaid Services [CMS], 2021). The HITECH Act laid the foundation to operationalize infrastructure to support the conversion of a paper intensive system to a more digital platform. The HITECH Act was defined by the expectations outlined in Meaningful Use. Now that this foundation of technology has been accomplished, there is a movement towards improved value and quality.

To transform current episodic medical care into innovative health care, HITECH's Meaningful Use and the existing Physician Quality Reporting System, as well as Value-Based Payment Modifiers have all been harmonized under the Merit-Based Incentive Payment System (MIPS) (Office of the National Coordinator for Health Information Technology [ONC], 2019). MIPS has the potential to bring about unprecedented change in systems of care through the combined use of targeted technology and data collection, as well as analysis to drive innovation. This drive to provide digitally supported innovative care has widespread implications on training and competency expectations of all health professionals. The expectations of the health care workforce to manage and lead in a technology-saturated, data-rich environment has implications not only for those who provide care, but also for those who educate the student and those who provide professional development for the practicing healthcare professional.

DRIVERS OF INFORMATICS AND INFORMATION TECHNOLOGY INFUSION IN HEALTHCARE

Understanding the discipline of informatics and how those working in healthcare are affected by informatics processes and information and communication technology (ICT), is essential to recognize the national, regional, and local drivers of the use of health information and the political agenda for the use of health IT. The use of medical data and health information is not new, nor is the use of an electronic medical record. The 1950s ushered in the use of mainframe computer systems to automate the financial and accounting functions of hospitals. This automation made the generation of hospital bills more efficient as reimbursement rules increased in complexity. The massive computer hardware filled entire rooms and was solely process oriented. Computer infrastructure and the EHR are discussed throughout this book, but an emphasis and recap are helpful as it relates to the appropriateness of health informatics in the curriculum.

Recapping the Beginning of Digitization

Hospitals in the 1960s began the design and development of patient care applications to accomplish single processes in specialty units. The first electronic medical records appeared in the 1960s. An early version of an electronic medical record was developed and implemented in the Mayo Clinic in Rochester, Minnesota in the 1960s (Becker's Hospital Review, 2015). By 1965, approximately 73 hospitals and clinical information projects and 29 projects for the storage and retrieval of medical document and clinical data were under development (Becker's Hospital Review, 2015). In the 1970s, public health departments worked with vendors to develop software to automate the reporting of vital events and to generate statistical data for state and federal agencies. Birth and death vital records, causes of death, and maternal and infant mortality incidence reporting are all generated from data from individual hospitals, providers, funeral directors, and others. The data is sent to State health departments from hospitals and care providers for review and analysis before being sent to the Centers for Disease Control and Prevention (CDC). Prior to the 1970s, this process was totally done on paper. After the 1970s, this process was moved to mainframe processing and then, ultimately, to personal computers. When computer hardware became more compact in size, the speed of processing exponentially increased. Business sectors automated their data collection and analysis processes. The conversion of medical and healthcare processes lagged.

The Impact of Information Technology on Healthcare

The impact of information technology on the healthcare sector has been a subject of interest, discussion, and evaluation and has received significant federal strategic attention for more than three decades. Various Institute of Medicine (IOM) reports since 1999 have linked health IT to healthcare improvement. The overarching goal of IOM reports across decades was to support the point of care infusion of informatics processes and information technology as they have been in other business sectors such as service, finance, and retail.

One main conclusion in *To Err is Human*, the first IOM report, is that the majority of medical errors are caused by faulty systems, processes, and conditions that lead people to make mistakes or fail to prevent them at some part of the process (Kohn et al., 2000). The report pointed to health IT as a solution for reducing medical errors and increasing patient safety through automation of processes, reduction of duplication, and the creation of databases for system evaluation (Becker's Hospital Review, 2015).

The next IOM report, *Crossing the Quality Chasm*, addressed the importance of health IT and noted how crucial it is to clinical decision making, delivering population-based care, consumer education, professional development, and research (Committee on Quality of Health Care in America, 2001). A third IOM report, published in 2003, was *Health Professional Education: A Bridge to Quality* (Greiner & Knebel, 2003*)*. This report specifically listed informatics as one of five core competencies in the educational programs of all health professionals so that all clinicians can communicate, manage knowledge, mitigate error, and support decision making using information technology (Greiner & Knebel, 2003).

President Obama signed into law the American Recovery and Reinvestment Act (ARRA) on February 17, 2009, after a slow but steady decade long progression to convert paper-based health records to electronic delivery (American Recovery and Reinvestment Act [ARRA], 2009). The HITECH Act, among other initiatives, enacted as part of ARRA, provided resources to the Office of the National Coordinator for Health IT (ONC). The HITECH Act provided financial and technical support through the Centers for Medicare and Medicaid Services (CMS) and the ONC to healthcare facilities, fueling the rapid implementation of certified EHRs within acute and ambulatory care services.

In 2010, the ONC commissioned the IOM to summarize the existing knowledge of the effects of health IT on patient safety and to make recommendations for both federal and private sector organizations to maximize health IT and patient safety. The resulting report, *Health IT and Patient Safety: Building Safer Systems for Better Care* ("IOM Report"), was released in 2012 (IOM Report Institute of Medicine, 2012). Building upon the 2012 IOM Report, in July 2013, the ONC published the Health IT Patient Safety Action and Surveillance Plan and established ONC's Health IT Safety Program to coordinate activities related to the plan (IOM Report Institute of Medicine, 2013). The Health IT Patient Safety Action and Surveillance Plan laid out specific steps to: (1) increase the quantity and quality of data and knowledge about health IT safety; (2) target resources and corrective actions to improve health IT and patient safety; and (3) promote a culture of safety related to health IT (IOM Report Institute of Medicine, 2013).

Health IT Adoption

Nationally, progress has been made in the adoption and use of health IT to improve outcomes and care across the nation but work still needs to be done to see that every person and their care provider can get appropriate health information when and how they need it. The Office of the National Coordinator (ONC) reported in 2021, that in 2017, 96% of all hospitals had a certified EHR and this is an improvement from 2011 when the ONC reported that only 72% of hospitals had a certified EHR (Office of the National Coordinator [ONC], 2021). In June 2014, the ONC released *Connecting Health and Care for the Nation: A 10-Year Vision to Achieve an Interoperable Health IT Infrastructure (ONC)*. This report described ONC's broad vision and framework and was the springboard for the Shared Interoperability Roadmap and the ONC Strategic Plan, both released in 2015.

President Obama signed the bipartisan 21st Century Cures Act (Cures Act) in 2016. The Cures Act represents a significant shift in how electronic health information is managed, which affects how health IT is used, how data is shared, and importantly, how healthcare providers interact with patients and their data. Among the provisions, the Cures Act promotes data

sharing through expanded interoperability of that data within and outside of the specific healthcare enterprise in which the patient receives care (ONC). The Cures Act prohibits data blocking and mandates immediate access and portability of personal electronic health information for patients, providers, and payers (ONC).

In summary, EHRs are not new. The use and development of the technology extends back to the 1960s, but the spread of the technology was limited. It was the HITECH Act and its funding that positioned informatics and health IT at the forefront of all healthcare sectors that the implementation of health IT exploded across the country. Through this explosion, it became apparent, early in the process, that health professionals lacked the education, competency, and capability to take full advantage of the data and technology that was at their fingertips. Without a level of competency and capability beyond basic data entry into fields in an EHR, healthcare providers are unable to grasp the full potential of informatics processes and the technologies that are used to change systems to support and extend care. Healthcare clinical leaders are unable to envision all the changes that are required to bring about improved care processes and outcomes without basic competency. Leaders continue to be unfamiliar with the details of quality measures, interoperability, patient engagement, and data analytics, terms which are frequently cited but often misunderstood. Providers need to be capable of understanding how to obtain information to support a learning health system (LHS). An LHS, as first discussed in Chapter 3, (also referred to as a Learning Healthcare System) is defined as one with "goal-oriented feedforward and feedback loops that create actionable information with the potential to effect marked improvements in population health and decreases in the cost of evidence-based care if implemented correctly" (Kohn et al., 2000).

EDUCATION REFORM INITIATIVES THAT SUPPORT THE DRIVERS OF TRANSFORMATION

The drivers that pushed information technology into medicine and healthcare, and into the hands of care givers and providers, have had an impact on the academic landscape. One resulting action is the call for education reform. The need to ensure informatics processes, and that the best practice use of information technology occurs during care, demands competent graduates who are capable of using the data and informatics processes and technologies within redesigned workflow processes in whichever way and with whomever care is practiced. This need for reform is not new. Findings from a 1999 American Medical Informatics Association (AMIA) Spring Conference workgroup highlight that, even with the minimal use of EHRs in most healthcare facilities at that time and before the drivers pushed forward more technology infusion into healthcare, there was a need for all health professions educational programs to add teaching on informatics processes and information technology use to the academic pathways of the non-informatician health professional (American Nurses Association, 2022). The American Association of Medical Colleges (AAMC); the American Association of Colleges of

Nursing (AACN); the National Advisory Council on Nursing Education and Practice (NAC-NEP); the Medical Library Association (MLA) Task Force for Knowledge and Skills; and the International Medical Informatics Association (IMIA) Group on Health and Medical Informatics Education drafted broad guidelines during this meeting for the development of health informatics competencies and informatics education for all health professionals to include. These comprise the optimization of information systems in practice; storing these tools in a personalized manner; integration of tools into workflows and organizations; and the design of systems to permit critical information detection (American Nurses Association, 2022). Move forward two decades, and the educational requirements have not changed drastically and neither has the low level of informatics education in health professions curriculum despite an environment totally infused with technology and awash in data. Educationally focused healthcare professional associations, practice leaders, and special interest groups are once again calling for reforms in education so that learners and graduates can be competent and capable of using the full potential of data and information technology to radically transform care to influence the health of a nation. For all health professionals, calls for the inclusion of health informatics training and for the best evidence for the use of health IT in any care setting are not new but have become pressing over time. As the United States continues to transform its healthcare system to be safe, efficient, patient centered, timely, equitable, and effective, it must invest in the education of individuals to ensure that the workforce is poised to meet the challenges of an integrated health system that is built on digital and technological platforms. The demand for an increasingly technological and integrated health system requires educators to use an interprofessional approach to education while continuing to meet the specific needs of the different health workers.

Two decades ago, the IOM produced five core competencies that all health professionals should possess regardless of discipline to meet the needs of the 21st-century healthcare system (Greiner & Knebel, 2003). They are:

1. Provide patient centered care,
2. Work in interdisciplinary teams,
3. Employ evidence-based practice,
4. Apply quality improvement, and
5. Utilize informatics.

These remain important competencies despite the passage of time. So, how have the various healthcare professions associations responded? The following sections will briefly address the current expectations.

The American Nurses Association Scope and Standards of Nursing Informatics Practice

Nursing has played an early leading role in crafting informatics roles, responsibilities, and knowledge, skills, and attitudes (KSAs) to bring about transformation for nurses with patient care responsibilities and for those who are specializing in Informatics. In 1992, the American Nurses Association (ANA) recognized nursing informatics as a nursing specialty

that integrates nursing science, computer science, and information science to manage and communicate data, information, and knowledge in nursing practice. The viewpoint was helping nurses to understand how to use the new hardware and software that was being made available. The definition was further refined, and roles and responsibilities were defined in the first editions of *The Scope of Practice for Nursing Informatics* (ONC) and *The Standards of Practice for Nursing Informatics* (American Nurses Association, 1995). As technology and informatics developed over time, these documents were combined into the ANA's *Scope and Standards of Nursing Informatics Practice* (American Nurses Association, 2001) and expanded in 2008 and again in 2015 as *Nursing Informatics: Scope and Standards of Practice* (American Nurses Association, 2008, 2015) to reflect the growing changes in nursing informatics roles and responsibilities brought about by the dramatic bolstering of the nation's health IT agenda. In 2021, a group of expert informatics nurses with experience as practitioners and educators was convened with the purpose of updating the Scope and Standards of Nursing Informatics to meet demand today. One of the first tasks of this group was to collaboratively develop a new definition of nursing informatics that moved the purpose beyond just the technology design and implementation to the potential for transformation. The new definition as approved is:

Nursing informatics is the specialty that transforms data into needed information and leverages technologies to improve health and healthcare equity, safety, quality, and outcomes (American Nurses Association, 2022).

This new edition describes the competency expectations of nurses who provide care at all levels and informatics nurses regarding:

1. The creation of data to information to knowledge to wisdom,
2. The development and use of clinical decision support and expert systems,
3. Management and use of big data, data storage, and analytics,
4. Artificial and augmented intelligence, machine learning, natural language processing, and deep learning,
5. Using data for forecasting and predictive analytics, and
6. Refining the user experience (American Nurses Association, 2022).

Each edition of the ANA Scope and Standards of Nursing Informatics Practice describes the necessary competencies of practicing nurses at all levels and provides the informatics and information technology competency expectations of both the nurse informatician and the Informatics Nurse Specialist who is a nurse holding a graduate degree in informatics and a nursing informatics certification. Each new edition considers the level of informatics sophistication, technology development, and healthcare need and adjusts the competency expectations accordingly. The earliest edition focused on a basic understanding of hardware and software and how the nurse could lead the use of these in the care setting. Currently, the focus of the newest edition asks nurse leadership to consider the development of competent nurses who can use big data, data science, and analytics to drive change and improve outcomes (American Nurses Association, 2022).

The American Association of Colleges of Nursing

From 2019 to 2021, the AACN responded to external drivers to change healthcare and to the expressed needs of practice partners by forming a broad team of subject matter experts, nurse education leadership, and leadership from practice partners to refine the Essentials of Nursing Practice. Over this time, the team thoughtfully and with evidence developed foundational elements, ten domains and concepts, competencies and measurable and actionable sub competencies, a new model for nursing education, and implementation strategies. The Domains of the Essentials include: (1) Knowledge for Nursing Practice, (2) Person Centered Care, (3) Population Health, (4) Scholarship for Nursing Practice, (5) Quality and Safety, (6) Interprofessional Partnerships, (7) Systems-Based Practice, (8) Informatics and Healthcare Technology, (9) Professionalism, and (10) Personal, Professional and Leadership Development (American Association of Colleges of Nursing [AACN], 2021). Domain 8 calls out competency expectations in Informatics and Healthcare Technology. The AACN Essential topic of informatics and health care technologies is not new and dates to 2006 to 2008, but those essential lists did not explicitly describe measurable sub competencies for which educational facilities could be held accountable (AACN, 2006, 2008).

The 2021 edition of the Essentials, Domain 8, Informatics and Healthcare Technologies contains actionable and measurable competency expectations for graduates of US nursing schools that schools will be responsible to provide to the students. The competencies in Domain 8 are:

1. Understanding how the various ICT tools are used in the care of patients, communities, and populations;
2. Demonstrating the use of information and communication technologies and informatics processes to deliver safe nursing care to diverse populations in a variety of settings;
3. Using ICT to support chronicling of care and communication among providers, patients, and all system levels; and
4. Using information and communication technologies in accordance with ethical, legal, professional, and regulatory standards, and workplace policies in the delivery of care (AACN, 2021).

The revised AACN Essentials requires that all nurses will require an understanding of the informatics process of data to information, to knowledge, to wisdom, and how to use health IT to achieve this within a legal and ethical context and in an efficient workflow. These competencies should serve as a solid foundation for the graduate level nurse informatician.

American Association of Medical Colleges

Physicians need to interact competently with an interprofessional team using information technology and informatics processes. Although no unified documentation on expected informatics competency for medical education could be located on the AAMC site, Hersh et al. documented specific learning objectives and milestones to support developing informatics competent medical practitioners (Association of American Medical Colleges and the Howard Hughes Medical Institute,

2009). These competencies were developed through a consensus agreement between a group of six faculty.

Hersh et al. (2014) offer multiple competencies across the continuum of medical education (Association of American Medical Colleges and the Howard Hughes Medical Institute, 2009). Among them are:

1. Find, search, and apply knowledge-based information to patient care,
2. Use and guide implementation of clinical decision support,
3. Provide care using population health management approaches,
4. Protect patient privacy and security,
5. Use information technology to improve patient safety,
6. Engage in quality measurement selection and improvement,
7. Use Health Information Exchange (HIE) to identify and access patient information across settings,
8. Engage patients to improve their health and care delivery using personal health records and patient portals,
9. Maintain professionalism using information technology tools.
10. Provide clinical care via telemedicine,
11. Apply personalized/precision medicine, and
12. Participate in practice-based research.

Implementing these competencies into medical school curriculum would help to ensure that physicians could lead change with data and technology.

The American Council on Graduate Medical Education

Like their nurse informatician partners, physician education oversight does describe informatics competency expectations for physicians seeking fellow training and board certification in clinical informatics. Fellowship is advanced graduate medical education that extends competency beyond knowledge attained in residency (The Clinical Informatics Milestone Project, 2015). Five levels of milestones are described with specific sub competencies. Patient Safety and Unintended Consequences, Technology Assessment, Clinical Decision Support Systems, Impact of Clinical Informatics on Patient Care, Project Management, and Information System Lifecycle, and Assessing User Needs are all described under the specific levels (The Clinical Informatics Milestone Project, 2015; Triola et al., 2010; Hersh et al., 2014). The levels, from 1 to 5, represent an increasing complex set of demonstrable skills from those one would expect of an incoming fellow to what one would expect of a practitioner who has advanced beyond performance targets for a fellow and into what one would expect of a practitioner with years of experience (The Clinical Informatics Milestone Project, 2015).

The American Academy of Colleges of Pharmacy

Pharmacies in hospitals and in community settings are also fully automated with information technology from computers to robotics. Pharmacists and pharmacy technologies are expected to demonstrate competency using information technology and informatics processes to effect better outcomes. Retrospectively, it was noted that the education provided for the student to achieve competence, despite inclusion in the 2007 Accreditation Council for Pharmacy Education Standards and Guidelines, as a requirement was found to be inconsistent (Fox et al., 2011). In 2019, work was done to refine and revise those competencies. The pharmacist informatics task force of the American Academy of Colleges of Pharmacy (AACP) used 11 sources and faculty feedback to create a revision (Martin et al., 2019). This revision lists the following domains with detailed competencies aligned (Fox et al., 2011; Martin et al., 2019). The domains are:

1. Legal and regulatory,
2. Interoperability and Standardization,
3. Patient Outcomes,
4. Health Care and Clinical Biomedical Informatics,
5. Practitioner Development and Education, and
6. Emerging Technologies.

THERE IS A COMPETENCY GAP

While competency expectations of a health professions student are reasonable and explicit, there is a gap. Those responsible for educating or training health professions students or current providers, often lack informatics KSAs so there is often not an adequate transfer of competence to students. For example, the AACN reports that the average age of nursing faculty with a doctoral degree in positions of professor, associate professor, and assistant professor were 62.4, 57.2, and 51.2 years (AACN, 2020). Given the age of faculty, they were not educated about informatics during their own time in school and not even during clinical practices. This results in an informatics skill and competency gap among graduates. For nursing, this significant gap has been identified by the HIMSS TIGER, the HIMSS EU*US eHealth Work Project, and Nursing Knowledge Big Data Science Education Workgroup (Blake et al., 2018). To substantiate and justify the size of the gap, in 2017, the EU*US Work Project team issued a survey to over 1000 targeted respondents to measure the need, supply, and trends that support necessary workforce skills and competencies (Blake et al., 2018). Over 870 responses were returned from the US and the EU. Respondents represented all the health care professions involved in health IT and represented the full spectrum of the healthcare workforce. A synthesis of results pointed to five major gaps related to training and skills: lack of knowledge and skills of providers and caregivers; lack of knowledge and skills of faculty and educators; availability of courses and programs; quality and quantity of training materials. Moreover, research by Brunner et al identified the pressure placed on universities to deliver eHealth education in a curriculum wide approach for which the universities are struggling to meet the needs for applicable and novel learning opportunities (Blake et al., 2018).

Supporting the Educators

Given the external drivers for change and the mandates from the various professional associations that oversee the competencies of healthcare professional graduates, informatics organizations have stepped forward and are developing professional education opportunities, toolkits, and resources for faculty and educators. Among those organizations are:

1. The American Association of Colleges of Nursing. The AACN has tools to assist with the infusion of the sub competencies into the curriculum. Some are still under development (https://www.aacnnursing.org/AACN-Essentials/Implementation-Tool-Kit).
2. The Nursing Knowledge Big Data Science Initiative Education Workgroup (https://bigdata.dreamhosters.com). The goal of this group is to ensure sharable and comparable nursing data through standardized data, data science, social determinants of health, and expanded understanding of health IT.
3. HIMSS Technology Guiding Education Reform (TIGER) Virtual Learning Environment (VLE) (https://www.himss.org/tiger-virtual-learning-environment). The VLE is a digital interactive learning environment powered by HIMSS. HIMSS offers learning resources (https://www.himss.org/resources-all).
4. HIMSS Accelerate (https://www.himss.org/news/accelerate-announces-digital-platform-launch). This is a digital platform that provides professional development tools, networking, and curated content.
5. American Medical Informatics Association (AMIA) (https://amia.org/education-events/education-catalog). AMIA is a preeminent professional informatics association. AMIA offers education resources.

Accreditation, Certification, and Credentialing

Accreditation, certification, and credentialing are quality indicators for ensuring accountability in a specific field of study. Every academic program producing health professionals is overseen by an accrediting body who conducts a formal evaluation of the educational program, institution, or system against defined standards for the purpose of quality assurance and enhancement (Brunner et al., 2018).

In addition to the general education of a health professional, several specializations have their own accreditation. Informatics is one of those specializations. As the field of informatics expands, it is imperative to ensure a standard of education, training, and continuing the endorsement of informatics professionals. This standard of excellence is accomplished through three activities: educational program accreditation, individual certification, and organization/individual credentialing. These three activities, while working independently, work synergistically to achieve the goal of quality. Table 25.1 lists these activities and examples of various professional associations involved in these activities in health informatics.

Accreditation of educational programs and institutions in the United States is a means to ensure and improve the quality of higher education through the use of a set of standards developed by peers (Frank et al., 2020). An institution or program that has successfully completed an accreditation review has the needed curriculum, qualified faculty, student support, and other services in place to assist students in achieving their educational goals (Frank et al., 2020). Accreditation of a program is extremely important in that this designation denotes not only quality but assures the student that the school and program are aligned with professional standard setting organizations and that the school is in good standing with state and federal agencies.

TABLE 25.1   Quality Indicators

Quality Indicator	Definition	Organizations	Scope
Accreditation	Accreditation in the United States is a means to ensure and improve higher education quality, assisting institutions and programs using a set of standards developed by peers. An institution or program that has successfully completed an accreditation review has in place the needed instructional, student support, and other services to assist students to achieve their educational goals.	Commission on Accreditation for Health Informatics and Information Management Education (CAHIIM), www.cahiim.org	Health informatics
		Liaison Committee on Medical Education (LCME), www.lcme.org	Medicine
		Commission on Collegiate Nursing Education (CCNE), www.aacn.nche.edu/ccne-accreditation	Nursing
		Accreditation Commission for Education in Nursing (ACEN), www.acenursing.org	Nursing
		Commission on Accreditation in Physical Therapy Education (CAPTE), www.capteonline.org	Physical therapy
		American Occupational Therapy Association (AOTA), www.aota.org/education-careers/accreditation.aspx	Occupational therapy
		Accreditation Council for Education in Nutrition and Dietetics, www.eatrightacend.org/ACEND/content.aspx?id=73	Nutrition
		Council on Social Work Education (CSWE) Commission on Accreditation, www.cswe.org/accreditation.aspx	Social work
		Council on Academic Accreditation in Audiology and Speech-Language Pathology (CAA), www.asha.org/academic/accreditation	Speech pathology and audiology
		Commission on Dental Accreditation, www.ada.org/en/coda	Dentistry and oral hygiene
		Accreditation Council for Pharmacy Education, www.acpe-accredit.org	Pharmacy
Certification	A person is certified as being able to competently complete a job or task, usually by the passing of an examination and/or the completion of a program of study.	American Nurses Credentialing Center, www.nursecredentialing.org/InformaticsNursing	Nursing informatics
		American Board of Medical Specialties, www.abms.org/board-certification	Medical informatics
		Certified Professional in Health Information and Management Systems (CPHIMS), www.himss.org/health-it-certification/cphims	Chief information officers and other health professionals
		College of Healthcare Information Management Executives (CHIME) Certified Healthcare CIO (CHCIO), www.chimecentral.org/chcio	Chief information officers and information technology executives only
Credentialing	Credentialing is the process of establishing the qualifications of licensed professionals, organizational members, or organizations, and assessing their background and legitimacy. Healthcare institutions and provider networks conduct their own credentialing, granting, and reviewing specific clinical privileges and allied health staff membership.	No official organization for this effort; conducted by the organization concerning their employees	–

Health professions schools are accredited based on their specialty. For example, academic nursing programs are accredited by The Commission on Collegiate Nursing Education (CCNE). Specialties also have a separate accreditation. For example, Nurse Anesthetist programs are accredited by The Council on Accreditation of Nurse Anesthesia Education Programs (COA). The primary accreditation organization for accrediting health informatics programs is the Commission on Accreditation for Health Informatics and Information Management Education (CAHIIM). As accreditation moves to a student outcomes focus, the development of health informatics competencies is critical. Competencies are developed by professional organizations, such as the AMIA, and then used by the accrediting organization. The CAHIIM standard concerning curriculum states that the curriculum must build on health informatics competencies. However, now, informatics-related programs exist within university programs that are accredited as part of the specialty accreditation for that program. For example, a nursing informatics tract offered as part of a school of nursing graduate program could be accredited by either Accreditation Commission for Education in Nursing Inc. (ACEN), the Commission on Collegiate Nursing Education (CCNE), or the NLN Commission for Nursing Education Accreditation (CNEA). What should occur is that the nursing program overall is accredited by CCNE, and the Informatics graduate program is also accredited by CAHIIM.

Certification is a process that indicates that an individual or institution has met predetermined standards. Specialty areas, such as informatics, have professional organizations that provide certification to individual practitioners to ensure that the individuals are qualified in terms of knowledge and skills. A person is usually certified as being able to competently complete a job or task by passing an examination. Certification examinations are developed from job analyses and professional competencies.

Credentialing is the process of establishing the qualifications of licensed professionals, organizational members, or organizations, and assessing the professional's and/or organization's background and legitimacy (Eaton, 2015). In this process, the individual or the organization presents evidence that they are prepared to practice in a competent and safe manner. The evidence may be graduation from an accredited program, individual certification, demonstration of continuing education, and other forms of scholarship.

These three quality indicators of health informatics practice depend on the professional association to develop practice competencies. The professional organization describes the discipline through these competencies. Accreditation defines standards and peer review to determine standard achievement. Certification is accomplished through examination of the individual's ability to demonstrate competency and job proficiency. Credentialing requires evidence that includes accreditation and certification. These activities form a three-legged stool that defines and promotes the knowledge and skills for the discipline of health informatics.

One of the primary professional organizations engaged in activities to support accreditation and certification in health informatics is the AMIA. AMIA became a member of CAHIIM in 2015 and, in cooperation with CAHIIM, established the Health Informatics Accreditation Committee to coordinate the development of health informatics competencies to be used in the accreditation of health informatics programs.

AMIA established the Advanced Interprofessional Informatics Certification (AIIC) task force to develop a certification process for professionals who practice clinical/health informatics at an advanced level (National Academies of Sciences, Engineering, Medicine, 2014). The first cohort of non-physician informatics professionals have now achieved that certification. AMIA also collaborated with the American Board of Medical Specialties (ABMS) and American Board of Pathology (ABP) to develop a certification examination for physicians to earn a board certification in the subspecialty of clinical informatics.

CHALLENGES OF TECHNOLOGY-ENHANCED EDUCATION

The nation has been challenged to create digitally supported, data driven, and innovative models of care. This requires health professions students to be competent and capable to participate in and lead this work. To do this there has to be faculty, educators, and mentors who are also competent and capable to teach and guide. This requires administration leadership with understanding and vision. Several challenges must be overcome to teach informatics and assist students at all levels to develop appropriate competencies because there is an acknowledged gap that exacerbates the gap in informatics competency among new health professional graduates. The paucity of faculty prepared to teach informatics competencies is well documented (AACN, 2020; Blake et al., 2018). Although advanced informatics education programs are accelerating, finding qualified faculty to teach in these programs is extremely difficult. At the same time, health IT tools and applications in the curriculum are no longer a luxury but a necessity. Teaching informatics requires knowledge of the content, experience in the use of informatics skills in clinical practice, and access to health IT tools for the curriculum.

Faculty Expertise

Any strategy to include informatics and technology in health professionals' education must involve attention to faculty informatics expertise. The ability for the faculty to teach informatics competencies at the appropriate level depends on: (1) faculty's recognition of their own competency level and to recognize that to teach this content requires knowledge beyond basic functions of an EHR; (2) faculty's understanding of the informatics competencies needed by their students; (3) faculty's ability to understand the parallels of health, healthcare, and health IT, as well as quality and safety; (4) faculty's ownership of the need for informatics; and (5) support from their schools and department leadership, including infrastructure and help with technology needs as they arise.

All health professionals must be ground in a similar set of competencies. This is supported by AMIA, which considers informatics when used for healthcare delivery to be the same regardless of the health professional group involved (whether dentist, pharmacist, physician, nurse, or other health professional) (AMIA, 2016). The focus is not the profession but improving the use of information with the assistance of technology within a team context. Health informatics is a new subject in healthcare and recently has received more recognition as a specialty area, but all practicing healthcare providers need a fundamental set of competencies. A growing number of health professions' associations understand the importance of and the need for students to learn the concepts and competencies of health informatics and have started including this information in their national exams.

Given the existing informatics competency gap among current faculty and the lack of informatics trained and clinically educated faculty, existing faculty need to be trained. As is not unusual for a newer specialty, the only alternative is often to recruit willing but untrained personnel from the existing faculty or healthcare team and appoint them to cover informatics. These practitioners or faculty are then expected to instruct students and/or colleagues clinical informatics concepts and methodologies or to begin building or optimizing an EHR and other technologies.

All programs educating direct and indirect care providers at the various competency levels need to prepare professionals to be able to synthesize knowledge; integrate evidence into practice; work collaboratively and in interdisciplinary teams; use clinical information and decision support systems and provide safe and ethical care. Faculty in all healthcare education programs need formal informatics education or faculty development that aligns with the expected level of learner (entry to practice, advanced, practice doctorate or research doctorate) they teach. The Competencies Matrix of Health IT and Informatics Skills is displayed in Box 25.1.

Despite these efforts to bring informatics to the forefront and increase informatics knowledge and competencies in the curriculum, a number of studies demonstrated slow progress on integrating these competencies in the curriculum (Skiba & Rizzolo, 2011; Staggers et al., 2002; Billings, 2007). As described earlier, faculty have been cited as the largest barrier to greater IT integration in education because they lack the knowledge and skills regarding new technologies and their potential (Billings, 2007). Associations, such as the American Association of Colleges of Nursing (AACN) and other professional organizations have developed initiatives to ensure informatics processes and the use of information technology knowledge, skills and attitudes are covered in the curriculum. AACN is currently in process of developing a ToolKit 9 (https://www.aacnnursing.org/AACN-Essentials/Implementation-Tool-Kit) and the Education Workgroup of the Nursing Knowledge Big Data Initiative is developing Resources.

Health IT Tools

In addition to experienced faculty, many academic institutions do not have the infrastructure to support and maintain the integration of health IT tools, such as an academic electronic health record (AEHR) or barcode medication administration (BCMA), essential for informatics competencies in the curriculum (Herbert & Connors, 2016). AEHR and BCMA are adapted versions of clinical information systems used in acute and ambulatory care facilities, with modifications that customize the product for the learning environment. To be competent, students need to use the tools that they will use in clinical practice and connect the data and information to decision making, communication, and teamwork during the workflow. One such tool is an AEHR that incorporates point-of-care, evidence-based practice information. The cost of these tools may be prohibitive in academic environments or, if the tools are available, faculty members often lack the knowledge and expertise needed to strategically incorporate the tools in their teaching. Successful implementation requires integration in the curriculum and a change in workflow. Teaching students to be competent with health IT tools and practices cannot be an add-on to an already overcrowded curriculum. Faculty need to adjust their teaching practices to integrate the technology into teaching and learning across the curriculum and they need to know where to find the evidence and best practice for the technology use during care. In addition, if the health professions specific standard, competency, or essential setting organization has other domain expectations for the learner, those must be integrated with the informatics domain. For example, the AACN 2021 Essentials has ten domains that include these categories of competency: (1) knowledge for nursing practice; (2) person centered care; (3) population health; (4) scholarship for nursing practice; (5) quality and safety; (6) interprofessional partnership; (7) systems-based care; (8) informatics and health care technology; (9) professionalism; and (10) personal, professional and leadership development (AACN, 2021). A faculty member teaching clinical content could build an unfolding case in which several of these domains are addressed. One could envision students debating the interprofessional team needs to support cancer patient engagement in understanding their genomic information and the impact that information has on personalized, patient-centered care that can occur within the system in which the patient is receiving care.

To achieve this goal, faculty need to critically examine what content is taught and how it contributes to a workforce that supports the evolving LHS using informatics and information technology. For example, if one of the goals of the LHS is to achieve the best outcome for every patient, we need better evidence at point of care on which to base healthcare decisions. However, with the current pace of change, the problem is the health professional's ability to acquire the needed evidence in a timely manner. While knowledge of the importance of evidence-based practice is apparent in faculty publications, it has not yet found its way extensively into the curriculum framework of health professional programs. As evidence-based healthcare practice evolves, educators need to be ready to transform curriculum to ensure that graduates have a new skill set that is recognized and used in the healthcare setting. However, curriculum is not readily adaptable to change, thus creating a gap between education and practice that needs to be resolved in this rapidly changing healthcare environment. Curriculum that is agile, flexible, and up to date with employers' needs in a shifting healthcare environment will serve graduates well.

BOX 25.1 Competencies Matrix of Health Information Technology and Informatics Skills

Direct Patient Care

Generalist (All students and health professionals need this information.)

- Demonstrate skills in using patient care technologies, information systems, and communication devices that support safe practices.
- Use telecommunication technologies to assist in effective communication in a variety of healthcare settings.
- Apply safeguards and decision-making support tools embedded in patient care technologies and information systems to support a safe practice environment for both patients and healthcare workers.
- Understand the use of CIS to document interventions related to achieving positive outcomes.
- Use standardized terminology in a care environment (e.g., functional independence measures, nursing diagnosis terminology).
- Evaluate data from all relevant sources, including technology, to inform the delivery of care.
- Recognize the role of IT in improving patient care outcomes and creating a safe care environment.
- Uphold ethical standards related to data security, regulatory requirements, confidentiality, and clients' rights to privacy.
- Apply patient care technologies to address the needs of a diverse patient population.
- Advocate for the use of new patient care technologies for safe, quality care.
- Recognize that redesign of workflow and care processes should precede implementation of care technology to facilitate practice.
- Participate in evaluation of information systems in practice settings through policy and procedure development.

Direct and Indirect Patient Care

Graduate Level

Master's

- Analyze current and emerging technologies to support safe practice environments and optimize patient safety, cost effectiveness, and health outcomes.
- Evaluate outcome data using current communication technologies, information systems, and statistical principles to develop strategies to reduce risks and improve health outcomes.
- Promote policies that incorporate ethical principles and standards for the use of health and information technologies.
- Provide oversight, guidance, and leadership in the integration of technologies to document patient care and improve patient outcomes.
- Use information and communication technologies, resources, and principles of learning to teach patients and others.
- Use current and emerging technologies in the care environment to support lifelong learning for self and others.

Practice Doctorate (DPT, DDS, DNP, MD, DOT, PharmD, etc.)

- Design, select, use, and evaluate health IT programs, including consumer use of healthcare information systems.
- Analyze and communicate critical elements necessary to the selection, use, and evaluation of healthcare information systems and patient care technology.
- Demonstrate the conceptual ability and technical skills to develop and execute an evaluation plan involving data extraction from practice information systems and databases.
- Provide leadership in the evaluation and resolution of ethical and legal issues within healthcare systems relating to the use of information, IT, communication networks, and patient care technology.
- Evaluate consumer health information sources for accuracy, timeliness, and appropriateness.

Indirect Patient Care

Health IT Support

Workflow and Information Management (IM) Specialist

- Document workflow and IM models of practice.
- Conduct user requirements analysis.
- Develop revised workflow and IM models based on Meaningful Use of a certified electronic health record (EHR) product.
- Develop a set of plans to keep the practice running if the EHR system fails.
- Work directly with practice personnel to implement the revised workflow and IM model.
- Evaluate the new processes, identify problems and solutions, and implement changes.
- Design processes and information flows that accommodate quality improvement and reporting.

Implementation Support Specialist

- Install hardware and software to meet practice needs.
- Incorporate usability principles in software configuration and implementation.
- Test the software against performance specifications.
- Interact with the vendors to rectify technical problems that occur during the deployment process.
- Proactively identify software or hardware incompatibilities.
- Assist the practice in identifying a data backup and recovery solution.
- Ensure that the mechanism for hardware and software recovery and related capabilities is appropriately implemented to minimize system downtime.
- Ensure that privacy and security functions are appropriately configured and activated.
- Document IT problems and evaluate the effectiveness of problem resolution.
- Assist end users with audits.

Technical and Software Support Staff

- Interact with end users to diagnose IT problems and implement solutions.
- Document IT problems and evaluate the effectiveness of solutions.
- Support systems security and standards.
- Assist end users with the execution of audits and related privacy and security functions.
- Incorporate usability principles into ongoing software configuration and implementation.
- Ensure that the hardware and software "fail-over" and related capabilities are appropriately implemented to minimize system downtime.
- Ensure that privacy and security functions are appropriately configured and activated in hardware and software.
- Interact with the vendors as needed to rectify technical problems that occur during the deployment process.
- Work with the vendor and other sources of information to find the solution to a user's questions or problems as needed.

Informatics Specialists

Consultant

- Analyze and recommend solutions for health IT implementation problems in clinical and public health settings.
- Advise and assist clinicians in taking full advantage of technology, enabling them to make best use of data to drive improvement in quality, safety, and efficiency.
- Assist in selection of vendors and software by helping practice personnel ask the right questions and evaluate answers.
- Advocate for users' needs, acting as a liaison between users, IT staff, and vendors.

- Ensure that the patient and consumer perspective is incorporated into the EHR, including privacy and security issues.
- Train practitioners in best use of the EHR system, conforming to the redesigned workflow.
- Provide leadership, ensuring that implementation teams function cohesively.

Implementation Project Manager

- Apply project management and change management principles to create implementation project plans to achieve the project goals.
- Interact with diverse personnel to ensure open communication across end users and with the support team.
- Lead implementation teams consisting of workers in the roles described previously.
- Manage vendor relations, providing schedule, deliverable, and business information to health IT vendors for product improvement.
- Coordinate implementation-related efforts across the implementation site and with the health information exchange partners, troubleshooting problems as they arise.
- Apply an understanding of health IT, Meaningful Use, and the challenges practice settings will encounter in achieving Meaningful Use.

Trainer

- Be able to use a range of health IT applications, preferably at an expert level.
- Clearly communicate both health and IT concepts as appropriate, in a language the learner or user can understand.
- Apply a user-oriented approach to training, reflecting the need to empathize with the learner or user.

- Assess training needs and competencies of learners.
- Accurately assess employees' understanding of training, particularly through observation of use both in and out of the classroom.
- Design lesson plans, structuring active learning experiences for users and creating use cases that effectively train employees through an approach that closely mirrors actual use of the health IT in the patient care setting.
- Maintain accurate training records of the users and develop learning plans for further instruction.

Data Scientist

- Prepare the dataset using advanced analytics.
- Select appropriate analytics.
- Describe the dataset.
- Create and provide a visualization of the data.

Researcher and Innovator

- Conduct research on design, development, implementation, and impact of informatics solutions.
- Conduct research on mobile health and telehealth technologies and the impact on informatics.
- Conduct research on emerging patterns of care and outcomes.
- Analyze outcomes leading to new evidence-based guidelines.
- Develop new methods of organizing data to enhance research capacities.
- Design and develop informatics solutions.
- Develop new ways to interact with computer systems and access data.
- Assist in setting the future agenda for health informatics.
- Disseminate process and outcomes of research and product development.

Note: Competencies apply to both students and their faculty in each category.

TEACHING AND LEARNING IN AN EVOLVING HEALTHCARE AND TECHNOLOGY ENVIRONMENT

Reports and white papers published in the past decade suggest paradigm shifts in health professional education. As the technology-driven healthcare system continues to evolve, it is only right that we overhaul the educational platforms to prepare graduates who are the core of the healthcare environment. Health professionals, in all domains of practice and at all levels, must be "technology competent" to be able to participate in decision making and evaluation of health IT systems and their meaningful use. These systems are patient centered and support healthcare providers in information management, knowledge development, and evaluation of evidence-based innovative practice strategies that support value-based care. Currently, the United States is facing transformative changes in healthcare and living through one of the most dynamic ages in the history of healthcare. Through technology advancements, drug discoveries, and new medical device innovations, along with the ability to communicate worldwide and deliver healthcare in different settings, graduates will witness more change in healthcare within the next few years than ever before. Awareness of the continued transformation in the healthcare environment is essential for practice.

The Role of Informatics in the Curriculum

The term *informatics* as it relates to healthcare is ubiquitous and ambiguous, largely because of the various health professionals and related disciplines that use health IT and health data. AMIA

and its classification of informatics domains—translational bioinformatics, clinical informatics, clinical research informatics, consumer health informatics, and public health informatics—provide one structure to the overall categories of health informatics.

As new health IT evolves to meet the demands of the healthcare system, informatics competencies need to be addressed at all levels of health professional curricula. Informatics competencies should be considered along a continuum from basic to advanced competencies. All health professionals will need some level of basic informatics knowledge and skills introduced in their curriculum, while certain clinicians and informaticians will need advanced specialty education.

The History of Informatics Competency Development

Health-related disciplines have completed foundational work on needed competencies: nursing, public health, and medicine. The Delphi work in 2002 by Staggers et al. spurred additional work on informatics competencies (e.g., for advanced practice nurses and BSN students) (Staggers et al., 2002). The initial list of competencies was updated in 2011, and a review of informatics competencies was completed in 2012 and updated in 2021 (Connors et al., 2012; Chang et al., 2011; Goncalves et al., 2012; Quality and Safety in Nursing Education [QSEN], 2020). This work augmented through QSEN and the TIGER Informatics Competency Collaborative (QSEN, 2020; Technology Informatics Guiding Education Reform [TIGER], (n.d.); American Medical Informatics Association [AMIA], 2008). In 2007, the American Health Information Management Association (AHIMA) and AMIA convened a joint task force to identify basic core competencies expected of a healthcare workforce that uses EHRs in their daily work (AMIA, 2008). The results of this work is a matrix tool that addresses cross-cutting core competencies required of all health professionals regardless of discipline (AMIA, 2008).

Public health experts completed a consensus list of informatics competencies in the mid-2000s, and their most current work from 2009 is available online at http://www.mhsinformatics.org/CI-Fellowship/Workforce-Development/Competencies/PHI_Competencies.pdf. In 2018, the Horizon 2020 Project in collaboration with HIMSS TIGER developed a synthesis of competencies from the US and the EU. From this, the team developed a tool to explore and extract competencies by role. The tool is HITComp (http://ehealthwork.org) (EU*US eHealth Work, 2020). This tool is available for faculty use and may help to clarify the discrete informatics tasks by role: clinician, administration, and leader.

More recently, AMIA released a list of informatics competencies for health/clinical informatics professionals to be certified in clinical informatics. Information is available on the AMIA's general website and at https://brand.amia.org/m/4bc4471348808af7/original/AHIC_cert_guide_appendix_A-pdf.pdf. Unfortunately, there is not yet a consensus about informatics competencies despite the large amount of work in the area. Clearly, more work is needed to harmonize informatics competencies across disciplines and reach consensus about required core competencies.

The Science of Informatics and Curriculum Design

The science of informatics is inherently interprofessional, drawing on (and contributing to) other component fields, including computer science, decision science, information science, management science, cognitive science, data science, and organizational theory. Discipline-specific sciences and practices, such as nursing, medicine, dentistry, and pharmacology, are what differentiate how informatics is applied. Knowledge of the interprofessional approach to informatics; the science that underpins informatics; the relationship among the elements of data, information, knowledge, and wisdom; and the corresponding automated support systems drive the framework for curriculum development (American Nurses Association, 2022). Working in teams across disciplines provides a better understanding of the various roles of the informatics team and assists in placing the right competencies with the right role and educational level. In addition, providing informatics education in an interprofessional environment will assist in ensuring that health professionals in different disciplines understand and appreciate the various levels and types of competencies across disciplines.

FRAMEWORK FOR INFORMATICS CURRICULUM

The Learning Health System

The term *LHS* refers to the cycle by which the global health system learns from itself. In broad terms, the health system starts by absorbing information about patient treatment, then evaluates and applies the results to similar patients and researches this data to create clinical guidelines and policy. Finally, the health system incorporates the resulting recommendations into the electronic system to support clinical decisions in real time. The cycle continuously repeats and improves itself. In more specific terms, the LHS encompasses much more than the healthcare experience and more than individual or patient-specific information. It incorporates the macro system where all stakeholders (patients, healthcare professionals, private payers, employers, public payers, researchers, population health analysts, quality measure stewards, technology developers, HIE, standards development organizations, hospitals and hospital systems, government (federal, state, tribal, and local) contribute, share, and/or analyze data to create information and new knowledge to benefit patient care. This knowledge is then consumed by stakeholders and becomes a continuous learning cycle. The product of a successful LHS is the emergence of healthcare data that informs clinical decisions, reports on conditions or events, and measures the quality of care while providing evidence for the care of individuals and populations (Fig. 25.1).

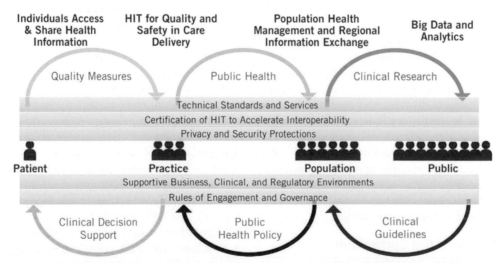

Fig. 25.1 The Learning Health System. Source: ONC. Connecting health and care for the nation: A 10-year vision to achieve an interoperable health IT infrastructure. https://www.healthit.gov/sites/default/files/ONC10yearInteroperabilityConceptPaper.pdf.

As the LHS unfolds, this is an opportunity for health professional education to be guided by this national model. Since the release of the IOM's LHS series, the ONC has become one of the prime promoters of the LHS. The ONC released two important documents for public in 2015: the interoperability roadmap and the strategic plan for 2015 to 2020 (Office of the National Coordinator [ONC], 2015). The roadmap contains the ONC's interoperability goal and is ONC's "vision for a future Health IT eco system where electronic health information is appropriately and readily available to empower consumers, support clinical decision-making, inform population and public health and value-based payment, and advance science" (Warren et al., 2010). In this document, the ONC focuses on achieving interoperability for health IT. The purpose of the interoperability goal is to "support a broad scale LHS by 2024." The LHS is a critical element in meeting the goals and outcomes in the proposed ONC strategic plan. In a system that increasingly learns from data collected at the point of care and applies lessons learned to improve patient care, health professionals will be the cornerstone for assessing needs, directing approaches, ensuring integrity of the tracking and quality of the outcomes, and leading innovation (Office of the National Coordinator [ONC], 2015). However, practitioners and health professional educators need to know that how and what they learn will dramatically change as technology, evidence-based practices, and innovations evolve over time. Orienting the education system to meet the needs of an evolving LHS requires new ways of thinking about how we can create and sustain a healthcare workforce that recognizes the by-products of an LHS and uses these by-products to adjust curriculum and address lifelong learning needs. Therefore, it is essential to have a nimble curriculum that can readily adapt to change.

Pedagogy

Pedagogy is a broad term that includes multiple theories of behavior based on the learning process. Modern pedagogy has been strongly influenced by three major categories of theory: behaviorist, cognitive, and constructivism. Behaviorists believe that learning is a change in behavior caused by external stimuli—the "know what." Early computer programs were based on behaviorist theory. This theory is useful in learning basic content and concepts. Cognitive psychology claims that learning involves memory, motivation, thinking, reflection, and abstraction. It is concerned with how to apply content, access, and synthesize information, think critically, and make decisions—the "know how." Constructivism asserts that learners interpret information and the world according to their personal reality and that they learn by observing, processing, and interpreting information and then customizing the information into personal knowledge for immediate application. Learners use previous knowledge to create new knowledge and act on it—the "know why." The LHS model is built on the theory of constructivism.

Teaching Tools and Learning Strategies

Today's information age students are calling for learner-driven education environments that provide access to powerful learning tools, knowledge bases, and scholarly exchange networks for the delivery of learning. New tools and novel approaches must be incorporated to teach fundamental concepts and methods that can be applied in different situations. For example, there is no doubt that health professional students will encounter EHRs in clinical practice; however, students in clinical practice settings are denied access to documenting in this record. This is a common but unsafe practice, since it forces the faculty, students, and staff to develop workarounds for documenting care that was provided by students. Integrating an AEHR in the curriculum as a teaching tool provides students a nonthreatening approach to interacting with health IT while learning discipline-specific content and processes. The interactive learning approach with this technology includes viewing and entering clinical documentation, viewing diagnostic results (lab, diagnostic imaging, reports), performing chart reviews, order management, medication administration and reconciliation, and developing plans of care. It is through these and other learning activities that the student begins to use evidence-based clinical practices, critical-thinking skills, and data-driven decision making.

The AEHR can also be used to promote learning about decision support tools, safety alerts, clinical workflow, population management, quality improvement, and interprofessional learning. Education programs can emphasize the importance of the EHR in healthcare, but unless there is an opportunity for students to use the EHR in the clinical setting, they will not develop the competencies required for practice in a progressive, technology-enriched healthcare environment (Chickering & Gamson, 1987). Yet, using an EHR alone is not sufficient for health professional students to learn the capabilities of the clinical information system. Health professional students need a theoretical base, often provided via lectures, reading, and discussion to completely understand the full potential of an EHR and HIE and how both technologies can empower providers to be meaningful users of these systems. The AEHR provides a technology teaching platform that supports higher-order, evidence-based teaching strategies such as active learning, time on task, rapid feedback, collaboration (Chickering & Gamson, 1987; Chickering & Ehrmann, 1996), and interprofessional education (IPE) when it is integrated across the health professional's curriculum. IPE is education that provides students within the health disciplines "with opportunities to learn and practice skills that improve their ability to communicate and collaborate. Through the experience of learning with and from those in other professions, students also develop leadership qualities and respect for each other, which prepares them to work in teams and in settings where collaboration is a key to success (IOM Institute of Medicine, 2013). Other examples of teaching and learning strategies that should be incorporated in the curriculum are collaborative practice, knowledge management, simulation, and web tools. An example of a *collaborative practice tool* is TeamSTEPPS (Agency for Healthcare Research and Quality [AHRQ], 2016), an evidence-based teamwork system that improves communication and teamwork skills among health professionals. TeamSTEPPS is an established system for improving patient safety as well as the efficiency and effectiveness of the healthcare team. Because graduates are expected to work in interprofessional teams, this skill needs to be part of all health professional curricula. Additional information on TeamSTEPPS is located at http://www.ahrq.gov/professionals/education/curriculum-tools/teamstepps/index.html.

Similarly, *knowledge management tools* build individual and organizational intelligence by enabling people to improve the way in which they capture, share, and use knowledge. Knowledge management involves not only building your own knowledge repository (personal knowledge management) but also using the knowledge, ideas, and experience of others to improve the organization's performance. An LHS incorporates knowledge-based decision support tools to build on what works well and discover which evidence leads to better practice, strategy, and policy.

Simulation is a tool used to assist in resolving the patient safety issue while enhancing student learning. During the past decade, simulation in health professional programs has increased exponentially. Simulation is an educational process that replicates the clinical work environment, including informatics, and requires students to demonstrate an identified skill set. Simulation-based IPE is a new phenomenon with increasing evidence to support outcomes. Qualitative feedback regarding IPE indicates that participants report feeling comfortable learning with students from other professions and find value in the interprofessional simulation sessions.

Web tools are on the rise in all aspects of our lives, including healthcare and education. The emergence of new classes of web-based applications has introduced new possibilities for healthcare delivery as well as new environments for teaching and learning. A variety of web tools is available, and the menu continues to grow. Some of these tools are blogs, vlogs, podcasts, social media networks (e.g., Facebook, Twitter, YouTube), virtual worlds (https://www.iste.org/explore/classroom/explore-these-virtual-worlds-learning), and virtual reality (https://www.med-technews.com/medtech-insights/vr-in-healthcare-insights/virtual-reality-a-medical-training-revolution-during-covid-1/).

Mobile and connected health technologies are changing the way in which consumers and healthcare providers access information and learn. The LHS is a multi-stakeholder collaboration across the public and private sector, including patients, consumers, caregivers, and families. Fundamental to the LHS is the full engagement of patients and the public. New mobile technologies and emerging health apps allow more patients access to healthcare than ever before and allow for on-demand treatment and health management. As the momentum for patient engagement builds, it will be imperative that we prepare health professionals in this world of connected health (Chickering & Ehrmann, 1996). Seamlessly integrating mobile and digital technologies (smartphones, iPads, robots, patient portals, secure messaging, personal health records, mobile apps, social media, and patient-generated health data tools) in the curriculum is an efficient and effective mechanism for bringing health professional education into the digital age and assisting students to gain the competencies they need in practice. Table 25.2 shows examples of suggested learning strategies to integrate the teaching tools in the curriculum.

INFORMATICS ROLES AND COMPETENCIES

A standard list of informatics competencies does not exist for all health care professionals. What is clear is that all undergraduate, graduate, and practicing health professionals need to have a certain level of knowledge about competency in informatics and its impact on an LHS that supports evidence-based practice, quality care, and safety. In addition, informatics specialists are needed to work in interprofessional teams to provide vision, leadership, and management and to advance the science of health informatics through wisdom, research, and innovation. Informatics specialists, educated in informatics specialty programs at the master's or doctoral level (both the research doctorate [PhD] and the practice doctorate) will continue to be in high demand. Currently there are not enough health professionals in this specialty area of practice. In addition, subspecialties within health informatics with their own additional education needs are beginning to evolve. For example, a more recent key player on the informatics team is the "data scientist." These individuals bring structure to big data generated by the LHS. Data scientists analyze large volumes of health data, often from various sources, to identify trends, extract knowledge, make discoveries, and visually communicate the data in a clear, competent, and meaningful manner. The goal is to leverage the power of analytics to improve care and lower cost. These subspecialists within informatics needed to be well prepared in the discipline of health informatics but must also receive additional education for their role as a data scientist.

Health IT Workforce Roles

Over the past decade, the HITECH Act programs have had a significant impact on health IT roles and competencies. In 2010, the U.S. Department of Health and Human Services (HHS) estimated a shortfall of 51,000 qualified health IT workers over the next 5 years based on data from the Bureau of Labor Statistics, the Department of Education, and independent studies. To address this shortfall, the ONC awarded grants totaling $84 million to 16 universities and junior colleges to help support the training and development of more than 50,000 new health IT professionals. A total of 12 key health IT workforce roles were identified. Each role has specific required educational preparation and outcomes. Six roles require 1-year university-based training and the remaining six roles require 6 months of intense training in a community college or distance-learning organization. As of October 2013, 20,777 graduates were reported to have completed the university-based (1704) and community college programs (19,773). This is not even close to the 51,000-shortfall projected in 2010. Health IT staffing shortages continue. The crunch will continue to grow due to the aging population of workers, the expansion of digital platforms, security risks placing priority on cybersecurity, and a larger job market outside of healthcare (Gue, 2019; ONC, 2021). In 2016, ONC issued $6.4 million in new funding to continue to train the health IT workforce. Specifically, awardees updated training materials from the original Workforce Curriculum Development Program and were to train 6000 incumbent healthcare workers to use new health information technologies in a variety of settings:

TABLE 25.2   Examples of Teaching Tools and Strategies

Tools	Strategies
Academic Electronic Health Record (AEHR)	Integrate throughout the curriculum to teach informatics competencies from basic to complex, including documentation, navigation, best practice guidelines, quality measures, clinical decision support at point of care, order management, medication administration and reconciliation, data collection, data mining, privacy and security issues, population management, quality improvement, and more. • Warren, J. J., Manos, E. L., Meyer, M., & Roche, A. (2012). Integrating an academic electronic health record into simulations. In Campbell, S., & Daley, K. (Eds.), *Simulation scenarios for nursing educators*. New York, NY: Springer. Build case studies within the AEHR to use across disciplines to foster interprofessional education (IPE) and collaborative practice.
Collaborative practice	Make Team STEPPS a part of your curriculum. Can be incorporated at all levels, basic to advanced. http://www.ahrq.gov/professionals/education/curriculum-tools/teamstepps/index.html • The National Center for Interprofessional Practice and Education: https://nexusipe.org Work with others to develop IPE case studies for education and practice.
Knowledge management	Engage students in communities of practice (CoP) to share clinical evidence and new knowledge among the various healthcare team members. Teach students to evaluate and/or develop clinical practice guidelines and clinical decision support tools.
Web tools	Web tools provide a rich set of technologies for engaging students and remove the logistical barrier for IPE. 1. Sabus, C., Sabata, D., & Antonacci, D. M. (2011). Use of a virtual environment to facilitate instruction of an interprofessional home assessment. *Journal of Allied Health, 40*(4), 199–205. 2. Antonacci, D. M., & Modaress, N. (2008). Envisioning the educational possibilities of user-created virtual worlds. *AACE Journal, 16*(2), 115–126. 3. https://text4baby.org
Simulation	1. Society in Healthcarehttps://www.ssih.org
Mobile/connected health	1. HIMSS Resources https://www.himss.org/resources-all 2. Mobile App for Healthcare https://guides.library.kumc.edu/c.php?g=451707&p=3084693
Virtual Reality	1. Virtual Reality and Simulation https://blog.carlow.edu/2021/05/10/virtual-reality-for-health-science-education/

team-based care environment, long-term care facilities, patient-centered medical homes, accountable care organizations, hospitals, and clinics. The workforce efforts focused on four key topic areas: population health, care coordination, new care delivery and payment models, and value-based care.

Box 25.1 organizes the competencies derived from the ANA's *Nursing Informatics: Scope and Standards of Practice*, QSEN, TIGER, and the ONC work role descriptions and categorizes the competencies across curriculum levels. It also includes health IT support professionals, recognizing that these individuals work closely with informatics specialists, researchers, and innovators. Organizational informatics specialists may subsume these support roles.

Community College Training Overview

The educational training materials developed for the community college training program were supported by the ONC Curriculum Development Centers Program's grants. The complete set of teaching materials for the curriculum components is available on the ONC website (https://www.healthit.gov/topic/onc-hitech-programs/workforce-development-programs) (Skiba, 2015). This is a great resource and foundation for a strong, short-term training program, but it should not replace the integration of the content and competencies across health professional curriculum or the need for advanced education

in health informatics. Since the ONC workforce development plan is designed to rapidly increase the number of healthcare IT professionals, these competencies need to be cross mapped in higher education programs to reach the goal of an LHS. As academic institutions, healthcare organizations, and accrediting agencies establish competencies for health IT and health professionals, they need to look to these nationally defined workforce roles and competencies for guidance. For a health informatics curriculum to be relevant, it must encompass both current and future roles of health IT professionals in all types of health organizations. As the LHS continues to evolve, these roles and competencies will adjust to better align with the market demands of students, communities, and employers. The problem is that healthcare organizations are looking for seasoned health IT professionals, and those individuals are rare currently. Specific roles designed for community college training include the following:

Implementation and support specialist. Individuals in this role provide support before and during implementation of health IT systems in clinical and public health settings. They execute implementation plans by installing hardware and software, incorporating usability principles, testing software against performance specifications, and interacting with vendors to resolve issues during deployment. Backgrounds for these individuals include IT and information management.

Implementation managers. Individuals in this role provide on-site management of adoption support teams before and during implementation of health IT systems. Backgrounds for this role include experience in health and/or IT environments as well as administrative and management experience. These individuals apply project management and change management skills to create implementation plans to achieve project goals, lead implementation support teams, and manage vendor relations.

Technical and software support staff. Individuals in this role maintain health IT systems in clinical and public health settings. Previous backgrounds include IT and information management. Workers interact with end users to diagnose and document IT problems as well as implement solutions and evaluate their effectiveness.

Trainer. Individuals in this role design and deliver training to employees in clinical and public health settings. Backgrounds for these workers include experience as a health professional or health information specialist. Experience as an educator or trainer is also valued.

University-Based Education Overview

Specific health IT roles requiring university-based education and training include the following:

Clinician and public health leader. Individuals in this role are expected to lead the successful deployment and use of health IT to achieve transformational improvement in the quality, safety, outcomes, and value of health services. Training appropriate to this role will require at least 1 year of study, leading to a university-issued master's level certificate or master's degree in health informatics or health IT as a complement to the individual's prior clinical or public health academic training. The individual entering this program may already hold a master's or doctoral degree, or the program may be part of his or her existing program of study, leading to an advanced clinical practice or public health professional degree. Career opportunities include chief information officer and chief informatics officer.

Health information management and exchange specialist. Individuals in this role support the collection, management, retrieval, exchange, and analysis of electronic information in healthcare and public health organizations. These individuals would require a bachelor's degree in health information management (HIM) but would not enter leadership or management roles unless they had graduate-level or master's education in HIM or health informatics.

Health information privacy and security specialist. Individuals in this role are charged with maintaining trust by ensuring the privacy and security of health information as an essential component of any successful health IT deployment in healthcare and public health organizations. Education for this role requires a computer science specialization within baccalaureate-level programs or a certificate of advanced studies or post-baccalaureate training in HIM or health informatics. Individuals in this role would be qualified to serve as institutional and organizational information privacy or security officers.

Research and development specialist. Individuals in this role support efforts to create innovative models and solutions that advance the capabilities of health IT. They conduct studies on the effectiveness of health IT and its impact on healthcare quality. Education required for this role is a doctoral degree. Career opportunities include faculty roles as well as data science, enterprise-wide analytics, and research and development positions.

Program and software engineer. Individuals in this role will be the architects and developers of advanced health IT solutions. They need to have knowledge and understanding of health domains to complement their computer and information science expertise. This knowledge will enable them to work with the healthcare team (including the patient) to develop solutions that address their specific concerns. Training appropriate to this role is specialization within a baccalaureate program or a certificate of advanced studies or a post-baccalaureate education in health informatics. A certificate of advanced study or a master's in health informatics may be very appropriate for individuals with IT backgrounds.

Health IT subspecialist. A small subset of specialized individuals with a general knowledge of healthcare or public health and in-depth knowledge of disciplines that inform health IT policy or technology is critical to the success of the health IT initiative. Such disciplines might include ethics, economics, business, policy and planning, cognitive psychology, and industrial and systems engineering. These individuals might expect to find employment in research and development organizations or teaching. These positions would require at least a master's degree but more likely a doctoral degree.

Practice workflow and information management redesign specialist. Individuals in this role assist in reorganizing the work of a healthcare provider to take full advantage of meeting the MU/MIPS criteria. These individuals may have backgrounds in healthcare or IT, but they are not licensed clinical professionals.

Clinician or practitioner consultant. This role is like the redesign specialist discussed previously; however, these individuals have backgrounds and experience as licensed clinical or public health professionals. In addition to the responsibilities discussed previously, they address workflow and data collection issues, including quality outcomes and improvement, from a clinical perspective. They serve as a liaison between users, IT staff, and vendors.

Educating the Generalist

All health professionals at the generalist level need KSAs related to informatics. According to QSEN, nurses at the prelicensure level, as well as other health professionals at the entry level, should be able to use information and technology to communicate, manage knowledge, mitigate error, and support decision making in a caring and secure environment (National League for Nursing [NLN], 2008). These QSEN competencies, as well as some of the ONC health IT role competencies, are further delineated in the NLN position statement titled *Preparing the Next Generation of Nurses to Practice in a Technology-Rich Environment: An Informatics Agenda* (NLN, 2008). Upon examination of these basic competencies, it is obvious that integrating an EHR into the academic environment is essential to fully prepare healthcare workers to use EHRs in clinical practice. Colleges and universities use academic versions of EHRs in the classroom and simulated case scenarios to create powerful high-fidelity learning environments that promote informatics competencies (Chang et al., 2011; Warren et al., 2010; Fauchald, 2008; Jeffries et al., 2011; Warren & Connors, 2007; American Association of Health Centers [AAHC], 2016). Just as pilots are trained in simulators to fly airplanes, simulation, including the use of an EHR, can be used to teach health professionals IPE and informatics skills.

Educating Healthcare Specialists at the Graduate Level

While there is variation across the healthcare disciplines, the overall pattern is that increased levels of education correlate with increased specialization as well as advanced management and leadership. As the use of technology expands, all master's- or doctorate-prepared health practitioners, regardless of specialty, must have the knowledge and skills to meaningfully use current technologies to innovate, deliver, and coordinate care across multiple settings and with an interprofessional team. They must be able to consider appropriate technologies and analyze data that impacts point-of-care outcomes. In addition, they must have the expertise required to communicate with the media, the public, policy makers, and health professionals regarding health IT and the secure and trusted use of HIEs. Integral to these skills is an attitude of openness to innovation and continual learning, since information systems and care technologies are constantly changing (AACN, 2021). The need for an informatics skill set across all levels of the curriculum further points out the importance of integrating informatics tools in the curriculum and a shift in teaching approaches to include collaboration and teamwork. At this level, students use EHR data to monitor open-loop processes, generate research questions, look for links to evidence-based decision making, detect unanticipated events, and support clinical workflow and population management. Clinicians at this level use a variety of digital technologies to advance their skills as integrators, aggregating information from patients and their health records, recognizing patterns, making decisions, and translating those decisions into action.

Educating the Health Informatics Specialist

Informatics specialists are formally prepared at the graduate level (master's or doctorate) in health informatics programs. Informatics specialists design, manage, and apply discipline-specific data and information to improve decision making by consumers, patients, nurses, and other healthcare providers (American Nurses Association, 2022). Informatics specialists must have effective communication and analytical skills, as well as clinical knowledge and technical proficiency. Most health informatics specialists work in a hospital or healthcare setting in management or administrative positions; however, a significant percentage hold positions with health-related vendors, suppliers, insurance companies, and consulting firms. As EHRs and other information and communication technologies become increasingly important, informatics specialists will become even more vital in bridging the gap between clinical care skills and technology. These specialists are expected to practice in interprofessional team environments, interact with health IT support professionals, and lead change. They need to be knowledgeable about clinical information systems and how they support the work of clinicians.

The healthcare industry is looking for informatics specialists to correctly design, build, test, implement, and maintain health IT systems to meet MU criteria. The specific job description and activities of an informatics specialist in any setting will, of course, be determined by the employing organization, but these activities can be expected to include responsibilities such as analysis, project management, software tailoring and development, designing and implementing educational programs, administration, management and leadership, consulting, and program evaluation and research.

Educating the Health Informatics Researcher and Innovator

The role of the informatics researcher is prominent in the emergence of an LHS that focuses on best care practices and the generation and application of new knowledge. Constant innovation is needed to keep pace with evolving technologies and ever-changing regulatory mandates. As new health technologies emerge, innovations will grow, and research and development will be essential to support commercialization. Preparation for the researcher and innovator role is at the doctoral level. Education for the researcher focuses on discovering knowledge and analyzing evidence; at the practice level, the focus is on evaluating, applying, and implementing evidence.

The role of an informatics researcher includes knowledge of research designs and applications to develop better and more efficient ways of entering, retrieving, and using health informatics to improve health outcomes and engage consumers. An informatics researcher plays a key role in developing new data collection methods and assisting with finding the appropriate data to collect for various projects and research grants. This research ranges from experimental research to process improvement and from informal evaluation to evidence-based practice (AACN, 2021). Informatics researchers must be effective written and oral communicators, as dissemination of their work through consultation, publication, and presentation is an important part of their role. They should have a clear understanding of research design and how to develop accurate and correct questions for surveys and research projects. The ability to work in a team environment with those both familiar and not as familiar with research is essential. Excellent computer skills and knowledge of databases and software programs available for research are important. A background or experience in patient focused healthcare and consumers is helpful. Knowledge of healthcare organizations, state and federal regulations and policies regarding healthcare practices, data collection, data stewardship, and confidentiality is critical. In addition, a spirit of entrepreneurship along with knowledge of commercialization and technology transfer are important to the innovator role.

Continuing Professional Development

Lifelong learning is a key component of an LHS. The acceleration of national efforts to increase adoption of health IT across all healthcare arenas (including consumer engagement, public health surveillance, and research) affects all health professionals. As practice changes and recent technology evolves, continuous learning is necessary to have competent, up-to-date, skilled professionals who can respond quickly to the needs of the system. Health professionals who are interested in expanding their education to include informatics have opportunities for learning through formal academic education as well as continuing education programs. The HITECH Act, federal and private initiatives, professional organizations, the health IT industry, and universities have increased opportunities for health IT and informatics in continuing education. A web search for health IT or health informatics seminars and webinars or conferences will provide a variety of opportunities to help meet the learner's specific needs.

CONCLUSION AND FUTURE DIRECTIONS

Health, healthcare, and education in this country are going digital, setting the stage for an LHS dependent on continuous learning and facilitated by information and communication technologies. This developing potential presents opportunities and challenges for health professional education. It is forcing educators to redefine and rethink how they educate health professionals.

Health informatics specialty programs will continue to expand, and core informatics competencies will be taught across all levels of the curriculum for health professionals. In the future, health informatics education will see a move to baccalaureate as entry level. The practice doctorate (DNP, MD, DOT, DPT) will dominate practice and leadership in health informatics. The LHS will require a new skill set that will necessitate a major redesign of educational programs for health professionals, including a focus on interprofessional collaborative education and practice. Informatics competencies and new workforce roles will continue to evolve as the continuous learning loop and recent technologies change the way in which healthcare and education are delivered. Continuous learning through formal academic programs, short-term courses, conferences, workshops, and seminars is at the core of ensuring that clinical practice reflects the current best evidence. In the future, one can expect to see continued learning and just-in-time learning incorporated directly into the information systems used to provide care. For example, as standards of care change, healthcare providers may not need to attend a workshop to learn about these new standards but will be brought up to date on these new standards through the decision support systems incorporated in the EHR.

ACKNOWLEDGMENTS

The author wishes to acknowledge the contributions of E. LaVerne Manos, Helen B. Connors, Judith J. Warren, and Teresa Stenner to the previous edition of this chapter.

▌ DISCUSSION QUESTIONS

1. Under the Medicare Access and CHIP Reauthorization Act of 2015 (MACRA) quality, value and accountability become the focus as opposed to fee for service. The meaningful use of information systems is part of this. How does data and information technology support this quality payment program? (https://qpp.cms.gov)
2. Compare and contrast informatics knowledge/competencies, information literacy, and computer literacy.
3. Compare and contrast the competencies in the Competencies Matrix of Health Information Technology and Informatics Skills (see Table 25.1)—generalists, advanced practice, health IT support, informatics specialist, and researcher/innovator. Differentiate between direct and indirect patient care roles.
4. Describe a set of strategies that could be used to integrate informatics competences within an undergraduate curriculum as opposed to teaching this content as a separate course. How would you align and interweave informatics competencies with other expected competency such as leadership, communication, or patient safety?
5. Describe how health informatics can be used to transform interprofessional education (IPE).
6. What resources would you need to integrate an academic electronic health record into healthcare simulations (with and without human patient simulators)? Include staff in the discussion.
7. Develop an action plan to improve informatics competencies for faculty; develop an action plan to improve informatics competencies for students.
8. Develop a plan of study for a researcher to be able to engage in Big Data analytics.
9. Discuss the Learning Health System in relation to developing a curriculum and assignments to assist students in gaining the competencies required for participating in this system.
10. The top health professional in your organization is challenged with implementing a healthcare information system for the organization and is putting together a committee for this purpose. The top health professional recognizes your talents and abilities to be a major contributor to this committee. What qualities, characteristics, intellectual strengths, and future ambitions would drive you to be influential in your role?

CASE STUDY

In affiliation with the University of Excellence Medical Center (UEMC), the University of Excellence (UE) is recognized as a major academic health center. As defined by Association of Academic Health Centers (AAHC), an academic health center "encompasses all the health-related components of universities, including their health professions schools, patient care operations, and research" (American Association of Health Centers AAHC, 2016). The UEMC includes schools of allied health, dentistry, medicine, nursing, pharmacy, and public health. The UEMC is a growing health system that consists of patient care operations ranging from small rural hospitals to large multiple-specialty tertiary referral hospitals.

- The health professional schools at UE have agreed to incorporate the five core competencies identified by the IOM in their report entitled *Health Professions Education: A Bridge to Quality* (Institute of Medicine, 2003). These core competencies include patient-centered care, interdisciplinary teams, evidence-based practice, quality improvement, and informatics. With this goal in mind, they are currently working together to integrate informatics throughout their revised curricula. The plan is to develop an interprofessional approach that incorporates informatics across the different educational programs within these schools. The schools have requested a meeting with clinical leaders from Best Memorial Hospital to gain a practice perspective on what information should be included in the curriculums. Best Memorial Hospital is part of the UEMC system. Best Memorial Hospital has a long history of association with local universities, functioning as a

site for student clinical experiences. Undergraduate students enrolled at the UE College of Health Professions often complete a portion of their clinical work at the hospital.

Each year the hospital hires healthcare graduates from this university.

Clinicians in first-level management positions at the hospital are enrolled in graduate programs at the university.

The vice president for clinical practice at Best Memorial Hospital, where you work, has included you on the list of leaders to attend the meeting with UE. In preparation for this meeting, complete the tasks below.

Discussion Questions

1. Prepare a list of key references for using an interprofessional approach to integrating informatics into the curricula of healthcare professionals.

2. Prepare a list of competencies, concepts, and/or skills that should be included in the educational preparation of graduates of the healthcare educational programs at both the undergraduate and graduate levels. Give examples that include an interprofessional approach to the practice of informatics.

3. Describe how informatics competencies could be incorporated into the clinical experiences of students. Be specific. For example, how should student access to Best Memorial Hospital's clinical information systems be developed? Who should provide the needed instruction for orienting each group of students?

REFERENCES

AACN. (2020). Nursing shortage. https://www.aacnnursing.org/News-Information/Fact-Sheets/Nursing-Shortage.

AACN. (2008). The Essentials of Baccalaureate Education for Professional Nursing Practice. https://www.aacnnursing.org/portals/42/publications/baccessentials08.pdf

AACN. (2006). The Essentials of Doctoral Education for Advanced Nursing Practice. https://www.aacnnursing.org/DNP/DNP-Essentials

Agency for Healthcare Research and Quality (AHRQ). TeamSTEPPS: Strategies and tools to enhance performance and patient safety. http://teamstepps.ahrq.gov/. Accessed July 6, 2016.

American Association of Colleges of Nursing [AACN]. (2021). The Essentials: Core Competencies for Professional Nursing Education. https://www.aacnnursing.org/AACN-Essentials

American Association of Health Centers (AAHC). About AAHC. http://www.aahcdc.org/About.aspx. Accessed August 29, 2016.

American Medical Informatics Association (AMIA). (2008). Joint Work Force Task Force: Health Information Management and Informatics Core Competencies for Individuals Working With Electronic Health Records. https://bok.ahima.org/PdfView?oid=104073

American Nurses Association. (2022). *Nursing informatics: Scope and standards of practice* (3rd ed.). Washington, DC: American Nurses Publishing. in press.

American Nurses Association. (2008). *Nursing informatics: Scope and standards of practice.* Washington, DC: American Nurses Publishing.

American Nurses Association. (2015). *Nursing informatics: Scope and standards of practice* (2nd ed.). Washington, DC: American Nurses Publishing.

American Nurses Association. (2001). *Scope and standards of nursing informatics practice.* Washington, DC: American Nurses Publishing.

American Nurses Association. (1995). *The standards of practice for nursing informatics.* Washington, DC: American Nurses Publishing.

American Recovery and Reinvestment Act (ARRA). (2009). http://www.gpo.gov/fdsys/pkg/PLAW-111publ5/html/PLAW-111publ5.htm.

AMIA. Advanced Interprofessional Informatics Certification (AIIC). https://www.amia.org/advanced-interprofessional-informatics-certification. Accessed July 6, 2016.

Association of American Medical Colleges and the Howard Hughes Medical Institute. (2009). Scientific Foundation for Future Physicians Committee. Report of the AAMC-HHMI Committee. Washington, DC. https://www.hhmi.org/news/aamc-hhmi-committee-defines-scientific-competencies-future-physicians.

Becker's Hospital Review. (2015). A history of EHRs: 10 things to know. https://www.beckershospitalreview.com/healthcare-information-technology/a-history-of-ehrs-10-things-to-know.html.

Billings, D. (2007). Foreword. In P. Jefferies (Ed.), *Simulation in nursing education*. New York, NY: National League for Nursing.

Blake R., Blake A., Shaw T., Hubner U., Thye, J., & Varri A. et al. (2018). The EU*US eHealth Work Project: Project Overview. Measuring, Informing, Educating, and Advancing eHealth. http://www.promisalute.it/upload/mattone/documentiallegati/R.Blake-TheEU- USeHealthWorkProjectMeasuringInformingEducatingan dAdvancingaSkilledeHealthWorkforce_13660_2983.pdf

Brunner, M., McGregor, D., Keep, M., Janssen, A., Spallek, H., Quinn, D., et al. (2018). An ehealth capabilities framework for graduates and health professionals: Mixed-methods study. *Journal of Medical Internet Research*, 20(5), e10229. https://doi.org/10.2196/10229.

Buchanan, C., Howitt, M. L., Wilson, R., Booth, R. G., Risling, T., & Bamford, M. (2021). Predicted influences of artificial intelligence on nursing education: Scoping review. *JMIR Nursing*, 4(1), 1–11..

Centers for Medicare and Medicaid Services [CMS]. (2021). Health Information Technology for Economic and Clinical Health. https://www.cms.gov/Medicare/Compliance-and-Audits/Part-A-Cost-Report-Audit-and-Reimbursement/HITECH-Audits

Chang, J., Poynton, M. R., Gassert, C. A., & Staggers, N. (2011). Nursing informatics competencies required of nurses in Taiwan. *International Journal of Medical Informatics*, 80(5), 332–340. https://doi.org/10.1016/j.ijmedinf.2011.01.011.

Chickering, A. E., & Gamson, Z. F. (1987). Seven principles for good practice in undergraduate education. *AAHE Bulletin*, 39(7), 3–6.

Chickering, A. W., & Ehrmann, S. C. (1996). Implementing the seven principles: Technology as lever. *AAHE Bulletin*, 49, 3–6.

Committee on Quality of Health Care in America, (2001). *Institute of Medicine. Crossing the quality chasm: A new health system for the 21st century*. Washington, DC: The National Academies Press.

Connors, H., Warren, J., & Popkess-Vawter, S. (2012). Technology, and informatics. In J. F. Giddens (Ed.), *Concepts for nursing practice* (pp. 443–452). St. Louis, MO: Elsevier.

Eaton, J.S. (2015). An Overview of U.S. Accreditation. Council for Higher Education Accreditation (CHEA). https://www.chea.org/sites/default/files/other-content/Overview%20of%20US%20Accreditation%202015.pdf

EU*US eHealth Work. (2018). A Horizon 2020 Project. HITComp Tool. http://ehealthwork.org

Fauchald, S. K. (2008). An academic-industry partnership for advancing technology in health science education. *Computers, Informatics, Nursing*, 26(10), 4–8.

Fox, B. I., Flynn, A. J., Fortier, C. R., & Clauson, K. A. (2011). Knowledge, skills, and resources for pharmacy informatics education. *American Journal of Pharmacy Education*, 75(5), 93.

Frank, J. R., Taber, S., van Zanten, M., Scheele, F., Blouin, D., & International Health Professions Accreditation Outcomes Consortium. (2020). The role of accreditation in 21st century health professions education: Report of an International Consensus Group. *BMC Medical Education*, 20(Suppl 1), 305.

Goncalves, L., Wolf, L.G., & Staggers, N. (2012). Nursing informatics competencies: Analysis of the latest research. Paper presented at NI 2012: Advancing Global Health through Informatics. Montreal, Canada, June 2012.

Greiner, A. C., & Knebel, E. (Eds.). (2003). *Health professions education: A bridge to quality*. Washington DC: The National Academies Press.

Gue D. (2019). The Health It Staffing Shortage is a Problem Morphing Into a Crisis. HIT Consultant. https://hitconsultant.net/2019/10/16/health-it-staffing-shortage-crisis/

Herbert, V. M., & Connors, H. (2016). Integrating an academic electronic health record: Challenges and success strategies. *Computers, Informatics, Nursing*, 34(8), 345–354.

Hersh, W. R., Gorman, P. N., Biagioli, F. E., Mohan, V., Gold, J. A., & Mejicano, C. (2014). Beyond information retrieval and electronic health record use: Competencies in clinical informatics for medical education. *Advances in Medical Education and Practice*, 5, 205–212.

Institute of Medicine. (2003). *Health professions education: A bridge to quality*. Washington, DC: The National Academies Press.

IOM (Institute of Medicine). (2013). *Interprofessional education for collaboration: Learning how to improve health from interprofessional models across the continuum of education to practice: Workshop summary*. Washington, DC: The National Academies Press.

IOM Report (Institute of Medicine). (2013). Health information technology patient safety action surveillance plan. https://www.healthit.gov/sites/default/files/safety_plan_master.pdf

IOM Report (Institute of Medicine). (2012). Health IT and patient safety: Building safer systems for better care. http://www.nap.edu/catalog/13269/health-it-and-patient-safety-building-safer-systems-for-better.

Jeffries, P. R., Hudson, K., Taylor, L. A., & Klapper, S. A. (2011). Bridging technology: Academe and industry. In K. J. Hannah & M. J. Ball (Eds.), *Nursing informatics: Where technology and caring meet* (4th ed., pp. 167–188). New York, NY: Springer.

Kohn, L. T., Corrigan, J. M., & Donaldson, M. S. (Eds.). (2000). *To err is human: Building a safer health system*. Washington, DC: The National Academies Press.

Lundgren, A. S., Linberg, L., & Carlsson, E. (2021). "Within the hour" and "Wherever you are": Exploring the promises of digital healthcare apps. *Journal of Digital Social Research*, 3(3), 32–59.

Martin, L. G., Warholak, T. L., Hincapie, A. L., Gallo, T., Kjos, A. L., & AACP Joint Task Force on Informatics. (2019). Health informatics competencies for pharmacists in training. *American Journal of Pharmacy Education*, 83(2), 6512.

National Academies of Sciences, Engineering, Medicine. (2014). Future directions of credentialing research in nursing: A workshop. www.nationalacademies.org/HMD.

National League for Nursing (NLN) Board of Governors. (2008). Preparing the next generation of nurses to practice in a technology-rich environment: An informatics agenda. NLN. http://www.nln.org/docs/default-source/professional-development-programs/preparing-the-next-generation-of- nurses.pdf?sfvrsn=6.

Office of the National Coordinator (ONC). (2015). Federal Health IT Strategic Plan. Final Published Version. https://www.healthit.gov/topic/interoperability.

Office of the National Coordinator (ONC). (2015). Interoperability Roadmap. Final Published Version 1.0. https://www.healthit.gov/sites/default/files/hie-interoperability/nationwide-interoperability-roadmap-final-version-1.0.pdf.

Office of the National Coordinator (ONC). (2021). Workforce Development Programs Health IT Curriculum Resources for Educators. https://www.healthit.gov/topic/onc-hitech-programs/workforce-development-programs

Office of the National Coordinator [ONC]. (2021). Non-Federal Acute Care Hospital Electronic Health Record Adoption. https://www.healthit.gov/data/quickstats/non-federal-acute-care-hospital-electronic-health-record-adoption

Office of the National Coordinator for Health Information Technology [ONC]. (2019). Meaningful Use and the Shift to the

Merit-Based Incentive Program System. https://www.healthit.gov/topic/meaningful-use-and-macra/meaningful-use

Office of the National Coordinator (ONC). (n.d.). Connecting health and care for the nation: A 10-year vision to achieve an interoperable health IT infrastructure. https://www.healthit.gov/sites/default/files/ONC10yearInteroperabilityConceptPaper.pdf

Office of the National Coordinator (ONC). (n.d.). Empowering Patients with Their Health Record in a Modern Health IT Economy. https://www.healthit.gov/curesrule/overview/about-oncs-cures-act-final-rule

Quality and Safety in Nursing Education (QSEN). (2020). Competencies. https://qsen.org/competencies/pre-licensure-ksas

Skiba, D., & Rizzolo, M. A. (2011). Education and faculty development. In K. J. Hannah & M. J. Ball (Eds.), *Nursing informatics: Where technology and caring meet* (4th ed., pp. 65–80). New York, NY: Springer.

Skiba, D. J. (2015). Connected health: Preparing practitioners. *Nursing Education Perspectives, 36*(3), 198.

Staggers, N., Gassert, C. A., & Curran, C. (2002). A Delphi study to determine informatics competencies for nurses at four levels of practice. *Nursing Research, 51*(6). 383–39.

Technology Informatics Guiding Education Reform (TIGER). (n.d.). TIGER International Informatics Competency Synthesis Project. https://www.himss.org/tiger-initiative-international-competency-synthesis-project

The Clinical Informatics Milestone Project. (2015). https://www.acgme.org/globalassets/PDFs/Milestones/ClinicalInformaticsMilestones.pdf

Triola, M. M., Friedman, E., Cimino, C., Geyer, E. M., Wiederhorn, J., & Mainiero, C. (2010). Health information technology and medical school curriculum. *The American Journal of Managed Care, 16,* SP54–SP57.

Warren, J. J., & Connors, H. R. (2007). Health information technology can and will transform nursing education. *Nursing Outlook, 55*(1), 59–60.

Warren, J. J., Meyer, M. J., Thompson, T. L., & Roche, A. J. (2010). Transforming nursing education: Integrating informatics and simulations. In C. A. Weaver, C. W. Delaney, P. Weber, & R. L. Carr (Eds.), *Nursing and informatics for the 21st century: An international look at practice, trends, and the future* (2nd ed., pp. 145–161). Chicago, IL: HIMSS Press.

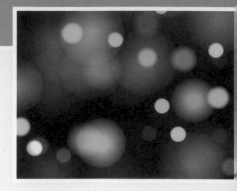

26

Distance Education—A New Frontier

Sarah C. Shuffelton and Vickie Bennett

OBJECTIVES

At the completion of this chapter, the reader will be prepared to:
1. Summarize the history of course delivery systems, including the terminology, types, and their impact on today's distance learning.
2. Summarize how to evaluate course delivery systems using appropriate criteria.
3. Summarize the key factors that should be considered in the design and support of eLearning experiences.

KEY TERMS

adult learners, 419

course delivery system, 415

course management system, 415

distance education, 414

learning management system, 413

ABSTRACT ❖

The changes in our educational environment reflect shifts in our demographics, economic conditions, and technological developments. Innovative technology tools, communication platforms and an increase in distance learning are enhancing educational opportunities for lifelong learning within a diverse global community. This chapter presents a brief history of distance education, defines related terms, and discusses course delivery systems, including issues related to the selection of these systems. It concludes with a discussion of issues related to the development and implementation of distance education and lifelong learning.

INTRODUCTION

Technology developments and the internet are providing opportunities to examine how institutions of higher learning and healthcare organizations deliver instruction or training and how this delivery may be improved. Since the late 1990s and early 2000s, distance education has become an increasingly important part of education. It is one of the "most complex issues facing higher education institutions today" (Oblinger et al., 2001). While this statement was written years ago, it holds true today (El Refae et al., 2021). Most colleges and universities are now beyond asking whether they should offer distance learning options. They are instead addressing how to manage these offerings in an effective, efficient, and economical way. These discussions focus on increasing enrollment, retaining students, staying competitive, addressing the needs of a changing student population, and improving quality. In addition to the educational institutions, healthcare institutions and organizations provide continuing education, mandatory training, and patient education through distance education options.

Given the current work environment and social distancing mandates, a growing number of health-related programs are offering part or all their program content through distance education. Increasingly students come to school with work and family obligations or live in areas distant from educational opportunities. Distance education is a viable option for this demographic of health professions students (National Council of State Boards of Nursing, 2021). It provides increased flexibility in meeting the educational needs of the changing student population while influencing how publishers deliver textbooks and how instructors facilitate all learning styles through creative use of interactive activities, social media, videos, podcasts, and other means.

COURSE DELIVERY SYSTEMS

Technological developments have an impact on institutions, student expectations, and how students learn. For example, most institutions or organizations provide wireless connections because students, patients, and families expect to be able to use their wireless devices in schools, hospitals, and outpatient facilities. Course delivery systems experience similar expectations from faculty, students, and staff. Systems are expected to be visually appealing, easy for students and faculty alike to navigate, and provide a stable platform on which to upload assignments and view course content. Additionally, Oblinger and Oblinger (2005) proposed that discussions about distance learning should not be about technology, but the activities that technology enables: working in teams or with peers, social networking, participatory learning, interaction, immediacy, and multimedia expression (Oblinger & Oblinger, 2005). Choosing the appropriate course delivery system will impact the success or failure of the educational material being presented. This chapter presents a brief history of distance education, defines evolving terms, examines course management and learning management systems (LMSs) for delivering distance education, and presents issues related to development and implementation of distance education in colleges, universities, and organizations.

Historical Development

The historical development of distance education in the United States can be divided into four phases. The first phase, *correspondence courses*, came about in the mid-to-late 1800s and utilized printed material delivered to students by the Pony Express or railroads. Prospective students spent self-directed time reading materials, completing assignments and examinations. Once completed the assignments or examinations were returned by the postal service to be evaluated. Depending on the distance between the school and the student, evaluation of assignments could take weeks.

The founding of the Boston Society to Encourage Studies at Home in 1873 by Anna Ticknor (Agassiz & Eliot, 2011) and the Chautauqua Correspondence College in 1881 (Moore et al., 2003) were two instrumental events that moved correspondence education forward as both schools responded to the need for a more educated workforce. The Boston Society to Encourage Studies at Home focused on providing higher education for women by women, a unique and groundbreaking concept at the time (Bergmann, 2001). An inexpensive postal service facilitated this development. While the number of offered courses grew along with enrollment, so too did the concerns about quality education and the effectiveness of this means of delivery—a theme that continues today. Phase 2, encompassing the 1920s through the early 1980s, enhanced the delivery method for distance education by involving the *broadcast media*: films, radio, and television (Bianchi, 2008). The terms changed from correspondence to telecourses and then from correspondence education to distance education during this time.

In the 1920s radio quickly swept the United States delivering music, entertainment, and education. Benjamin Darrow founded the School of the Air in Chicago in the late 1920s. Darrow used real students and teachers to deliver content over the airwaves to thousands of in-class students (Bianchi, 2008). The lack of funding in Chicago encouraged Darrow to move back to his home state of Ohio and begin the Ohio School of Air in 1929. Ohio History Central stated:

"The National Committee on Education by Radio (NCER), also known as the Payne Fund, originally financed the Ohio School of the Air. Two radio stations broadcast the programs each day: The Ohio State University's station WEAO (now WOSU) and WLW in Cincinnati. The school gained the support of the Ohio Department of Education, and the Ohio General Assembly agreed to provide additional funding for the programs after months. The Ohio School of the Air reached more than 100,000 students in twenty-two states in its first year and created interest in radio education at the national level.

In 1937, the state legislature ended funding for the Ohio School of the Air. Without government support for its efforts, the Ohio School of the Air ended" (Ohio School of the Air, n.d.).

In the 1950's television's growing popularity found its way into the classroom, via closed circuit classroom content, eventually moving to larger scale broadcasting content on cable and satellite (Fabos, 2004). "In the late 1960s and early 1970s, the use of radio and television in education continued to grow, but not in terms of distance education. Educators were using television in the classroom as a tool to demonstrate and explain concepts, and families were tuning in at home to educational broadcasts (i.e., cable television, Public Broadcasting Service, and National Public Radio)" (Kentnor, 2015).

While students were ready to embrace the telecourses method of delivery because of family, work responsibilities, geographic challenges in accessing academic institutions, and disability issues, the academic institutions continued to question the effectiveness of this new delivery method and the changes required in teaching methods.

Phase 3, *Online education*, which took place in the mid to late 1980s and 1990s, found colleges and universities laying fiber optic cables on campus. This high-speed connection made live two-way video communication possible between local (main campus) classrooms and remote (branch campus) classrooms. Students and faculty at both sites could see and hear each other, although with a slight transmission delay. This was education at a distance but in real time (synchronous). In addition, developing technology made it possible for more people to purchase personal home computers with dial-up internet access, enabling students to access course materials from a distance and to interact with faculty and other students through email, telephone, or other communication systems.

In healthcare education, faculty have been providing distance education courses and programs for more than 35 years (Billings, 2007). Early programs relied on mostly print materials and audiotapes, with on-campus meetings during the semester. As time progressed education appeared as computer-aided instructional programs and interactive videodiscs ran on freestanding computers (Billings, 2007). With changing technology developments, delivery system formats changed from mostly printed materials to broadcast courses (e.g., distance learning classrooms that broadcast live classes to remote sites).

Phase 4, *User Generated content*, which began in the late 1990s and continues to the present, saw advances on the internet and the development of Web 2.0 tools, such as podcasts, wikis, blogs, and video conferencing. This moved the focus from information retrieval to user-generated content, interactive learning, and virtual communities. This phase saw a surge in development of distance education courses and programs to meet the needs of a mobile society concerned about costs, currency, and lifelong learning, as well as a need to stay competitive in the job market.

Terminology

Although the phrases in distance learning are used interchangeably, the nuances that can exist between these terms have broad implications for higher education and related institutions.

Asynchronous learning occurs when the learner views planned educational content at a *different time* than the educational content was presented. Asynchronous learning could include reading assigned articles, watching videos, or doing internet searches on predetermined topics. Note that *time* is the key factor when discussing this type of learning, the educational activity and the learning event take place at various times.

Synchronous learning occurs when the educational event and the learning take place at the same time. Synchronous learning can take place in a face-to-face classroom or through electronic means (webinars, internet-based communication platforms). If the educational event and the learning take place at the same time, it is considered synchronous learning.

Blended learning is a combination of asynchronous and synchronous learning. Often the asynchronous learning is done in preparation of a planned learning event. Learners are asked to view videos or read articles and plan to apply that knowledge or interact with other learners in a live environment (either in person or remotely).

Distance education is instruction and planned learning in which the teacher and the learner are separated by location, teaching, and learning occur at various times, and material is delivered electronically or in print. Others remove the time element, defining distance education as teaching and learning where the teacher and learner are only geographically separated and rely on technology for instructional delivery (Martin & Bolliger, 2018). Time is not a critical element in this definition of distance education, but distance and the use of communication technology are the critical elements. It is also critical to distinguish distance education from independent learning or programmed computer instruction in that distance education is planned, mediated instruction. This means that the teacher not only designs learning experiences to guide the student's learning but also provides direction, comments on coursework, and issues a grade on completion of the course. The National Council of State Boards of Nursing also provides an example of this definition. The Distance Learning Education Committee defines distance education as "instruction offered by any means where the student and faculty are in separate physical locations. Teaching methods may be synchronous or asynchronous and shall facilitate and evaluate learning in compliance with BON approval status/regulations" (Spector & Lowery, 2015). Note the focus on learning and expansion to include both views—at the same time (synchronous) or not at the same time (asynchronous). There are variations in the meaning; therefore, accrediting bodies are defining distance education within their regulations (Southern Association of Colleges and Schools Commission on Colleges Board of Trustees, 2020; Lowery & Spector, 2014).

Distributive (distributed) education is a type of distance education where one customizes the learning environment to the learning styles of the learners. The learners may be taking distance, hybrid (combination of online and face to face), or on-site courses (Benzie & Harper, 2019), defined distributed education as "products [that] can be inserted into the learning environment in a range of ways, either integrated into the online LMS, or hyperlinked to by course or learning resource sites" (p. 634). The primary goal of distributed learning is the customization of the learning environment to better meet the learner's needs at the *learner's own pace* using technologies and an interactive collaborative environment that can take place on or off campus. Distributed learning is more inclusive in its delivery methods (Farnsworth et al., 2012). Note the following advantages of distributive education in its mixed media learning style:

- Exposes learner to practical real-world settings
- Builds learning and social skills through collaboration
- Integrates learning into daily lives

Additional information concerning the next generation of learners, learning environments, personal learning assistant initiatives, and related research can be seen at the Office of the Undersecretary of Defense for Personnel and Readiness's Advanced Distributed Learning Network at https://www.adlnet.gov/adl-research/.

Three other useful terms one might encounter are online education, eLearning, and mLearning. Each will be defined here, but what is important is how these terms are used within the context of the content they are referencing.

Online education requires the use of the internet or an intranet to deliver educational materials.

"**E-learning** is a training system that involves only electronic means of education and Internet technologies" (Tyurina et al., 2021). There are three major elements that make eLearning different from face-to-face learning: asynchronous learning, a different location, and use of electronic devices that provide for interaction and communications (Koch, 2014). The consensus seems to be that eLearning requires a computer or other electronic device such as a smartphone or tablet. eLearning involves a greater variety of equipment than online resources or the internet in that any electronic device may be used: DVDs, CD-ROMs, and so forth. Currently, education can be accessed on any electronic device. eLearning has moved from desktops to laptops, to iPad, to Chromebooks (Apple books), to cellular devices. Additionally, Quick Response codes are becoming more prevalent to direct users to documents or websites to obtain more information.

mLearning is the use of a mobile device (smartphone, tablet, iPad) as an educational tool for meaningful, just-in-time learning at any place and time. Mobile devices refer to those devices that can be held in the hand. While mLearning is considered an extension of eLearning, there are differences between the two. These differences include information access, context, and layout (Benvin, 2016; Gutierrez, 2021). mLearning contains

---

BOX 26.1 Outline for a Strategic Plan for Distributive Education

Executive Summary

This section sets the background for the plan and includes the following subsections. *Introduction*. This subsection sets the stage for why universities and organizations are doing this. It addresses what is happening in the broader world, then locally, and then within the institution. It should answer the following questions: Why is the institution and faculty doing this? What are the goals? How will faculty and the institution define related terms? Some include a strengths, weaknesses, opportunities, and threats (SWOT) analysis in the introduction. Others place it within the Details section as a separate subsection called *SWOT analysis*. Others place it in an appendix to the plan.

- **Mission statement**. What is the mission for this initiative? How does that fit with the mission of the college or university? The mission statement should include the language of the school's mission.
- **Goals**. What are the specific goals for this initiative in terms of students, faculty, programs, and so forth? This can include goals such as providing flexibility in helping students achieve their educational goals, targeting the adult and second-degree populations, and developing faculty. Areas to address in the goals are as follows:
- **Students**. Who are the target students? What are the rules as to who can take these courses or enroll in the program? How will students be oriented to these means of learning?
- **Faculty**. How will faculty be trained? What training will faculty need? How will ongoing support be provided? How will this count toward faculty teaching loads? Who will monitor quality?

- **Courses and programs**. What programs and courses will be offered in this delivery method? Who makes these decisions? How are decisions approved? How do faculty address issues such as the Technology, Education, and Copyright Harmonization (TEACH) Act and copyright? What is the target class size? How will that decision be made?
- **Support issues**. What course management systems (CMS) will be used? Can it interface with the school's other systems? When will faculty have access to a shell for course development? What library changes will be needed to support remote students? How will access to other support services such as registration, paying tuition, and accessing tutoring be managed? What support services will students need?
- **Policy and procedures**. Who will develop and approve them? When?

Details

This section provides the details for each of the goals identified. *Goals*. List and number each goal. For example, 1a, 1b, 2a, 2b, 2c

- **Recommendations**. After careful review, comparison, and research, what is the recommendation for each goal? For example, after careful review, Blackboard is the recommended CMS. Recommendations should also include who will be responsible for moving each goal forward.
- **Budget items**. Include projected costs for achieving each goal.
- **Time frame**. Include a target date for achievement of each goal.

---

short learning sessions (microlearning), accessed when needed, driven by context, and applied immediately. As mobile devices continue to develop more capabilities, you will see more interactive, stimulating learning environments. What we need to focus on is the learning environment that mobile devices can facilitate. When developing education for the mobile platform the design of the educational content should be at the forefront of the developer's mind. The screen size of the mobile device is smaller than traditional computers and the use of viewable content is limited. Additionally, interactions like chat, response icons, videos, documents, and group work may take extra steps for those viewing on a mobile device or the functionality may not be available at all, decreasing the effectiveness of the educational content.

Faculty should discuss and define these terms during their strategic planning process when developing education courses and programs. Box 26.1 provides a sample outline for a strategic plan, and Box 26.2 provides an outline for a progress report. These same questions and processes also apply when implementing training initiatives in the work world. Questions to ask and answer during strategic planning include: What terms are faculty and the school using to describe the distance learning initiative? You can turn this question around to say, "Describe the distance training initiative." What terms do the accreditation agencies use? How are colleagues in other schools and accrediting agencies defining the terms? How will these definitions be conveyed to the learner?

Types of Systems Used in Distance Learning

Course delivery systems (CDS), also known as course management system (CMS) or LMS, are software programs or

---

BOX 26.2 Content for a Progress or Status Report on a Strategic Plan

- **Plan name and date**. For example, Distributive Education Plan 2016–2019.
- **Goal and objective**. List each goal and objective.
- **Tasks, actions, or activities**. What is needed to achieve the goal and objectives, coded to each goal and objective?
- **Persons responsible**. Who is held responsible for this task?
- **Budget**. Original or revised.
- **Due date**. May include original and revised dates for completion of the task.
- **Progress note or description**. Status of the task: what has been done and what needs to be done.

---

applications that permit the development and delivery of a course or training program without requiring knowledge of programming code. These programs provide the tools necessary to plan, implement, and assess the learning process by giving the professor/trainer the ability to create and deliver content, monitor learner participation and progress, provide for interactive communications, and assess learning outcomes. There are distinct differences between a CDS (CMS) and an LMS and that a CMS is a narrower term than an LMS. An LMS includes course management but also additional features that manage course registration, integration with HR systems, administrative features, and integration with other institutional information systems (Ninoriya et al., 2011; Behera et al., 2017; Krouska et al., 2018). In other words, an LMS manages all aspects of eLearning or corporate training, while a CMS focuses on content delivery and learner interaction and communication. This distinction, however, is blurring as CMS vendors incorporate more of the management aspect into their products.

Proprietary CMSs are software packages, purchased or licensed by organization (Nelson & Staggers, 2014). These vendors provide a license either to install the system on the customer's servers or to host the customer's license on their servers. Proprietary CMSs have been the dominant systems on the market. These original systems merged leaving a small number that make up the current market of proprietary systems.

Most CMSs provide content management, user management and enrollment, assessment of learners, communications such as e-mail and discussion forums, and social learning tools such as wikis, blogs, journals, and mobile features.

There are several CMS software programs available, and the market is constantly changing. See Table 26.1 for CMS usage rankings reported by NYC Design in 2021 (Bradley, 2021). Although Table 26.1 lists the most frequently used CMSs in the academic higher education world, the business world uses other CMSs for its training. More common examples include Canvas,

D2L Brightspace, Google Classroom, Blackboard, Docebo, Schoology, Talent LMS, Edmodo, TovutiLMS, and Moodle (G2.com, 2021). Other CMSs are popular with the K-12 institutions and still others with the international market.

Examples of LMS and CMS

Canvas LMS. Canvas LMS was launched in 2011 by Instructure Incorporated. Canvas LMS is part of an educational technology company that serves K-12 and Higher Education across the globe. Their mission is to "elevate student success, amplify the power of teaching, and inspire everyone to learn together" (Instructure, n.d.).

Blackboard. Blackboard was founded in 1997 as a small educational technology company and provides a full range of CMS service (Fig. 26.1). Blackboard is used across domestic and international markets that includes K-12, higher education, governments, and businesses (Blackboard, 2021).

Moodle. Moodle is popular among educators around the world as a tool for creating online websites for students. To work, Moodle must be on a web server, either on one of the school's servers or on a server at a web hosting company such as MoodleCloud which services small schools and Moodle Partners like ClassroomRevolution LLC and eLearningExperts (Moodle, 2021). There is a fee to use a hosting company, but the overall cost of this approach may be less because of free access to the code.

Google classroom. Google Classroom was launched in 2014 and designed with teachers' needs in mind. Google Classroom is offered in a free and paid format for K-12 and higher education faculty (Google, n.d.).

Partnerships. Book publishers often partner with software vendors to provide a package of tools to assist with the delivery

TABLE 26.1 NYC Design Profile of the Course Management Systems Market, January 2021	
CMS	**Market Share (%)[a]**
WordPress	41
Drupal	19
OmniUpdate	9.5
Cascade CMS	7
Adobe Experience Manager	4

[a]Rounded up.

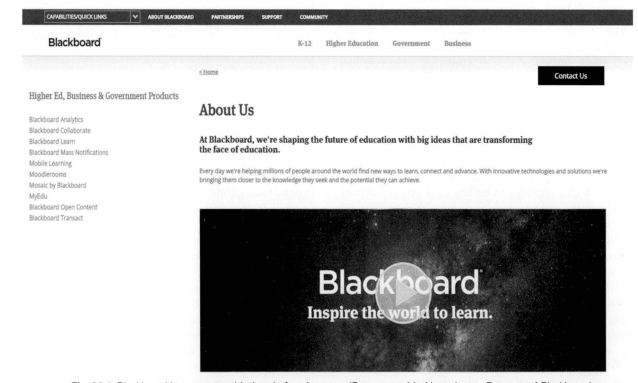

Fig. 26.1 Blackboard home page with the platform's menu. (From www.blackboard.com. Property of Blackboard and used with permission.)

of distance education. Elsevier's Evolve LMS and Pearson's learning environments (LearningStudio, MyLab, Mynursinglab) supply everything from customized, concept-to-completion LMSs to digital content. These online learning environments offer resources to both faculty and students (e.g., interactive grade book features, learning tools that simulate clinical experience and charting, cloud-based technology). In most cases, the disadvantage to using this approach is that they may require you to use their textbook or may require students to purchase an access code. When you change textbooks, you may lose access to these resources. If students try to resell their textbooks on the used-textbook market, the access code is not valid.

Portals. Portals are customized, personalized entries or gateways where users, including students and faculty, can access all the content they typically need. A portal is a user-centric web page that includes access to a CMS. The portal integrates and provides a secure access point to the data, information, and applications that users need in their roles as a student or faculty. Portals include enterprise resource systems (finance, human relations), community building communications, admissions, retention, web-based academic counseling, CMSs, and metrics to measure success. Two examples of vendor-based portals are Ellucian and Jenzabar.

Ellucian. Ellucian's focus is assisting educational institutions to grow by offering applications that integrate and interface the systems that faculty and students need. Fig. 26.2 presents the homepage of their website with the software submenu showing (Ellucian, n.d.).

Jenzabar. Jenzabar is another example of a portal system that supports a college or university across each department, including administrative offices and academic departments (Jenzabar, 2021). Jenzabar attempts to align the school's mission

and goals with technology investments. Fig. 26.3 shows the Higher Education Solutions menu on the homepage and the range of offerings that Jenzabar provides. Notice the Cloud services on the left side of the screen. These products are similar for most portal systems. Their eLearning software includes the typical features of CMS: content management, course copy, a gradebook, exams, e-mail, calendars, chat, discussion forums, online meetings, test analytics, and usage statistics.

Integrated campus LMSs, personal learning systems (PLS), and personal portals, these systems integrate learner functions such as registration, billing, courses, library, tutoring, and other related learner services.

SELECTING A COURSE MANAGEMENT SYSTEM

When starting the selection process, it is important to first decide on the type of system that will meet the needs of the institution and its students (Wright et al., 2014). The Course Management System (CMS) selection decision often rests with administrators, information technology (IT) personnel, and faculty, although institutions may have student representatives on the planning committee.

The process for the selection of a CMS should be an integral part of the strategic plan for university's distance education or the organization's continuing education training. CMS selection should never be delegated to the IT department with minor input from other stakeholders. Considerations for selection include the following:

- **Objectives or goals**. What are the goals/objectives for distance education or organizational training? How does a CMS fit with these goals/objectives? How does this fit with the school's philosophy and mission?

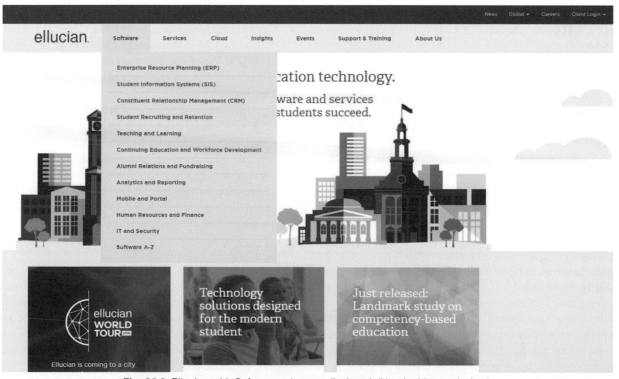

Fig. 26.2 Ellucian with Software submenu displayed. (Used with permission.)

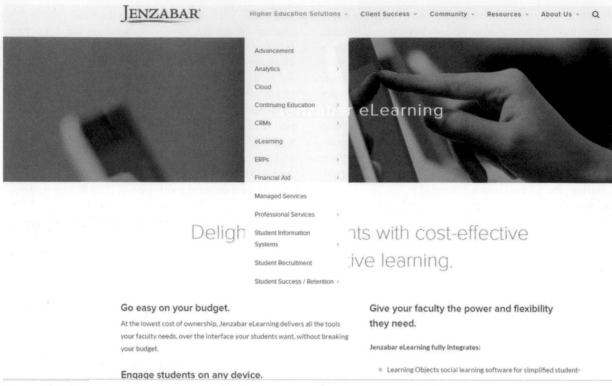

Fig. 26.3 Jenzabar products menu. (Copyright 2013 Jenzabar, Inc. All rights reserved. Used with permission.)

- **Features**. What features do faculty or trainers believe are essential to delivering the course or training? What are desirable features but not essential ones? How will the infrastructure be supported?
- **Integration with current institutional systems**. How important is the new system? Which other information systems need to be addressed? Does the CMS support interoperability with third-party products (e.g., registrar's applications, billing, registration)? If interoperability is limited, the organization should consider another CMS.
- **Compatibility with different student systems** such as operating systems, mobile devices, and related security programs like firewalls and antivirus programs.
- **User base**. How many institutions and end users will use the product? Is the installed user base important to your organization? Is there a local user group associated with the CMS? What type of support does it provide for the faculty, students, and IT department? How stable is the company offering the CMS? This question may require the financial department to investigate.
- **Customization/Maintenance**. Will the CMS require extensive custom programming or maintenance? Are sufficient staff and resources in place for that type of work?
- **Scalability**. How scalable is the CMS? Can it easily expand, or contract based on varying needs?
- **Usability**. How user friendly is the CMS? Does it have the tool set that faculty or trainers need to deliver the courses? Are there data tracking and report features? Are those tools intuitive to use for both learners and faculty or trainers to complete typical tasks?

- **Outcome measures**. Does the CMS support outcome measures? If so, does it support the outcome measures important to the organization?
- **Sharable Content Object Reference Model (SCORM) compliance**. Is the system SCORM compliant (encourages the standardization of LMSs)? Is that important? Are there other standards that are important?
- *Cost*. What does it cost to buy the CMS? What does it cost to own the CMS? What is the cost of hosting versus housing the CMS? What are the mechanisms for and frequency of upgrades? What are the costs of these upgrades?

There are additional criteria for the selection of a CMS that fall into these categories: ease of use, stability, tool set, and support. Other considerations may relate to compatibility, integration, or cost issues related to financial and technical support. Faculty and educators within healthcare organizations can provide valuable insights into system selection. Articles such as "Top Learning Management System (LMS) statistics for 2020 you need to know" can be helpful for the selection committee to gain a big picture perspective (Pappas, 2019).

Ease of Use

There is a learning curve to using CMS software. The interface should be intuitive to use. Does it use common educational terms to describe tools such as discussion forums or boards? Does its design support distance education or is it an adaptation of other products? Faculty should ask questions and complete typical educational tasks to assess ease of use for grading papers, projects, and tests; returning files; and setting up and using the grading center. Also important are tools such as wikis, blogs, conferencing, and chat that are available for collaboration activities for assignments such as group projects. How easy is it for students and faculty to learn to use these tools? This could include an analysis of the number of clicks it takes to upload content, what file formats are acceptable for upload, and what file size limits are enforced. Another area to analyze is the ease of content movement between courses and between semesters and the ease of archiving and exporting courses. Too many required clicks or difficulty in understanding the screen discourages faculty from using tools. Does the setup reduce time and effort or demand more time and effort in delivering the course?

Stability

How stable is the company offering the CMS? Will it be in business next year or will the school have to select another system next year if the company fails or another company acquires it? Stability also includes system reliability issues such as the frequency of system crashes and the turnaround time to restore the system after such a crash. Students and faculty require 24/7 access.

Tool Set (Features)

What are the bundled tools in the CMS, and which ones require additional funds to access? For example, is Blackboard's Collaborate tool bundled with the basic version of Blackboard, or does access to that tool increase the price? Do faculty want collaborative tools such as video conferencing, podcasting, blogging, wiki abilities, chatting, and so forth? What "smart" features do faculty need? This may include alerts that the system automatically sends to students and tools that remember who the user is and where he or she left off in doing work. Do faculty want mobile computing as part of the tool set? Do they want textbook cartridge capabilities or online testing tools? Cartridges are files that a textbook publisher provides faculty who select its textbook. Once uploaded, the cartridge sets up the course in the CMS. These cartridges contain lessons, PowerPoint slides, discussion forums, tests, and so forth. It is the role of faculty to identify what tools they need to teach a course.

Vendor Support

Is implementation training provided? Is that part of the start-up costs? What training materials does the CMS offer? Does it have a 24/7 help system, either by phone or by chat? What support does it offer students?

After considering these factors, faculty are responsible for determining the essential criteria or features necessary to deliver a quality course using appropriate technology as well as any "nice to have" but not essential criteria or features. CMS decisions are often made internally for the academic environment. Thus, knowing school- and profession-specific requirements is critical.

CMS products are improving with new technological developments and arrangements with partners that bring new tools to the product. For example, most products now provide access to Web 2.0 tools that facilitate collaboration efforts. These include tools such as wikis, blogs, conferencing, ePortfolio, and journaling. Most products now also offer mobile learning options.

INSTRUCTIONAL DESIGN FOR DISTANCE LEARNING

While most principles of instructional design hold true for distance education, the principal teaching change in a learning environment is the use of technology to engage and empower the learner. This section is not a comprehensive treatise about instructional design concepts but a discussion of key factors that should be considered in the design of eLearning experiences.

Adult Learners

The key to presenting any type of education, whether synchronous, asynchronous, or blended is to know your learners and their skill set. As the introduction to this chapter pointed out, there can be a different mindset among digital natives (learners who grew up with technology) and students who were schooled using more historical methods. Faculty will usually see a range of students with a varying degree of abilities. **Adult learners** come from all backgrounds, ages, and with varying levels of experiences in the real world and in the digital world. Rothwell, (2020) advises that adult learners want education to apply knowledge immediately to a specific situation and answer the question "why is this information to us at this moment?" For example, how can your education on conflict management be used immediately when faced with the problem of horizontal violence.

It is also important to understand the previous experiences the adult learner brings to the classroom or training room. Adult learners will draw on previous experiences when learning or applying new concepts or using new skills. When the adult learner applies their previous experiences to the latest information, it will give the current information a deeper connection and feel more immediately usable.

Adult learners may seem passive at first but allowing them to take responsibility for the education by giving them self-assessments and based on that assessment ask them what they would like to learn first. In eLearning modules, this could be as easy as having the user click one topic in a presentation to start learning first, then move to the next topic they find of interest. Setting expectations or learner responsibilities at the start of a class or training will allow the adult learner to feel more engaged and self-directed. For example, the educator or trainer directs the learner to listen to a specific podcast or read a particular article, then the learner has the responsibility to do an exploratory WebQuest activity that requires them to explore the web for quality resources and expands their knowledge about this content. A WebQuest is an inquiry-oriented lesson format in which most or all the information that learners work with comes from the web. See Google's Teaching with Technology website (https://sites.google.com/site/learnteachtech/webquest-projects) for examples. Additionally, providing tasks or checklists of what will be covered in the education and then demonstrating how the tasks are done will benefit the adult learner.

Learning Style

Every person has their own style or preferences when it comes to learning and understanding current information.

Understanding the various learning styles allows the educator or trainer to develop educational content that includes as various learning styles, thus increasing the ability of the learner to retain the knowledge. (Leite et al. (2010) found the VARK learning styles inventory to be both a valid and reliable instrument when determining preferred learning modalities. VARK stands for Visual, Aural, Read/Write and Kinesthetic and each learning modality focuses on preferences for that learning style. The VARK website defines the preferences for each learning modality as follows:

- **Visual learners** prefer graphical representations of information such as maps, diagrams, charts, and the like. "When a whiteboard is used to draw a diagram with meaningful symbols for the relationship between different things that will be helpful for those with a Visual preference."
- **Aural or auditory learners** prefer information that is heard or spoken. The VARK also states email and texting is included in this modality as "it is often written in chat-style with abbreviations, colloquial terms, slang and non-formal language." Auditory learners prefer to repeat what they've learned aloud to reinforce the concepts.
- **Read/Write** learners prefer to see words in all their forms— books, magazines, manuals, reports—and "people who prefer this modality are often addicted to PowerPoint, the Internet, lists, diaries, dictionaries, thesauri, quotations and words, words, words…"
- **Kinesthetic learners** prefer experiences or hands-on methods of learning. "It includes demonstrations, simulations, videos and movies of *"real"* things, as well as case studies, practice and applications."

The VARK questionnaire can be found at https://vark-learn.com/the-vark-questionnaire/, as well as strategies for using each modality (VARK, 2021).

Engagement

In early 2020, COVID-19 required organizations to rethink how they provided education, information, and communication to staff, communities, and students while maintaining physical distance and gathering restrictions. Various communication platforms found themselves as the hub for connecting organizations, teams, and classrooms. In addition to the logistical challenges presented with social distancing, audience engagement waned as they were now faced with the distraction of working or attending school from home. In this section we will discuss engagement tools and activities that can be used in the various learning environments.

Audience engagement is as important in the distance learning forum as it is for in person presentations. In person the educator can pick up visual clues of comprehension, questions, or distractions from physical clues from those in attendance. Determining engagement or understanding in a distance environment can be challenging. Unless attendees are using cameras, the educator is unable to use their facial expressions as visual cues. Often educators have used the communication platform's built-in response tools like polls, chat, Q&A, or a raise hand feature to engage attendees and confirm understanding. The common communication platforms include Zoom, Webcx,

Teams, GoToMeetings. Most communication platforms have **breakout rooms** incorporated into their platform for small group activities or discussions.

In addition to the built-in features in communication platforms, there are web-based **audience response applications** like **MentiMeter, Poll Everywhere**, or **Slido that will** provide engagement for even the shyest attendee. **MentiMeter, Poll Everywhere**, and **Slido** use quizzes, word clouds, multiple choice questions, graphics, and ranking systems to engage the learner. These applications offer free and subscription services. Slido and Poll Everywhere have a plug-in to use with PowerPoint, making these a feasible choice to use for in person meetings or in the synchronous or blended learning environment.

Providing breaks is as important in the virtual environment as it is in in-person, more so. It is harder to focus on the virtual environment than in an in-person environment. Our brains and our bodies get fatigued or give in to distractions around the 30-to-40-minute mark. Encouraging a 5-minute **movement** or **brain break**, especially for longer offerings, can be enough to re-energize your attendees. Physical movement, both virtually and in person allows the learner to walk away without missing vital content. Activities like an interactive coloring page, or word search, when used over a communication platform can extend the breaks for those who come back early.

Brain breaks can also be used in the asynchronous learning environment to provide learners with a temporary respite from content. Brain breaks work best when used between chunks of information. The brain break, a **photo, music, or unrelated content**, signals the learner that this piece of content is complete and can be filed away for recall or contemplation later.

Playing games in large or small groups can create a team atmosphere and improve group cohesion. **Kahoot** and **Quizlet** are web-based trivia games that can be used to reinforce the content you are presenting, while traditional games like **Pictionary** or **Charades** can provide a welcome distraction and improve engagement and can be done in person or in synchronous environments. Additionally, playing Bingo and using topics or key concepts from your presentation in the squares can help improve engagement. The games will take preparation and planning, but it will be worth the work. Games can also be used in the asynchronous learning environment, attaching points to knowledge checks, or providing positive feedback, through photos or graphics for correct responses can capture the gaming atmosphere. The asynchronous module can be designed as a game board moving the learning along the board, with each "square" representing updated content.

Outcomes and Evaluation

When presenting education, in any format writing clear, measurable goals, and outcomes is critical to ensure that students know the course expectations and how faculty will assess their learning. Each lesson, module, or activity should identify the purpose, goals, and objectives; provide clear directions for what students are to do; and provide a scoring rubric or guide for evaluation of students' achievement of the objectives or outcomes. These should also include due dates and time periods. Especially important to include in distance learning is how the learner will participate in the learning activities. Will they be required to attend virtual class meetings? Will they be expected to use specific software to complete the assignment or activity? Additionally, links to training or knowledge articles will be included for software that is unfamiliar to the learner.

Instructional and Learner Activities

Instructional and learner activities should provide learners with the skills, knowledge, and experience necessary to meet the course objectives. These activities or experiences should consider the learners' need for engagement, activity, and relevance to the content, objectives, and work world. This means that the professor will need to take advantage of the tool set available through the CMS software as well as tool sets available from outside sources. It may also mean that the professor must step outside their comfort zone in learning new ways to deliver the course and develop relevant learning experiences. Faculty and educators should have access to a wide variety of collaborative tools that encourage interaction with the content and with others. These tools include wikis, blogs, discussion forums, journals, and WebQuests. Other learner activities could include developing podcasts, videos, and group projects. When designing course activities, keep in mind that active participation facilitates learning better than does passive participation. For training, the same applies, making it relevant to the work tasks. As an example, teaching how to use Excel and related features with activities that demonstrate common uses from the work setting is much more effective than a basic, intermediate, and advanced perspective for organizing the learning.

To help guide the selection of learning activities, one should consider the use of a model like the Community of Inquiry Model, with its three main concepts of social presence, cognitive presence, and teaching presence. Social presence refers to establishing a support learning community where students can express themselves as real people and develop social relationships. Cognitive presence is the development of learning materials where students construct knowledge through reflection and discussions in a safe and supportive environment. Teaching presence is the last concept that deals with designing the learning experiences, guiding the learning, and moving the students to the desired student learning outcomes (Garrison et al., 1999). The educator's presence and personality can be crucial in making students feel connected and engaged (Conrad & Donaldson, 2011).

Evaluation

Regular and timely feedback to learners on their progress is important to learner success and engagement with the content/concepts/skills. Learners benefit from frequent feedback as they master updated content, but this can also be very time consuming for faculty or trainers.

Faculty members who design learning activities or projects where grading requires faculty judgment as opposed to "objective testing" should develop a grading rubric or guide for each activity and place it with the directions or guidelines file as well as attach it to the assignment in the CMS. These guidelines should also convey to learners when students will receive comments and grades on submitted work. When developing these guidelines, trainers should think carefully about how they will use these same guidelines during the grading process. Comments, suggestions, and feedback are crucial when evaluating assignments. The feedback provided by faculty aids in reinforcing important concepts, rectifying misconceptions, and ensuring understanding of the content.

Once the grading is completed, faculty will also need to enter scores in the CMS so that these scores can be viewed in the online student grade sheet. Online grade sheets now offer the students methods of sorting and analyzing their grades. Faculty should consider how students might interpret this information. For example, would a student learning current information be motivated or discouraged if they determine they have the lowest score in the class?

In addition to the evaluation of each learner's learning, faculty should consider course evaluation, learning activities and the faculty's teaching presence. On a course-by-course basis, faculty may develop activities that provide learner feedback to the professor. A student statement illuminating what the student learned from completion of the activity provides feedback as to what is working and what is not. For example, at the end of each blog entry, have the student identify up to three things that they have learned and why they found them to be important. As a final example, require the students to rate themselves on a scale of 1 to 5 on how well they achieved each course objective and to support that rating with data (an activity or a resource that helped them learn, a product that they produced).

Also, to consider, does the school have course evaluation or best practices guidelines? Are these guidelines appropriate for distance education courses? Course evaluation forms link to faculty contracts and will not necessarily help improve the course. Does the faculty member use something like Quality Matters, which is a peer review process to certify the quality of online and blended courses (Quality Matters, n.d.)? It might be helpful to use a guide like Quality Matters as the course is developed. There is no one best practice guide for distance education, but all guides consider these points as being critical to quality:

- Institutional commitment and resources
- Curriculum and instructional rigor with interactivity and regular communication between faculty and learners
- Faculty support services
- Student support services
- Evaluation of the course and programs

In the corporate world, the trainer needs to consider how a training session fits with the rest of the training provided by the corporation and the corporation's mission, goals, and values. For example, in a class on clinical documentation, will the employees be able to document in the electronic health record, effectively and avoid the common data entry errors at the completion of the training? Feedback on instructor presence, training content, and engagement of activities provides the instructor an opportunity to improve content for future use. Equally important to a well-designed and well-delivered course are the support services available to learners.

Learner Support Services

Student support services are important to the achievement of learner outcomes, learner satisfaction, and learner retention. In planning for learner support services, the faculty may need to assess what support services online learners expect. Nelson states, "putting all student services online will not eliminate the need for support services specifically designed for distance education students" (Nelson, 2007). That statement is still relevant today. All learners, both on and off campus, must have access to the same resources, but they may be delivered in a separate way.

Library

While most schools have online access to full text databases, interlibrary loans, and book borrowing, there is a wealth of other library resources of which the learner should be made aware. The following are two examples:

- Top Sites Blog contains a list of the top 10 free online libraries (http://topsitesblog.com/free-online-libraries). These online libraries contain mostly historical information but can assist students with their general education requirements as well as provide historical information about healthcare.
- Nursing on the Net: Health Care Resources You Can Use (https://nnlm.gov/training/nursing/sampler.html) includes a list of topics with links such as alternative medicine, drug information, evidence-based nursing, and mobile apps, to name a few. There is an extensive listing of links to resources under these categories. This site is maintained by the National Network of Libraries of Medicine and is updated regularly.

The Association of College and Research Libraries (ACRL) publishes a set of standards for libraries servicing the distance education population, initially approved on July 1, 2008, but referred to as a "living document" (Association of College & Research Libraries, 2008). Guidance in the use of these standards may be found at the DLS website (http://acrl.ala.org/DLS/). In addition, a bibliography of recent literature on distance learning library services can be accessed at https://distancelearningsection.wordpress.com/resources-publications/.

During the planning phase, the school should compare its services to those standards and develop a plan to acquire the services and materials that do not currently meet those standards. In addition, faculty must discuss what additional services online students may need that on-campus students do not. This can vary from institution to institution based on how the course is delivered. For example, do learners need a different user ID and password to access the school's online full text databases, or do they have one user ID and password to access all resources whether on or off campus? Do they have access to an online librarian who can help them with their search strategy?

Tutoring Services

All learners studying at a distance should have the same access to tutoring services as on-campus learners. There are online tutoring services that learners may use for a fee or that the school may provide. Some examples include Tutor.com (www.tutor.com), Smarthinking, Inc. (http://www.pearsoned.com/higher-education/products-and-services/services-and-solutions-for-higher-ed/services/smarthinking/), and Chegg Study (https://www.chegg.com/study). See also http://www.tutor.com/higher-education. The tutoring service must be like those that the school offers on campus and must have the same pricing structure. Faculty should ask questions about these services regarding the fees, live real-time help, hours of operation, and qualifications of the tutors. For example, does the service have tutors who can address the needs of healthcare students?

If there are peer tutoring services for on-campus learners, how will those same services be available to the distance education learner? What technology will be in place to provide for these services? For example, does the school provide a web-based video solution where the writing center peer tutor can interact with the student and the student's paper while talking about needed improvements? If a video conference system is not available, the learner could e-mail the paper to the tutor and arrange a phone conversation to discuss it.

Help Desk (Support Center)

Given the nature of technology and the potential for technical issues to arise during the semester, the school will need to address technical assistance for off-campus and on-campus learners. Should it provide for a university-based help desk, an outsourced help desk, or a combination? This is not an easy decision. It requires a cost analysis to assess staffing a help desk with staff and students versus outsourced staffing. Software will be necessary to run the help desk and a training budget allocated to train the staff. The school will need to make decisions about help desk staff's ability to reset passwords and access the CMS, with designated privileges for functions they can perform, such as configuring a student's browser and firewall and running virus checks. What is the range of help that a student working at the help desk can provide? Will more hours be allotted during the first few weeks of the semester when more help may be needed?

Because distance learning occurs at any time (24/7) and any place, schools are opting for outsourcing. Outsourcing can be offered by either the CMS vendor or be a freestanding service that is independent of the vendor. A key question to ask in the CMS selection process is whether a CMS provides a help desk service. Faculty may want to confirm that the school's CMS provider can effectively bundle a help desk product with its CMS product; CMSs are moving in this direction (to a portal or bundled product). If so, what is the fee and what is the advantage of using that service for the distance education program?

Another approach is to use a general help desk provider. The following are examples of a portal, CMSs, and LMSs help desk services.

- **BlackBeltHelp** (www.blackbelthelp.com) is a freestanding help desk service that has been working with higher education institutions for the past 5 years. It offers 24/7, 365 days a year support to students, faculty, and staff. Support includes LMS and ERP issues, general IT help, and so forth.
- **Ellucian** (http://www.ellucian.com/Support-and-Training/Ellucian-Client-Support/). This portal solution also offers help desk services. It helps 365 days per year to faculty, staff, and students. Since it knows the portal software, it may be in a better position to assist students than a freestanding help desk service.

- **Blackboard** (http://www.blackboard.com/higher-education/student-services-and-technology-support/index.aspx). On July 8, 2014, Blackboard acquired Perceptis to enhance its help desk support service.
- **Canvas** (https://community.canvaslms.com/t5/Instructor-Guide/tkb-p/Instructor). This portal provides instructor assistance in all areas of the Canvas infrastructure. It is an assistive portal for instructors to discover uses of each section of the Canvas LMS.

If outsourcing is the solution, then the college must ensure that it outsources the correct work and tasks. For example, will the help desk be able to reset passwords? Will it have remote access to see what the student is doing or to control the student's desktop? What should it know about the CMS or LMS? Will it have privileges to enter the CMS?

In summary, learners will need access to the help desk 24/7 or close to it, and this will necessitate a variety of communication channels: phone, chat, video conference, self-help website, and so forth.

Online Textbooks

The cost and acquisition of required textbooks in a timely fashion merits attention. How is the campus bookstore responding to the growing student population that may not reside on campus or live nearby? Does it provide online ordering and shipping to the student's residence? What does that do to the costs? Does it provide eText options? Can learners rent their textbooks through the bookstore? Will open textbooks (licensed under an open copyright license) be used that are free to the students? Other options that learners may use are the growing number of online textbooks such as Chegg, Ecampus, and CourseSmart. Of course, the student has the option to order from websites like Amazon and Barnes & Noble College, as well as from traditional booksellers. The following are examples of distributors in the higher education market:

- **Chegg** (www.chegg.com). Chegg provides students with the ability to rent textbooks as well as buy new and used textbooks at a reduced cost. Students can also sell their books back to Chegg. It also offers homework help for courses, scholarships, and course selection help.
- **VitalSource** (https://www.vitalsource.com/). VitalSource provides eTextbook and digital learning tools. It provides both online and off-line access. It has a partnership arrangement with more than 50 publishers and offers more than 90% of the textbook market in higher education.

What guidance should the school provide to learners in distance education courses regarding acquisition of textbooks? For example, are these books that the student will need throughout their time in college? Depending on the answer, the students then must ensure that they are renting or using digital forms of the textbook that are available to them for the duration of their time in college. The Higher Education Opportunity Act (HEOA), discussed later in this chapter, mandates that students be provided with information about the required textbooks when they register for a course. What should they know about older editions? Are they acceptable or not? When will students need access to the textbooks? They may need certain textbooks immediately but may not need others until later in the course. Knowing this may help students balance the cost of textbooks. Will students need a code to access the textbook website? If so, does a used textbook come with the code or will the student need to buy that separately? Buying codes separately is more expensive and may not save students money when the used book costs and new code costs are combined. What is the return policy of these online distributors?

Community and Academic Support

The retention rate for students who learn in their own space and time has been a problem. How should the school adjust certain traditional student services to provide for a feeling of connectedness and belonging for distance education students? Will this aid in retention and better student outcomes?

- **Administrative services.** These services include registration, financial aid, adds and drops, and admissions. Since most schools provide these services online, the procedures for accessing them should be the same as those used by on-campus students. The key institutional issue here is whether this should be a portal solution with one interface or stand-alone systems.
- **Academic support.** This includes advising and career services. These services are already extended to students through web portals or department websites and through social media tools such as Facebook and Twitter. The school may need to develop additional options for use of social media tools to extend the services in both time and space. For example, use of video conferencing or chat rooms for advising sessions with extended hours may be appropriate. It may also be important to put in place an alert and "job well done" system. to keep students on track and motivate them to finish. Questions to ask are: Does the software integrate with the CMS? What are the issues if it does integrate? What if it doesn't integrate? Schools also have as a part of the student information system an online audit for ease of scheduling courses, reminders for requirements they met, and links to appropriate content.
- **Community building.** This is an area that schools may neglect more than other learner support services. How does the institution build a sense of belonging and identification with the program or school? Faculty and the school should consider services such as a cyber cafe either in or outside the CMS program (CMSs have a community tab or feature separate from a course) or a blog that students can use to interact outside of the course. Faculty might also consider a regular newsletter or podcast that highlights an event, student, or opportunity. What about a webinar on an issue of concern to healthcare or nursing that is open to students in the program? What about an online student government community? There are other community-building options, but these must engage the students and help them identify with their online learning community.

Legal, Accessibility, Quality Considerations

This section addresses additional issues that relate to distance education—legal, disability, quality, and readiness.

Digital Millennium Copyright Act of 1998

The Digital Millennium Copyright Act (DMCA) addresses the demands of the digital and internet age and conforms to the requirements of the World Intellectual Property Organization (American Library Association, 2015). This is a complex act that is outside the scope of this chapter. This chapter highlights those areas of the law that might affect a distance learning program. DMCA protects any copyrightable work. Copyrightable work includes written text or literary works, visual works, graphic works, musical works, and codes that pass between computers (United States Copyright Office, 1998). Key sections that affect distance learning include the following:

- Prohibiting the circumvention of protection technologies, including encryption or password-cracking programs, and the manufacturing of devices that defeat such protection measures.
- Limiting liability of online service providers because of the content that users transmit over their services
- Expanding existing exemptions for making copies of computer programs under certain conditions
- Updating rules and procedures for archival preservations
- Mandating studies to examine distance education in a networked world

DMCA also established the Takedown Notice, through which copyright holders can demand removal of infringing content. This requires the copyright holder to follow the appropriate process and procedures.

Since this is a complex law, students and faculty should check with the school's legal counsel if they are in doubt about violating DMCA while preparing and posting educational materials for a distance course. Schools also have a checklist that can be used as a guide to maintain compliance with this law. This checklist is often posted on the library website.

Technology, Education, and Copyright Harmonization Act

The Technology, Education, and Copyright Harmonization (TEACH) Act, passed in 2002 and signed into law by President George W. Bush, addresses issues that require attention when planning and delivering distance education. The purpose of this act was to clarify acceptable use of copyrighted materials as it relates to distance education. Responsibilities for compliance with this act are placed on the institution and its IT staff. The TEACH Act permits the performance and display of copyrighted materials for distance education under the following conditions: (Turkewitz & Kenneally, 2020)

- The institution is an accredited, nonprofit educational institution.
- Only students who have enrolled in the course can have access to these materials.
- The use must be for either "live" or asynchronous sessions (permits storage of the materials on a server).
- The institution must provide information to faculty and students stating that course materials may be copyrighted and provide access policies regarding copyright.
- The institution must limit access to the materials for the period necessary to complete the session or course.

- The institution must prevent further copying or redistribution of copyrighted materials.
- No part of the use may interfere with copy protection mechanisms

For professors, the law includes the following: (Gassaway, 2001)

- The materials must be part of mediated (systematic) instructional activities (i.e., relevant to the course).
- The use must not include the transmission of textbook materials or other materials purchased or works developed specifically for online uses.
- Faculty can use only reasonable and limited portions of such materials, as they would typically use in a live classroom.
- The materials must be available *only* to registered students and not to guests or observers.
- Faculty must post a notice or message in the CMS that identifies the copyrighted materials and therefore precludes the student from copying or distributing these materials to others, as that would be a breach of copyright law.
- Faculty must pay attention to "portion" limitations (how much one can use).

The latest attempt at revisions to the TEACH Act is H.R. 3505, introduced on November 15, 2013, for the purpose of developing accessibility guidelines for electronic instructional materials and related information technologies in higher education institutions. The Congress.gov website (https://www.congress.gov/bill/113th-congress/house-bill/3505) provides a copy of the bill, a summary of the bill, as well as information on the progress of this bill, which is still in the Subcommittee on Higher Education and Workforce Training as of October 14, 2016.

Consult the school's policy and legal and library authorities when in doubt about materials necessary for the course. The American Library Association has an excellent website that further explains the roles of the institution (administrators or policymakers and IT staff), faculty, and librarians.

Higher Education Opportunity Act

The Higher Education Opportunity Act (HEOA) of 2008 is a reauthorization of the Higher Education Act of 1965. It requires postsecondary institutions to be more transparent about costs and requires that the institution post a net price calculator as well as security and copyright policies on its website (EDUCAUSE, 2009). While many of the provisions in this act do not directly affect faculty (since they relate to administrative offices that deal with fees, growth, public relations, credits, etc.), the following do affect faculty: the textbook information provision, the definition of distance education, and the requirement to establish that students are indeed who they say they are (Middle States Commission on Higher Education, 2009, 2010).

HEOA compliance entails the following:

- Faculty must select and submit textbook requirements to the campus bookstore *before* posting the next semester's schedule and registration. Each institution establishes the process for this. Under certain circumstances, the institution may post a "to be determined" notice if textbook selection was not practical before the school posts the next semester's schedule.

- Schools must pay attention to the change in terminology from distance learning to distance education.
- Education describes the process from the institution's perspective; it includes the use of one or more technologies to deliver instruction to students who are in a separate location and to support regular and substantive interaction between faculty and students.
- Learning describes the process from the students' perspective; it focuses on how the student interacts with the course content, classmates, and instructor in mastering the course content.
- Institutions must have a process in place to verify that the enrolled student is the person completing the course. Faculty may assist in determining how this process will work and with the development of a policy to cover this provision.

There are periodic updates to HEOA and the related regulations. These changes can be found at sites such as https://www.naicu.edu/special_initiatives/hea101/publications/page/updates-on-regulations-and-regulatory-process. Most educational institutions keep abreast of these updates and notify faculty during faculty in-service days.

Intellectual Property

The issue of intellectual property is coming to the forefront as a major concern in the digital age. Faculty are increasingly concerned about the ownership of distributive course materials and the use of those materials. Faculty members assume these course materials are their creative property, meaning that a requirement exists for others to obtain permission to use them. Since these materials exist in digital form on a school's accessible server, others may have access to these materials with or without faculty consent. In today's world, these materials may have commercial value, and institutions are increasingly taking ownership of these materials. A clear institutional policy will convey to all persons involved who owns what and what constitutes allowable use of the materials. Questions to consider in developing an intellectual property policy are (Diaz, 2005):

- What works are included under the policy (e.g., artworks, writings, software, course learning objects, PowerPoint slides, podcasts)?
- To whom does the policy apply (e.g., all employees, professors, researchers, postdoctoral fellows, administrators, students)?
- Under what circumstances does the school own the materials?
- Under what circumstances does the faculty member own the materials?
- Can there be joint ownership?
- Is this a work for hire or within the scope of the faculty member's employment?
- What institutional resources did the faculty member use to create the materials?
- What keywords should the policy clearly define?
- Is there a clear, definitive written agreement between the faculty member and the institution as to ownership and rights?
- Who is responsible for obtaining copyrights, trademarks?

Family Educational Rights and Privacy Act

The Family Educational Rights and Privacy Act (FERPA) is a federal law that requires colleges and universities to give students access to their educational records. Colleges and universities must maintain the confidentiality of personally identifiable educational records. See www.ed.gov/policy/gen/guid/fpco/ferpa/index.html for the U.S. Department of Education's summary of FERPA. While distance education courses were not a direct concern to those who wrote the FERPA rules, any time a faculty member or a university generates student information electronically, you must take precautions.

Consider the following guidelines for distance education and student records:

- Only enrolled students and the faculty teaching the course should have access to the course. However, the CMS administrator also has access to the course to manage and troubleshoot problems in using the CMS. The school must make the administrator aware of FERPA policies.
- If a college uses a hosting client (someone off campus that maintains the CMS), this arrangement makes the hosting client a third-party vendor. While the client should not have access to information that links a student to a grade, the client's systems administrator does have access to the servers and to everything on them.
- Students should be able to view only their own grades in the online grade book. They should not be able to see other students' grades. Issues may arise regarding discussion forums, depending on how the faculty use them. Faculty should not post evaluative comments or grades for students' comments in the discussion forum.
- Faculty should also state in the course requirements that students are required to post to the discussion forum, share their papers.
- If faculty use Excel to keep a record of student grades, they should remove the students' ID numbers from the spreadsheet, leave no storage devices where others may access them, password protect the spreadsheet (but faculty must remember the password), and use an encryption program that comes with external drives. This will protect the confidentiality of student data.
- If faculty lose a portable device such as a thumb drive that contains student grade sheets where the student names and grades are identifiable, they must notify the proper college or university authorities to determine what additional action must be taken.
- If faculty require students to send or post information to sites outside the college (e.g., blogs; social networking sites such as LinkedIn, Facebook, and YouTube), a clear policy must be developed and followed. This type of assignment can be ripe for FERPA violations.

Accessibility

Distance learning opportunities can open doors for millions of Americans with disabilities. When planning for the delivery of distance education courses, faculty must not create access barriers for the disabled. Laws such as the Americans with Disabilities Act (ADA) prohibit discrimination due to disability, and sections

504 and 508 of the Rehabilitation Act provide protections to learners with disabilities (U.S. Department of Justice, n.d.). What constitutes a reasonable accommodation for a particular learner will depend on the situation and the type of program. The accommodation, however, may not be unduly costly or disruptive for the school or be for the student's personal use only. In colleges and universities, the student has the primary responsibility to identify and document the disability and to request specific support, services, and other accommodations. Most schools have a person responsible for assessing students with disabilities and providing an accommodation letter to faculty. Each accommodation letter details modifications for each student with a disability. The modifications may include the following items:

- Providing extended time to turn in assigned work
- Providing extra time for timed exams
- Administering an exam in an alternative format, such as a paper exam when others will take the exam on a computer through the CMS
- Allowing spelling errors on papers or exams without deduction of points

Given the disability of the student and the nature of distance education, the student may need computer assistive devices. Students with disabilities may need adapted keyboards; magnification software; screen reader programs, such as Job Access With Speech (JAWS) (http://www.freedomscientific.com/products/fs/jaws-product-page.asp) or Dolphin's SUPERNOVA (http://www.yourdolphin.com/products.asp), that convert the text and images to speech; voice recognition; and alternative communication programs. Most operating systems support persons with disabilities by incorporating accessibility utilities into the system. Organizations can incorporate close captioning into training modules or provide transcripts for podcasts or videos to enhance retention and engagement (Gernsbacher, 2015; Stefaniak et al., 2021).

For faculty, this may mean providing alternative experiences for a student with a disability (e.g., use of a captioned video for the hearing-impaired student). Faculty that teaches distance education courses should review the tutorial titled Ten Simple Steps toward Universal Design of Online Courses (located at https://ualr.edu/pace/tenstepsud/) that addresses these issues. It lists 10 steps and provides examples and details for each one.

Quality

The traditional model of quality evaluation is site based, but distance and distributive education are not site based (Baer & Easton, 2002). Distance education is changing the thinking about quality assessment methods. Pond suggests that this new paradigm creates opportunities and challenges for quality assurance and accreditation (Pond, 2002). Pond further suggests that the traditional items of quality assurance, such as physical attendance, contact hours, proctored testing, and library holdings, are impractical or simply not rational in a distance education course. Pond makes the following three suggestions:

- Use a consumer-based means of judging quality like Amazon or eBay.
- Accredit the learner by having the learner demonstrate competencies rather than earn credits or certify the teacher's competencies.

- Move quality assurance toward an outcomes- or product-based model.

This new model will look at quality indicators such as continuity between "advertising" and reality, personal and professional growth of the learner, relevance, and multidirectional interactions. Eaton states that accreditation institutions or agencies need to do the following (Eaton, 2002):

- Identify the distinctive features of distance learning delivery.
- Modify accreditation guidelines, policies, or standards to meet the needs of this distinctive environment.
- Pay attention to student achievement and learning outcomes.

In the Eaton article, Appendix A features guidelines for quality assurance in distance education, and Appendix B includes 12 important questions about external quality review that are worth examining. Faculty must answer these questions: How will they evaluate quality in the distance education environment? How will the approach be the same as or different from that used for on-campus courses or programs? What are the current criteria that educational accrediting agencies will use to accredit or review the program? How do faculty address these criteria? What issues arise when states serve as the primary arbiters of policy and governance issues in U.S. education, but the student population resides in one state and does not physically go to the campus in another state where the student is taking distance education courses (Levine & Sun, 2002)?

Readiness

This section examines both the institution's readiness and the learner's readiness for teaching and learning in a distance education model. Institutions may enter the distance education market to maintain competitiveness; others may do so because their recruitment staff identified a market need. This movement may be seen as increasing revenues in these difficult financial times without the need for brick-and-mortar facilities. Regardless of the reason, the critical issues for readiness are as follows:

- Does the movement to distance education fit with the institution's missions and goals?
- Is the institution ready to invest in the technologies necessary to produce a quality program?
- Does the institution have the resources—people, money, and time—to develop and implement the program?
- Does the institution have faculty buy-in?
- Does it have administrative commitment?
- Does it have staff buy-in?
- Are faculty ready and prepared?
  - Some institutions, such as Pennsylvania State University (PSU) and SUNY, have developed a faculty readiness assessment; the SUNY document is available at https://hybrid.commons.gc.cuny.edu/teaching/getting-started/faculty-self-assessment-preparing-for-online-teaching/.

Without this readiness and commitment, distance education will not work or at best will result in a program of marginal quality. Just as the institution needs to be ready, it also needs to assess the students and potential student population for their readiness. The move to this method is moot for institutions because competition is forcing distance education solutions and most universities have already made this transition. In the corporate world (i.e., hospitals), it is also moot because of the need to provide mandatory training that considers employees working all shifts and all days. What is essential is the assessment of technologies necessary to deliver the training, resources necessary to make it happen, and trainer readiness to prepare the training materials.

Students who enter distance education courses need to consider their interest and ability to succeed in this learning environment. Inappropriate expectations about requirements for succeeding in these types of courses can lead to frustration and failure. Key questions include:

- What information does the institution provide to these learners to assess their readiness to learn in distance courses?
- Does the institution provide learners with a self-assessment tool such as Kizlik's readiness assessment (http://www.adprima.com/dears.htm) or Cypress College's readiness assessment (http://www.cypresscollege.edu/DistanceEdquiz/CCDERQ.aspx)?
- How will the institution make learners aware of the requirements for learning in this manner?
  - For example, do learners know that distance courses require discipline and organization in setting aside time to complete the learning, as well as reading and comprehension skills to understand the concepts and develop the skills necessary for this program or course?
- Can students follow directions, ask questions, and can work on their own under the guidance of a faculty member?
- How does the institution make eLearners aware of their responsibilities?
  - For example, students will have to meet course deadlines, check in to the course regularly, interact with faculty and classmates, ask questions as necessary, and conduct themselves in a professional manner in all interactions.

The institution should list or outline learner requirements in a policy and procedures document and make this document available to students to ensure that they understand their responsibilities.

The Future of Course Management Systems

What is the future of CMS software? Saini (2020) presents eLearning trends for 2020 and 2021. These include mobile and wearable access to eLearning materials; more peer-to-peer learning; microlearning; personalized learning using pull technologies putting the learner in control; and augmented and gaming learning environments providing practical experiences. What will this mean to faculty and students? What will this mean for the selection of CDSs? Institutions need to consider how adding mobile ability in the criteria for selection of CMS software. Does this mean that colleges, universities, and organizations that make this decision will require students to have a tablet or wearable device like glasses, watches, or bracelets? Think about how this might affect education of patients with articles like "Wearable Enhanced Learning for Healthy Ageing: Conceptual Framework and Architecture of the 'Fitness MOOC'" (Buchem et al., 2015). What will this mean for the design of learning materials and learning experiences? What will this mean for educating our learners in how to collaborate with patient educational experiences?

Another area of growing technological development is collaborative tools that are smarter (i.e., remember who users are, what they like, and what they are doing and provide relevant information to each user. Users should also see more lifelike virtual 3D worlds integrated into the CMS software. Imagine a time when bathroom mirrors remind students that work is due, when students can interact with their world on their TV screens, and when students can chat with classmates and the professor through their kitchen counter. What will this mean for the design and teaching of distance education and the new wave of distributive courses?

Web 3.0, first appearing in 2006, is adding another level of integration to higher education. This iteration of online information access includes a semantic (allowing sharing and understanding the meaning of words), artificial intelligence (computer understanding of human language), dimensionality (computer three-dimensional ability), and use of metadata (Morris, 2011). Web 3.0 changes the online educational ecosystem from a one-dimension *information posting* to a higher level of ontology allowing increased educational methodologies like multimedia content, data acquisition and use, and simulations. This type of learning expands a student's ability to experience a personalized education including the ability to look, touch, and visualize an educational topic (Miranda et al., 2014). Web 4.0 is already identifying methods to increase theoretical abilities of education creating a *spatial* web (https://digitalcommunications.wp.st-andrews.ac.uk/2021/03/11/how-web-3-0-will-impact-higher-education/).

CONCLUSION AND FUTURE DIRECTIONS

The changes in our educational environment are reflective of shifts in our demographics, economic conditions, and technological developments. Web 2.0 tools opened educational opportunities for lifelong learning to a diverse global community. Web 3.0, with its spatial and semantic technologies, will now add emerging terms, course management and LMSs, and issues related to the development and implementation of distance education and distributive learning are all elements resulting from these budding educational opportunities.

The next generation of CMSs and LMSs will be integrated portals that are smarter, track more information, and analyze learner data across functions such as e-mail, wikis, chats, forums, and so forth. They will include personal learning environments (PLEs), immersive, 3D learning worlds with better communication channels and collaboration for any time and any place learning with tablets and mobile devices (Brown et al., 2015). This will result in just-in-time, customized learning environments where the focus is on outcomes rather than traditional credit hours. This emerging environment is about the learners, the learners' needs, and the integration and use of appropriate technologies.

ACKNOWLEDGMENT

The authors wish to acknowledge the contribution of Irene Joos to the previous edition of this chapter.

DISCUSSION QUESTIONS

1. Research how constant connectivity affects you socially, cognitively, and physically. Ask yourself how technology is changing the way you think and focus, and how this affects your learning style. Provide two examples and resources that support how technology is changing how we socialize.
2. From a student or faculty perspective, develop criteria to use in comparing and evaluating two course management systems (CMS) or learning management systems (LMS) delivery systems. Select two systems and compare them using the developed criteria. Discuss what you learned in developing these criteria and in comparing two products against them. Include answers to the following questions: How useful were these criteria, what was missing, and how would you revise the criteria next time?
3. Think of a situation where distance education might be appropriate. Identify three technology tools that might be useful for the specific audience and how they would be used. What skills would the learner need to use them? What skills would the instructor/trainer need?
4. Research the future of higher education, distance learning, and the movement toward personal learning environments (PLEs). What will a day in the life of a nursing student be like in 2030? What impact will technologies have on license renewal?

CASE STUDY

You are a faculty member serving on the online learning committee. The university requires an assessment of which learning strategies are working and which are not and an examination of the current standards, emerging trends, and how the school should plan for an increase in distance education. The committee is charged with setting the course for this initiative for the next 2 years. Subcommittees may exist, each with a specific charge. You are serving on the subcommittee charged with developing the stakeholder matrix, a document identifying all "stakeholders"—those who have an interest in this initiative, how they fit in the organizational structure, what influence they exert, and so forth. These are the people from whom you will collect data and who you will involve in the process and occasionally in the decision making.

Create a five-column table with the following headings for the columns: Stakeholder Name and Organization; Organizational Role; Influence and Power; Unique Information About This Person/Organization; and Strategies for Communicating and Working With This Person. Each stakeholder will be entered as a new row in the matrix.

Once you design the stakeholder matrix, analyze its importance and how it will be used. Using what you learned in this chapter, create a strategy for each column. For example, determine how you would systematically identify each stakeholder. Develop up to three questions to guide your collection of the data for each column and complete this matrix.

Discussion Questions

1. Discuss the pertinent laws that should be considered for this initiative.
2. Describe next steps in the process that would help assure the success of the initiative.
3. Using what you learned in this chapter and by searching the web for distance learning materials, list two future directions.

REFERENCES

Agassiz, L., & Eliot, S. (2011). *Society to encourage studies at home: Founded in 1873 by Anna Eliot Ticknor: Born June 1st, 1823, died October 5th, 1896.* Nabu Press.

American Library Association (2015). *DMCA: The Digital Millennium Copyright Act.* http://www.ala.org/advocacy/copyright/dmca.

Association of College & Research Libraries (2008). *Standards for distance learning library services.* https://www.ala.org/acrl/standards/guidelinesdistancelearning.

Baer, M.A., & Easton, J.S. (2002). Forward. In *Maintaining the delicate balance: Distance learning, higher education accreditation, and the politics of self-regulation (Distributed education: challenges, choices, and a new environment).* Foreword, American Council on Education.

Behera, P. C., Mohapatra, S., & Dash, C. (2017). Comparative study on LCMS, LMS and CMS. *International Journal of Information Science and Computing, 4*(2), 79. https://doi.org/10.5958/2454-9533.2017.00008.4.

Benvin, B. (2016). Mlearning: The revolution changing elearning. *Training & Development, 43*(3), 18–19.

Benzie, H. J., & Harper, R. (2019). Developing student writing in higher education: Digital third-party products in distributed learning environments. *Teaching in Higher Education, 25*(5), 633–647. https://doi.org/10.1080/13562517.2019.1590327.

Bergmann, H. F. (2001). "The Silent University": The society to encourage studies at home, 1873–1897. *The New England Quarterly, 74*(3), 447. https://doi.org/10.2307/3185427.

Bianchi, W. (2008). Education by radio: America's schools of the air. *TechTrends, 52*(2), 36–44. https://doi.org/10.1007/s11528-008-0134-0.

Billings, D. M. (2007). Distance education in nursing: 25 years and going strong. *Computers, Informatics, Nursing: CIN, 25*(3), 121–123. https://doi.org/10.1097/01.NCN.0000270044.67905.4a.

Blackboard. (2021). *About us.* https://www.blackboard.com/about-us

Bradley, P. (2021, January 23). *The state of university and college content management systems in 2021.* NYC Design. https://medium.com/nyc-design/us-university-and-college-content-management-systems-2021-6196c29d337a.

Brown, M., Dehoney, J., Millichap, N. (2015, July/August) What's next for the LMS. *Educause Review.* https://er.educause.edu/articles/2015/6/whats-next-for-the-lms.

Buchem, I., Merceron, A., & Kreutel, J. (2015). Wearable enhanced learning for health ageing: conceptual framework and architecture of the "fitness MOOC". *Interact Des Architect Journal, 24,* 111–124.

Conrad, R. M., & Donaldson, J. A. (2011). *Engaging the online learner activities and resources for creative instruction.* San Francisco: Jossey-Bass.

Diaz, V. (2005). Distributed learning meets intellectual property policy: Who owns what? *Campus Technology.*

Eaton, J. (2002). Maintaining the delicate balance: Distance learning, higher education accreditation, and the politics of self- regulation. *American Council on Education, Center for Policy Analysis.* http://www.chea.org/pdf/Maintaining-the-Delicate-Balance-Distance-Learning-Higher-Education-Accreditation- and-the-Politics-of-Self-Regulation-2002.pdf.

EDUCAUSE. (2009) *Implementing the Higher Education Opportunity Act: A checklist for business officers.* http://www.educause.edu/Resources/ImplementingtheHigherEducation/192839.

El Refae, G. A., Kaba, A., & Eletter, S. (2021). Distance learning during COVID-19 pandemic: Satisfaction, opportunities and challenges as perceived by faculty members and students. *Interactive Technology and Smart Education* https://doi.org/10.1108/ITSE-08-2020-0128.

Ellucian. (n.d.). *About us.* https://www.ellucian.com/about-us.

Fabos, B. (2004). Giddy prophecies and commercial ventures: The history of educational media. In *Wrong turn on the information superhighway: Education and the commercialization of the internet. essay.* Teachers College Press.

Farnsworth, T. J., Frantz, A. C., & McCune, R. W. (2012). Community-based distributive medical education: Advantaging Society. *Medical Education Online, 17*(1). https://doi.org/10.3402/meo.v17i0.8432.

G2.com. (2021) *Best Learning Management Systems.* https://www.g2.com/categories/learning-management-system-lms

Garrison, D. R., Anderson, T., & Archer, W. (1999). Critical inquiry in a text-based environment: Computer conferencing in higher education. *The Internet and Higher Education, 2*(2–3), 87–105. https://doi.org/10.1016/S1096-7516(00)00016-6.

Gassaway, L. (2001) Balancing copyright concerns: The TEACH Act of 2001. EDUCAUSE. http://er.educause.edu/~/media/files/article-downloads/erm01610.pdf.

Gernsbacher, M. A. (2015). Video captions benefit everyone. *Policy Insights From the Behavioral and Brain Sciences, 2*(1), 195–202. https://doi.org/10.1177/2372732215602130.

Google. (n.d.). *Classroom: Google for education.* https://edu.google.com/products/classroom/.

Gutierrez, K. (2021, April 14). Understanding the difference between eLearning and mLearning [web log]. https://www.shiftelearning.com/blog/difference-between-elearning-and-mlearning.

Instructure. (n.d.), *Canvas LMS.* https://www.instructure.com/canvas

Jenzabar. (2021). *Higher education institutions rely on Jenzabar solutions to navigate covid-era challenges and build the digital campus of tomorrow.* https://jenzabar.com/pressrelease/higher-education-institutions-rely-on-jenzabar-solutions-to-navigate-covid-era-challenges-and-build-the-digital-campus-of-tomorrow.

Kentnor, H. (2015). Distance education and the evolution of online learning in the United States. *Curriculum and Teaching Dialogue, 17,* 21–34. https://doi.org/10.52966/ctd.2021.

Koch, L. F. (2014). The nursing educator's role in e-learning: A literature review. *Nurse Education Today, 34*(11). https://doi.org/10.1016/j.nedt.2014.04.002.

Krouska, A., Troussas, C., & Virvou, M. (2018). *Comparing LMS and CMS platforms* supporting social e-learning in higher education. [Conference session]. 2017 8th International Conference on Information, Intelligence, Systems and Applications, Institute of Electric and Electronic Engineers, Zakynthos, Greece. https://doi.org/10.1109/IISA.2017.8316408

Leite, W. L., Svinicki, M., & Shi, Y. (2010). Attempted Validation of the Scores of the VARK: Learning styles inventory with multitrait–multimethod confirmatory factor analysis models. *Educational and Psychological Measurement, 70*(2), 323–339. https://doi.org/10.1177/0013164409344507.

Levine, A., & Sun, J. (2002). Barriers to distance education. *American Council on Education, Center for Policy Analysis* http://www.acenet.edu/news-room/Documents/Barriers-to-Distance-Education-2003.pdf.

Lowery, B., & Spector, N. (2014). Regulatory implications and recommendations for distance education In prelicensure nursing programs. *Journal of Nursing Regulation, 5*(3), 24–33. https://doi.org/10.1016/s2155-8256(15)30046-6.

Martin, F., & Bolliger, D. U. (2018). Engagement matters: Student perceptions on the importance of engagement strategies in the online learning environment. *Online Learning, 22*(1), 205–222. https://doi.org/10.24059/olj.v22i1.1092.

Middle States Commission on Higher Education. (2009, Fall). *New HEOA regulations impact distance education programs, substantive change & monitoring growth, transfer of credit.* http://www.msche.org/news_newsletter.asp.

Middle States Commission on Higher Education. (2010, January). *Distance education and the HEOA.* http://www.msche.org/news_newsletter.asp.

Miranda, P., Isaias, P., & Costa, C.J., (2014). The impact of web 3.0 technologies in e-learning: emergence of e-learning 3.0. In Proceedings of the 6th International Conference of Educatino and New Learning Technologies, Barcelona, Spain, EDULEARN14 Proceedings, pp. 4139–4149.

Moodle. (2021, August 9). *Moodle US.* https://moodle.com/partners/moodle-us/.

Moore, M. G., Pittman, V. V., Anderson, T., & Kramarae, C. (2003). *From Chautauqua to the virtual university: A century of distance education in the United States.* Center on Education and Training for Employment, College of Education, the Ohio State University.

Morris, R. D. (2011). Web 3.0: Implications for online learning. *TechTrends, 55*(1), 42-46. Retrieved from https://go.libproxy.wakehealth.edu/login?url=https://www.proquest.com/scholarly-journals/web-3-0-implications-online-learning/docview/851367699/se-2?accountid=14868 National Council of State Boards of Nursing. (2021, August 9). Distance Education. Retrieved from https://www.ncsbn.org/6662.htm.

Nelson, R. (2007). *Student support services for distance education students in nursing programs.* In K. T. Heinrich, & M. H. Oermann (Eds). Challenges and new directions in nursing education annual review of nursing education (v. 5). Springer.

Nelson, R., & Staggers, N. (2014). *Health Informatics: An interprofessional approach.* Elsevier, Mosby.

Ninoriya, S., Chawan, P., Meshram, B., Department of Computer Entineering, & Vjti, M. (2011). CMS, LMS and LCMS For eLearning. *International Journal of Computer Science Issues, 8*(2), 644–647.

Oblinger, D. G., Barone, C. A., & Hawkins, B. L. (2001). *First in a series distributed education and its challenges: An overview.* 202, 785–2990. www.acenet.edu/bookstore

Oblinger, D., & Oblinger, J. L. (2005). Is it age or IT: First steps toward understanding the net generation. In *Educating the net generation* (2nd ed., Vol. 29, pp. 8–16). EDUCAUSE.

Ohio School of the Air. (n.d.). Ohio School of the Air—Ohio History Central. http://ohiohistorycentral.org/w/Ohio_School_of_the_Air.

Pappas, C. (2019, November 29). *Top learning management system (LMS) statistics for 2020 you need to know.* https://elearningindustry.com/top-lms-statistics-and-facts-for-2015?__cf_chl_jschl_tk__=pmd_34f1806692cfef085ad42ac2903159d967195cf4-1628729311-0-gqNtZGzNAfijcnBszQfO

Pond, W. (2002). *Distributed education in the 21st century: Implications for quality assurance.* Online Journal of Distance Learning Administration. https://www.westga.edu/~distance/ojdla/summer52/pond52.html.

Quality Matters. (n.d.) *Why QM? About.* https://www.qualitymatters.org/why-quality-matters/about-qm

Rothwell, W. (2020). *Adult learning basics* (2nd ed.). ATD Press.

Saini, J. (2020, September 3). 5 eLearning trends for 2020 (and 5 predictions for 2021). eLearning Industry. https://elearningindustry.com/5-elearning-trends-dominating-2020-predictions

Southern Association of Colleges and Schools Commission on Colleges Board of Trustees. (2020). *Distance education and correspondence courses* [Policy Statement]. Southern Association of Colleges and Schools Commission on Colleges. https://sacscoc.org/app/uploads/2019/07/DistanceCorrespondenceEducation.pdf

Spector, N., & Lowery B. (2015) *NCSBN's distance education guidelines for prelicensure nursing programs.* [Conference session]. NCSBN's virtual conference on distance education in pre licensure programs; https://www.ncsbn.org/7451.htm.

Stefaniak, J.E., Conklin, S., Oyarzun, B., & Reese, R.M. (2021). *A practitioner's guide to instructional design in higher education.* EdTech Books. https://edtechbooks.org/id_highered

Turkewitz, N., & Kenneally, C. (2020, December 14). *Copyright and distance learning: Lessons from the teach act.* Copyright Clearance Center. https://www.copyright.com/blog/copyright-and-distance-learning-lessons-from-the-teach-act/.

Tyurina, Y., Troyanskaya, M., Babaskina, L., Choriyev, R., & Pronkin, N. (2021). E-learning for SMEs. *International Journal of Emerging Technologies in Learning, 16*(2). https://doi.org/10.3991/ijet.v16i02.18815.

U.S. Department of Justice. (n.d.). *Americans with Disabilities Act (ADA).* A guide to disability rights laws. https://www.ada.gov/cguide.htm#anchor62335.

United States Copyright Office. (1998). *The Digital Millennium Copyright Act of 1998.* United States.

VARK. (2021). *The VARK modalities.* https://vark-learn.com/introduction-to-vark/the-vark-modalities/.

Wright, C.R., Montgomerie, T.C., Reju, S.A., & Schmoller, S. (2014). Selecting a learning management system: Advice from an academic perspective. *Educause Review.* https://er.educause.edu/articles/2014/4/selecting-a-learning-management-system-advice-from-an-academic-perspective.

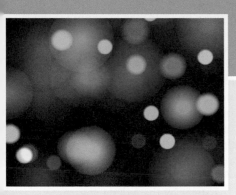

27

Legal Issues, Federal Regulations, and Accreditation

Jonathan M. Ishee and Michael J. Paluzzi

OBJECTIVES

At the completion of this chapter, the reader will be prepared to:
1. Describe the U.S. governmental processes and structure that regulate health information technology (health IT).
2. Explain the difference between laws, regulations, and sub-regulatory guidance.
3. Interpret laws to prevent fraud and abuse prior to using electronic health records.
4. Summarize accreditation measures and agencies in the United States.
5. Discuss how new technology and digital health are driving changes in health IT.

KEY TERMS

accreditation, 431
Anti-Kickback statute, 435
cybersecurity donation safe harbor, 436
EHR donation safe harbor, 436

False Claims Act, 436
liability, 434
mHealth, 440
privacy, 432

Stark law, 435
wearable devices, 440

ABSTRACT ❖

This chapter provides (1) a brief synopsis of the legal system of the U.S. government as a basis for understanding how healthcare and specifically informatics is regulated; (2) an overview of selected laws and regulations impacting health informatics; (3) an overview of the accreditation process for healthcare entities, focusing specifically on health information systems management; and (4) insight on emerging uses of technology in the healthcare arena, with the potential for new or increased regulations.

INTRODUCTION

The U.S. healthcare system functions within the context of the legal system of the U.S. government. Healthcare, and in turn health informatics, is heavily regulated by federal and state governments. Therefore, understanding health informatics-related legal issues, federal regulations, and accreditation begins with an understanding of the basic structure of the legal system in the United States.

The federal government consists of the three branches of government: legislative, executive, and judicial. Each branch plays a role in health information technology (health IT) laws and regulations. Bills (proposed laws) are passed by the U.S. legislature and become law. Administrative agencies within the executive branch implement these laws by establishing regulations or rules. Disagreements about how those laws and regulations should be interpreted are settled by the courts, the judicial branch. These judicial interpretations become precedent and are

binding on future actions. Through these processes each of the three branches of the U.S. government has significant impact on the day-to-day operations within the American healthcare system and health IT. In addition to laws and regulations, healthcare systems must also meet accreditation requirements to be eligible for participation in healthcare programs administered by the government. While there are a variety of accrediting agencies in healthcare, the two primary agencies that accredit hospitals and other healthcare-related institutions are The Joint Commission (TJC) and Det Norske Veritas (DNV) Healthcare.

LEGAL SYSTEM

Federalism and the Constitution

The government of the United States functions as a federal system. There is a distribution of power between the federal government and the state and municipal governments. The U.S. Constitution, the supreme law of the land, defines the basic composition of the three branches of government and sets forth the powers of each branch. It also provides the state governments with governing authority. State governments have their own rule-making authority and do not need to have federal approval before passing a state law. However, any laws or regulations that states pass must comply with the Constitution and be within the scope of power granted to them by the Constitution. The states and municipal governments are subject to both the federal government and the Constitution, despite having some autonomy.

Categories of Power

Within the Constitution, there are two types of grants of powers, express or implied. *Express*, or enumerated powers, are powers explicitly granted to Congress. Examples of express powers include the powers to regulate interstate commerce, to create requirements for states or individuals who receive federal funding, or to levy taxes. *Implied powers* do not define the exact scope of the authority granted. An example of an implied power is the necessary and proper clause, which gives Congress the power to enact any laws "necessary and proper" to execute its responsibilities under the Constitution. Congress has used both express and implied powers to implement laws that ultimately impact informatics and health IT, including Health Information Portability and Accountability Act (HIPAA), Meaningful Use requirements for EHRs, and the Patient Protection and Affordable Care Act (PPACA).

Powers expressly delegated to the federal government may not be exercised by the state governments (McCulloch v. Maryland, 2016). Any law a state passes that encroaches upon the federal government's scope of authority would be preempted by the federal law, and the state law would be invalid. For example, a state could not pass a law to establish its own system to patent new health IT. The federal government alone has the power to issue patents and trademarks, so the state law would be overturned.

There are also powers that are given both to the federal government and to the state governments. These are called *concurrent powers*. For instance, both the federal government and the state government could regulate the privacy of personal health information in EHRs. When both the federal and the state governments have the authority to regulate a particular industry, the question is which is the controlling law if state and federal laws conflict becomes more complex. Typically, a federal law will control and preempt a conflicting state law absent special circumstances. An example of when federal law would not preempt state law occurs when a state enacts a health privacy law that provides more privacy protections than HIPAA, such as California's Confidentiality of Medical Information Act (California Civil Code §§ 56 et seq).

The state and federal governments also occasionally collaborate so that laws passed in various states do not create a hostile environment for health IT nationwide where different states have conflicting regulations that make the use of health IT across states impractical. Two current examples of collaboration are the Health Information Exchange (HIE) Consensus Project and the Health Information Security and Privacy Collaboration (Office of the National Coordinator for Health Information Technology, 2015). Both of these projects seek to minimize the differences in laws and regulations between the states that govern HIE and health IT privacy and security. Regulations with different requirements in every state for the same subject matter can be burdensome to comply with for an entity that operates nationwide. It should be noted that while collaborations may produce model laws (a proposed series of laws pertaining to a specific subject), it is still up to individual state legislatures to pass legislation implementing the model law.

State governments have significant regulatory power related to healthcare and health informatics. Sometimes this power has been expressly granted to the states by the federal government through legislation, as is the case with Medicaid (42 U.S.C. §§ 1396 et seq, 2016). In other cases, the state derives its power to regulate the healthcare industry through the Tenth Amendment (that of reserved powers) and the state police power to establish laws to protect the health and safety of the public. For example, state governments may pass stricter regulations for health IT security and privacy than what the federal government mandates through HIPAA.

FEDERAL HEALTHCARE REGULATORY FRAMEWORK

The healthcare regulatory system, on a federal level, is shaped like a pyramid (Fig. 27.1). At the base, on the broadest level, are laws passed by Congress. On the next level are regulations, or rules, which are promulgated by administrative agencies (Administrative Procedure Act, 1946). Finally, at the top of the pyramid are advisory opinions and subregulatory guidance documents issued by administrative agencies.

Laws

Laws passed through Congress are often written in broad terms and establish only general objectives that must be met. For an overview of the process of passing a law through Congress, see Table 27.1. Congress does not typically provide the specific means to implement the law. As part of the legislative process, Congress may choose to delegate authority to implement those laws to the executive branch. This delegation may carry with it

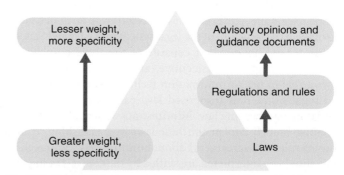

Fig. 27.1 The healthcare regulatory system at the federal level.

TABLE 27.1 The Legislative Process

Bill is introduced in the Senate.	Bill is introduced in the House.
Bill is sent to committee or subcommittee for hearing, debate, and amendment. Health information technology (Health IT) bills would typically be sent to the Senate Committee on Health, Education, Labor, and Pensions.	Bill is sent to committee or subcommittee for hearing, debate, and amendment. Health IT bills would typically be sent to the House Committee on Commerce and Energy, which has a Health Subcommittee.
Bill is sent to the floor of the Senate for a vote.	Bill is sent to the floor of the House for a vote.

Bill goes to a conference committee to reconcile the Senate and House versions of the bill to form one compromise bill.

Compromise bill goes back to both the House and Senate floors for a vote.

Compromise bill is sent to the president for a signature.

If the president vetoes the bill, it may still become a law if two-thirds of Congress vote in favor of the bill.

TABLE 27.2 Administrative Agencies

Agency	Purpose
Food and Drug Administration (FDA)	• Regulates and approves new drugs and medical devices. Issues regulations about drug interactions, safe storage, and handling of drugs, and counterfeiting of drugs or devices. • Responsible for producing a new report proposing a new risk-based regulatory framework for health IT.
Centers for Medicaid and Medicare Services	• Issues regulations for Medicaid and Medicare, including information about appropriate billing and coding. • Issues the Conditions of Participation, which govern the accreditation standards. • Responsible for enforcement of Stark and Anti-Kickback laws.
Office of the National Coordinator for Health Information	• Responsible for establishing programs and regulations to improve safety, quality of care, and efficiency through health IT. • Establishes standards and certification criteria for EHRs.
Office of Civil Rights	Enforces HIPAA and HITECH compliance.
Department of Justice	Enforces False Claims Act and Anti-Kickback statutes.
Federal Trade Commission	• Regulates development of new health IT devices. • Responsible for enforcement of competition in the healthcare market.
National Labor Relations Board	Issues regulations that can govern the interaction of healthcare and social media.

EHRs, Electronic health records; *FDA*, Food and Drug Administration; *health IT*, health information technology; *HIPAA*, Health Information Portability and Accountability Act; *HITECH*, Health Information Technology for Economic and Clinical Health.

the power to pass separate, legally binding regulations, or rules, to facilitate compliance with the laws.

For example, Congress may pass a law that states that healthcare entities need to establish a quality control system. The law that Congress passes may not provide the specifications that such a system must meet or determine a specific timeline to implement such a system, but the law does mandate participation in the quality control program. Congress, to fully execute the law, turns to administrative agencies. For the executive branch of the government to assist with what would ordinarily be a legislative duty, Congress must first grant the administrative agency a specific authority to create regulations. Once an agency has been granted authority to pass regulations under a particular law, it can begin the rule-making process (5 U.S.C. §§ 551 et seq, 2016).

Regulations and Rule Making

The burden of creating regulations to carry out legislation often falls on the executive branch and the administrative agencies because they are more experienced than Congress in working within a particular industry or regulatory system. There are several agencies that play significant roles in regulating health IT. Table 27.2 provides examples.

The rule-making process starts with the drafting of a proposed rule. The agency is required to submit that proposed rule for publication and a comment period. This comment period is open to anyone who might have an interest in the proposed rule. A key responsibility of health informaticians either working through their professional organizations and/or as individuals is to take advantage of this opportunity to participate in the rule-making process. Comments are made through a government website. The agency reads the comments and either publishes a final rule or issues another proposed rule if significant changes will be made to the initial rule. A final rule is typically published with responses to comments submitted during the proposed rule's comment period. Through its response to the comments, the agency provides insight into how it will be enforcing the rule or what result is expected from a particular regulation. This

commentary is not binding authority, but it does provide valuable information for entities looking to fulfill their obligations under newly promulgated rules. Once a final rule is passed and published, it becomes a regulation, which is legally binding.

Guidance and Advisory Opinions

In addition to rule making, agencies also provide *advisory opinions* and *guidance documents* on regulations they enforce. Advisory opinions are responses to a written request by a regulated party for an interpretation of whether its action complies with a particular regulation. These advisory opinions are only legally binding on the particular entity that has asked for the opinion and involve a very narrow issue. Agencies publish advisory opinions to provide assistance and information on the application of a regulation to particular facts. These advisory opinions are another way to understand the agency's rationale behind enforcement.

Guidance documents are official agency publications designed to help subjects understand and comply with specific regulations. Guidance documents are often significant and can appear similar to rule making in their scope. Typically, guidance is issued to clarify potentially ambiguous sections of a rule or to explain how an agency intends to enforce a rule. Guidance documents are much narrower in scope than rules, and there may be several guidance documents that relate to different subsections, or even words, of a single rule.

Guidance documents may be issued by the administrative agency without a specific authorization from Congress because they are not legally binding. This means that guidance documents may be issued at any time by the administrative agency without having to comply with the formal requirements of the rule-making process. Despite their informal nature, guidance documents can have as much impact on an industry as a rule because, in practice, agencies tend to treat the two similarly.

Enforcement

The last step of the healthcare regulatory process is enforcement. There are two mechanisms for regulatory enforcement. The first is through the administrative agencies that promulgate the regulations. The second mechanism is through the court system.

Administrative Enforcement

Administrative enforcement can be initiated in several ways. Oftentimes enforcement mechanisms will be built into the law or regulation. The Health Information Technology for Economic and Clinical Health (HITECH) Act, passed in 2009, called for the Office for Civil Rights to implement an audit program to evaluate compliance with HIPAA standards. Compliance issues that are identified during the audit program may then trigger an initiation of a formal investigation. Similarly, the Physician Self-Referral (Stark) law now contains a mechanism for healthcare entities to self-disclose violations of the law once the entity discovers a potential compliance issue. Another way an enforcement action may be initiated is through a complaint from an individual.

Once an enforcement action has been initiated, an administrative agency investigates the allegations of noncompliance. The administrative agency investigating the complaint may be the same agency that issued the regulation, or it may be a separate agency that is tasked with enforcement, like the Department of Justice, the Office of the Inspector General, or the Office for Civil Rights. The agencies have the authority to enact a wide range of penalties, from monetary penalties to exclusion from participating in federal programs to a demand for corrective action. Examples of penalties for HIPAA-related violations can be seen in Chapter 28.[1]

Typically, an agency will negotiate and try to reach a settlement with a potentially noncompliant entity before initiating a formal proceeding. If the entity reaches a settlement agreement with the agency, there will be no finding of liability against the entity. However, settlement agreements may still result in monetary penalties or expulsion from federal programs.

If a settlement agreement cannot be reached, then a formal proceeding will be initiated. Once a formal proceeding is initiated, the entity has a right to have a hearing in front of an administrative law judge if monetary penalties are involved. An administrative law judge is a decision maker who is independent

from the agency and has authority under the agency's procedural rules to issue a binding decision. An administrative proceeding in front of an administrative law judge is typically less formal and less strict procedurally than a comparable proceeding in front of a federally appointed judge. The exact nature of the proceedings will be governed by the agency's rules. Once a final decision is issued, a formal appeal of the decision is permitted. Before the appeal may go before a federal court, it must be appealed through the agency, usually in front of a review board.

Court System

An enforcement proceeding may also be initiated in the federal court system, either at the beginning of the process or as an appeal of an administrative decision. If the allegations involve a criminal indictment, then the proceedings must be started in the federal court system. The federal court system is composed of three levels of courts. A case is initially brought in a district court. If a case is appealed, it is appealed to the circuit court that oversees the district court. It is possible to petition for an appeal from the circuit court to the Supreme Court through a writ of certiorari, but the Supreme Court hears very few appeals during a year because it has the sole discretion whether to grant any appeal.

A court proceeding is more formal than an administrative proceeding. In addition, a court proceeding, and an administrative proceeding may follow different procedural rules. Another significant difference between a court and an administrative hearing is the length of time it takes to reach a decision. Bringing an action in a federal court takes much longer to resolve than would be the case in an administrative proceeding.

A court and an administrative proceeding are functionally equivalent. The federal court judge and the administrative law judge have the same remedies available if the entity is found guilty of noncompliance. The administrative law judge and the federal court judge issue binding decisions, although there is an additional route to appeal if the decision is issued in an administrative proceeding as opposed to a federal court proceeding.

FRAUD AND ABUSE AND BILLING ISSUES RELATED TO ELECTRONIC HEALTH RECORD USE

Although the federal government has incentivized the use of EHRs, there are pitfalls for the unwary user. EHRs can make clinical documentation easier for users, but use of an EHR can lead to fraud and abuse claims by the federal government that may include hefty fines and jail time if violations are proven. Chief among the potential pitfalls is EHR purchase transactions. EHR systems are expensive. Hospitals and healthcare systems are usually able to cover these expenses within their budget, but it is often financially difficult for independent practitioners including medical group practices to purchase these systems. The systems purchased by these practitioners need to be interoperable with other healthcare entities such as hospitals, long-term care facilities, laboratories, and other healthcare institutions. It may seem logical for these practitioners

[1] NTD: Is this internal reference still correct

to approach hospitals, laboratories, and other large corporations to ask them to help fund these purchases. However, legal, and regulatory hurdles must be understood, and purchasers need to be wary before moving forward with these types of transactions.

In the area of fraud and abuse, there are three laws that should be considered before providers purchase EHR systems—the Stark law, the federal Anti-Kickback statute, and the federal False Claims Act (FCA). It is important to have a general understanding of what these laws prohibit, and to examine transactions related to and within the EHR while keeping these laws in mind.

Stark Law

The Stark law, passed in 1992, is named after its sponsor, U.S. Congressman Peter Stark. It is a combination of statutes and regulations that were promulgated in three phases (National Mining Association v. Jackson, 2016). The Stark law governs physician self-referral for Medicare and Medicaid patients (Section 1877 of the Social Security Act, 2016). This law prohibits a physician from referring patients for certain designated health services (DHS) to entities with whom the physician has a financial relationship. DHS includes the following services (other than those provided as emergency physician services furnished outside of the United States):

Clinical laboratory services
  Physical therapy services
  Occupational therapy services
  Outpatient speech-language pathology services
  Radiology and certain other imaging services
  Radiation therapy services and supplies
  Durable medical equipment and supplies
  Parenteral and enteral nutrients, equipment, and supplies
  Prosthetics, orthotics, and prosthetic devices and supplies
  Home health services
  Outpatient prescription drugs
  Inpatient and outpatient hospital services (42 U.S.C. § 1395nn).

The Stark law's central tenet is that there is a conflict of interest created when referring physicians or their families can benefit from the referral. It is believed that allowing self-referrals encourages over-utilization of services, increasing healthcare costs. Therefore, healthcare providers must be careful when they enter business relationships with family members, or with companies where the physician has a financial interest.

There are two types of financial relationships that trigger the Stark law. The first is when there is physician or family "ownership or investment interest" in the entity furnishing the DHS (42 U.S.C. § 1395nna2A). The second type of arrangement is a compensation arrangement with the physician or the physician's immediate family (42 U.S.C. § 1395nna2B). This relationship can be either direct or indirect. The only way to avoid the requirements of Stark law is to fall under an exception or a "safe harbor." The penalties for not complying with the Stark law are discussed in more detail later, but may include civil monetary penalties, denial of payment, or exclusion from the federal healthcare program.

Federal Anti-Kickback Statute

The federal Anti-Kickback statute is a criminal statute that prohibits the exchange or offer to exchange anything of value to induce referral of a federal healthcare program beneficiary (42 U.S.C. § 1320a-7b). Because this is a criminal statute, the government must prove its case beyond a reasonable doubt. A typical situation where a violation of the Anti-Kickback statute might occur is when physicians lease/sublease space within their office to another provider who is able to refer business to the landlord/sublessor physician. Another situation often arising in the Anti-Kickback context is when physicians receive remuneration from a drug company when they are able to prescribe a drug manufactured by that company. In the EHR context, the Anti-Kickback statute could be triggered when a hospital or other healthcare provider offers to purchase or to help fund an EHR for a provider who refers patients to the hospital or other healthcare provider for testing, surgery, lab work, or another clinical services.

The statute requires a knowing and willful offer of payment, solicitation, or receipt of any remuneration to induce someone to refer patients or to purchase, order, or recommend any item of service that may be paid for under a federal healthcare program (42 U.S.C. § 1320a-7ba). The PPACA added a provision clarifying the intent requirement of the Anti-Kickback statute. Under the PPACA, actual knowledge of an Anti-Kickback statute violation or the specific intent to commit a violation of the Anti-Kickback statute is *not* necessary for conviction under the statute (Section 6402f2 of the Patient Protection and Affordable Care Act, 2010).

Remuneration and inducement involve exchanges that are direct or indirect, overt, or covert, or cash or in kind. The threshold for triggering the Anti-Kickback statute is low. "If one purpose of the payment was to induce future referrals, the Medicare statute has been violated" (U.S. v. Greber, 760F.2d 68, 69 3rd Cir. 1985, cert. denied, 474 U.S. 988, 1985).

The penalties for violating the Anti-Kickback statute apply to those on both sides of the transaction. A single violation can result in a fine of up to $25,000 and up to 5 years imprisonment. Additionally, a violation can result in mandatory exclusion from the federal healthcare program. The government may also assess civil monetary penalties, which could result in treble damages plus an additional $50,000 for each violation (78 Fed. Reg. 79202, 2013).

Safe Harbors

The Office of Inspector General and the U.S. Department of Health and Human Services (HHS) have been given the authority to adopt safe harbors that protect against criminal and civil prosecution for Stark law and Anti-Kickback statute violations in certain situations. To qualify for safe harbor protection, the arrangement must cover all parameters of the safe harbor as written. There are common criteria that must be met to meet safe harbor requirements under the Anti-Kickback statute. These criteria include the following:

- Written and signed agreements are in effect for more than 1 year.

- Agreement specifies all services, products, and space to be provided.
- Agreement specifies part-time intervals and/or charges.
- Payment is set in advance, is fair market value, and does not consider the volume or value of referrals.
- Agreement terms do not exceed commercially reasonable terms.
- Agreement does not involve counseling or promotion of illegal activity.

Health and Human Services Donation Safe Harbors

In 2006, an EHR donation safe harbor exception was created, allowing certain referral recipients to donate an EHR system to referral sources. This safe harbor was originally scheduled to end in 2014 but was revised and extended until 2021 (78 Fed. Reg. 79202, 2013). In 2021, the safe harbor was extended again and revised to reflect the changing landscape of advances in EHR technology. This safe harbor was designed to facilitate physician adoption of EHR technology, as many physician practices were unable to purchase and support the technology due to its excessive cost.

Under this exception, a donor may donate EHR technology and services to persons in a position to refer to the donor. The donor may only pay up to 85% of the cost to purchase and implement the technology. This allows hospitals and other large healthcare entities to transfer or assist with the purchase of EHRs for physicians and other practices that refer patients to them at a large discount without violating the Stark law or the Anti-Kickback statute. Under the latest iteration of the safe harbor, the list of protected donors has been expanded to include entities that have an indirect responsibility for patient care (e.g., parent companies of hospitals, healthcare systems and accountable care organizations). To qualify for the safe harbor, the EHR must meet current EHR certification criteria as of the date of the donation. This means the EHR must be certified by a certifying body authorized by the National Coordinator for Health IT. This certification process is further explained in Chapter 20. Table 27.3 includes the basic safe harbor requirements.

In the 2021 final rule, the Anti-Kickback statute and Stark law added a related cybersecurity donation safe harbor exception that protects the donation of cybersecurity software *and* certain hardware (importantly, the donation of hardware is not protected by the EHR safe harbor and exception discussed above) with no contribution requirement (i.e., the donor can cover the entire cost of the donated item or service).

False Claims Act

The False Claims Act (FCA) imposes civil liability on any person who submits a claim to the federal government that he or she knows or should know to be false and imposes certain monetary penalties for violations of the act. The FCA prohibits fraudulent or false claims submitted to the government for payment and fraudulent or false claims that would decrease an amount owed to the government. Monetary penalties are imposed by the FCA, including a penalty of three times the amount of the claim submitted to the government for payment

TABLE 27.3   Electronic Health Record Donation Safe Harbor

Type of Expense	Hospital or MA Donor	Physician Recipient
Software (includes training costs and internet connectivity)	85%	15%
Hardware	0%	100%

Additional Requirements:

Donor cannot finance any portion of the costs required to be paid by the physician.

Donor cannot impose any additional requirements that would hinder the software being interoperable with other community providers.

Will cover replacement technology if such technology qualifies as necessary and used to create, maintain, transmit, receive, or protect electronic health records.

Cannot consider the volume or value of referrals.

Cannot be a condition for doing business with the donor.

Must be documented in writing.

EHR, Electronic health record; *MA*, Medicare Advantage.

plus $11,000 per claim (31 U.S.C. § 3729a1). In the healthcare arena, the FCA creates an issue with EHRs because each clinical encounter generates a bill. If that bill is not accurate and is sent to a governmental payor (such as Medicare, Medicaid, or the military's health insurance program Tricare) for payment, it is considered a false claim. This can present an added challenge with coding systems being changed, such as the recent move from International Classification of Diseases (ICD)-9 to ICD-10. Each individual bill would be a separate violation of the FCA, and the fines and penalties can add up very quickly. No intent to defraud the government is required to violate the law. Although the statute uses the word "knowingly," it does not require that a person submitting a claim have actual knowledge that the claim he or she is submitting is false. Acting in reckless disregard, or in deliberate ignorance of the truth or falsity of the information, can also lead to liability under the statute (31 U.S.C. § 3729b1).

The PPACA expanded the scope of the FCA. Medicare and Medicaid providers may discover that they have received payment on a mistaken claim that they submitted to Medicare or Medicaid. The claim may have been improperly coded, or there was a clerical error, resulting in an overpayment to the provider. Under the PPACA, a provider receiving a Medicare overpayment has 60 days to report and return the money before facing civil charges once the overpayment has been identified, or should have been identified (42 U.S.C. § 1320a-7kd1). If providers retain overpayments past the 60-day deadline, this creates an "obligation" under the FCA, and the provider faces liability under the FCA as well. Each individual overpayment is a separate false claim and triggers the penalties and fines discussed previously. When an overpayment situation occurs, it is very important to act quickly to return the money to the government to avoid the FCA fines and penalties.

Private citizens may also bring suits to enforce the FCA. These suits are called *Qui Tam* suits, and the person who brings them is referred to as the *Qui Tam* relator. These *Qui Tam* relators can potentially recover a portion of any judgment or settlement. The U.S. Department of Justice reviews all cases brought by *Qui Tam* relators and determines whether the government should join in the lawsuit. When the government joins, the amount that is recoverable by the *Qui Tam* relator is diminished but is still significant.

In addition to civil penalties (42 U.S.C. § 1320a-7a), the federal government can also prosecute and fine those engaging in healthcare fraud from a criminal perspective. An example of this is the general Healthcare Fraud statute. This statute provides that any person who knowingly and willfully executes, or attempts to execute, a scheme or artifice to (1) defraud any healthcare benefit program, or (2) obtain, by means of false or fraudulent pretenses, representations, or promises, any of the money or property owned by, or under the custody or control of, any healthcare benefit program in connection with the delivery of or payment for healthcare benefits, items, or services shall be fined under this title or imprisoned not more than 10 years, or both (18 U.S.C. § 1347). It is important to note that this criminal statute applies to any healthcare payor, public or private, and is not just limited to federal healthcare programs. Additionally, there is a criminal FCA statue that can be used against healthcare providers, but unlike the general healthcare fraud discussed previously, the criminal FCA only applies to a claim for payment from the federal government (18 U.S.C. § 287).

Wire/Mail Fraud

Mail fraud and wire fraud are additional issues that need to be considered during claims submission by providers. Mail fraud includes healthcare fraud that occurs through use of the U.S. mail system or common delivery services such as FedEx or UPS. Mail fraud can occur when paper claims with improper coding are sent to patients or their insurers. If these paper-based claims for payment contain fraudulent information, charges of criminal mail fraud can be brought against the provider (18 U.S.C. § 1341).

Improper computerized claims submission can lead to charges of wire fraud. The statute addressing wire fraud provides criminal penalties for devising a scheme to defraud or "for obtaining money or property by means of fraudulent or false pretenses" (18 U.S.C. § 1343). Wire fraud involves interstate use of wire, radio, or TV communication to commit fraud, and would clearly encompass computerized claim submission. Each claim submitted would create a separate count of wire fraud. Both mail and wire fraud are punishable by fines of up to $1000 and up to 5 years imprisonment per violation. For example, assume a physician upcoded 50 claims and submitted those claims electronically to Medicare via the EHR billing module. In addition to the civil penalties any physicians would face through the FCA, they may face criminal charges for 50 counts of wire fraud and one or more counts of Medicare fraud.

Fraud and Abuse and the Electronic Health Record

Each entry in an EHR helps determine what a healthcare provider will bill to an insurer or to Medicare or Medicaid. When these entries are inaccurate, fraudulent billing may occur. Each time a fraudulent claim is submitted to a government payor, there is a separate claim of fraud the government can make. Therefore, it is very important that those who use EHRs are educated regarding steps they can take to ensure that fraud does not occur.

Healthcare fraud can include such things as billing for services not rendered, billing for services that were unnecessary, or unbundling services that are billed as one Current Procedural Terminology (CPT) code to increase revenue. Over-documentation is the practice of inserting false or irrelevant documentation to create the appearance of support for billing at a higher level of service. Some EHRs auto populate fields when using templates that may be inaccurate if not appropriately edited. For example, if a provider reviews an order set for a particular diagnosis and the orders are prechecked, including procedures that have already been performed, this may lead to additional testing that is not necessary.

Most EHRs allow providers to create macros and templates for documentation. These macros and templates should be edited each time they are used to accurately reflect what occurred at each visit. Providers often do not take the time to edits these templates. For example, pediatricians may have a template they use for an adolescent well-child visit. The template may say that a mental health screening was done when it was not done at a particular visit. The physician then bills for the mental health screening, resulting in fraudulent billing. Features in the EHR resulting in over-documentation to meet reimbursement requirements can cause problems for providers when the services were not medically necessary or were not delivered.

One of the biggest fraud and abuse issues the government is targeting within the EHRs is the use of copy and paste functionality. When used appropriately, copy and paste can be a valuable tool. However, it can also result in creating a flawed medical record that could result in poor patient care. Consider a situation where the phrase "family history of breast cancer" is copied and pasted into a medical record as "history of breast cancer." This history is then reviewed by providers on each additional visit, which could lead to unnecessary care and testing that would not otherwise be needed by this patient.

The Centers for Medicare and Medicaid Services (CMS) published a toolkit that advises providers about ways they can ensure EHR fraud and abuse detection. Key recommendations are as follows: (Centers for Medicare and Detecting and Responding to Fraud, 2015)

- Providers should purchase systems that incorporate anti-fraud features.
- Software should have operational audit logs that always remain operational.
- Systems should have the ability to show who modified a record and when.

- Providers utilizing EHRs should have robust compliance programs that include standards of conduct that ensure that employees act in an appropriate and lawful manner.
- Employees should be trained regarding risks associated with EHRs. The training should emphasize the importance of accurate record-keeping and the potential criminal and disciplinary issues that can arise if there are issues with the integrity of the health record.
- Providers should audit their EMRs or EHRs to ensure that audit logs are functioning appropriately, and users are appropriately utilizing the system. Fraud detection software is available to perform pattern matching that would identify text that is cloned or copied from other sections. Unusually high usage of these features should be addressed with employees. If issues are identified, an appropriate investigation should occur.

A 2013 report issued by the Department of HHS Office of Inspector General found that most hospitals with EHR technology had audit functions in place, but not all were using them to the full extent (U.S. Department of Health and Human Services, 2013). This report noted that although most hospitals were analyzing audit log data, their efforts were aimed at HIPAA privacy issues, and not on the prevention of fraud and abuse.

It is important for those who are utilizing EHRs to recognize and understand the risks they face related to fraudulent billing. Audit controls should be in place to help providers ensure that the records they are creating are accurate.

State Law

In addition to federal law, each state has its own laws regarding fraud and abuse in the healthcare system. When providers are billing their states through Medicaid, they must also be cognizant of their local laws related to fraud and abuse, and how those laws might impose civil or criminal penalties on unwary healthcare providers.

ACCREDITATION

CMS has designated TJC and DNV as third-party agencies able to accredit hospitals for participation in Medicare and Medicaid programs (Centers for Medicare & Medicaid Services, 2012, 2014). TJC and DNV each have separate accreditation programs, but both accreditation programs use the Medicare Conditions of Participation as baseline requirements for hospitals to achieve accreditation (Kenney, 2015). TJC uses a survey and audit program called TJC Standards that it developed specifically for the healthcare industry. It provides more detailed, care-based requirements that a hospital must satisfy (The Joint Commission, 2016). Additionally, TJC provides guidance documents on the implementation of its care requirements and publishes alerts and recommendations for coping with new issues that may impact the quality of patient care in the future (The Joint Commission, 2015).

DNV uses the National Integrated Accreditation for Healthcare Association Organization program, which evaluates hospitals based on compliance with the Medicare Conditions of Participation and the International Organization of Standard's (ISO) 9001 Quality Management Program, an internationally recognized quality control program that is used across many industries (DNV GL Healthcare, 2015). DNV does not set specific care-based requirements, instead requiring only the satisfaction of the Medicare Conditions of Participation. It then uses the ISO 9001 program to evaluate other quality metrics.

While both TJC and DNV offer accreditation programs, only TJC provides a specific health information management chapter (The Joint Commission, 2014). DNV addresses health IT only through the broader Medicare Conditions of Participation. The remainder of this section will take a closer look at TJC standards and its specific recommendations for health information management.

The Joint Commission Health Information Management Standards

TJC has developed a specific chapter of its accreditation standards dealing with information management. The goal of TJC's information management standards is to ensure that healthcare providers have a well-planned information management system that assists practitioners with the provision of safe and high-quality care. There are four primary categories of responsibilities a hospital will have to address to ensure full performance of the TJC Standards for information management:

1. Planning for management of information,
2. Using health information,
3. Using knowledge-based information, and
4. Monitoring the data and health information process.

Included within those broader categories are provisions for protecting the privacy of health information and managing the capture, storage, and retrieval of health data.

Each larger category is divided into separate elements of performance that TJC uses to evaluate hospitals' compliance when it performs accreditation surveys. The elements of performance are specific actions that a hospital must take to satisfy the overall standard. For example, within the planning for management of information category, elements of performance include the organization identifying the information needed to provide quality, safe care; the organization identifying how data and information will flow through the organization; the organization using that identified information to develop a process to manage information; and staff and practitioners participating in the assessment, integration, and use of information management systems in the delivery of care. In other examples, elements of performance related to patient privacy and security of patient information track the HIPAA standards, requiring specific privacy and security policies and procedures to be in place. For a summary of TJC's standards relating to information management, see Table 27.4.

During an accreditation survey, TJC surveyors evaluate the hospitals on each element of performance to determine whether the overall standard is met. Every element of performance is given a scoring category, and the elements of performance are ranked based on the threat to patient safety and quality of care

TABLE 27.4 The Joint Commission Information Management Accreditation Standards

Category	Examples of Standard
Planning for Management of Information	Organization plans for managing information.
	Organization plans for continuity of its information management processes.
Using Health Information	Organization protects the privacy of health information.
	Organization protects the security and integrity of health information.
	Organization effectively manages the collection of health information.
	Organization retrieves, disseminates, and transmits health information in useful formats.
Using Knowledge-Based Information	Knowledge-based information resources are available, current, and authoritative.
Monitoring Data and Health Information Processes	Organization maintains accurate health information.

© Joint Commission Resources: Information Management. 2016 Comprehensive Accreditation Manual for Ambulatory Care (CAMAC). Oakbrook Terrace, IL: Joint Commission on Accreditation of Healthcare Organizations, Accessed August 1, 2016. Reprinted with permission.

(The Joint Commission, 2015). Whether or not a hospital fails to meet the standard for accreditation, based on its failure to meet an element of performance, depends on the nature of an incomplete element of performance.

Sentinel Event Alerts

The TJC also issues Sentinel Event Alerts, describing potential hazards to the quality of care and patient safety. TJC will identify actions that may serve to minimize the risk associated with those hazards. Since 2008, TJC has issued two major Sentinel Event Alerts related to health IT.

The earlier of the two, Sentinel Event Alert 42, was issued in December 2008 (The Joint Commission, 2008). In Alert 42, TJC identified the two primary factors that led to preventable adverse events related to, or caused by, health IT. The first factor was the human–machine interface and the second was the overall organization and design of the health IT system. Contributing to these factors was a general failure to perform adequate due diligence before investing in and implementing health IT—including failing to involve practitioners in the discussion on the best uses of and the care-related needs for health IT, an overreliance on vendor advice regarding health IT, and an inability to integrate feedback from providers into the end user experience. TJC advised hospitals to take more time to receive input from providers before investing into any health IT, to continuously monitor the use of the health IT, and to implement adequate training programs prior to initiating the use of any new IT programs.

Sentinel Event Alert 54 was issued in March 2015 (The Joint Commission, 2015). This alert built upon the conclusions of Alert 42. Again, TJC found that the use of health IT had inherent risks for preventable adverse events after they analyzed over 3375 adverse events reports. TJC identified eight areas of weakness that contribute to adverse events within health IT. The three largest areas of weakness came from (1) the human–computer interface (a full one-third of health IT–related events), (2) workflow and communication issues relating to health IT support, and (3) design issues related to clinical content and decision support. To understand more about health IT design, usability, and interaction outcomes, readers are referred to Chapter 22. To help resolve these issues, TJC recommended action through three pathways.

The first pathway is an increased culture of safety. A safety-minded culture includes active internal reporting and identification of health IT hazards. In addition to internal reporting, hospitals should not hesitate to make reports to external organizations, such as patient safety organizations, to reduce the aggregate risk throughout the healthcare system. The focus in reporting should be identifying risks rather than apportioning blame to individuals involved in any adverse events. Hospitals should also conduct an analysis of any adverse event to determine if health IT had been involved in the adverse event. Any analysis or identification of an adverse event or risk of an adverse event should be communicated globally, including with vendors, so that the overall hazard related to health IT is decreased.

The second pathway is process improvement. This involves implementing strategies to make the health IT programs themselves safer and free from malfunction, as well as using the health IT programs to monitor patient safety. TJC recommends using the SAFER (Safety Assurance Factors for EHR Resilience) guides, an EHR checklist produced by the Office of the National Coordinator (ONC) to address the safety of the installed IT programs. The SAFER checklist includes items such as backing up hardware systems, conducting extensive testing of systems before implementation, and using standardized codes across all platforms. TJC also recommends ensuring that providers and other health IT users have adequate training on the use of IT programs and that IT programs are structured to be user-friendly and to minimize the effect of human error.

The third and final pathway is through hospital and facility leadership. The leadership of the hospital should encourage the culture of safety and responsibility related to potential adverse events caused or contributed to by health IT. The identification and reporting of adverse events should be done in a manner to encourage reporting and not assign blame. Additionally, leadership should be proactive in engaging health IT users to provide feedback and recommendations for improvements to IT interfaces and hazard identification. Furthermore, leadership should be proactive about evaluating IT programs for safety risks and inefficiencies. If leadership believes a change to IT programs is in the best interest of patient safety and quality of care, any modifications or improvements to the system should be implemented only after appropriate due diligence and training of all end users.

THE INTERSECTION OF NEW TECHNOLOGY AND REGULATION

Digital Health Tools

The explosion of mobile health (mHealth) technology and consumer-driven health applications has taxed an outdated regulatory framework that was never designed for these new types of technologies. This section presents a discussion of the current regulatory framework and recent efforts to update this framework, given the impact of exploding innovate technology in healthcare. Currently, no single agency is tasked with regulating health IT or applications. Regulatory authority is spread over agencies such as the Food and Drug Administration (FDA), Federal Trade Commission (FTC), state medical boards, Federal Communications Commission (FCC), CMS, and ONC for health IT.

Food Drug and Cosmetic Act

The FDA has authority over the Food Drug and Cosmetic Act (FDCA). As the title of the FDCA suggests, the FDA has regulatory authority over foods, drugs, cosmetics, herbal supplements, and medical devices (including certain health IT and embedded medical device software). The FDA is also tasked with assuring the safety and effectiveness of medical devices. Specifically, Section 201(h) of the Act defines a "Device" as an instrument, apparatus, implement, machine, contrivance, implant, in vitro reagent, or other similar or related article, including a component part, or accessory which is: recognized in the official National Formulary, or the United States Pharmacopeia, or any supplement to them, intended for use in the diagnosis of disease or other conditions, or in the cure, mitigation, treatment, or prevention of disease, in man or other animals, or intended to affect the structure or any function of the body of man or other animals, and which does not achieve its primary intended purposes through chemical action within or on the body of man or other animals and which is not dependent upon being metabolized for the achievement of any of its primary intended purposes (21 U.S.C. § 201h).

Table 27.5 illustrates the various classes of medical devices and FDA oversight.

Initially it appears the FDCA regulates any type of health IT because the majority, if not all, of health IT is intended to be used "in the diagnosis of disease or other conditions, or in the cure, mitigation, treatment, or prevention of disease, in man." (Food and Drug Administration) However, FDA has taken a risk-based approach and not exercised its authority over certain health information technologies such as EHRs, even if such EHRs have computer decision support (CDS) or computerized physician order entry (CPOE) functionality.

Congress passed the Food and Drug Administration Safety and Innovation Act (FDASIA) in 2012 in recognition of the need for federal agencies to work together to come up with a new regulatory framework related to emerging health IT (Section 618 of the Food and Drug Administration Safety and Innovation Act). Specifically, Section 618 of the FDASIA required that the FDA in consultation with ONC and FCC create "a report that contains

TABLE 27.5 Food and Drug Administration Classes of Medical Devices

	Class I	Class II	Class III
Patient safety risk	Low	Medium	High
FDA requirements	General controls	General controls and special controls	General controls and premarket approval
Percentage of medical devices that fall into this category	47%	43%	10%
Examples	Dental floss	Power wheelchair	Replacement heart valve

FDA, Food and Drug Administration.

a proposed strategy and recommendations on an appropriate, risk-based regulatory framework pertaining to health IT, including mobile medical applications, that promotes innovation, protects patient safety, and avoids regulatory duplication" (Food and Drug Administration). In issuing its final report, the agencies divided health IT into three categories: (1) administrative health IT functions, (2) health management health IT functions, and (3) medical device health IT functions, with corresponding recommendations on each (FDASIA Health IT Report, 2014).

The report suggests no additional FDA oversight on technology primarily engaged in administrative health IT functions, and no increased oversight activities for technology classified as a medical device serving a health management health IT function outside of the FDA's current focus "on medical device health IT functionality, such as computer aided detection software, remote display or notification of real-time alarms from bedside monitors, and robotic surgical planning and control" (FDASIA Health IT Report, 2014). The report recommended setting up a Health IT Safety Center in which federal agencies could convene stakeholders to discuss patient safety issues and the other topics described in Fig. 27.2. Since the report does not recommend that the FDA regulate any new technologies that are not currently the focus of FDA regulation, the practical results of the recommendation is that new consumer-focused mHealth technologies discussed later are in effect unregulated from a patient safety standpoint.

mHealth Wearable Devices

The development and use of mHealth applications and wearable devices has exploded with the advent of smartphones and broadband cellular technology. Patients can now open an application on their phone and be immediately connected to a physician for treatment or ask the mHealth app a question about a health issue and be immediately given an answer, including a course of treatment. Insurers now provide premium discounts to individuals who use wearable devices and agree to share the information collected with the insurer. While these applications provide convenience to patients, they also raise potential regulatory and liability issues.

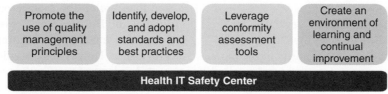

Fig. 27.2 Food and Drug Administration Safety and Innovation Act recommendation for health IT safety center. From Food and Drug Administration Safety and Innovation Act, Pub. Law 112-144.

As discussed previously, regulators seem to have taken a hands-off approach when it comes to mHealth applications and wearable devices. This perception was reinforced in January 2015 when the FDA issued draft guidance titled "General Wellness: Policy for Low-Risk Devices" (Food and Drug Administration, 2019). This guidance reaffirmed the idea that the FDA will not regulate wearable devices used for general wellness under the FDCA. The FDA uses a two-part test in determining whether a wearable device is a low-risk general wellness product and not subject to regulation: (1) the project makes only general wellness claims, and (2) the product does not present inherent risks to a user's safety. Under the first part of the test, the FDA examines whether the device is designed and intended to maintain healthy lifestyles or promote healthy activities and does not make any reference to diseases or conditions unless it is well understood that healthy lifestyle choices may help reduce the risk of or help living with a certain disease or condition (such as making a claim that a wearable device will cure or mitigate diabetes). If a device uses an intervention or technology that requires device controls such as implants or raises novel questions of biocompatibility, the second part of the two-part test may trigger FDA scrutiny.

Telehealth

mHealth applications have the functionality of connecting a patient in real time to a physician who may be physically located in a different state and may not be licensed in the same state of the patient. The novel Coronavirus pandemic of 2019 (COVID-19) prompted a series of changes to federal and state policies that quickly allowed telehealth to meet patient demand. These changes impact how states regulate interstate licensure for out-of-state physicians and other healthcare practitioners providing **telehealth** services. For example, in Idaho, pursuant to a medical board proclamation, out-of-state physicians, and physician assistants with a license in good standing in another state did not need an Idaho license to provide telehealth to patients located in Idaho during the response to COVID-19. Other states promulgated similar rules set to expire with the public health emergency resulting from COVID-19 (Federation of State Medical Boards, 2022). The question remains as to how states will make permanent or expire the temporary waivers and rules used to promote telehealth services across state lines.

In addition to state law changes, states have entered state licensing compacts, like the Interstate Medical Licensure Compact (IMLC) (Physician license, 2022) and the Enhanced Nurse Licensure Compact (eNLC) (National Council of State Boards of Nursing, Inc, 2022). These compacts were created to preserve state regulation of medical practice while making it easier for physicians to provide care remotely to patients in other states. The use of these compacts rose dramatically because of COVID-19.

All states will fall into three buckets: (1) those that outright prohibit out-of-state physicians from practicing in their state; (2) those that have more flexibility (like those that enter the above compacts); and (3) those that offer limited scope telehealth licenses for specialists and other unique circumstances or services.

For more traditional telehealth applications, interstate licensure issues continue to be a challenge to the broader use of this form of health IT.[2]

Privacy and Ownership of Data Collected by mHealth and Wearable Devices

The privacy of health data that is collected by mHealth applications and wearable devices is also an issue of intense debate. Since these applications are not covered entities under HIPAA, there is no healthcare specific federal prohibition on the collection, use, and disclosure of personal health information that is collected by the app. Recently, the FTC has recognized the need for more transparency regarding how information collected by mobile applications is used by application developers and has published some subregulatory guidance on this issue, but such guidance does not have the force of law (Federal Trade Commission, 2015). This does not mean that there are no regulations related to the privacy of data collected by these types of applications and devices. State privacy laws expand the prohibition of the collection and use of personally identifiable information related to health information, but most states do not have these types of protections (Tex).

Another unresolved issue involves the ownership of data collected by mHealth applications and wearable devices in the era of Big Data and data analytics. The data collected by these devices are valuable to both the developer of the device or application and to third parties such as researchers or pharmaceutical companies (Business Insider, 2014). This has led developers to monetize the sale of aggregated data to third party researchers as part of the developer's business plan. Patients should read the terms and conditions that accompany a particular device before use to determine whether the device manufacturer will share users' personal information with third parties.

---

[2] NTD: Is this internal reference still correct

Liability Issues

Finally, only mHealth applications that are regulated by the FDA are those considered medical devices, such as electrocardiograms or physiologic monitoring. The majority of the more than 165,000 available health apps are not considered medical devices, and they are not regulated by the FDA (or any other federal agency) from a patient safety perspective. This can be problematic when there is incorrect or grossly false data in the application and a patient relies on this information in lieu of seeking professional medical advice and suffers an injury. Adding to this problem is that developers of mHealth applications are in foreign countries, with varying legal systems making it difficult for an injured patient to recover damages from a developer.

Furthermore, the data collected by mHealth applications and wearable devices are becoming increasingly combined with patient data stored in EHRs, which can lead to reliance on the accuracy of this data by providers when creating a treatment plan or treating a chronic disease (Mobile & Device Integration, n.d.). If a provider relies on this information and such reliance results in harm to the patient, should the developer be held accountable, in addition to the provider? Also, if a developer is held liable, should the developer now be able to argue that it should have the benefit of the monetary caps states have enacted related to medical malpractice tort reform?

Alternatively, if this type of information is available to a provider but is not reviewed, is the provider liable? These issues all play into whether the standard of care owed a patient should take technology into account. For a more detailed discussion about these issues and current research, see Chapter 14 on Digital Health.

Social Media and Informatics

Another hot button issue in healthcare and informatics is the role that social media plays in balancing the rights of employees and free speech against the privacy rights of patients. More recently the National Labor Relations Board (NLRB) made this balancing act more difficult by publishing model social media policies for employers that might, if enforced, effectively prohibit employers from implementing social media policies that protect patient privacy.

Historically, employers would protect patient privacy on social media by creating and enforcing employment policies prohibiting employees from posting patient information on social media. These types of policies were enacted after a spate of high-profile incidents in which employees posted patient information to social media. Here are examples:

- A 2012 *Chicago Daily Herald* article detailed incidents such as a physician who on his blog called a patient "lazy" and "ignorant" because the patient made several visits to the emergency room after failing to monitor her sugar levels (Being Facebook Friends and Doctors May Cross Line, 2012).
- In yet another case, a medical student filmed a doctor inserting a chest tube into a patient, whose face was clearly visible,

and then posted the footage on YouTube (Being Facebook Friends and Doctors May Cross Line, 2012).
- In another incident, a temporary employee assigned to the Providence Holy Cross Medical Center in Los Angeles posted a photo of a patient's medical record (clearly showing the patient's name), accompanied by the comment, "funny but this patient came in to cure her VD and get birth control." (Patient Info on Facebook Traced to Temp Staff. Same-Day Surgery, 2012)

Section 7 of the National Labor Relations Act (NLRA) protects the right of employees to "engage in… concerted activities for the purpose of… mutual aid or protection" and gives the NLRB authority to investigate such behavior even if the employee filing a claim is not a union member or the employer is located in a right-to-work state (29 U.S.C. §§ 151-169). On May 30, 2012, NLRB's Acting General Counsel published a memo that disapproved of a social media policy that prohibited employees "from posting information… that could be deemed material non-public information or any information that is considered confidential or proprietary" (The National Labor Relations Board, 2016). Similarly, the NLRB found unlawful a social media policy that prohibited an employee from sharing "confidential information with another team member unless they have a need to know the information to do their job." These memos (if they were to be enforced) would effectively prohibit healthcare employers from implementing prudent social media policies that prohibit employees from engaging in activities that might expose the employer to violations of HIPAA or state privacy laws. After widespread condemnation by healthcare providers, the NLRB may revise these memos and guidance documents, but this has not been finalized.

CONCLUSION AND FUTURE DIRECTIONS

The healthcare system in the United States is highly regulated, and these regulations have a significant impact on the practice of health informatics. As a result, for their own safety, health professionals, health informaticians, the providers they serve, and the patients who depend on the healthcare system must understand and utilize the regulatory framework associated with health IT and informatics. This is especially important as the use of the technology becomes more widespread in the delivery of healthcare and the implementation of new consumer-focused technologies. Additionally, health informaticians must become proactive as the law and regulators struggle to catch up with health technology–related innovations as well as providers' and patients' reliance on these new technologies.

ACKNOWLEDGMENT

The authors wish to acknowledge the contributions of Shannon Majoras and Robin L. Canowitz to the previous edition of this chapter.

DISCUSSION QUESTIONS

1. How does the U.S. regulatory framework work to ensure patient safety?
2. Describe two express powers and one implied power given to the federal government in the Constitution that has implications for health-related technology.
3. Name two federal agencies and describe their role in the regulatory oversight of health IT.
4. What are the different types of healthcare fraud and abuse statutes?
5. What are three key issues with mHealth applications and wearable devices?
6. How are patient privacy rights impacted by labor and employment regulations?

CASE STUDY

A 50-member multispecialty medical practice has decided to implement a new EHR system. The practice chooses the new EHR system based on both clinical functionality and the practice management and billing functionality that is demonstrated specifically because the EHR sales representative repeatedly states that the new EHR can reduce patient visit times (thus increasing the number of patients a provider can see in a day) and increase reimbursement to the practice by helping the practice "correctly code" to the highest E/M (evaluation and management) code available. While the healthcare providers and practice administrator are impressed with the new EHR, the new system will cost $2,000,000 for the EHR software and $250,000 for the associated hardware, plus yearly maintenance fees of $125,000. These costs exceed the practice's budget. One day, while meeting with the vice president of a community hospital, the practice administrator mentions this issue and how the practice will have to delay purchasing an EHR due to the budget constraints. The VP states that the hospital will be happy to cover 85% costs for the new EHR system if the practice agrees to (1) consider their hospital first before sending a patient to any other potential competitors including not just ER or inpatient admission but outpatient diagnostic services and hospital-owned specialty practices, (2) include the hospital's logo on patient education materials printed from the system, (3) use the hospital's template for designing data entry pages for practitioners, and (4) use the hospital's template for the patient portal in the design of their patient portal.

Discussion Questions

1. Explain the basic requirements for a hospital to help finance the purchase of an EHR system by a provider.
2. Discuss whether the proposed course of action would be permissible under current fraud and abuse regulations.
3. If the structure of the proposed donation is not permitted under current fraud and abuse regulations, explain what steps the parties would need to take to make the transaction compliant.
4. Explain common issues related to use of EHR and healthcare fraud.
5. Discuss how the proposed new EHR could potentially facilitate healthcare fraud.

REFERENCES

18 U.S.C. § 1341.
18 U.S.C. § 1343.
18 U.S.C. § 1347.
18 U.S.C. § 287.
21 U.S.C. § 201(h).
29 U.S.C. §§ 151-169.
31 U.S.C. § 3729(a)(1).
31 U.S.C. § 3729(b)(1).
42 U.S.C. § 1320a-7a.
42 U.S.C. § 1320a-7b(a).
42 U.S.C. § 1320a-7b.
42 U.S.C. § 1320a-7k(d)(1).
42 U.S.C. § 1395nn(a)(2)(A).
42 U.S.C. § 1395nn(a)(2)(B).
42 U.S.C. § 1395nn.
42 U.S.C. §§ 1396 et seq. http://www.gpo.gov/fdsys/pkg/USCODE-2010-title42/pdf/USCODE-2010-title42-chap7-subchapXIX-sec1396d. pdf. Accessed July 5, 2016.
5 U.S.C. §§ 551 et seq. http://www.archives.gov/federal-register/laws/administrative-procedure/. Accessed July 5, 2016.
78 Fed. Reg. 79202 (December 27, 2013).
Administrative Procedure Act, Pub. L. 79-404, 60 Stat. 237; 1946. http://legisworks.org/sal/60/stats/STATUTE-60-Pg237.pdf.
Being Facebook friends and doctors may cross line. (2012, July 9). *Chicago Daily Herald.*
Business Insider. Senator warns Fitbit is a 'privacy nightmare' and could be 'tracking' your movements; 2014. http://www.businessinsider.com/senator-warns-fitbit-is-a-privacy-nightmare-2014-8#ixzz3A5M2nn17.
California Civil Code §§ 56 et seq.
Centers for Medicare & Medicaid Services. (2012, September 26). Continued approval of Det Norske Veritas Healthcare's (DNVHC) Hospital Accreditation Program. 77 Federal Register 51537.
Centers for Medicare & Medicaid Services. Continued approval of the Joint Commission's (TJC) hospital accreditation program. 79 Federal Register 36524. June 26, 2014.
Centers for Medicare & Medicaid Services. (2015). Detecting and responding to fraud, waste and abuse associated with the use of electronic health records (July 2015). https://www.cms.gov/Medicare-Medicaid-Coordination/Fraud-Prevention/Medicaid-Integrity-Education/ Downloads/ehr-detect-fwabooklet.pdf.
DNV GL Healthcare. (2015). DNV GL's pioneering NIAHO program integrates ISO 9001 with the Medicare conditions of participation.

http://dnvglhealthcare.com/accreditations/hospital-accreditation. Accessed November 2, 2015.

FDASIA Health IT Report. (2014). Proposed strategy and recommendations for a risk-based framework. http://www.fda.gov/AboutFDA/CentersOffices/OfficeofMedicalProductsandTobacco/CDRH/CDRHReports/ ucm390588.htm.

Federal Trade Commission. (2015).https://www.ftc.gov/news-events/blogs/business-blog/2015/02/location-location-location?utm_source=govdelivery.

Federation of State Medical Boards. (2022). *U.S. states and territories modifying requirements for telehealth in response to COVID-19.* https://www.fsmb.org/siteassets/advocacy/pdf/states-waiving-licensure-requirements-for-telehealth-in-response-to-covid-19.pdf.

Food and Drug Administration Safety and Innovation Act. (2018). Pub. Law 112-144. https://www.fda.gov/regulatory-information/selected-amendments-fdc-act/food-and-drug-administration-safety-and-innovation-act-fdasia.

Food and Drug Administration. (2019). General wellness: Policy for low risk devices. Draft Guidance for Industry. https://www.fda.gov/regulatory-information/search-fda-guidance-documents/general-wellness-policy-low-risk-devices.

Kenney, L. (2015). American Society for Healthcare Engineering. Hospital accrediting organizations offer different approaches to the survey process. http://www.ashe.org/resources/ashenews/2013/hosp_ao_article_131011.html#.Vjd2-t_lupo. Accessed November 2, 2015.

McCulloch v. Maryland, 17 U.S. 316 (1819). JUSTIA: U.S. Supreme Court; 2016. https://supreme.justia.com/cases/federal/us/17/316/.

Mobile & Device Integration. (n.d.). http://www.cerner.com/Solutions/Workplace_Health/Wellness_Solutions_and_Services/Mobile_and_Device_ Integration/.

National Council of State Boards of Nursing, Inc. (2022, March 30). *Nurse licensure compact (NLC).* NCSBN: Leading Regulatory Excellence. https://www.ncsbn.org/nurse-licensure-compact.htm.

National Mining Association v. Jackson, 816F.Supp. 2d 37 (D.D.C. 2011). JUSTIA: U.S. Law; 2016. http://law.justia.com/cases/federal/district-courts/district-of-columbia/dcdce/1:2010cv01220/143120/167/.

Office of the National Coordinator for Health Information Technology. (2015). Policymaking, regulation, & strategy. Federal-State Health Care Coordination. https://www.healthit.gov/policy-researchers-implementers/federal-state-health-care-coordination/. Accessed December 7, 2015.

Patient info on facebook traced to temp staff. (2012, May 1). Same-Day Surgery.

Interstate Medical Licensure Compact. (2022, March 21). Physician license. Retrieved March 25, 2022, from https://www.imlcc.org/

Section 1877 of the Social Security Act. https://www.ssa.gov/OP_Home/ssact/title18/1877.htm. Accessed July 5, 2016.

Section 618 of the Food and Drug Administration Safety and Innovation Act, Pub. Law 112-144.

Section 6402(f)(2) of the Patient Protection and Affordable Care Act, Pub. L. No. 111-148, 124 Stat 119 (2010).

Tex. Health and Safety Code § 181.100 et seq.

The Joint Commission. (2008). Sentinel Event Alert 42: Safely implementing health information and converging technologies. http://www.jointcommission.org/sentinel_event_alert_issue_42_safely_implementing_health_information_and_ converging_technologies/.

The Joint Commission. (2014). The Joint Commission standards edition: Information management. http://foh.hhs.gov/tjc/im/standards.pdf.

The Joint Commission. (2015). Benefits of Joint Commission accreditation. http://www.jointcommission.org/about_us/accreditation_fact_sheets.aspx.

The Joint Commission. (2015). Facts about scoring and certification decision. http://www.jointcommission.org/facts_about_scoring_and_certification_decision/.

The Joint Commission. (2015). Sentinel Event Alert 54: Safe use of health information yechnology. http://www.jointcommission.org/assets/1/18/SEA_54.pdf.

The Joint Commission. (2016). Facts about Joint Commission standards. http://www.jointcommission.org/facts_about_joint_commission_accreditation_standards/.

The National Labor Relations Board. (2016). The NLRB and social media fact sheet. https://www.nlrb.gov/news-outreach/fact-sheets/nlrb-and-social-media; Accessed on July 5, 2016.

U.S. Department of Health and Human Services, Office of Inspector General (December, 2013). Not all recommended fraud safeguards have been implemented in hospital EHR technology. http://www.oig.hhs.gov/oei/reports/oei-01-11-00570.pdf.

U.S. v. Greber, 760F.2d 68, 69 (3rd Cir. 1985), cert. denied, 474 U.S. 988 (1985).

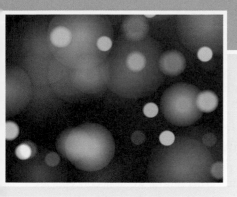

28

Privacy and Security

Paul DeMuro and Henry Norwood

OBJECTIVES

At the completion of this chapter, the reader will be prepared to:

1. Describe foundational concepts related to privacy in the context of informatics.
2. Describe components and enforcement of HIPAA and related state laws pertaining to the privacy and protection of health information.
3. Describe the implications of the Patient Safety and Quality Improvement Act's key features in relation to health data privacy and security.
4. Explain the implications of the Genetic Information Nondiscrimination Act as it pertains to the protection of health information within the broader, national health information security framework.
5. Discuss the purposes of state biometric information privacy acts within the national health information privacy and security framework.
6. Describe how organizations protect against and litigate cybercrimes.
7. Describe the health information privacy and security frameworks of other nations.

KEY TERMS

availability, 446
biometric identifiers, 451
breach, 448
breach notification, 448
business associate, 449
confidentiality, 446
covered entities, 448

designated record set, 448
genetic information, 451
informed consent, 447
integrity, 446
Meaningful Use Program, 450
Patient Safety Organizations, 450
privacy, 446

protected health information, 448
research exception, 451
right of access, 448
risk assessment
   (risk analysis), 450
security, 446

ABSTRACT ❖

Health informatics is at the forefront of modern medicine as the abundance of health data allows health providers to analyze their practices with efficiency and accuracy unavailable in the past. The privacy and security of patient health information are vital to the success of health informatics as a field of practice. This chapter discusses how the concepts of privacy and security apply to electronic health information. National health data privacy and legal security structures are examined as well as an analysis of specific international legal considerations addressing health data privacy and security. The chapter concludes with an examination of security concepts and procedures necessary to ensure the safety and integrity of electronic health data.

INTRODUCTION

A primary responsibility of healthcare providers and their business associates is to ensure that the health data they are responsible for is held in the strictest confidence. The reality is that the risks to confidentiality are significant for electronic health data.

The importance of protecting and safeguarding protected health information (PHI) has grown exponentially as health-related device use has expanded into areas such as mobile devices, electronic health records (EHRs), sensors, biomedical devices, telehealth, personal health records (PHRs), personal health devices, and health information exchanges (HIEs). Increased usage brings increased risk for data breaches. The increase in the number of users, types of uses, and volumes of health IT-based data is directly proportional to the increased opportunities for privacy and confidentiality breaches. Patients and healthcare providers typically support concepts related to the use of data for research purposes, electronic health data storage, and communication. However, concerns regarding data security persist.

Lawmakers in the United States and worldwide have sought to provide for the privacy and security of health information through legislation. Understanding the major legal considerations within the United States and abroad is vital to engaging in the fields of healthcare and informatics.

THE RIGHT TO PRIVACY

"Whatever, In connection with my professional practice, or not In connection with It, I see or hear in the life of men, which ought not to be spoken of abroad, I will not divulge…" (Miles, 2004). The Hippocratic Oath, dated approximately to 400 BC, expresses the fundamental interest of privacy in the practice of medicine. This interest has only become more important as medicine has entered the modern, technological era. As health information is being generated as electronic data in greater quantities and the number of parties seeking access to this data, including patients, providers, insurers, and other third parties, the need for health information privacy and security increase proportionally.

What is Privacy?

Privacy is the right of individuals to control access to their person (body privacy) or information about themselves (information privacy), (Neuhaus et al., 2011). In informatics, the concern is focused primarily on the privacy of information. Designing systems to ensure the security of information privacy is one of the most difficult challenges for institutions and individuals living in our digital age. Health records can contain information on any or all aspects of an individual's life and may contain extremely sensitive information (e.g., sexually transmitted diseases, behavioral health information, or financial information) (Privacy Policy Guidance, 2021). Health data and information must be kept private if such data are considered trusted

information and a primary resource for building new knowledge. Also, the information must be protected from access and misuse by unauthorized persons. Moreover, specific policies and procedures must be implemented to prevent disclosures or breaches that encroach on the privacy of the data's primary owner—the patient.

Privacy, Confidentiality, and Security

The differences between privacy, confidentiality, and security can be difficult to pinpoint. Terms central to these concepts are defined in Table 28.1. Privacy pertains to the party with access to information, a patient's right to keep information private, and what constitutes inappropriate or unauthorized access. Confidentiality relates to protecting and safeguarding health information from inappropriate access, use, and disclosure. In short, privacy is about the *person*, while confidentiality is about the *information*. Privacy speaks to the rights of patients, as they have a right to their privacy. Confidentiality speaks to the responsibility of healthcare providers because they are responsible for keeping patients' information private. Security relates to the administrative, technical, and physical safeguards implemented to prevent privacy and confidentiality breaches and ensure information integrity and availability.

Fair Information Practice Principles

Recognition of the right to medical data privacy was recognized in the United States as early as the 1970s. Fair information practices (FIPs), also referred to as fair information practice principles (FIPPs), drafted in the 1970s, are a set of internationally recognized practices for addressing the privacy of information (Case C-131/12, 2014). The principles are the result of joint work by US, Canadian, and European government agencies over time and are available in reports, guidelines, and legal codes that ensure that information practices are fair and provide adequate privacy protection to individuals. Although these statements can vary according to the source, typical FIPPs are included in Table 28.2.

Since the original FIPPS was drafted, many government agencies have addressed the impact of the computerization of health records. Some industrialized countries codified FIPPs into a privacy law at the federal level, although this has not yet

TABLE 28.1   Distinctions Among Terms

Terms	Definitions
Accountability	The requirement for actions of an entity is traced uniquely to that entity.
Authenticity	Able to be verified and trusted; confidence in the validity of a transmission, a message, or message originator.
Availability	Data or information is accessible and useable on demand by an authorized person.
Confidentiality	Data or information is not made available or disclosed to unauthorized persons or processes.
Integrity	Data or information have not been altered or destroyed in an unauthorized manner.
Privacy	The practice of maintaining the confidentiality and security of protected health information.
Safeguards	Protective measures prescribed to meet the security requirements (i.e., confidentiality, integrity, and availability) specified for an information system. Safeguards may include security features, management constraints, personnel security, and security of physical structures, areas, and devices. Synonymous with security controls and countermeasures.
Security	Protecting information and information systems from unauthorized access, use, disclosure, disruption, modification, or destruction to provide confidentiality, integrity, and availability.

TABLE 28.2   Fair Information Practice Principles

Principle	Description
Transparency	Organizations should be transparent and notify individuals regarding collection, use, dissemination, and maintenance of personally identifiable information (PII).
Individual participation	Organizations should involve the individual in the process of using PII and, to the extent practicable, seek individual consent for the collection, use, dissemination, and maintenance of PII. Organizations should also provide mechanisms for appropriate access, correction, and redress regarding the use of PII.
Purpose specification	Organizations should specifically articulate the authority that permits the collection of PII and specifically articulate the purposes for which PII is intended to be used.
Data minimization	Organizations should only collect PII that is directly relevant and necessary to accomplish the specified purpose(s) and only retain PII for as long as is necessary to fulfill the specified purpose(s).
Use limitation	Organizations should use PII solely for the purposes specified in the notice. Sharing PII should be for a purpose compatible with the purpose for which the PII was collected.
Data quality and integrity	Organizations should, to the extent practicable, ensure that PII is accurate, relevant, timely, and complete.
Security	Organizations should protect PII in all media through appropriate security safeguards against risks such as loss, unauthorized access or use, destruction, modification, or unintended or inappropriate disclosure.
Accountability and auditing	Organizations should be accountable for complying with these principles, providing training to all employees and contractors who use PII, and auditing the actual use of PII to demonstrate compliance with these principles and all applicable privacy protection requirements.

occurred in the United States. Instead, in the United States, FIPPs are the basis of many individual laws at the federal and state levels. The value of the FIPPs is that they provide a framework for privacy laws and can form the foundation for an organization or an industry privacy policy. For example, although the Health Insurance Portability and Accountability Act of 1996 (HIPAA) does not formally codify FIPPs in the legislation, it implements all FIPPs in some form.

The Right to be Forgotten

An individual's right to restrict or eliminate personal information on the internet is currently the subject of much debate. The "right to be forgotten" as to which this right is often referred, has become popularized in the European Union (EU) and is gaining support among policymakers in other countries. A right to be forgotten had already been established to a certain degree, having received judicial recognition in *Google Spain SL v. Agencia Espan ola de Proteccion de Datos* (EU General Data Protection Regulation GDPR, 2016a). In *Google Spain*, a case in Spain, the European Union's Court of Justice held that the right to be forgotten on the internet is a right held by all members of the EU. This right, however, must be balanced against the public right to freedom of information. For matters which are more private in nature (e.g., information regarding an individual's health), the information should be deleted by the data controller pursuant to the right to be forgotten. The right to be forgotten would also be codified into the EU's overarching data protection law, the General Data Protection Regulation (GDPR) (Schloendroff v, 1914). The decision in *Google Spain* focused on internet search engines, such as Google, but the decision has ramifications for other data controllers as well, including health data controllers.

Health data sharing has expanded in modern times, and it is no longer the case that an individual will only share their personal health information with a medical provider in furtherance of receiving medical treatment. Patients themselves are entering their health information into health apps and electronic programs, which are operated by organizations collecting their health data. If these organizations are collecting health data from members of the EU, then once these organizations receive an individual's data, they become data controllers under the EU's right to be forgotten. EU members have the right to demand that health data controllers delete the health information in possession of an organization, assuming the organization held the information subject to the individual's consent or that the purpose for which the organization held the individual's health information is no longer necessary.

The right to be forgotten is an emerging area of law and has not yet gained global acceptance. The United States, where many of the larger internet search providers are based, has not yet formally accepted the right to be forgotten. The major implications of the right to be forgotten in the healthcare industry remain to be seen.

Informed Consent

"Every human being of adult years and sound mind has a right to determine what can be done with his own body, and a surgeon who continues to operate without his patient's consent commits an assault for which he is liable for damages" (Murray, 2012). The doctrine of "informed consent" was first recognized as the right of a patient to control the healthcare the patient received. The doctrine has since been extended to include the right of a patient to control their health information.

Over the years, several elements have been held to encompass a patient's informed consent (The Health Insurance Portability, 2014). The patient must have the capacity to make decisions on their own behalf, which includes the mental capacity to understand the decision the patient is making. A patient must be given sufficient information that would enable a reasonable patient to understand the decision the patient must make and to understand the possible consequences of that decision. Further, a patient's consent must be voluntarily given and not obtained through some form of fraud or duress.

There are exceptions to the requirement and necessity of informed consent in the healthcare context. There are generally exceptions to this prohibition, involving the incapacity of the patient, such that the patient would be unable to comprehend the information communicated to them and where the potential harm caused by delivering the information would outweigh the benefits. In certain circumstances, the right to informed consent may also be waived by the patient.

HIPAA AND STATE PRIVACY LAWS

The Scope of HIPAA

The Health Insurance Portability and Accountability Act (HIPAA) is the primary legal authority in the United States regarding health information privacy (45 CFR Part 160 and Subparts A and E of Part 164). Importantly, HIPAA only applies to "covered entities," which include healthcare providers, health care clearinghouses, and health plans. HIPAA can be divided into three broad rules: the Privacy Rule, the Security Rule, and the Breach Notification Rule.

The HIPAA Privacy Rule creates national standards designed to protect private health information (45 CFR Part 160 and Subparts A and C of Part 164). The Privacy Rule applies to a certain type of information, known as "protected health information." PHI is information relating to an individual's physical or mental health condition, the healthcare provided or recommended for that individual, or the payment information regarding the provision of healthcare to the individual, which either identifies a specific person or which can reasonably identify that person.

PHI cannot be used by entities covered by HIPAA for any reason other than treatment-related reasons allowed in the Privacy Rule or if the individual whose information is at issue authorizes the information to be used for specific purposes in writing. PHI cannot be disclosed by covered entities unless it is disclosed to the individuals, upon request, or to certain government agencies if there is an ongoing investigation. Covered entities also may use or disclose PHI for the organization to treat, pay, and conduct other healthcare activities.

The HIPAA Security Rule requires that "covered entities" implement measures that can lower an entity's risk of a cyberattack (45 CFR §§ 164.400-414). Specifically, the Security Rule applies to a particular type of PHI, referred to as "electronic PHI." Electronic PHI is PHI transmitted by the organization using electronic means.

The Security Rule requires covered entities to conduct regular risk analyses to detect potential vulnerabilities to electronic PHI being stored by the organization. Covered entities then must work to minimize these vulnerabilities and must have protocols in place to detect and prevent malicious software from infecting their computer systems. Users of the covered entity's computer systems must be trained on how to protect against malicious software and report any suspicions that malicious software has infected their computer system(s).

The Security Rule also requires covered entities to use access controls, allowing only necessary users to access electronic PHI. The Security Rule requires covered entities to conduct risk analyses of all threats to any electronic PHI generated by the covered entities or its "business associates" to determine if any electronic PHI is in jeopardy of theft, exposure, or loss. Covered entities must also demonstrate that their workforce complies with the Security Rule.

As an additional incentive to avoid putting electronic PHI at risk and to put those negatively affected on alert, HIPAA provides several rules requiring covered entities to notify different parties in the case of a breach. These provisions are in HIPAA's Breach Notification Rule, which applies to all PHI, not only electronic PHI (45 CFR 164.402).

Under Title 45 Section 164.402 of the Code of Federal Regulations, a breach is defined as: "the acquisition, access, use, or disclosure of protected health information in a manner not permitted. which compromises the security or privacy of the protected health information" (45 CFR 164.524). Any impermissible use of PHI is presumptively a breach requiring notification unless the covered entity can demonstrate there is a low likelihood that the PHI was compromised. If a covered entity commits a breach that involves unsecured PHI, the entity is required to perform a "breach notification," disclosing the breach to the US Department of Health and Human Services, any individuals who may be affected by the breach, and depending on the circumstances, to the public through the media.

The HIPAA Right of Access Rule

A particular rule within the HIPAA Privacy Rule that has been the focus of several HIPAA investigations in recent years is the "Right of Access Rule" (HHS). The Privacy Rule requires healthcare providers to comply with requests by individuals for access to their health information. The right of access includes the right to inspect and copy an individual's health information and to request that the provider release their information to a third party.

When a request for health information is made by an individual, the provider is required to allow access to the information in what is referred to as a "designated record set." A designated record set is a set of records maintained by the provider consisting of (1) medical and billing records; (2) health insurance or claim management information; and (3) other records not listed in the first two categories that are utilized by the provider in the provider's decision-making process regarding the individual. The information an individual is entitled to within the designated record set includes diagnostic results, imaging scans, and provider notes.

Not included in the designated record set are records not used by the provider in the decision-making process regarding the individual requesting access. These details include information that the provider uses in making decisions regarding the provider's business, but that is not used in making decisions regarding the individual. Further, psychotherapy notes and information prepared regarding a legal proceeding are specifically excluded from the designated record set.

Providers are required to comply with the right of access requests within 30 calendar days of receipt of the individual's request. Providers are permitted to obtain one extension of time to comply with a valid right of an access request if the provider conveys, in writing, to the requestor the need for additional time, the reason for the necessary extension, and the date by which the individual will be granted access to their records. It should be noted that on December 10, 2020, The Department of Health & Human Services (HHS) proposed modifications to the HIPAA Privacy Rule, including the right of access provision.

The Right of Access provision generally requires providers to provide the designated record set in the form requested by the individual. If the record set is not readily capable of being transmitted in this form, the record set must be either provided in a format agreed to by the individual and the provider or in hard copy. The provider is required to maintain the capacity to transmit health information electronically in at least a basic form. Of note, providers must also comply with the provisions of the HIPAA Security Rule while providing individuals access to their health information.

An individual's request for access to his or her health information may be properly denied by the provider under a select set of circumstances. If the grounds for denial exist, this denial may be the entirety of the records requested or merely a portion of the records requested. In the event the provider denies the individual access, it must provide a written denial describing the reasoning behind the denial and notifying the individual of his or her right to have the denial reviewed (if permitted), along with the review process. The denial must also explain the OCR complaint process to the individual. This written denial must be provided to the individual within 30 days of receipt of the individual's initial request for access—or within the extension, period if applicable. If the provider does not possess the information requested, the provider must inform the individual of the location of the health information if the provider is aware of the location.

Business Associate Agreements Under HIPAA

A "business associate" is an individual or organization, separate from a covered entity, which performs services for the covered entity involving PHI. HIPAA requires covered entities to enter into "business associate agreements" with any outside organization providing services for the covered entity that involves access to PHI (Department of Health & Human Services, 2021).

Business associate agreements must delineate the permissible uses and disclosures of PHI by the business associate. Business associate agreements also must provide that the business associate will implement technical security measures to protect electronic PHI. The business agreement limits how the business associate is able to use and disclose PHI. Business associates are separately liable from covered entities under HIPAA and can be subject to civil or criminal penalties if they use or disclose PHI beyond what is permitted by the business associate agreement.

The HIPAA Enforcement Role of HHS's Office of Civil Rights

The US Department of Health and Human Services' Office of Civil Rights ("OCR") is tasked with enforcing HIPAA Privacy, Security, and Breach Notification Rules (45 CFR). OCR enforces HIPAA requirements by investigating HIPAA complaints, performing compliance reviews, and providing covered entities with compliance guidance. OCR is only permitted to act on complaints if: the allegedly at-fault party is a covered entity or a business associate; the alleged misconduct involves a violation of either the HIPAA Privacy or Security Rule; any complaints are filed within 180 days of the time when OCR knew or should have reasonably known of the alleged violation.

Once an investigation is undertaken, OCR will send a notice of determination to the covered organization and provide it an opportunity to submit evidence in its defense. The organization has thirty days following notification to submit such evidence (Cal). If OCR determines that a penalty should be imposed on the organization, OCR will inform the organization by sending a notice of proposed determination, which will state the applicable statutory authority, the underlying findings of fact and circumstances justifying the penalty, OCR's reasoning in reaching its conclusions, the penalty amount and justification for same, and instructions for payment/responding to the notice. The covered organization does have the option of requesting a hearing in front of an administrative law judge, but more often a settlement agreement is reached between the organization and OCR. Any civil penalty imposed on the organization must be deposited into the US treasury.

There are four categories of penalties based on the level of awareness of the HIPAA violation by the organization. Category 1 applies where the organization did not know and reasonably should not have known of the violation and carries a minimum penalty of $100 per violation and a maximum of $50,000, with an annual penalty limit of $25,000. Category 2 applies where the violation was not due to willful neglect and carries a minimum penalty of $1,000 per violation and a maximum of $50,000, with an annual penalty limit of $100,000. Category 3 applies when the violation results from willful neglect but is remedied within 30 days from the violation's discovery, carrying a minimum penalty of $10,000 per violation, and a maximum of $50,000, with an annual penalty limit of $250,000. Category 4 applies where the violation is due to willful neglect and is not remedied, carrying a minimum penalty of $50,000 per violation, with an annual penalty limit of $1,500,000. OCR is permitted to consider aggravating or mitigating factors in making its determination regarding the monetary penalty amount, including the nature of the violation, the length of time the violation occurred, the harm posed to others, and whether the violation was intentional or could have been avoided, the organization's history of compliance or violations, and the financial stability of the organization.

State Laws Regulating Health Information Privacy

Most states in the US have enacted individual laws regulating health information privacy within their states. These laws vary regarding the scope and degree of protection provided, but state health information privacy laws are generally consistent with the scope of HIPAA.

In California, the PHI privacy and security state law is the California Confidentiality of Medical Information Act (Tex). Under the California Act, it is improper for a healthcare provider, healthcare service plan, or a contractor in connection with a healthcare provider or healthcare service plan to disclose a patient's medical information without the patient's advance, written authorization. There are certain exclusions to the general prohibition on disclosure, including disclosure according to a court order, subpoena, order by an administrative body, or valid search warrant. The California Act further provides for a patient right of access consistent with the requirements of HIPAA.

The Texas Medical Records Privacy Act (Fla, 2021) is Texas's state-based health information privacy law. Under the Texas Act, patients have the right to know the manner their health information will be used. This general requires healthcare providers to provide written notice to patients regarding uses, disclosures, and breaches of their health information. Written consent by the patient is required for the uses of health information outside of uses regarding the provision of health services, payment for health services, or administrative tasks necessary to health services. The Texas Act also provides for a right of access to a patient's health information.

Florida Statute § 456.057 is the primary health information privacy state law in Florida (Pub). The statute prohibits the disclosure of patient health information by healthcare providers absent written consent by the patient. Providers are required to provide patients with copies of their health records upon request by the patient, consistent with the HIPAA right of access provision. Providers in possession of health information are required to implement safeguards to ensure the privacy and security of the information.

In New York, Public Health Law § 4165 is the state-based health information privacy and security law serving as the equivalent to HIPAA (HITECH, 2009). The New York Public Health Law requires providers to maintain the privacy and security of patient health information, including preventing the unauthorized disclosure of health information. Patients are granted a right of access to their health information. Further, written consent by patients is required for disclosure of health information to parties aside from the patient and aside from disclosures within the provider's facility.

State health privacy laws reflect the scope of HIPAA regarding health information privacy and security. While state laws cannot allow for less stringent standards than HIPAA, they may allow for more stringent standards and, therefore, providers should consult the state health privacy laws within their state to ensure compliance.

Health Information Technology for Economic and Clinical Health Act

The Scope of HITECH

The Health Information Technology for Economic and Clinical Health Act ("HITECH") was enacted in 2009. However, HHS did not enact its Final Rule to implement HITECH until 2013 (42 USC, 2009). HITECH is intended to drive forward the use of electronic health technology while providing for privacy and security during this use.

The Final Rule implementing HITECH regulations sought to assimilate the new health information technology requirements

into the existing legal framework created by HIPAA. In support of its goal to encourage the use of electronic health information technology, the Final Rule implemented the "meaningful use program" (Patient Safety, 2005). The meaningful use program provided monetary incentives to healthcare providers to implement EHRs within their practice, including the use of electronic patient files, electronic prescriptions, and administrative data. Note, at the time HITECH was written and promulgated, "meaningful use" was the term identified to ensure proper use of funds for standing up an EHR. That program is no longer in use; therefore, the term "meaningful use" by the Centers for Medicare and Medicaid Services was replaced with "promoting interoperability."

Enhancement of HIPAA Provisions

HITECH also extended the HIPAA privacy and security rules to business associates of covered entities. HITECH enhanced the "risk assessment" and "breach notification" HIPAA requirements. The risk assessment requirement mandates organizations review their data security protocols, prepare cyber threat assessments, and implement a plan of action for ensuring the privacy and security of PHI. Individuals are further provided with a right to obtain their PHI in electronic form, as implemented by the HIPAA Right of Access Rule.

PATIENT SAFETY AND QUALITY IMPROVEMENT ACT

The Patient Safety and Quality Improvement Act and Patient Safety Organizations

The Patient Safety and Quality Improvement Act of 2005 (PSQIA) is federal legislation intended to enhance patient safety by creating a repository of de-identified patient health data for research and review of potential errors during medical care. Participation by health organizations is voluntary.

Under PSQIA, HHS is required to maintain a network of patient safety databases, housing the anonymized medical data collected, and to ensure the database is manageable and accessible to providers for safety and quality purposes. The organizations that create the patient safety databases are referred to as "patient safety organizations."

The network must have the ability to collect, store, and analyze anonymized patient data.

The information stored is intended to be used to analyze statistics and patterns regarding health care patient safety and errors. Patient safety organizations are required to publish annual reports reflecting the conclusions from this analysis.

Protection of Health Information Collected Under PSQIA

The patient data collected and stored pursuant to PSQIA is established under the law as privileged work product for purposes of state or federal litigation and criminal legal matters, subject to exceptions regarding court-ordered disclosures (Public Law, 2008). PSQIA also provides for the privacy and security of the patient data stored under the act. Patient safety organizations may not disclose patient data unless the data has been de-identified and the purpose of the disclosure is in furtherance of patient safety or mitigation of medical errors. Unauthorized disclosures may result in civil monetary penalties.

GENETIC INFORMATION NONDISCRIMINATION ACT

The Scope of GINA

Enacted into law in 2008, the Genetic Information Nondiscrimination Act ("GINA") prohibits discrimination in health insurance coverage and employment based on an individual's genetic information (Public Law, 2008). "Genetic information" is defined under GINA as information about an individual's genetic tests, genetic tests of the individual's family members, genetic tests of any fetus of an individual or family member who is a pregnant woman, and genetic tests of any embryo legally held by an individual or family member utilizing assisted reproductive technology. The manifestation of a disease or disorder in family members, any request for, or receipt of, genetic services, or participation in clinical research that includes genetic services by an individual or family member (Shifrin & Tobin, 2021).

Title I of GINA, prohibits discrimination based on genetic information regarding health insurance. Health insurers and health plan administrators are not permitted to request or require individuals to provide their genetic information. They are not permitted to rely on an individual's genetic information in the decision-making process regarding whether to ensure the individual, set rates on insurance, or establish the insurance terms. Title I provides civil monetary penalties and corrective action in enforcement actions by HHS or the Department of Labor ("DOL").

Title II of GINA pertains to employment and prohibits employers from relying on genetic information in the decision-making process regarding hiring, firing, promoting, or any other decision pertaining to employment. Title II provides a private right of action along with civil monetary penalties and corrective action in enforcement actions by the U.S. Equal Employment Opportunity Commission (EEOC).

Exceptions to the Use of Genetic Information Under GINA

There are three primary exceptions or limitations to GINA's restrictions regarding reliance on genetic information. The "research exception" provides that health plan administrators may request a plan participant take a genetic test for the purpose of research, but the administrator may not require the participant to take part in the genetic testing. To satisfy the research exception, the following elements must be met: (1) the request for testing must be made in writing and not otherwise in violation of applicable state or federal law; (2) the administrator must expressly state that the testing is voluntary and noncompliance will have no impact on the participant's insurance status; (3) the genetic information may not be used for purposes of underwriting; and (4) the health plan must notify HHS in writing that the research will be performed and is permitted under the research exception.

The second major exception of GINA pertains to its scope, in that GINA does not apply regarding life insurance, disability insurance, or long-term care insurance. The final limitation to GINA is that its prohibition on discrimination does not apply to an individual's diagnosis of a health condition or display of symptoms but only applies to discrimination based on genetic information itself.

BIOMETRIC INFORMATION PRIVACY ACTS

Biometric Information Privacy Acts

Comprehensive state laws regulating the collection and use of individuals' biometric information, often referred to as "biometric information privacy acts" (BIPAs), have been gaining interest throughout the United States, and many states have proposed legislation regarding biometric information privacy. BIPAs generally regulate the collection and use of biological data used to identify an individual, referred to as "biometric identifiers," which include fingerprints, facial geometry, retinal and iris scans, and voiceprints (740 ILCS, 2021).

BIPAs are intended to be enforced across all industries within the jurisdictions to which they apply. The acts apply to private individuals, private entities, as well as public or governmental entities. Many concerns and litigation regarding BIPAs have arisen in the employment context as employers seek to use biometric information to increase workplace efficiency as well as for security purposes.

Specific State Legislation Providing Biometric Information Protection

Only three states, Illinois, Texas, and Washington, have passed BIPAs (Davis, 2019). Generally, BIPAs provide that a person may not capture, use, or sell biometric identifiers without the individual's consent. Biometric identifiers that have been lawfully obtained must be stored and maintained with reasonable care. Within a reasonable time after collection and use of lawfully obtained biometric identifiers, the holder is required to destroy the identifiers. Similarly, Illinois' BIPA features a private right of action, but all three permit state attorneys general to enforce violations. Some states, including New York, California, and Arkansas, provide for the protection of biometric information through more general laws, such as consumer protection statutes.

Concern over the capture of biometric information has only grown in recent years, and it can be expected that additional states will soon enact their BIPAs to meet the concerns of their constituents.

CYBERCRIME AND CYBERSECURITY

The Threat of Cybercriminal Activity

Because health information is predominantly stored in electronic form, it can be compromised by cybercriminals (Ingalls, 2021). Cybercrime involving PHI threatens to undermine the level of trust between patients and the health organizations maintaining their information. The growing market for health data ensures health data will be shared with an increasing number of parties, spanning far from the original party with whom the individual's health information was shared—likely, the individual's healthcare provider. This increased sharing leads to a larger threat that the shared data will be compromised through a cyberattack as cybersecurity safeguards and measures will not be uniformly stringent among the multiple actors possessing valuable health data. A brief overview of the various threats cybercriminals employ demonstrates the varied threat posed by cybercrime to the safety of health information.

Phishing is a method of cyber hacking involving e-mails sent to a member of an organization or to several members of an organization that appear to be sent from a credible source (What is keystroke logging and keyloggers, 2021). The hacker who sent the e-mail attempts to induce the recipient to disclose sensitive information regarding the organization, such as login or password information. The hacker may also attempt to lure the member into opening a fraudulent webpage, resulting in the installation of malware onto the organization's computer. *Spear phishing* is a specific form of phishing in which a message is targeted to a specific employee of an organization.

Keylogging refers to the activity of covertly logging a computer user's keystrokes on the computer's keyboard by infecting the target computer (DeMuro, 2016). The user is generally unaware their keystrokes are being logged and, therefore, may willingly be transmitting sensitive information to the hacker.

Ransomware is a type of computer malware designed to extort ransom payments from its targets (HIPAA Journal, 2017). Ransomware acts by infecting a computer, disabling the entire computer, or disabling specific functions of the computer, and presenting a message on the computer screen demanding a ransom payment in exchange for regaining the computer's functionality. Ransomware has taken on many different forms and continues to evolve since its inception.

Healthcare organizations are appealing targets to ransomware hackers. In recent years, the volume of U.S.-based ransomware attacks focusing on the healthcare industry has increased. Healthcare organizations may be appealing to hackers because every minute could be a matter of life and death, and every minute the organization does not have full access to its electronic healthcare information, patients are at risk, increasing the pressure on healthcare organizations to recover access to their systems by paying the ransomware hackers. All healthcare organizations need to be prepared to prevent, protect against, and manage a ransomware attack to ensure the privacy of their patients and others who have entrusted the organization with their data as ransomware attacks increase in frequency.

Denial of service attacks occurs when hackers disrupt an organization's computer systems by flooding them with multiple, unnecessary requests, overwhelming the system. Denial of service hackers often make use of several, internet-connected devices to send the target system unnecessary requests in a coordinated manner. The use of a network of devices in this manner is often referred to as a "botnet."

Malware is a general term referring to software designed to cause damage to a computer system. *Adware* is a specific form of malware designed to automatically generate advertisements for specific companies onto the infected computer. *Spyware* is a form of malware that tracks the information stored onto a computer as well as the computer's activity and transmits the information to an outside source.

Data Breach Litigation

While HIPAA is the primary law in the United States regulating health information privacy, the healthcare industry has been the subject of more class action lawsuits regarding data breaches than any other industry in recent years, utilizing different theories of liability (Mulligan & VonderHaar, 2016). To date, there is no commonly recognized theory of liability to hold healthcare organizations accountable for stolen or jeopardized personal healthcare information (In re Barnes & Noble Pin Pad Litig, 2006).

An often-used theory of liability has been the common law of negligence. The two varieties of negligence theory often used in this context are: (1) the healthcare organization owes a non-delegable duty to protect the health information it holds, and any attack that jeopardizes this information constitutes a breach of that non-delegable duty; and (2) the healthcare organization provided negligent security increasing the risk of a cyberattack.

The first theory of liability is grounded in the same context as a premises liability case, in which a property owner owes a duty of care to those on their property (Hackett, 2015). This theory is often hamstrung by the requirement in negligence cases requiring foreseeable and actual harm. Cases brought under this theory often fail because it is difficult or impossible to determine what damage has been sustained by a healthcare consumer whose private health information has been jeopardized.

The second negligence theory is more akin to a negligent security theory, under which the healthcare organization is viewed as having a duty to provide adequate security in protecting private health information, and a hack that jeopardizes this information can be the basis of negligence suit. This theory has found traction in the recent "Ashley Madison" case (Krebs, 2015). Ashley Madison is the name of a company hosting a website for adults committing marital infidelity (Kravets, 2017). Hackers were able to breach the company's servers and threatened to leak users' information unless the site was shut down. Ashley Madison refused, and the hackers released the private information of approximately 32 million users. Users whose information had been released sued Ashley Madison under several theories, including a negligence theory, and pled to negligent data security. The case survived several legal hurdles and resulted in a settlement between the affected consumers and Ashley Madison for $11.2 million. While this theory of negligence has been tested, it is still unclear if it will be accepted by most courts in the cyber breach context.

It is also worth noting that, while there is no federal legislative scheme for cyber-liability in hacking cases, California has passed such a law, specifically in the private health information context, based on breach of privacy, called the Confidentiality of Medical Information Act. Similarly, common law causes of action based on invasion of privacy may also present valid remedies to consumers whose health information has been put at risk by hackers.

Cybersecurity Methods to Prevent and Mitigate Cyberthreats

The techniques hackers use to compromise sensitive data, including health data, are constantly evolving. A strong cybersecurity framework and consistent anti-hacking practices can reduce the risk of cybercrime.

Backing up all electronic data to a secured backup location can prevent a terrible situation from becoming a nightmare. A healthcare organization with a secured, isolated backup at a remote location can restore its computer systems in approximately four hours. Those backups should be tested and assessed annually to ensure that they can protect against a cyber threat. Once a computer is infected with a virus, the virus can move between computers using the same network, which is why it is imperative to store backup data outside of the original network to ensure it also would not be exposed to the virus. External backups can be stored in a cloud-based system or stored in physical form.

Not every healthcare organization staff member requires access to the organization's shared network to perform their tasks, and, therefore, access to the network can be limited based on priority. Administrative access to shared networks should only be granted if necessary and limiting the use of access can reduce the window of opportunity that a ransomware hacker has to infiltrate the network. Access controls can also be used to limit the files a user can access, thus controlling the potential danger zones a user can access.

Some versions of cyber viruses require an authorized computer user to open a malicious email called *phishing e-mails*. These e-mails only pose a threat if they are opened by an employee. While training and awareness programs can be effective at reducing the risk of an employee opening these false emails, some hackers are very skilled at making the emails appear authentic and important. Along with a prevention training program, healthcare organizations should take efforts to ensure these emails never reach their employees in the first place. Spam filters can be enabled to detect these malicious emails, and authentication technologies are available to detect emails being sent from unknown locations. System administrators should also monitor inbound and outbound emails for suspicious activity.

Although not all versions of a cyber virus depend on human action, many versions infect computers by deceiving computer users into clicking links or opening emails. One of the simplest preventive steps a healthcare organization can take to defend itself from a hacking attack is to inform its personnel of the risk posed by malicious cyber viruses. Common methods by which viruses are used to infect computers; and actions to avoid while using a healthcare server are clicking on advertisements, browsing unnecessary websites, or opening e-mails that seem suspicious. A training and awareness program regarding the threats of hacking, along with periodic reminders, can go a long way toward preventing an attack.

The risks of certain malware that operates by taking advantage of a network's existing vulnerabilities can be mitigated by employing a *patch management system* to detect and prevent holes in the system's network. Other more common methods of defending computer systems include setting up firewalls that block unknown IP addresses and ensuring anti-virus and anti-malware settings are set to scan for threats.

INTERNATIONAL INFORMATION PRIVACY AND SECURITY ACTS

Data privacy laws currently exist in most nations worldwide. Most national data privacy laws provide for the protection of health information as well as other forms of sensitive information. A brief survey of select nations illustrates the commonality of issues and solutions identified by lawmakers approaching data privacy regulation.

The European Union

The General Data Privacy Regulation (GDPR) is a regulation passed by the EU in 2016 (GDPR, 2016). More than any other national data privacy law, the GDPR has served as a model data privacy law for other nations. The GDPR applies to all EU member states, and many EU member states have passed their own data privacy laws implementing the GDPR.

Under the GDPR, organizations maintaining personal health information must inform patients of the organization's use of the patient's information and may only use such information for a legitimate purpose. Organizations may only retain health information until its purpose is completed and may only use the health information necessary to complete its purpose.

Patients have the right to know what information is being used and the purpose for the use, as well as to amend incorrect information. Informed consent from the patient is required if their health information will be used by the organization outside of its original purpose.

The GDPR also contains several information security provisions. Organizations must establish minimum, documented procedures to safeguard the health information in their possession. Information security trainings are also required to be conducted by the organization for any employees maintaining the information. It is recommended, under the GDPR, that organizations assign a data protection officer, whose role it is to oversee the organization's compliance with the GDPR and to ensure the security of the stored information. The GDPR also features breach notification provisions, requiring an organization to notify those negatively impacted by an information security breach within 72 hours.

Information-sharing by the organization with third parties is permitted under the GDPR. However, the sharing organization retains responsibility for any compromise of the shared information and is further responsible for ensuring the third party complies with the GDPR in relation to the shared information.

The "right to be forgotten" is featured in Article 17 of the GDPR and provides that health organizations must erase any health information in their possession upon the individual's request if the purpose for which the organization held the information has been accomplished. The organization only used the information for marketing purposes, or if the organization only used the individual's information subject to the individual's consent, that consent has now been revoked.

Canada

In Canada, the Personal Information Protection and Electronic Documents Act (PIPEDA) is the primary health data protection law applying to Canada (Canada, 2021). PIPEDA applies to Canadian organizations maintaining, collecting, and using personal information, including personal health information.

The provinces of Alberta, British Columbia, Labrador, New Brunswick, Newfoundland, Nova Scotia, and Quebec have their own privacy laws as well, which are substantially similar to PIPEDA. Organizations with similar privacy laws are exempt from PIPEDA regarding the maintenance, storage, and use of health information within a specific province.

PIPEDA generally requires organizations in possession of patients' health information to abide by ten equitable principles regarding the organization's handling of the health information.

The principle of Accountability requires organizations to appoint an information privacy official responsible for the organization's compliance with PIPEDA and for maintenance. The organization must further maintain the health information in its possession and implement reasonable measures to protect the information in its possession.

The principle of Identifying Purposes requires organizations to identify the purposes for the organization's collection and use of a patient's personal health information. If the organization seeks to fulfill a new purpose, it is required to obtain the patient's consent to the new purpose.

The principle of Consent requires the organization to obtain informed consent from the patient upon collecting, using, and disclosing the patient's personal health information. Consent can be withdrawn by the patient at any point in time. There is not a strict rule under PIPEDA regarding the form of consent, but instead the form of consent should be commensurate with the sensitivity of the information or transaction involved.

The principle of Limiting Collection requires organizations only to collect the amount of patient health information that is necessary for the organization to fulfill its consented-to purpose. It is further required that organizations only collect information using legitimate, lawful methods.

The principle of Limiting Use, Disclosure, and Retention, similar to the previous principle, requires organizations to limit the information used, disclosed, and retained only to the extent necessary to fulfill its stated purpose. The organization must also be capable of explaining the reasoning behind its use, disclosure, and retention of health information.

The principle of Accuracy requires organizations to make reasonable efforts to ensure the patient health information in its information is accurate and current. The organization is recommended to implement policies regarding regularly updating certain categories of information.

The principle of Safeguards requires organizations to put into practice security policies designed to protect patient health information. These policies are required to be regularly reviewed and updated. Employees accessing health information must be trained and made aware of the organization's safeguard policies. The level of protection offered by an organization's safeguards should be commensurate with the value, sensitivity, and risk posed to the information in the organization's possession.

The following principle, Openness, requires organizations to make their information management and privacy policies available to the general public, clear, and reasonably understandable.

The principle of Individual Access grants individuals the right to access their health information in possession of an organization. The organization must respond to patient requests to access their information within thirty days upon receipt of the patient's request. This thirty-day limit may only be extended in circumstances under which it would be unreasonable for the organization to respond within 30 days. In addition to patient information itself, the organization must also disclose how a patient's information has been used by the organization. This principle also gives patients the right to have their information amended for accuracy.

The final principle, that of Challenging Compliance, gives individuals the right to challenge an organization's Compliance with PIPEDA. A successful challenge alleging an organization has failed to comply with the PIPEDA principles will require the organization to come into PIPEDA compliance. Organizations must have procedures regarding the handling of PIPEDA compliance challenges.

Brazil

On August 14, 2018, Brazil passed its signature legislation providing for the protection of individual data, including health data. The Lei Geral de Protecao de Dados (LGPD) was modeled after the GDPR and defines personal data to include health, genetic, and biometric data (Federative Republic of Brazil, 2018).

The LGPD provides 10 bases for which and organization may collect health data, which includes collecting data with the consent of the individual. Consent to the collection of an individual's health data must be informed and provided in writing. An individual's consent to the collection and use of their health data must provide for the purpose of the collection and the permitted uses of the individual's health data. The organization must remain within the permitted purpose and permitted use to which the individual gave their consent. The individual has the right to revoke their consent at any point in time.

The individual has the right to access their health information upon request and may also request that the organization cease using their health information even if the organization remains within the permitted use of the information. The LGPD also provides requirements for the security of health information in possession of organizations. Organizations are required to adopt reasonable security measures to protect an individual's personal health information. Further, organizations are required to notify an individual if their health information has been compromised. Organizations must also notify the regulatory agency tasked with enforcing the LGPD of any comprises of personal health information.

Mexico

Mexico has recognized the privacy of personal data as a constitutional, fundamental right. In 2010, Mexico passed the Federal Law on Protection of Personal Data Held by Private Parties (United Mexican States, 2010). In 2013, the National Institute for Access to Information and Protection of Personal Data (INAI) issued the Guidelines on Privacy Notices, establishing the primary information privacy framework applicable to health information in Mexico.

Under the guidelines, an organization must obtain a patient's written, informed consent before possessing their health information. Certain exceptions apply to the consent rule, such as in situations where consent cannot be given due to the health condition of the patient and medical care is necessary to prevent additional harm.

Generally, an organization is bound by the principles of legality, consent, quality, loyalty, proportionality, and accountability in its obligations to maintain a patient's personal health information. Organizations are required to implement security measures intended to safeguard personal health information from loss, unauthorized use, or unauthorized access. Further, organizations must only use health information in accordance with the purpose stipulated by the patient and the information may be altered or destroyed at the direction of the patient. Patient health information may only be possessed by an organization for as long as necessary to fulfill its stated purpose.

The guidelines permit transfers of health information to third parties. Transfers of health information require the execution of data transfer agreements. Further, the informed consent of the patient must be granted as well.

Organizations maintaining health information are required to appoint a data protection officer. The data protection officer is tasked with ensuring the organization's compliance with the guidelines, ensuring the protection of health information, and responding to patient inquiries regarding their information.

The guidelines provide for a breach notification requirement. Organizations maintaining health information are required to disclose, immediately, the existence of any breach, unauthorized disclosure, or unauthorized use of a patient's health information to the patient. The nature of the incident, the information at risk, recommendations, remedial actions, and a method of obtaining additional information must, at a minimum, be included in the organization's disclosure.

Japan

Japan passed one of the earliest privacy laws in Asia. Passed in 2003, the Act on the Protection of Personal Information (APPI) is Japan's primary personal health data privacy law (Japan, 2003). It has been amended and enhanced in recent years to keep pace with technological developments. The recent changes make the APPI more like the GDPR.

Like the GDPR, the APPI requires the individual's informed consent prior to the collection and use of personal health information. Personal health information may only be transferred to third parties upon the organization's obtaining written, informed consent from the individual. As with most data privacy laws, the organization is only permitted to obtain a reasonable amount of information to further the organization's proper purpose, and the individual has the right to access, amend, or supplement its data.

The APPI established a Personal Information Protection Commission (PPC), the governing authority regarding data protection in Japan. The APPI contains breach notification provisions, under which an organization in possession of personal health information must notify the PPC and the individual involved, in the event of a compromise or breach of personal health information.

Organizations are required to maintain the security of personal health information. The APPI requires reasonable steps be taken to ensure the accuracy, security, privacy, and supervision of personal health information. Unlike other data privacy laws, the APPI does not require the appointment of a data protection officer. Organizations are tasked with ensuring their own compliance with the APPI and for maintaining the security and privacy of the health data in their possession. Even though the APPI does not require the appointment of a data protection officer per se, the APPI does require organizations to name an individual who will control the personal health information in their possession of the organization.

Importantly, the more recent amendments to the APPI allow organizations to avoid many of the individual rights provisions of the APPI if the organizations anonymize the health data in their possession to the extent that the data cannot reasonably be traced to the individual. This provision was not part of the original APPI.

China

On November 6, 2016, China passed its Cybersecurity Law of the People's Republic of China ("PRC"), which became effective in June 2017 (People's Republic of China, 2016). The Cybersecurity Law is broad in scope, applying to personal information, information regarding the country's critical infrastructure, and the cross-border transfer of information.

Organizations maintaining personal information are prohibited from disclosing, altering, or destroying personal information in their possession without the authorization of the individual whose personal information has been collected. Individuals have the right to request their information be amended, deleted, or released to them. An individual's informed consent is needed to allow an organization to disclose the individual's information to a third party. It should be noted, however, that these privacy and consent provisions do not apply where the organization has de-identified the individual's personal information. The PRC Cybersecurity Law establishes a breach notification requirement where personal information has been improperly disclosed or improperly accessed by an unauthorized third party. The Cybersecurity Law further establishes a penalty structure for non-compliant organizations. Penalties are assessed by regulatory agencies and range from monetary penalties to licensure suspension.

On August 20, 2021, the PRC passed new, sweeping information privacy and security law, the Personal Information Protection Law (PIPL). The PIPL's new text has not been released at the time of this writing but is scheduled to enter into effect on November 1, 2021. Organizations in noncompliance with the PIPL at that time will be penalized for noncompliance. While the full text of the PIPL remains to be seen, the law is intended to serve as the primary data protection law in the PRC.

CONCLUSION AND FUTURE DIRECTIONS

Confidentiality, integrity, and availability are critical to patient care and for improving outcomes. Practitioners and patients need to be confident that patient data are accurate and accessible when needed.

Given record privacy breaches in recent years, the need for information security will continue to be an urgent topic in the future. Currently the healthcare system is heavily dependent on legislation and regulations to ensure health information privacy, confidentiality, and security. However, this approach presents its own set of problems. Innovations in technology constantly offer the opportunity to improve healthcare delivery. However, until these innovations are available and in use, it is impossible to develop legislation or regulation ensuring their adherence to ethical principles. Thus, safeguards can lag behind innovations. Legislative attempts to prevent these irresponsible behaviors can act to limit the development of new and innovative approaches to improve healthcare delivery. Health informaticians can play a vital role in the development of responsible legislation that limits market development as little as possible, but first need a solid grounding in the concepts and solutions for these important principles.

ACKNOWLEDGMENTS

The authors wish to acknowledge the contributions of David L. Gibbs, Nancy Staggers, Ramona Nelson, and Angel Hoffman to the previous edition of this chapter.

DISCUSSION QUESTIONS

1. Hospitals usually have policies and related procedures for responding when patients request a copy of their records. Select a procedure from your current place of employment or a local hospital. Compare and contrast the selected procedure with the requirements of the HIPAA Right of Access Rule and with the principles of FIPs.
2. What are the challenges and resources for creating an agreement to share health data across the borders of countries near you (e.g., Canada and the United States or Mexico and the United States)?
3. Providing access to healthcare providers and securing a system from inappropriate access can be a difficult balancing act. In many cases, the more secure a system is, the more restricted access to that system becomes. Discuss situations where this balancing act has created conflict or might create conflict within the clinical area and how that conflict was (or could be) managed.
4. Increasingly, patients are creating and maintaining PHRs with data from a variety of healthcare providers, as well as data they have generated about their health. What provisions should be included in the model privacy and security policy that patients might use in making decisions related to their privacy and the security of their PHRs?

CASE STUDY

Last month, you were hired with the title *Health Informatics Privacy and Security Specialist* at an independent community care hospital with 350 beds. The hospital includes a comprehensive outpatient clinic, a rehabilitation center with both inpatient and outpatient services, a cardiac care center, and an emergency room. In addition, four family health centers are located throughout the community. More than 930 primary care and specialty physicians are associated with the hospital, which has a staff of just over 2000 employees. The hospital has an EHR in place.

The hospital has a working relationship with a major academic medical center located 23 miles away. Acute care patients who need more extensive treatment are usually transferred to the medical center. These are often emergency situations, and data are freely shared among the institutions with the best interests of the patient in mind.

Located directly beside the hospital is a 194-bed skilled nursing home. While the nursing home has its own medical staff consisting of a physician and two nurse practitioners, patients needing consults or additional care are usually seen at the hospital with follow-up at physicians' offices. While the nursing home, most physicians' offices, and the hospital are independent institutions, there is a long history of sharing health-related data when treating patients who live at the nursing home and are seen at the hospital or in the physicians' offices. This coordination is seen as a general benefit for many patients. It appears that most patients have signed a form giving the hospital permission to send information to the nursing home. However, these forms have been stored in individual offices, so it is difficult to determine who has signed what forms and what permission has or has not been given to share information among the nursing home, hospital, and independent medical practices.

DISCUSSION QUESTIONS

1. What additional information is needed to clarify what problems may exist and what changes may be needed in terms of data that are shared among the institutions?
2. Can the EHR system and/or email be used to share data among these different institutions more effectively and securely?

If yes, how would this be done? For example, what agreements, policies, and procedures might need to be developed?
3. In your position as Health Informatics Specialist, how would you go about determining whether there are other potential security issues that now need to be managed by the hospital?

REFERENCES

Canada, *Personal Information Protection and Electronic Documents Act, SC* 2000, c 5. Available at: https://canlii.ca/t/541b8. Accessed August 2, 2021.

Case C-131/12, *Google Spain SL v. Agencia Espanola de Proteccion de Datos* (May 13, 2014), http://curia.europa.eu/juris/document/document.jsf?text=&docid=152065&doclang=EN [http://perma.cc/ED5L-DZRK].

Davis, J. *Third-party vendors behind 20% of healthcare data breaches in 2018*, Health IT Security, Available at: https://healthitsecurity.com/news/third-party-vendors-behind-20-of-healthcare-data-breaches-in-2018. Accessed. April 15, 2019.

Department of Health & Human Services, *Enforcement process*, https://www.hhs.gov/hipaa/for-professionals/compliance-enforcement/enforcement-process/index.html. Accessed August 2, 2021.

DeMuro, P.R. Keeping internet pirates at bay: Ransomware negotiation in the healthcare industry, 41 Nova Law Review 347, 352 (2017); 10-Minute Guide to Healthcare Ransomware Protection, XTIUM 2. Available at: http://www.xtium.com/beta/wp-content/uploads/2016/07/Xtium_10-Minute-Guide-to-Ransomware-Protection.pdf. Accessed August 2, 2021.

Dunbrack, L. (2016). IDC Health Insights, Providing Outside-In and Inside-Out Protection Against Ransomware and Other Intensifying Cyberthreats 2.

EU General Data Protection Regulation (GDPR): Regulation (EU) 2016/679 of the European Parliament and of the Council of 27 April 2016 on the protection of natural persons with regard to the processing of personal data and on the free movement of such data, and repealing Directive 95/46/EC (General Data Protection Regulation), OJ 2016 L 119/1.

EU General Data Protection Regulation (GDPR): Regulation (EU) 2016/679 of the European Parliament and of the Council of 27 April 2016 on the protection of natural persons with regard to the processing of personal data and on the free movement of such data, and repealing Directive 95/46/EC (General Data Protection Regulation), OJ 2016a L 119/1.

Federative Republic of Brazil. (2018). *Lei Geral de Protecao de Dados.*

Hackett, R. *What to know about the Ashley Madison Hack.* Fortune.com. http://fortune.com/2015/08/26/ashley-madison-hack/. Accessed August 26, 2015.

HIPAA Journal. (2017, September 13). *Healthcare Industry Tops List for Class Action Data Breach Lawsuits.* https://www.hipaajournal.com/healthcare-industry-tops-list-class-action-data-breach-lawsuits-8963/.

HITECH Act § 13410, Pub. L No. 111-5, 123 Stat. 226 (2009).

HHS. *What OCR considers during intake & review.* https://www.hhs.gov/hipaa/for-professionals/compliance-enforcement/examples/what-ocr-considers-during-intake-and-review/index.html.

Ingalls, S. *Types of malware & best malware protection practices*, eSecurity Planet. Available at: https://www.csecurityplanet.com/threats/malware-types/#phishing. Accessed February 16, 2021.

In re Barnes & Noble Pin Pad Litig., No. 12-cv-8617, 2013 WL 4759588, at *5 (ND Ill. September 3, 2013); Reilly v. Ceridian Corp., 664 F.3d 38, 42 (3d Cir. 2011); Forbes v. Wells Fargo Bank, 420 F. Supp. 2d 1018, 1020-21 (D. Minn. 2006); Bell v. Acxiom Corp., No. 4:06CV00485-WRW, 2006 WL 2850042, at *2 (ED Ark. October 3, 2006).

Japan, *The act on the protection of personal information*, 2003. Available at: https://www.cas.go.jp/jp/seisaku/hourei/data/APPI.pdf. Accessed August 2, 2021.

Kravets, D. *Lawyers score big in settlement for Ashley Madison cheating site data breach.* ARS Technica https://arstechnica.com/tech-policy/2017/07/sssshhh-claim-your-19-from-ashley-madison-class-action-settlement/. Accessed July 17, 2017.

Krebs, B. *Online cheating site Ashley Madison hacked.* Krebs On Security. http://krebsonsecurity.com/2015/07/online-cheating-site-ashleymadison-hacked/. Accessed July 15, 2015.

Miles, S. H. (2004). *The hippocratic oath and the ethics of medicine.* Oxford; New York: Oxford University Press.

Murray, B. (2012). Informed consent: What must a physician disclose to a patient? *AMA Journal of Ethics.* Available at: https://journalofethics.ama-assn.org/article/informed-consent-what-must-physician-disclose-patient/2012-07#:~:text=If%20disclosure%20is%20likely%20to,to%20refuse%20a%20specific%20treatment.

Mulligan, J., & VonderHaar, M. (2016). Health hackers: Questioning the sufficiency of remedies when medical information is compromised. *Health Law, 29*(1), 29–31.

Neuhaus, C., Polze, A., & Chowdhuryy, M. (2011). *Survey on health care IT systems: Standards, regulation and security.* Potsdam, NY: Potsdam University.

Patient Safety and Quality Improvement Act of 2005, Pub. L. No. 109-41, §§ 921-26, 119 Stat. 424 (2005).

People's Republic of China. (2016). *Cybersecurity Law of the People's Republic of China.*

Privacy Policy Guidance. The fair information practice principles: framework for privacy policy at the Department of Homeland Security. Available at: http://www.dhs.gov/xlibrary/assets/privacy/privacy_policyguide_2008-01.pdf. Accessed August 2, 2021.

Public Law 110-233—Genetic Information Nondiscrimination Act of 2008.

Public Law 110-233—Genetic Information Nondiscrimination Act of 2008, Title I(d)(6).

Schloendroff v. *Society of New York Hospital*, 211 NY 125 (1914).

Shifrin, D., & Tobin, M.B. Past, present and future: What's happening with Illinois' and other biometric privacy laws. *The National Law Review, XI*(289). Available at: https://www.natlawreview.com/article/past-present-and-future-what-s-happening-illinois-and-other-biometric-privacy-laws. Accessed August 2, 2021.

The Health Insurance Portability and Accountability Act of 1996. Pub. L. 104-191. Stat. 1936. Web. August 11, 2014.

United Mexican States, *Federal Law on Protection of Personal Data held by individuals (LFPDPPP)*, 2010.

What is keystroke logging and keyloggers, Kaspersky (Accessed: August 5, 2021), Available at: https://usa.kaspersky.com/resource-center/definitions/keylogger.

45 CFR Part 160 and Subparts A and E of Part 164.

45 CFR Part 160 and Subparts A and C of Part 164.

45 CFR §§ 164.400-414.

45 CFR §§ 164.402.

45 CFR §§ 164.524.

45 CFR § 160.312.

Cal. Civ. Code § 56.

Tex. Health & Safety Code § 181.001-207.

Fla. Stat. § 456.057 (2021).

NY Pub. Health Law § 4165; 10 NYCRR § 405.10.

42 USC sec 139w-4(0)(2) (2009), sec 13301, subtitle B: Incentives for the Use of Health Information Technology.

740 ILCS § 14 (2021); Tex. Bus. Com. Code § 503.001 (2021); RCWA § 19375 (2021).

29

HITECH and MACRA

Jonathan M. Ishee and Amanda Ray

OBJECTIVES

At the completion of this chapter, the reader will be prepared to:
1. Describe the purpose of the Interoperability and Patient Access and explain its main provisions.
2. Summarize efforts to access and exchange of health information.

KEY TERMS

information blocking, 459

interoperability programs, 459

ABSTRACT ❖

Healthcare reform legislation continues to evolve to improve the health of Americans. Previous legislation led to the financing of health information systems to create a digital ecosystem to facilitate the provision and financing of healthcare. This chapter will provide information related to the continued improvement of health access, management, and finances.

PROMOTING INTEROPERABILITY AND INTRODUCTION

In 2011, Centers of Medicare and Medicaid Services (CMS) established the Medicare and Medicaid electronic health record (EHR) Incentive Programs (now known as the Promoting Interoperability Programs) to encourage eligible medical practitioners, eligible hospitals, and critical access hospitals (CAHs) to adopt, implement, upgrade, and demonstrate meaningful use of certified electronic health record technology (CEHRT) (The Centers for Medicare & Medicaid Services CMS, 2022). Since then, CMS EHR Incentive Programs have evolved into Promoting Interoperability, through Medicare Access and CHIP Reauthorization Act (MACRA), Merit-based Incentive Payment System (MIPS), and its most recently enacted Information Blocking Rule. Table 29.1, Promoting Interoperability Programs Milestones, provides an overview of the stages to establish data sharing within systems.

Medicare Access and CHIP Reauthorization Act

The Medicare Access and CHIP Reauthorization Act of 2015 (MACRA) established the Quality Payment Program to reward eligible clinicians who provide higher-value care. Clinicians took part in the Quality Payment Program in one of two ways: (1) the MIPS and (2) Advanced Alternative Payment Models (Advanced APMs). In MIPS, the Promoting Interoperability category focuses on meaningful use of certified EHR technology, while Advanced APMs include their own requirements for participants to use certified EHR technology. Table 29.2, MACRA Payment Programs: MIPS and APMs, describes the revised healthcare payment legislation.

In addition to the Quality Payment Program, the nature and extent of information blocking has come into focus in recent years. In 2015, at the request of the Congress requested, the Office of the National Coordinator for Health Information (ONC) observed that prevailing market conditions created incentives for some individuals and entities to exercise control over electronic health information in ways that limit its availability and use. ONC and other divisions of the U.S Department of Health and Human Services (HHS) made intense efforts and strides to prevent adverse incentives that remain and continue to undermine progress toward a more connected health system. Based on economic realities and first-hand experience working with the health IT industry and stakeholders, the ONC concluded in its 2015 "Information Blocking Congressional Report," that information blocking was a serious problem and recommended that the Congress prohibit information blocking and provide penalties and enforcement mechanism to deter harmful practices (Fig. 29.1) (The Office of the National Coordinator for Health Information Technology, 2015).

TABLE 29.1   Promoting Interoperability Programs Milestones

In 2011, CMS established the Medicare and Medicaid EHR Incentive Programs (now known as the Promoting Interoperability Programs) to encourage EPs, eligible hospitals, and CAHs to adopt, implement, upgrade, and demonstrate meaningful use of certified electronic health record technology (CEHRT)	
Stage 1	Stage 1 set the foundation for the Promoting Interoperability Programs by establishing requirements for the electronic capture of clinical data, including providing patients with electronic copies of health information.
Stage 2	Stage 2 expanded upon the Stage 1 criteria with a focus on advancing clinical processes and ensuring that the meaningful use of EHRs supported the aims and priorities of the National Quality Strategy. Stage 2 criteria encouraged the use of CEHRT for continuous quality improvement at the point of care and the exchange of information in the most structured format possible.
Stage 3	In October 2015, CMS released a final rule that established Stage 3 in 2017 and beyond, which focused on using CEHRT to improve health outcomes. In addition, this rule modified Stage 2 to ease reporting requirements and align with other CMS programs (85 FR 25584).

TABLE 29.2   MACRA Payment Programs: MIPS and APMs

Merit-Based Incentive Payment Systems (MIPs)	• Incentivized providers to focus on "meaningful use" of Certified EHR technology (or, referred to as the "Medicare EHR Incentive Program." • Clinicians were expected to (1) demonstrate "meaningful use", use certified EHR technology, (3) and comply with privacy and security Federal laws to receive incentive payments (The American Medical Association, 2022).
Advanced Alternative Payment Models (APMs)	• In addition to meaningful use, required additional EHR technology requirements for participants • Another track providers could pursue to engage in high-quality, coordinated care. • Purpose to meet targets for the use of certified health information technology; no two APMs have the same requirements (HealthIT.gov, 2019).

Individuals' Perceptions of the Privacy and Security of Medical Records and Health Information Exchange

A majority of individuals are confident their medical records are safe from unauthorized viewing, but have concerns when health information is electronically exchanged

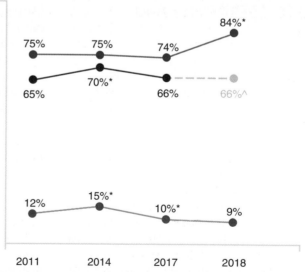

Fig. 29.1 Many individuals (84%) are confident their medical records are safe from unauthorized viewing but have concerns (66%) when health information is electronically exchanged. More individuals are now confident their records are safe from unauthorized viewing, compared to 2017. Less than ten percent of individuals reported withholding information from their healthcare provider due to privacy and security concerns regarding their medical record. This is down from 15% of individuals in 2014. Source: Office of the National Coordinator for Health Information Technology. (2019, June). "Individuals perceptions of the privacy and security of medical records and health information exchange" Health IT Quick-Stat #58. https://www.healthit.gov/data/quickstats/individuals-perceptions-privacy-and-security-medical-records-and-health.

TABLE 29.3   The ONC's Comprehensive Approach to Deter Information Blocking

Point 1:	Continue public and private sector collaboration to develop and drive the consistent use of standards and standards-based technologies that enable interoperability.
Point 2:	Establish effective rules and mechanisms of engagement and governance for electronic health information exchange.
Point 3:	Foster a business, clinical, cultural, and regulatory environment that is conducive to the exchange of electronic health information for improved healthcare quality and efficiency.
Point 4:	Clarify requirements and expectations for secure and trusted exchange of electronic health information, consistent with privacy protections and individuals' preferences, across states, networks, and entities (HealthIT.gov, 2019).

Notably, in the ONC's Information Blocking Congressional Report, the ONC argued a need for a more comprehensive approach to address targeted actions to deter and remedy information blocking as well as boarder strategies to address the larger context in which information blocking occurs (The Office of the National Coordinator for Health Information Technology, 2015). The ONC identified that the following policy actions should be considered to address broad challenges, noted in Table 29.3, that prevent and impede progress toward information sharing and systematic barriers to interoperability and health information exchange.

Years after the ONC's Informational Blocking Congressional Report, ONC and CMS enactment of the Information Blocking Rule addressed overarching policy concerns by implementing standards and accompanying policies requiring and/or encouraging the implementation of technical safeguards to prevent information blocking, while promoting patient data integration and uploading the integrity of data privacy and security.

The ONC primarily achieve this in its Final Rule by adopting Application Programming Interfaces (APIs) to improve the electronic exchange of healthcare data, optimizing interoperability, and managing information flow using a standardized application programming format. Through API, the ONC and CMS hope that sharing information with patients or exchanging information between a payer and provider or between two payers allowing information to be shared in a safe and less restrictive format. APIs will also allow patients to connect to mobile apps or to a provider EHR or practice management system to enable a more seamless method of exchanging information.

Information Blocking Rule Summary

The 21st Century Cures Act, enacted by Congress on March 9, 2020, allowed HHS and CMS to enact its own Final Rule, the CMS Interoperability and Patient Access Rule and (referred to herein as the "Information Blocking Rule"). The ONC issued a Final Rule, the ONC's Cures Act Final Rule, to advance interoperability by guaranteeing that patients have access to their own electronic health information (85 FR 25510-25640).

The Information Blocking Rule formed several initiatives to prevent a practice known as "information blocking," by removing information access barriers and empowering patients to access their electronic health information. "Information blocking" is the interference with, prevention of, or materially discouragement of access, exchange or use of electronic health information and can occur in many forms. For example, physicians can experience information blocking when trying to access patient records from other providers, connecting their EHR systems to local health information exchanges (HIEs), migrating from one EHR to another, and linking their EHRs with a clinical data registry. Patients can also experience information blocking when trying to access their medical records or when sending their records to another provider (Fig. 29.2).

Specifically, the Information Blocking Rule creates and implements new mechanisms and standards, for healthcare software developers, healthcare providers, and healthcare insurers to enable patients to access their own healthcare information through third-party software applications, so they can decide how, when, and with whom to share their information. The Information Blocking Rule was adopted on May 1, 2020 and requires all requirements and implementations to be made by either January 1, 2021 or January 2022. The Information Blocking Rule applies to Medicare Advantage (MA) organizations, Medicaid Fee-for-Service ("FFS") plans, Medicaid managed care plans, Children Health Insurance Plan (CHIP) managed care plans, CHIP FFS programs, QHP issuers of FFEs (collectively referred to herein as (applicable health plans); healthcare providers, such as hospitals, and healthcare IT or software developers. Table 29.4 provides definitions incorporated into the final rule.

Information Blocking Rule Provisions

Requirements for Health Insurers—Qualified Health Plan (QHPs), at a minimum, must make available Patient Access API including, adjudicated claims information; including provider remittances and enrollee cost-sharing, encounters with capitated providers and clinical data, including laboratory results (when maintained by the impacted payer). Data must be made available no longer than one (1) business day after a claim is adjudicated or encounter data is received.

Requirements for a Provider Directory API—Applicable health plans are required to maintain standardized information about their provider networks and make them available to patients through a Provider Directory API. Provider Directory API's must meet the following requirements:

i. Be accessible via a public-facing digital endpoint on the payer's website to ensure public discovery and access.

ii. Make available provider names, addresses, phone numbers, and specialties.

iii. Make available, at a minimum, pharmacy directory data, including the pharmacy name, address, phone number, number of pharmacies in the network, and mix (specifically the type of pharmacy, such as "retail pharmacy").[a]

---

[a]This requirement is for MA organizations that offer MA–PD plans.

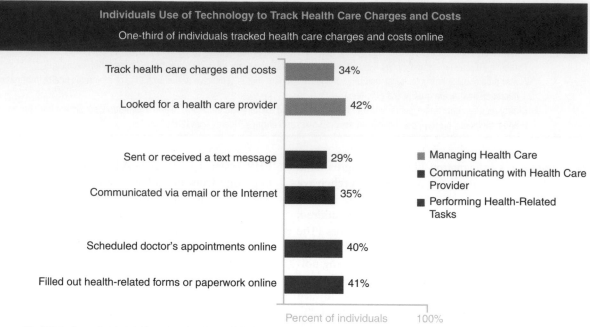

Individuals Use of Technology to Track Health Care Charges and Costs

One-third of individuals tracked health care charges and costs online

Track health care charges and costs — 34%

Looked for a health care provider — 42%

Sent or received a text message — 29%

Communicated via email or the Internet — 35%

Scheduled doctor's appointments online — 40%

Filled out health-related forms or paperwork online — 41%

■ Managing Health Care
■ Communicating with Health Care Provider
■ Performing Health-Related Tasks

Percent of individuals   100%

Fig. 29.2 Overall, 1 in 3 individuals tracked healthcare charges and costs with a computer, smartphone, or other electronic means in the past 12 months. About 4 in 10 individuals filled out paperwork related to their healthcare or made healthcare appointments online. Over one-third communicated with their provider online, while 3 in 10 individuals communicated with their healthcare provider via text message Just over 4 in 10 individuals looked for a healthcare provider online. From Office of the National Coordinator for Health Information Technology. (2018, April). "Individuals use of technology to track health care charges and costs" Health IT Quick-Stat #57. https://www.healthit.gov/data/quickstats/individuals-use-technology-track-health-care-charges-and-costs.

TABLE 29.4   Key Final Rule Definitions

"API"s	Application Programming Interface.
"Interoperability"	means with respect to health IT, means such health IT that enables the secure exchange of electronic health information with, and use of electronic health information from, other health IT without special effort on the part of the user; allows for complete access, exchange, and use of all electronically accessible health information for authorized use under applicable state or federal law; and does not constitute information blocking as defined in section 3022(a) of the PHSA, which was added by section 4004 of the Cures Act.
"Information Blocking"	**What:** In general, information blocking is a practice by a health IT developer of certified health IT, health information network, health information exchange, or healthcare provider that, except as required by law or specified by the Secretary of Health and Human Services (HHS) as a reasonable and necessary activity, is likely to interfere with access, exchange, or use of electronic health information (EHI)
	Who: Applies to applies to healthcare providers, health IT developers, exchanges, and networks (85 FR 25575).

---

iv. Make all directory information available to current and prospective enrollees and the public through the Provider Directory API within 30 calendar days of a payer receiving provider directory information or an update to the provider directory.

v. Meet technical safeguards codified at 45 C.F.R. 170.215.

Payer-to-Payer Data Exchange

The Final Rule requires applicable health plans to coordinate care between payers by exchanging, at a minimum, United States Core Data for Interoperability (USCDI) version 1.[b] This

payer-to-payer data exchange requires applicable health plans to send, at a current or former enrollee's request, specific information they maintain with a date of service on or after January 1, 2016 to any other payer identified by the current enrollee or former enrollee. Applicable health plans are only obligated to share data requests from another payer in the electronic form and format it was received. Unlike other provisions of the Final Rule, the payer-to-payer data exchange must be fully implemented by applicable health plans by January 1, 2022 (Fig. 29.4).

Exchange of Buy-In Data—The Final Rule requires all states participate in daily exchange of buy-in in data, which includes both sending data to CMS and receiving responses from CMS daily, and that all states submit the MMA file data to CMS daily by April 1, 2022.

---

[b]Office of the National Coordinator. U.S. Core Data for Interoperability (USCDI). https://www.healthit.gov/isa/us-core-data-interoperability-uscdi

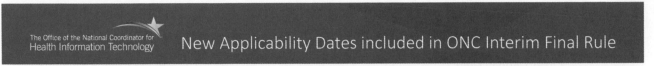

New Applicability Dates included in ONC Interim Final Rule

Information Blocking and the ONC Health IT Certification Program:
Extension of Compliance Dates and Timeframes in Response to the COVID-19 Public Health Emergency Interim Final Rule

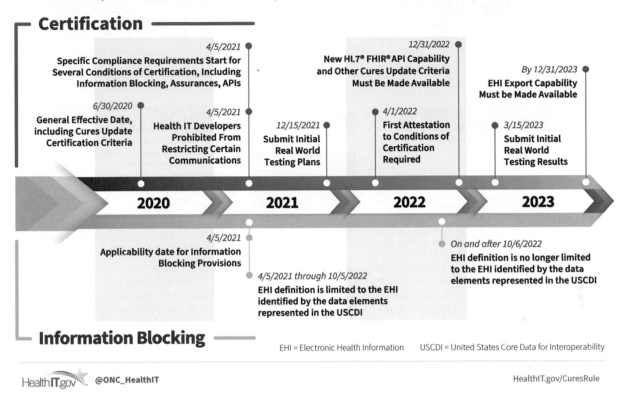

EHI = Electronic Health Information   USCDI = United States Core Data for Interoperability

HealthIT.gov @ONC_HealthIT   HealthIT.gov/CuresRule

Fig. 29.3 This graphic displays regulatory dates for the ONC's Cures Act Final Rule. Its scheduled publication date in the Federal Register was May 1, 2020, however, CMS' postponement of several provisions of its "interoperability and patient access" rule may affect ONC's timeline. From Office of the National Coordinator for Health Information Technology. (2019, June). https://www.healthit.gov/curesrule/resources/fact-sheets.

Requirements for Hospitals—To further advance electronic the exchange of electronic information, hospitals, including psychiatric hospitals and CAHs, that utilize electronic medical records systems must demonstrate:

i. Its system's notification capacity is fully operational and that it operates in accordance with all state and federal statutes and regulations regarding the exchange of patient health information;

ii. Its system sends notifications that must include the "minimum patient health information;" and

iii. Its system sends notifications directly through an intermediary that facilitates exchange of health information, and at the time of a patient's registration in the emergency department or admission to inpatient services, and at the time of, a patient's discharge and/or transfer from the emergency department or inpatient services, to all applicable post-acute care services providers and suppliers, primary care practitioners and groups, and other practitioners a groups identified by the patient as primarily responsible for his or her care, who needs to receive notification of the patient's status for treatment, care coordination, or quality improvement.

Public Attestations—CMS will publicly post on its website, any eligible hospital or CAH attesting under the Medicare FFS Promoting Interoperability Program that submits a "no" response to any of the attestation statements related to the prevention of information blocking.

Additionally, under the Final Rule, the names, and National Provider Identifier (NPI) of providers who do not have digital contact information included in the National Plan and Provider Enumeration System (NPPES) will be publicly reported until the information in included in the data base (Fig. 29.3).

Information Blocking Rule Exceptions

There are eight exceptions to the Information Blocking Rule, which include the following:

1. Preventing Harm: Under this exception, providers are permitted to engage in practices that are reasonable and necessary to prevent or reduce the risk of harm to a patient or another person. Table 29.5 provides detailed information related to the objectives and conditions to this rule.

2. Privacy: When this exception applies, a provider does not have to fulfill a request to access, exchange or use electronic

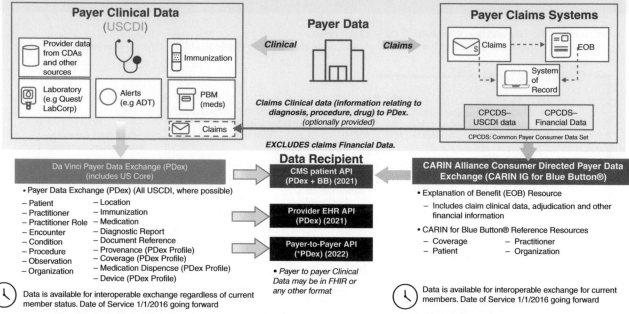

Fig. 29.4 CMS Guidance defines two sets of data to be made available by payers in the Patient Access API: Claims and Encounter Data and Clinical data. They provide links to specific implementations guides for the Patient Access API to provide guidance. Use of these implementation guides is not required, but if used these guides will provide information payers can use to meet the requirements of the policies being finalized. The CARIN Consumer Directed Payer Data Exchange IG (CARIN IG for Blue Button) defines how Claims and Encounter Data are to be provided. This DaVinci Payer Data Exchange IG (PDex) and the US Core IG define how Clinical Data is to be provided. This IG uses the same Member Health History "payload" for member-authorized exchange of information with other Health Plans and with Third-Party Applications. It describes the interaction patterns that, when followed, allow the various parties involved in managing healthcare and payer data to more easily integrate and exchange data securely and effectively. From FHIR.HLZ.org. "Data associated with payers meeting the administrative/ financial and clinical requirements of the interoperability exchange." HL7.FHIR.US.DAVINCI-PDEX\Home - FHIR v4.0.1

TABLE 29.5 Preventing Harm Exception

Objective of the Exception

This exception recognizes that the public interest in protecting patients and other persons against unreasonable risks of harm can justify practices that are likely to interfere with access, exchange, or use of EHI.

Key Conditions of the Exception • The actor must hold a reasonable belief that the practice will reduce a risk of harm;

- The actor's practice must be no broader than necessary;
- The actor's practice must satisfy at least one condition from each of the following categories: type of risk, type of harm, and implementation basis; and
- The practice must satisfy the condition concerning a patient right to request review of an individualized determination of risk of harm.

From The Office of the National Coordinator for Health Information Technology. "Cures Act Final Rule: Information blocking exceptions. https://www.healthit.gov/sites/default/files/cures/2020-03/InformationBlockingExceptions.pdf.

---

health information (EHI). The purpose of this exception is to protect an individual's privacy and ensure providers don't use or disclose EHI in a manner prohibited by state or federal privacy laws. For this exception to apply, the actor's privacy practices must satisfy at least one of four sub-exceptions: (i) a precondition to disclosure is not satisfied, such as obtaining patient consent or authorization where required by state or federal law; (ii) the actor is a developer of certified health information technology (IT) that is not required to comply with the HIPAA Privacy Rule; (iii) the actor is permitted to deny the individual's request for their EHI consistent with 45 CFR 164.524(a)(1) and (2) of the HIPAA Privacy Rule; or (iv) the actor chooses not to provide access, exchange or use of the individual's EHI if the individual requests the information not be shared, provided certain conditions are satisfied. Providers may deny an individual's request for access to EHI as permitted under 45 C.F.R. 164.524 of the HIPAA Privacy Rule or may choose not to provide access, exchange, or use of EHI if the individual has requested the information not be shared. Table 29.6 provides the objectives and conditions for privacy exception.

3. Security: The security exception covers risks to the integrity and security of the EHI and the system/software in which it is stored. It is intended to cover all legitimate security practices by actors but does not prescribe a maximum level of security or dictate a one-size-fits-all approach. The denial of access must be directly related to safeguarding the confidentiality, integrity, and availability of EHI; tailored to specific security risks; and implemented in a consistent and non-discriminatory manner. Examples of when a denial would be appropriate include a situation where there is an active or known virus or ransomware attack; the individual requesting the EHI can't prove their identity; or the request for EHI is received from a patient-facing application or website that the actor's system identifies as potentially malicious software. Table 29.7 provides objectives and conditions for this exception.

4. Infeasibility: This exception applies when legitimate practical challenges limit the ability to comply with requests for access, exchange, or use of EHI. If a provider lacks the required technology, legal rights, or other means necessary to enable EHI access, exchange, or use, they are not required to fulfill the request. For this exception to apply, the provider must meet one of the following conditions: (i) uncontrollable events prevent the actor from fulfilling a request, including but not limited to natural disaster, public health emergency, or public safety incident; (ii) the actor cannot divide the requested EHI; or (iii) the actor demonstrates, with a written record or documentation that certain factors led to the determination, that complying with the request is infeasible under the circumstances. Table 29.8 provides objectives and conditions for the infeasibility exception.

5. Health IT Performance Exception—This covers cases where a health IT system is offline for scheduled or unscheduled reasons. Table 29.9 provides objectives and conditions for this exception.

6. Content and Manner Exception—Until October 2022, physicians are only required to release data in the USCDI. This exception covers data requests outside of that set. Physicians should discuss this exception with their EHR vendor. Table 29.10 provides objectives and conditions for this exception.

7. Fees Exception—Practices are allowed to charge reasonable fees for providing data. This applies mostly to EHRs and HIEs. Table 29.11 provides objectives and conditions for this exception.

8. Licensing Exception—This exception applies mostly to EHRs. It allows vendors to license technology without it constituting information blocking. Table 29.12 provides objectives and conditions for this exception.

TABLE 29.6 Privacy Exception

Objective of the Exception	Key Conditions of the Exception
This exception recognizes that if an actor is permitted to provide access, exchange, or use of EHI under a privacy law, then the actor should provide that access, exchange, or use. However, an actor should not be required to use or disclose EHI in a way that is prohibited under state or federal privacy laws.	To satisfy this exception, an actor's privacy-protective practice must meet at least one of the four sub-exceptions: 1. Precondition not satisfied: If an actor is required by a state or federal law to satisfy a precondition (such as a patient consent or authorization) prior to providing access, exchange, or use of EHI, the actor may choose not to provide access, exchange, or use of such EHI if the precondition has not been satisfied under certain circumstances. 2. Health IT developer of certified health IT not covered by HIPAA: If an actor is a health IT developer of certified health IT that is not required to comply with the HIPAA Privacy Rule, the actor may choose to interfere with the access, exchange, or use of EHI for a privacy-protective purpose if certain conditions are met. 3. Denial of an individual's request for their EHI consistent with 45 CFR 164.524(a) (1) and (2): An actor that is a covered entity or business associate may deny an individual's request for access to his or her EHI in the circumstances provided under 45 CFR 164.524(a)(1) and (2) of the HIPAA Privacy Rule. 4. Respecting an individual's request not to share information: An actor may choose not to provide access, exchange, or use of an individual's EHI if doing so fulfills the wishes of the individual, provided certain conditions are met.

From The Office of the National Coordinator for Health Information Technology. "Information Blocking Exceptions. Cures Act Final Rule: Information Blocking Exceptions. https://www.healthit.gov/sites/default/files/cures/2020-03/InformationBlockingExceptions.pdf.

TABLE 29.7 Security Exception

Objective of the Exception	Key Conditions of the Exception
This exception is intended to cover all legitimate security practices by actors but does not prescribe a maximum level of security or dictate a one-size-fits-all approach.	The practice must be: 1. Directly related to safeguarding the confidentiality, integrity, and availability of EHI, 2. Tailored to specific security risks, and 3. Implemented in a consistent and non-discriminatory manner. 4. The practice must either implement a qualifying organizational security policy or implement a qualifying security determination.

From The Office of the National Coordinator for Health Information Technology. "Information Blocking Exceptions. Cures Act Final Rule: Information Blocking Exceptions. https://www.healthit.gov/sites/default/files/cures/2020-03/InformationBlockingExceptions.pdf.

TABLE 29.8 Infeasibility Exception

Objective of the Exception

This exception recognizes that legitimate practical challenges may limit an actor's ability to comply with requests for access, exchange, or use of electronic health information (EHI). An actor may not have—and may be unable to obtain—the requisite technological capabilities, legal rights, or other means necessary to enable access, exchange, or use

Key Conditions of the Exception

The practice must meet one of the following conditions:

- Uncontrollable events: The actor cannot fulfill the request for access, exchange, or use of electronic health information due to a natural or human-made disaster, public health emergency, public safety incident, war, terrorist attack, civil insurrection, strike or other labor unrest, telecommunication or internet service interruption, or act of military, civil or regulatory authority. Segmentation: The actor cannot fulfill the request for access, exchange, or use of EHI because the actor cannot unambiguously segment the requested EHI.
- Infeasibility under the circumstances: The actor demonstrates through a contemporaneous written record or other documentation its consistent and non-discriminatory consideration of certain factors that led to its determination that complying with the request would be infeasible under the circumstances.
- The actor must provide a written response to the requestor within 10 business days of receipt of the request with the reason(s) why the request is infeasible.

From The Office of the National Coordinator for Health Information Technology. "Information Blocking Exceptions. Cures Act Final Rule: Information Blocking Exceptions. https://www.healthit.gov/sites/default/files/cures/2020-03/InformationBlockingExceptions.pdf.

TABLE 29.9 Health Information Technology Performance Exception

Objective of the Exception

This exception recognizes that for health IT to perform properly and efficiently, it must be maintained, and in some instances improved, which may require that health IT be taken offline temporarily. Actors should not be deterred from taking reasonable and necessary measures to make health IT temporarily unavailable or to degrade the health IT's performance for the benefit of the overall performance of health IT.

Key Conditions of the Exception

The practice must:

1. Be implemented for a period of time no longer than necessary to achieve the maintenance or improvements for which the health IT was made unavailable or the health IT's performance degraded,
2. Be implemented in a consistent and non-discriminatory manner, and
3. Meet certain requirements if the unavailability or degradation is initiated by a health IT developer of certified health IT, HIE, or HIN.

An actor may act against a third-party app that is negatively impacting the health IT's performance, provided that the practice is:

1. For a period of time no longer than necessary to resolve any negative impacts,
2. Implemented in a consistent and non-discriminatory manner, and
3. Consistent with existing service level agreements, where applicable.

If the unavailability is in response to a risk of harm or security risk, the actor must only comply with the Preventing Harm or Security Exception, as applicable.

From The Office of the National Coordinator for Health Information Technology. "Cures Act Final Rule: Information blocking exceptions. https://www.healthit.gov/sites/default/files/cures/2020-03/InformationBlockingExceptions.pdf.

TABLE 29.10 Content and Manner Exception

Objective of the Exception

This exception provides clarity and flexibility to actors concerning the required content (i.e., scope of EHI) of an actor's response to a request to access, exchange, or use EHI and the way the actor may fulfill the request. This exception supports innovation and competition by allowing actors to first attempt to reach and maintain market negotiated terms for the access, exchange, and use of EHI.

Key Conditions of the Exception

Content Condition: Establishes the content an actor must provide in response to a request to access, exchange, or use electronic health information (EHI) to satisfy the exception.

1. Up to 24 months after the publication date of the Cures Act final rule, an actor must respond to a request to access, exchange, or use EHI with, at a minimum, the EHI identified by the data elements represented in the United States Core Data for Interoperability (USCDI) standard.
2. On and after 24 months after the publication date of the Cures Act final rule, an actor must respond to a request to access, exchange, or use EHI with EHI as defined in § 171.102.

Manner Condition: Establishes the way an actor must fulfill a request to access, exchange, or use EHI to satisfy this exception.

- An actor may need to fulfill a request in an alternative manner when the actor is:
  - Technically unable to fulfill the request in any manner requested; or
  - Cannot reach agreeable terms with the requestor to fulfill the request.
- If an actor fulfills a request in an alternative manner, such fulfillment must comply with the order of priority described in the manner condition and must satisfy the Fees Exception and Licensing Exception, as applicable.

From The Office of the National Coordinator for Health Information Technology. "Cures Act Final Rule: Information blocking exceptions. https://www.healthit.gov/sites/default/files/cures/2020-03/InformationBlockingExceptions.pdf.

TABLE 29.11 Fees Exception

Objective of the Exception

This exception enables actors to charge fees related to the development of technologies and provision of services that enhance interoperability, while not protecting rent seeking, opportunistic fees, and exclusionary practices that interfere with access, exchange, or use of EHI.

Key Conditions of the Exception

The Practice Must:

- Meet the basis for fees condition. For instance, the fees an actor charges must: —Be based on objective and verifiable criteria that are uniformly applied for all similarly situated classes of persons or entities and requests. —Be related to the actor's costs of providing the type of access, exchange, or use of EHI. —Not be based on whether the requestor or other person is a competitor, potential competitor, or will be using the EHI in a way that facilitates competition with the actor.
- Not be specifically excluded. For instance, the exception does not apply to: —A fee based in any part on the electronic access by an individual, their personal representative, or another person or entity designated by the individual to access the individual's EHI. —A fee to perform an export of electronic health information via the capability of health IT certified to § 170.315(b)(10).
- Comply with Conditions of Certification in § 170.402(a)(4) (Assurances—certification to "EHI Export" criterion) or § 170.404 (API).

From The Office of the National Coordinator for Health Information Technology. "Cures Act Final Rule: Information blocking exceptions. https://www.healthit.gov/sites/default/files/cures/2020-03/InformationBlockingExceptions.pdf.

TABLE 29.12 Licensing Exception

Objective of the Exception

This exception allows actors to protect the value of their innovations and charge reasonable royalties to earn returns on the investments they have made to develop, maintain, and update those innovations

Key Conditions of the Exception

The practice must meet:

The negotiating a license conditions: An actor must begin license negotiations with the requestor within 10 business days from receipt of the request and negotiate a license within 30 business days from receipt of the request.

- The licensing conditions:
- Scope of rights, Reasonable royalty, Non-discriminatory terms, Collateral terms, and Non-disclosure agreement
- Additional conditions relating to the provision of interoperability elements.

From The Office of the National Coordinator for Health Information Technology. "Cures Act Final Rule: Information blocking exceptions. https://www.healthit.gov/sites/default/files/cures/2020-03/InformationBlockingExceptions.pdf.

Penalties for Non-Compliance

Congress established, through the Cures Act, stated that developers of certified health IT and health information networks and exchanges, would be subject to civil monetary penalties of up to $1 million dollars per violation for engaging in information blocking, the penalties for healthcare providers that fail to comply are still unclear. The Cures Act provides that healthcare providers who engage in information blocking may be subject to "appropriate disincentives" as set forth by the HHS Secretary. It is anticipated that regulations will be proposed soon to create these "disincentives." For current participants in the Centers for Medicare and Medicaid's (CMS) Merit-based Incentive Payment System (MIPS), attestations with respect to information blocking have been included for several years. As the definition of information blocking is now set through the ONC rules, failure to comply with the ONC rules could be viewed as a breach of the MIPS attestations (85 FR 25510-25640).

Technical Approach and Standards

CMS requires the use of standards-based APIs, which will allow patients to use software applications of their choice to access and use their own electronic health information and other related information to manage their health. Software developers and healthcare providers using API interfaces must follow CMS and ONC technical standards, to streamline patient data. The ONC 21st Century Cures Act outlines technical standards in its Final Rule, which are as follows:

- Requires the use of the HL7 FHIR (FHIR release 4) standard along with a set of implementation specifications.
- Requires Certified APIs to implement the SMART Application Launch Framework Implementation Guides (based on the OAuth 2.0 security standard).
- Establishes the USCDI standard as the scope of patients' electronic health information that must be supported via certified API technology.
- Puts in place an application registration process to help ensure secure connections that include authentication and authorization capabilities.
- Requires health IT developers to support API-enabled services for data on a single patient and multiple patients.
- Requires API technology suppliers to publish the terms and conditions applicable to their API technology.
- Requires Certified API Developers to publish specific business and technical documentation necessary to interact with their certified API technology and make such documentation publicly accessible via a hyperlink.

CMS's view is that these requirements will ensure that a uniform, secure, and trusted API is established across the healthcare industry. To meet the criteria, entities covered by the rule, including applicable health plans, must implement technologies that support APIs capable of using the FHIR standard, which would allow for seamless sharing of EHI.

EXPANDING THE AVAILABILITY OF HEALTH INFORMATION AND PATIENT ACCESS

Individual Access to Standardized Healthcare Data

CMS indicated in its Final Rule the numerous benefits associated with individuals having access to standardized healthcare data. The patient access API widely used standard will tell providers and patients the full story, far greater than the information that claims and encounter data that EHR data can provide alone. Standardized data will offer a broader and more holistic understanding of an individuals' interactions with the healthcare system and identify and expand opportunities to understand a patient's access to healthcare (Fig. 29.5).

For instance, standardized date can illuminate inconsistent benefit utilization patterns in an individual's claims data, such as a failure to fill a prescription or receive recommended therapies, which may indicate that the individual has had difficulty financing a treatment regimen and may require less expensive prescription drugs or therapies (85 FR 25523). It also provides opportunity to identify and find opportunities to address an individual's non-adherence to a care plan, which is critical to keeping people with chronic conditions healthy and engaged so they can avoid hospitalizations (85 FR 25523). While a health plan can use claims and encounter data to help it identify which enrollees could benefit from an assessment of why they are not filling their prescriptions or who might be at risk for particular problems, putting this information into the hands of the individual's chosen care provider—such as the doctor or nurse practitioner prescribing the medications or the pharmacist who fills the prescriptions—helps them to engage the patient in shared decision making that can help address some of the reasons the individual might not be willing or able to take medications as prescribed or fully participate in treatments.

Additionally, the Information Blocking Rule aligns with the HIPAA Privacy Rule, by permitting patients' rights to request access to their records with the Patient Access API format. The API format is beneficial to patients, who so choose to exercise their HIPAA right of access to receive their PHI, by giving them a simple and easy electronic way to request, receive, and share data they want and need, including with a designated third party. However, some types of PHI, including for example, x-ray images, which are not formattable to the API standard, must be shared in another appropriate format to stay compliance with the HIPAA Privacy Right of Access provision.

Health Information Exchange and Care Coordination Efforts Across Payers

The Information Blocking Rule required applicable health plans to adopt and implement the standards-based API to meet

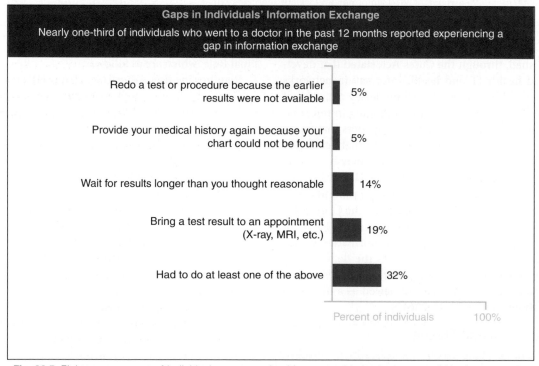

Fig. 29.5 Eighty-one percent of individuals went to a healthcare provider at least once within the past year. Overall, 32% of individuals who went to a doctor in the past 12 months reported experiencing a gap in information exchange. About 1 in 20 individuals who had been to the doctor in the last year reported having to redo a test or procedure because their prior data was unavailable. About 1 in 5 individuals had to bring prior test results to an appointment. From Office of the National Coordinator for Health Information Technology. (2019, June). "Gaps in individuals' information exchange" Health IT Quick-Stat #56. https://www.healthit.gov/data/quickstats/gaps-individuals-information-exchange.

enrollees' HIPAA right of access PHI requests. using common technologies and without special effort. As a result of this adoption of API standards across applicable health plans, such health plans would support the patient's directed coordination of care. The Rule identified and implemented the requirements below that these health plans are required to execute when requested by an enrollee, to coordinate care across other payers:

1. Receive the data set from another payer that had covered the enrollee within the previous 5 years;
2. Send the data set at any time during an enrollee's enrollment and up to 5 years later, to another payer that currently covers the enrollee; and
3. Send the data set at any time during enrollment or up to 5 years after enrollment has ended to a recipient identified by the enrollee (85 FR 25564).

CMS also required applicable health plans to form and participate in trusted exchange networks that meet the following criteria:

1. The trusted exchange network must be able to exchange PHI, defined at 45 CFR 160.103, in compliance with all applicable state and federal laws across jurisdictions.
2. The trusted exchange network must be capable of connecting both inpatient EHRs and ambulatory EHRs.
3. The trusted exchange network must support secure messaging or electronic querying by and between patients, providers, and payers (85 FR 25567).

CMS noted these requirements were implemented to help both enrollees and healthcare providers coordinate care and reduce administrative burden to ensure that payers provide coordinated high-quality care in an efficient and cost-effective way that protects program integrity.

Information Blocking Rule Conditions of Participation for Hospitals and Critical Access Hospitals

Conditions of Participation (CoPs) are health and safety standards developed by CMS that healthcare organizations, such as hospitals must meet to begin and continue participating in the Medicare and Medicaid programs. Under the Information Blocking Rule, hospitals must have a medical record service that has administrative responsibility for medical records and medical record must be maintained for every individual evaluated or treated in the hospital. While this is not a new practice for hospitals, they are required to meet the following conditions: (85 FR 25584)

1. Organization and staffing. The organization of the medical record service must be appropriate to the scope and complexity of the services performed. The hospital must employ adequate personnel to ensure prompt completion, filing, and retrieval of records.
2. Form and retention of record. The hospital must maintain a medical record for each inpatient and outpatient. Medical records must be accurately written, promptly completed, properly filed, and retained, and accessible. The hospital must use a system of author identification and record maintenance that ensures the integrity of the authentication and protects the security of all record entries.

a. Medical records must be retained in their original or legally reproduced form for a period of at least 5 years.
b. The hospital must have a system of coding and indexing medical records. The system must allow for timely retrieval by diagnosis and procedure, to support medical care evaluation studies.
c. The hospital must have a procedure for ensuring the confidentiality of patient records. In-formation from or copies of records may be released only to authorized individuals, and the hospital must ensure that unauthorized individuals cannot gain access to or alter patient records. Original medical records must be released by the hospital only in accordance with Federal or State laws, court orders, or subpoenas.

3. Content of record. The medical record must contain information to justify admission and continued hospitalization, support the diagnosis, and describe the patient's progress and response to medications and services.
4. Electronic notifications. If the hospital utilizes an electronic medical records system or other electronic administrative system, which is conformant with the content exchange standard at 45 CFR 170.205(d)(2), then the hospital must demonstrate that:

a. The system's notification capacity is fully operational and the hospital uses it in accordance with all State and Federal statutes and regulations applicable to the hospital's exchange of patient health information.
b. The system sends notifications that must include at least patient name, treating practitioner name, and sending institution name.
c. To the extent permissible under applicable federal and state law and regulations, and consistent with the patient's expressed privacy preferences, the system sends notifications directly, or through an intermediary that facilitates exchange of health information, at the time of:
i. The patient's registration in the hospital's emergency department (if applicable).
ii. The patient's admission to the hospital's inpatient services (if applicable).
iii. To the extent permissible under applicable federal and state law and regulations and consistent with the patient's expressed privacy preferences, the system sends notifications directly, or through an intermediary that facilitates exchange of health information, either immediately prior to, or at the time of the patient's discharge:
iv. The hospital has made a reasonable effort to ensure that the system sends the notifications to all applicable post-acute care services providers and suppliers, as well as to any of the following practitioners and entities, which need to receive notification of the patient's status for treatment, care coordination, or quality improvement purposes:
v. The patient's established primary care practitioner;
vi. The patient's established primary care practice group or entity; or
vii. Other practitioner, or other practice group or entity, identified by the patient as the practitioner, or practice group or entity, primarily responsible for his or her care.

CONCLUSION AND FUTURE DIRECTIONS

The Information Blocking Rule was implemented in efforts to put patients first by giving them access to their health information in a seamless fashion. The historical lack of seamless data exchange in healthcare has historically detracted from patient care, leading to poor health outcomes, and higher costs. The CMS Interoperability and Patient Access final rule establishes policies that break down barriers in the nation's health system to enable better patient access to their health information, improve interoperability and unleash innovation, while reducing burden on payers and providers. The rules established standards for patient access API, provider directory API, payer-to-payer data exchange, public reporting and information blocking, digital contact information, and admission, discharge, and transfer event notifications for hospitals.

ACKNOWLEDGMENT

The authors wish to acknowledge the contribution of Michele P. Madison to the previous edition of this chapter.

DISCUSSION QUESTIONS

1. How did interoperability and patient access in MACRA differ from the main provisions of the Information Blocking Rule? What were some of the policy reasons for each piece of legislation that were accomplished by each rule?
2. What does "information blocking" mean and what are some examples of information blocking?
3. What are Application Programming Interfaces (APIs) and what role do they play in preventing the frequency of information blocking and/or increasing access to patient information?
4. Summarize the main provisions of the Information Blocking Rule. What are some mechanisms that the Information Rule puts in place to prevent instances of "information blocking?"
5. What is the payer-to-payer data exchange? Which payers are required to participate and by which date does the data exchange require full implementation?

6. There are eight exceptions to the Information Blocking rule. What are those exceptions? Briefly explain each exception and the objection of each exception.
7. Who is subject to penalties for failure to comply with the Information Blocking Rule? What are those penalties?
8. What are standards-based APIs and why are they important? Who is subject to implementing API-standards?
9. How do the HIPAA Privacy and Security rules impact the provisions of the Information Blocking Rule?
10. Which types of providers are required to comply with the Information Blocking Rule? What rules are in place to ensure that providers comply with applicable provisions of the Information Blocking Rule.

CASE STUDY

Case Study: Determining when the Information Blocking Rule Applies

You were recently hired as the Chief Information Officer (CIO) for a regional hospital system. The Chief Compliance Officer is having trouble determining whether the information blocking rule should be implemented at the regional hospital system's newly acquired facility. Before it was acquired, the facility maintained paper medical records only and did not use an EMR. While the hospital system has a sophisticated EMR system, the IT staff is having trouble implementing the EMR system at the new facility. Using the information in the chapter, answer the following questions

Discussion Questions

1. Is the hospital system responsible for ensuring that the newly acquired facility complies with provisions of the Information Blocking Rule?
2. Could any of the Information Blocking Rule exceptions apply, considering the facilities history of maintaining a paper medical records system? If yes, what exceptions could apply?
3. If an exception likely does not apply, what information blocking provisions would apply the facility as a part of the hospital system?

REFERENCES

85 FR 25510-25640.

85 FR 25510-25640.

85 FR 25523.

85 FR 25523.

85 FR 25564.

85 FR 25567.

85 FR 25575.

85 FR 25584.

85 FR 25584.

HealthIT.gov. (2019) Advanced alternative payment model. https://www.healthit.gov/topic/meaningful-use-and-macra/advanced-alternative-payment-model.

The American Medical Association. (2022). Meaningful use: Electronic health record (EHR) incentive programs. https://www.ama-assn.org/practice-management/medicare-medicaid/meaningful-use-electronic-health-record-ehr-incentive.

The Centers for Medicare & Medicaid Services (CMS). (2022). *Promoting interoperability programs.* https://www.cms.gov/Regulations-and-Guidance/Legislation/EHRIncentivePrograms.

The Office of the National Coordinator for Health Information Technology. (2015, April). Report to Congress: Report on health information blocking. https://www.healthit.gov/sites/default/files/reports/info_blocking_040915.pdf.

30

Health Policy and Health Informatics

Todd B. Taylor and Lynda R. Hardy

By understanding HIT-related health policy, the role of professional organizations, federal infrastructure supporting HIT, and specific approaches for participating in the advocacy process, health informatics leaders can significantly affect health policy and in turn healthcare itself.

OBJECTIVES

At the completion of this chapter, the reader will be prepared to:
1. Describe the basic premise of policy characteristics and rationale for creating them.
2. Discuss the basic role of the federal government and its agencies in healthcare policy.
3. Summarize the steps required for development and implementation of an effective health information technology policy.
4. Describe interdisciplinary competencies and certifications available for informatics practitioners.
5. Discuss the major regulations that affect health informatics policies.

KEY TERMS

health information technology, 472
health policy, 472
HITECH Act, 475
Institute of Medicine, 474

Office of the National Coordinator for
   Health Information Technology
   (ONC), 474
patient safety, 482

public policy, 473
regulation, 477

ABSTRACT ❖

To improve healthcare delivery and health outcomes, informaticians (Box 30.1) and healthcare leaders require an understanding of health policy and how to influence the process. These leaders must also be knowledgeable about current and emerging technology-related public policy initiatives impacting healthcare practice and care delivery through informatics principles and technology.

This chapter begins by outlining the basics of policy in general, then informatics policy specifically. Examples of health information technology (HIT) policy are then described, including trends in local hospital, regional, and national public (government)

policy. Understanding the driving forces and resulting initiatives offers a foundation for understanding the leadership role of healthcare professionals seeking to influence health policy.

Healthcare professionals understand that effective and efficient use of HIT, when combined with best practices and evidence-based care, improve health and healthcare. As leaders, informaticians can help maximize the utility of HIT to bring practice standards and evidence-based decision-making to the point of care. Increasingly, this is accomplished by empowering patients and healthcare consumers as partners in this process.

INTRODUCTION

Health Policy defines health goals at the international, national, or local level and specifies the decisions, plans, and actions to be undertaken to achieve these goals (World Health Organization, 2021).

Health Informatics focuses on technology as a tool with the goal of an efficient, cost-effective healthcare system that ensures health for individuals, families, groups, and communities.

Taken together, these two disciplines drive the development, adoption, application, priorities, and direction of digital assets applied to healthcare. Put another way, health information

---

BOX 30.1 Definitions

Informaticians (Hersh, 2006): Informatics is the science of information. Informaticians identify, define, and solve information problems.

Healthcare Informatics (Saba & McCormick, 2015): "the integration of healthcare sciences, computer science, information science, and cognitive science to assist in the management of healthcare information."

Health Policy (World Health Organization, 2021): Defines health goals at the international, national, or local level and specifies the decisions, plans, and actions to be undertaken to achieve these goals. An explicit health policy can achieve multiple objectives: it clarifies the values on which a policy is based; it defines a vision for the future, which in turn helps to establish objectives and the priorities among them; and it facilitates setting targets and milestones for the short and medium term.

---

technology (HIT) policy identifies the values upon which such policy is based; defines a vision for the future, which in turn helps establish objectives and priorities among them; and facilitates setting targets and milestones for the short and medium term (World Health Organization, 2021).

Local (Private) Policy

"Policy" has multiple forms. Health professionals are very familiar with "Hospital Policy and Procedures" that define various aspects of hospital operations and staff behavior. Often lesser known are policies related to HIT that range from general to focused.

An example of a general HIT policy is a "single source" Electronic Health Record (EHR) vendor policy, contrasted with a "Best-In-Breed" multi-source EHR vendor strategy.

An example of a focused HIT policy is "acceptable password criteria," that is, length, character types, and refresh frequency as part of identity and access management to secure applications like an EHR.

Healthcare leaders, and particularly informaticians, must be prepared to address policy considerations related to informatics in response to internal and external factors. Public policy often drives local policy and external threats (e.g., cybersecurity) require careful and frequent management of local policies.

Public Policy

Unlike most public policy, HIT policy tends to be driven by necessity rather than ideology. Nevertheless, similar processes are used to develop and influence public policy related to informatics.

General healthcare public policy in the United States is unique as compared to other countries, including policies related to informatics. For example, while most of the world has adopted universal government-sponsored healthcare, the United States continues to maintain a hybrid system of private and public funding. While there are advantages and disadvantages, this situation tends to make HIT policy more challenging. Further, US policy on many fronts tends to change frequently depending on the party in power. As a result, healthcare leaders in the United States are challenged by an ever-changing healthcare landscape, as are HIT leaders.

Informatics Policy Challenges

While most espouse the desire for cost-effective, efficient, and safe healthcare delivery, often the biggest challenge is in establishing what these terms even mean, let alone the best way to achieve them. As a result, despite assertions to the contrary, healthcare policy tends to be more reactive than proactive and often driven by ideology.

The result? To be effective in influencing and managing healthcare policy, stakeholders and healthcare leaders within the American healthcare system must have a broad understanding of healthcare, the political milieu, and the drivers behind US healthcare policy, in addition to a deep understanding of informatics.

In this chapter, the basics of policy are described, and recent HIT policy initiatives are explored illustrating how to be effective policy mavens.

The chapter concludes by describing the leadership role of healthcare professionals and informaticists in influencing the development and implementation of healthcare policy. Included are specific actions known to be effective in moving healthcare policy forward. These actions are foundational competencies that healthcare leaders should possess to achieve the goal of providing safe, quality, and competent healthcare.

DESCRIPTION OF POLICY TYPES AND APPLICATION

The word "policy" has various meanings, depending on the context. In its simplest form, "policy" can be defined as "(noun) a course or principle of action adopted or proposed by a government, party, business, or individual" (Oxford Languages Dictionary, n.d.).

For example, one might purchase an "insurance policy," which is a legal contract between an insurance company (insurer) and the person(s), business, or entity being insured (beneficiary) that outlines benefits and responsibilities, including exclusions. Retail stores have "return policies," businesses have "employee policies," and even families have "policies," such as "no TV until homework is done." In short, polices are what create a civil society, acting like "paved roads" at times, and "fences" at others.

Nevertheless, "policy" is not "law." Policy guides or outlines *what to do* (vs. *how*) to achieve an objective, for the good of all. "Laws" are standards, principles, and procedures that must be followed, and in certain instances are used to implement or enforce policy (Law vs policy, 2021).

HIT policy assumes multiple forms. Healthcare software, devices, personnel, patient care, and other aspects have policy implications that have been addressed in other chapters and will not be addressed here. Local (private) HIT policy that guide IT departments will be addressed only as they relate to public policy.

Finally, few policies (of any type) stand by themselves. Most are interdependent with a broad range of other policies, laws, regulations, and even cultural norms. For example, federal economic policies often have a significant impact on healthcare, even when not directly related. And every healthcare policy will have implications for HIT. Therefore, one must be aware of a broad range of healthcare policy initiatives at all levels to successfully manage and react specifically to HIT policy initiatives.

Effective Policy Characteristics

Ideally, a policy is clear, concise, and manageable, with objectives, defined terms, realistic processes, appropriate incentives, and desired vision. In developing policy, established targets, priorities, and points of reference for both short- and medium-term planning should be considered.

Identifying and engaging relevant stakeholders leads to success by helping to inform, build consensus and identify potential untoward consequences. An unfortunate reality is that the expressed objective of certain policies may be considered by some to be "untoward consequences." Further, public policies are often largely based on ideology, leaving data, historical facts, and at times even rational thinking behind. Even at their best, public policies fail 25% to 50% of the time, depending on the definition of success (Andrews, 2018).

Impetus for Policy Initiatives

Research and comprehensive reports have, for decades, identified health and healthcare delivery issues in the US impacting the health of individuals, families, communities, and the country.

As early as 2001, an Institute of Medicine (IOM) report outlined concerns of decreased quality, excess costs, and avoidable errors, calling for new tools and methods to manage healthcare processes and knowledge (Committee on Quality of Health Care in America, 2001). This led some to recommend universal adoption of HIT, in particular EHR systems (Tang, 2003). Advanced interconnected EHRs promised improved care coordination, personalized healthcare, improved processes and safety, resulting in increased overall efficiencies in care and quality, and reductions in cost. Nevertheless most of these promises have been unrealized (Patel, 2021). There is no clear consensus on how to address many of the major healthcare issues or perhaps a better question is, should we (NEWPORT, 2021). Further, major ideological differences exist regarding the responsibilities and rights of individuals, families, groups, and institutions related to these issues. As a result, healthcare policy in the United States tends to be reactive and change with the political winds.

The challenge for healthcare informatics is how best to navigate these turbulent waters and use technology innovation to impact America's health and healthcare delivery. As noted, the first step toward consensus is to identify and engage relevant stakeholders. Fig. 30.1 lists traditional stakeholders that impact HIT policy in the US, where government plays a primary role. Other stakeholders include patients and patient organizations; physicians and physician organizations; nurses and nurse organizations; hospitals and hospital organizations; employers; insurance companies; and pharmaceutical companies. HIT-specific stakeholders include the Healthcare Information and Management Systems Society (HIMSS); American Medical Informatics Association (AMIA); the American Health Information Management Association (AHIMA); Association of Medical Directors of Information Systems (AMDIS); Alliance for Nursing Informatics (ANI); Joint Public Health Informatics (JPHIT); and various EHR and technology vendors.

Public Policy

Public Policy is what is meant when referring to "healthcare policy" and will be the focus of the remainder of this chapter.

In the book *Policy Paradox*, the author states, "The 'paradox' is that it is possible to define the same policies in contradictory ways" (Stone, 2011). And so, public policy has the potential for peace or war; economic boom or bust; incentives for right or wrong; even good or evil. Whether one is creating, influencing, implementing, or complying with healthcare policy, great care must be taken to assure positive outcomes are achieved.

DEVELOPING AND IMPLEMENTING HEALTH INFORMATION POLICY

A clearly stated policy provides a clear vision for the future and identifies reference points for planning. The federal government maintains a pivotal role in managing healthcare policy.

Role of Federal Government in Healthcare Policy

Federal agencies are purchasers, regulators, developers, and users of HIT. In these various roles, government agencies set policy and insure, pay for care, or provide direct patient care for tens of millions of Americans. They also protect and promote population and community health by investing in health and human services and in infrastructure. Additionally, federal agencies develop and implement policies and regulations to advance innovation, support research, promote competition, and protect individual and community safety, privacy, and security (The Office of the National Coordinator [ONC], 2021).

Federal Health IT Strategic Plan 2015–2020
The Office of the National Coordinator for Health Information Technology

Government		Universities
Federal: executive, legislative, and judicial State Local		Weill Cornell Medical College Center for Health Informatics and Policy (CHiP)

Foundations	Informatics	Payers
HIMSS: Institute for e-Health Policy	Associations AMIA HIMSS ANI	Insurance companies Employers Labor unions Individuals Government

Industry and Business	Organizations
Vendors with informatics applications Hardware vendors Vendors with support services	Consumers/patients/citizens Voluntary associations Medical Professional Societies

Fig. 30.1 Examples of health informatics stakeholders. *AMIA*, American Medical Informatics Association; *ANI*, Alliance for Nursing Informatics; *HIMSS*, Healthcare Information and Management Systems Society.

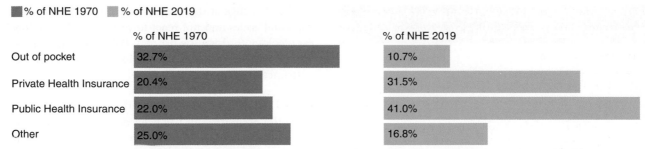

Fig. 30.2 National expenditures, 1970–2019. ("How has U.S. spending on healthcare changed over time?," Peterson-KFF Health System Tracker, accessed October 27, 2021, https://www.healthsystemtracker.org/chart-collection/u-s-spending-healthcare-changed-time/)

In 1970, the public funding percentage of total US healthcare spending was 22% and nearly doubled to 41% by 2019. Notably, out-of-pocket spending decreased by 22% over the same period (Fig. 30.2) (KFF analysis of National Health Expenditure [NHE], 2021).

Beyond substantial funding of healthcare, the federal government regulates virtually every aspect of it through mandates, funding incentives, and accreditation proxies (e.g., The Joint Commission [The Joint Commission]). So, while about 60% of healthcare spending remains in the private sector, federal and state governments have substantial regulatory control over all healthcare. For example, the Emergency Medical Treatment and Labor Act (EMTALA) (Consolidated Omnibus Budget Reconciliation, 1986) regulates nearly every aspect of emergency department (ED) care for Medicare-participating hospitals. The Affordable Care Act (ACA) (Patient Protection and Affordable Care Act [PPACA], 2010) mandates various benefits for both public and private insurance plans in the US (e.g., prohibition of exclusion for pre-existing conditions and mental health coverage parity, amongst others).

The U.S. Department of Health and Human Services (HHS) is the government's principal agency for protecting the health of all Americans and providing essential human services. Among its duties, HHS oversees healthcare coverage through Medicare, Medicaid, the Children's Health Insurance Program, and the ACA Health Insurance Marketplace. The HHS Strategic Plan FY 2018–2022 identifies current HHS programs, including implications for HIT (Box 30.2) (U.S. Department of Health & Human Services, 2022).

HHS has, in addition to its overall strategic plan, an internal "Information Technology Strategic Plan FY 2021–2023," that "represents the Department's future ambitions to deliver its core functions with greater agility, security, and effectiveness amidst an evolving public health landscape." (Information technology strategic plan, 2021)

The work of HHS is conducted by 11 divisions and 14 offices, including the Office of the National Coordinator for Health Information Technology (ONC), (HHS, 2021) which serves as the HHS Secretary's principal HIT advisor.

While the federal government HIT initiatives are now under the ONC, other federal agencies are also involved in health informatics projects. For example, the Center for Surveillance,

---

BOX 30.2   HHS FY 2018–2022 Strategic Goals, Objectives, and Strategies

Strategic Goal 1: Reform, Strengthen, and Modernize the Nation's Healthcare System.

Strategic Goal 2: Protect the Health of Americans Where They Live, Learn, Work, and Play.

Strategic Goal 3: Strengthen the Economic and Social Well-Being of Americans Across the Lifespan.

Strategic Goal 4: Foster Sound, Sustained Advances in the Sciences.

Strategic Goal 5: Promote Effective and Efficient Management and Stewardship.

HHS, U.S. Department of Health and Human Services. Data from 10 Ways Technology Is Changing Healthcare. The Medical Futurist, 3 March 2020. https://medicalfuturist.com/ten-ways-technology-changing-healthcare/# Accessed October 27, 2021.

Epidemiology, and Laboratory Services (CSELS) is under the direction of the CDC (https://www.cdc.gov/csels/index.html).

Office of the National Coordinator for Health Information Technology

The position of National Coordinator for HIT was created in 2004 (via Executive Order), and later codified in the Health Information Technology for Economic and Clinical Health Act (HITECH Act) of 2009 (American Recovery and Reinvestment Act of, 2009).

The ONC remains focused on two strategic objectives: (1) advancing the development and use of health IT capabilities, and (2) establishing expectations for data sharing.

The Office of the National Coordinator for Health Information Technology (ONC) is at the forefront of the administration's health IT efforts and is a resource to the entire health system to support the adoption of health information technology and the promotion of nationwide, standards-based health information exchange to improve health care. ONC is organizationally located within the Office of the Secretary for the U.S. Department of Health and Human Services (HHS). ONC is the principal federal entity charged with coordination of nationwide efforts to implement and

BOX 30.3 ONC 2020–2025 Federal Health IT Strategic Plan: Goals and Objectives

1. Promote Health and Wellness
   A. Improve individual access to usable health information
   B. Advance healthy and safe practices through health IT
   C. Integrate health and human services information
2. Enhance the Delivery and Experience of Care
   A. Leverage health IT to improve clinical practice and promote safe, high-quality care
   B. Use health IT to expand access and connect patients to care
   C. Foster competition, transparency, and affordability in healthcare
   D. Reduce regulatory and administrative burden on providers
   E. Enable efficient management of health IT resources and a nationwide workforce confidently using health IT
3. Build a Secure, Data-Driven Ecosystem to Accelerate Research and Innovation
   A. Advance individual- and population-level transfer of health data
   B. Support research and analysis using health IT and data at the individual and population levels
4. Connect Healthcare with Health Data
   A. Advance the development and use of health IT capabilities
   B. Establish expectations for data sharing
   C. Enhance technology and communications infrastructure
   D. Promote secure health information practices that protect individual privacy

use the most advanced health information technology and the electronic exchange of health information (About the ONC, 2021).

Currently, the ONC is the focal point for US HIT policy as outlined in its ***2020–2025 Federal Health IT Strategic Plan** (*ONC, 2021*)*. "This Plan is outcomes-driven, with goals focused on meeting the needs of individuals, populations, caregivers, healthcare providers, payers, public health professionals, researchers, developers, and innovators" (Bloomrosen et al., 2011). This (and subsequent versions) are must-reads for those who wish to delve into HIT policy (Box 30.3).

DEVELOP AND IMPLEMENT EFFECTIVE HIT POLICY

Political science is the academic discipline where policy development is most often taught and studied. However, an individual does not need a degree in political science to be successful in policy endeavors. Whether you are developing policy for the nation, a state government, a hospital, or an organization, the process is the same. The following describes the typical steps in that process.

Step One: The Agenda (Defining the Desired Result)

Public policy is typically intended to address problems; establish a common purpose or standard; or improve upon aspects of society or an organization. The first, and most important task, is to define the end objective or desired result. This is sometimes referred to as "what itch are we trying to scratch"—or put another way, first ask "why," then "how."

The challenge at this stage is to remain focused on the fundamental issues and not react to recent events or allow political ideology to drive the process. Policy driven by emotion or impure motives invariably results in untoward, even disastrous, outcomes.

Step Two: Policy Formulation

Once the desired result has been determined, a detailed analysis of the necessary approach to achieve that result must be performed. Depending on the issue, this can range from simple to very complex. Legal issues, economic barriers, public sentiment, political ideology, and technical barriers must be considered. One challenge frequently missed is simple human behavior, including incentives. For complex policies, behavioral experts, particularly behavioral economists, may be valuable in consultation. This may involve focus groups, polling, surveys, and other methods to predict how the subjects of the policy may respond.

Care must be taken to avoid untoward consequences, defined as something that is unexpected and undesirable. Therefore, while it is natural to focus on positive outcomes a policy might engender, it is equally important to consider potential untoward consequences of the adoption of HIT, particularly when implementations are accelerated (Bloomrosen et al., 2011).

Finally, these various actions are interdependent, such that if anyone fails, the entire policy may fail. It is prudent to consider potential failure points and create alternative actions should failure ensue.

Step Three: Establish Stakeholder Consensus

Stakeholder consensus is important for several reasons. First, it engages a variety of experts from various sectors helping to identify potential weaknesses and flaws, as well as identify innovative solutions. Consensus leads to support and even champions of the policy effort. Minimizing detractors goes a long way toward success.

Unfortunately, this step is often skipped for a variety of reasons and is the most frequent cause of policy failure. In today's political milieu, policy consensus may not even be possible and the party in power may simply force their policy agenda through. Obviously, as political winds change, so do those policies. Nevertheless, HIT policy is often immune from political ideology allowing consensus to be achieved more readily.

The process for establishing stakeholder consensus may take many forms and depends on the type of policy being considered. For healthcare at the federal level, the stakeholder list is quite extensive, even for HIT policy. But the avenues of stakeholder participation are well established as most individuals and local organizations funnel their policy actions through a nationally affiliated organization. For example, physicians often rely on the American Medical Association (AMA) or their specialty society. Hospitals may rely on the American Hospital Association (AHA), although with hospital consolidation into large networks, some hospital networks oversee advocacy directly.

Step Four: Policy Adoption and Approval

Even the best policy idea is useless if there is no avenue for adoption. At the federal level, adoption usually occurs in three ways: congressional action, regulation, or administrative Executive Order.

Congressional action typically means passing legislation into law. This is often necessary when funding is required but can be used for any sosrt of policy adoption. It can be a long and arduous process depending on the issue and the description of that process is well beyond the scope of this chapter.

Regulation is a much less cumbersome mechanism for policy adoption. Existing legislation may have already resulted in prior regulation in which new policy may seek simply to modify. Nevertheless, for HIT, working with the ONC may result in new or modified regulations for policy assigned or forwarded to that agency. For an organization wishing to impact regulation based on its own internal policy, a significant advocacy effort may be necessary. For regulation at the federal level (and often state level as well), there is a defined and often arduous process of publishing draft regulations with a comment period. This is often the only opportunity for stakeholders to impact the final regulations, although at times there may be several rounds of interim regulations followed by a new comment period before the regulation is finalized. This process is called "rulemaking."

Executive Order is often used by the administration in power to rapidly implement policy, and thereby circumvent Congressional approval. There are certain limitations to this method and such actions may be open to court challenges. In recent years, Executive Orders have been used extensively, due to a lack of ability (or willingness) to work with Congress. Nevertheless, Executive Orders may eventually find their way into legislation (see Box 30.4).

Adoption of policy at the state government level is similar to the federal level, although local hospital policy is quite different and straightforward. However, hospital policy that impacts personnel, and especially the medical staff, may require significant due diligence to avoid untoward consequences. An example is the recent trend of hospital IT departments to adopt a sole source EHR vendor policy, which eliminates well-established beloved best-in-breed departmental IT systems.

The final policy approval process will depend on the type of policy. The federal and state process is described above, but organization and hospital policy usually start in a committee, followed by a recommendation to the board of directors, who make the final decision. Policy that affects a hospital's medical staff may need approval by both the hospital governing board and the general medical staff. Once finalized, specific procedures to carry out the policy may be necessary and are often developed in tandem.

Step Five: Policy Implementation

As difficult as the first four stages may be, implementing a policy is often the most difficult of all. There is no effective way to implement bad policy. Likewise, a well-designed policy can be poorly implemented leading to the same failed outcome.

Jurisdiction determines who is responsible for the implementation stage; for federal HIT policy, that entity is typically the ONC. At this stage, the ultimate success and speed of the process is often determined by the leverage available to the regulating entity. This leverage frequently involves money, either through incentive payments or penalties that withhold Medicare funds or impose civil monetary penalties. Since most hospitals receive Medicare funds, over the years Congress has included requirements in the hospital "Conditions of Participation" (Medicare contract) to drive policy, even those unrelated to Medicare. Beyond this, however, federal agencies have little else they can do to drive adoption. Over time, the ONC has attempted to provide HIT guidance/education, promote IT standards, enable innovative technologies, and cajole the industry towards its mission. How successful the ONC has been a matter of opinion (and definition of "success") but considering the critical importance of HIT in modern healthcare, having a federal government agency in charge of the national HIT policy is well-deserved and prudent.

Step Six: Ongoing Evaluation and Termination of Policies

History has shown that once implemented, policies are difficult to terminate. And, when they are, it is usually because they became obsolete, failed to accomplish the desired outcome, or lost the support of those in power. For local policy, a "sunset" provision is sometimes used to force periodic reevaluation.

Nevertheless, certain policies become so entrenched they may be impossible to rescind. There are several examples in the social welfare realm, but an HIT example is what has been called "Note Bloat." This is an IT-enabled phenomenon (Wang et al., 2017) where it has become very easy to include increasing amounts of nonessential information (e.g., via templates or cut/paste) into the clinical chart, often leaving key aspects of the patient's record "buried" or omitted.

BOX 30.4 Adoption of Policy by Legislation and Executive Order (Example)

In 1982, the American College of Emergency Physicians (ACEP) adopted a policy called, "Bona Fide Emergency Defined." In 1994, this policy was renamed "Definition of an Emergency Service" which established the definition of the "prudent layperson standard" for an emergency.

With extensive advocacy efforts, the "prudent layperson standard" was eventually included in the Balanced Budget Act of 1997 requiring Medicare and Medicaid Managed Care plans to use this standard for determining medically necessary emergency care.

The standard was extended to all federal health plans in 1998 by the Executive Order of President Bill Clinton.

The Affordable Care Act (ACA) in 2010 extended this definition to all insurance plans regulated by the Employee Retirement Income Security Act (ERISA) and qualified health plans in the state ACA Exchanges. To date, 47 states (all except Mississippi, New Hampshire, and Wyoming) have also passed similar laws making the prudent layperson standard mandatory for state-licensed health insurance plans.

BOX 30.5   Elements of Good Policy Development

Write in clear, concise, simple language, using an active (action) voice

Title: Meaningful, concise title

Vision: Identify fundamental problem(s) and/or desired result (objective)

Data: Research, analysis, and review of prior similar policies

Identify the "owner"

Identify "stakeholders" (relevant actors and their interests)

Identify required resources (e.g., funding) and who might provide

Identify likely facilitators (supporters) and barriers (opposition)

Identify and develop policy instruments to address the problem and achieve objectives

Establish a reasonable time frame

Provide definitions

Address political and technical challenges

Consider untoward consequences

Clearly state the future vision

Establish a communication plan

Establish implementation plan

Establish evaluation process (e.g., sunset provision)

Routine evaluation should examine how well a policy is working towards its desired outcome, if there are better or more efficient ways to achieve the same objectives, or if it has become obsolete. Depending on the complexity, such evaluation may require substantial effort and further input from stakeholders.

It is often useful to include a "feedback loop" whereby ongoing comments and success measures can be monitored on a regular basis (Box 30.5).

Healthcare and Informatics associations participate in health policy development by working with multiple agencies and responding to requests for information to assist in the development of appropriate policy development (Table 30.1).

LEADERSHIP COMPETENCIES FOR DEVELOPING AND IMPLEMENTING HIT POLICIES

Healthcare professionals and informaticians have a responsibility to participate in the development and implementation of effective healthcare policies that maximize the utility of HIT and empower clinicians and patients as partners. Traditionally, physicians and nurses in collaboration with IT professionals and advocacy experts have shouldered these responsibilities. "No single profession, working alone, can meet the complex needs of patients and communities" (Institute of Medicine, 2021). To truly create cost-effective quality healthcare for all, each of the healthcare disciplines must "continue to develop skills and competencies in leadership and innovation and collaborate with other professionals in healthcare delivery and health system redesign" (American Academy of Nursing, 2021).

Ensuring Healthcare Practitioners Are Well-Positioned for Health Information Technology

Healthcare professionals and informaticians have, by necessity, become increasingly engaged with healthcare policy efforts.

Nursing HIT leaders have been recruited for key national appointments, as well as executive HIT positions. In 2014, The Nurses on Boards Coalition, comprised of The American Nurses Association (ANA), the American Academy of Nursing, and the American Nurses Foundation launched a national coalition to place 10,000 nurses on governing boards by 2020 (American Academy of Nursing, 2021). The goal was to bring nurses' valuable perspectives to governing boards as well as state-level and national commissions with an interest in health. This goal was met noting that 9,859 nurses are positioned on boards with another 13,978 wanting to serve (Nurses on Boards Coalition website: https://documentcloud.adobe.com/link/track?uri=urn:aaid:scds:US:2bca840a-26d4-4e48-ad0d-ad7fe5f5745e#pageNum=1). The Coalition provides information related to the state goal percent (from 42% in Oklahoma to 248% in Indiana).

Physicians have taken an increasingly active role in HIT, fulfilling a need for clinical informaticists at hospitals and in other healthcare-related industries. In 2013, the subspecialty of "Clinical Informatics" (American Board of Preventive Medicine Subspecialty in Clinical Informatics, 2021) was born with the administration of the first certifying exam administered by the American Board of Preventive Medicine. As of 2020, nearly 2300 physicians had been certified in Clinical Informatics and nearly 40 fellowship programs had been accredited by ACGME. Board certification is the natural outgrowth of the emerging roles of Chief Medical Information Officer (CMIO) and Chief Health Information Officer (CHIO), within hospital leadership teams (Ross et al., 2021). Physician informaticists also have taken larger roles within various IT-related industries, including innovation centers.

Currently, the health informatics discipline is being recognized through the AMIA with a professional certification. This certification, open to individuals with degrees and/or training in health informatics, is similar to the clinical informatics certification and provided an AMIA Certified Health Informatics Professional designation beginning in 2021.

Health Informatics Competencies

Many disciplines now mandate informatics as a part of core curriculum or competencies. Discipline-specific competencies are noted with some healthcare disciplines offering degrees specific for informatics, for example, nursing informatics, medical informatics, and public health informatics. The AMIA, in concert with Commission on Accreditation for Health Informatics and Information Management Education (CAHIM), created standards for master's level education related to informatics (Valenta et al., 2018).

Responding to Requests for Comments

With the increasing use of HIT, the number of related policies, legislation, and regulations has created a need for informaticists with policy experience to respond with comments on ensuing regulations and other related federal guidance documents. Legislation passed by Congress invariably requires further regulations to be written to guide implementation. This "rulemaking process" (Box 30.6) is used to clarify definitions, authority,

TABLE 30.1   Professional Association in Informatics Influencing Health Policy

Name	Mission Statement or Focus	Examples of Current Activities	Website
AMIA Public Policy Committee	To improve health in the United States and globally, we are engaging with policy-makers and other thought leaders to holistically improve health and healthcare with use of informatics' science, research, and practice ... AMIA Public Policy exists to improve the legislative and regulatory environment for health informatics research, practice, and education through AMIA member expertise. Priorities include: 1. Patient Empowerment 2. Health IT Safety 3. Workforce and Education Data Sharing in Research 4. Health IT Standards and Interoperability 5. Informatics-Driven Quality Measurement Population and Public Health 6. Health Data Privacy	• The American Health Information Management Association (AHIMA), the American Medical Informatics Association (AMIA), and the Electronic Health Record Association (EHRA) announced today the release of a preliminary report that examines key issues related to the operationalization of the definitions of electronic health information (EHI) and designated record set (DRS). (September 20, 2021) • In comments submitted to ONC's Recognized Coordinating Entity (RCE) for the Trusted Exchange Framework and Common Agreement (TEFCA), AMIA stressed that participants and subparticipants must be confident that participation in TEFCA will be a net benefit to their current exchange activities. AMIA further recommended that ONC scenarios to clarify how TEFCA will facilitate the various exchange purposes and how the participants and subparticipants will fit in (October 27, 2021).	https://www.amia.org/public-policy
HIMSS Policy Center	HIMSS believes that the appropriate use of IT and management systems can transform healthcare to save lives, improve outcomes of care, and reduce costs. Key issues include: 1. Health Information Exchange (Interoperability and Standards) 2. Meaningful Use 3. Privacy and Security 4. User Experience	• Weekly update via health IT policy newsletter • Annual HIMSS Policy Summit • 2014–2016 Policy Principles • HIMSS IT Value Suite • Policy Committee • Legislative Action Center • 2015–2016 Congressional Asks include expand access to telehealth services for Medicare beneficiaries, support for robust interoperability and health information exchange, and support for healthcare's efforts to combat cyber threats • Sent a letter to Senate HELP Committee outlining policy recommendations related to achieving interoperability, public process for certification of EHRs, and patient access to their personal health information along with a number of other topics	http://www.himss.org/library/health-it-policy

TABLE 30.1   Professional Association in Informatics Influencing Health Policy

Name	Mission Statement or Focus	Examples of Current Activities	Website
AHIMA The Advocacy and Public Policy Center	AHIMA's advocacy and public policy advocacy agenda seeks to transform health and healthcare by connecting people, systems, and ideas. At AHIMA, we've embraced three principles that underpin our work, our outlook, and our advocacy: access, integrity, and connection. As we work toward meaningful legislative and regulatory changes in 2021, AHIMA will work together with our members, national healthcare organizations, and other stakeholders to advance an advocacy agenda to realize our vision.	• AHIMA provided feedback on the Elements of the Common Agreement in support of the goal of establishing "a floor of universal interoperability across the country for health care" (October 11, 2021). • To empower individuals to become better informed and more involved in decisions that affect their health and healthcare, AHIMA believes that public policy must guarantee an individual's right to access their health information, regardless of where it is captured, stored, or exchanged (October 7, 2021).	http://www.ahima.org/about/advocacy
American Academy of Nursing Expert Panel on Informatics and Technology	The Expert Panel on Informatics and Technology gathers health policy data and information advises and represents the Academy on issues related to: health information management, implementation of informatics and technology through EHRs and PHRs (Electronic and Personal Health Records), HIPAA, patient safety initiatives, consumer and personal health, workforce issues and training, bioterrorism and bio surveillance, evidence-based practice, clinical decision support and other areas of concern related to the use of informatics and technology in nursing education, practice and research.	• Released a policy brief endorsing the improvement of nurses' well-being and joy in work (2019). • Released a policy noting support in sustaining and building on institutional and regulatory policies to ensure adequate infrastructure and workforce is in place for precision health implementation by nurses and other healthcare team members (June 2018).	https://www.aannet.org/expert-panels/ep-informatics--technology

AAN, American Academy of Nursing; *AHIMA*, American Health Information Management Association; *AMIA*, American Medical Informatics Association; *HIMSS*, Healthcare Information and Management Systems Society; Office of the National Coordinator for Health Information Technology.

BOX 30.6 Regulatory "Rulemaking" Process

Rulemaking is the policy-making process for Executive and Independent agencies of the Federal government. Agencies use this process to develop and issue Rules (also referred to as "regulations"). The process is governed by laws including but not limited to the Administrative Procedure Act (APA) (5 U.S.C. Chapter 5), Congressional Review Act, Paperwork Reduction Act, and Regulatory Flexibility Act and can lead to a new Rule, an amendment to an existing Rule, or the repeal of an existing Rule. Executive Orders such as 12,866, 13,563, and 13,579 also establish principles and guidance for the rulemaking process.

Once an agency decides that regulatory action is necessary or appropriate, it develops and typically publishes a proposed rule in the Federal Register, soliciting comments from the public on the regulatory proposal. After the agency considers this public feedback and makes changes where appropriate, it then publishes a final rule in the Federal Register with a specific date upon which the rule becomes effective and enforceable. In issuing a final rule, the agency must describe and respond to the public comments it received.

Data from 10 Ways Technology Is Changing Healthcare. The Medical Futurist, 3 March 2020. https://medicalfuturist.com/ten-ways-technology-changing-healthcare/#. Accessed October 27, 2021.

eligibility, benefits, and standards with input from professional societies, healthcare providers, third-party payers, consumers, and other special interest groups. Each organization's own internal policies may provide direction to guide these formal policy comments.

Developing Position Statements

Another common mechanism for advancing healthcare policy is through the development and publication of position statements (a.k.a. policy briefs). This may be an explanation or recommendation for a course of action that reflects an organization's stance on an issue. Position statements are typically developed after an internal discussion with content experts, then after consensus has been reached, advanced to the broader membership for review and input, and finally submitted to the oversight governance group or board for approval. For certain broad issues, a joint statement may be formulated by multiple organizations and then publicized in hopes of influencing national policy.

Healthcare Policy Advocacy

Healthcare informaticians working within professional associations bring a deep understanding of clinical processes, technology, and HIT systems in addition to experience as advocates for patients, groups, communities, and overall populations. Using contacts and infrastructure provided by a professional association, these leaders have a unique opportunity to share their knowledge in hopes of advancing healthcare HIT initiatives.

An understanding of healthcare policy principles may be gained through formal coursework, continuing education, literature review, and self-study available on the internet to be effective in the dual role of informatician and policy expert (Gillis, 2011). Most professional organizations have formal legislative and advocacy activities and committees where peer mentoring

can also be obtained. But there is no better way than getting involved with an actual policy initiative from beginning to end. If not ready for a national initiative, participating in state-level advocacy activities can provide adequate experience, including meeting with legislators and other policymakers.

Beyond this, leadership skills, communication skills, and leveraging one's professional network are key factors toward success. According to Alexander and Halley, to advocate, health professionals and informaticians must be strategists, leaders, and great communicators, and they must engage stakeholders across multiple spectrums to ensure that the needs of patients and professionals are met (Alexander & Halley, 2015). Communication skills are essential to craft and articulate "talking points" to engage and persuade. Using personal relevant stories (without violating HIPAA) are particularly effective. Exemplary leadership requires more than showing passion. It also requires connecting evidence (data) to the policy agenda and framing it in context. Collaboration and unified messaging among stakeholders are also keys to success.

EXAMPLES OF RECENT MAJOR HEALTH INFORMATION TECHNOLOGY POLICY INITIATIVES

Health Information Technology for Economic and Clinical Health Act (2009)

As previously noted, the IOM has had a significant impact on the adoption of HIT, particularly EHR systems. With the passage of the American Recovery and Reinvestment Act of 2009, Congress made a $49 billion (Burke, 2010) "bet," that increased implementation of HIT (including computers, software, and network connections throughout the healthcare system) would improve the quality and efficiency of healthcare in the United States. This effort became known as the HITECH Act with the express purpose to accelerate the adoption of HIT as a method of improving the quality, safety, and efficiency of healthcare (Blumenthal, 2009). It has also played a key role in informing the HHS Strategic Plan and, in turn, many of the programs and activities of the ONC.

HITECH has had more impact on healthcare informatics than any other legislation in US history. Its unprecedented amount of funding not only spawned a flurry of EHR implementations, but it also caused hospitals to replace aging and less well-connected systems. While expectations were high for achieving significant quality, safety, and cost benefits from this initiative, research shows that unplanned and unexpected consequences resulted from major policy and technological challenges (Ash et al., 2004; Koppel et al., 2005).

HITECH Methodology

HITECH started with monetary incentives via enhanced Medicare and Medicaid payments, then in 2016 began levying penalties for non-compliance. It required the use of EHRs certified to meet requirements set forth by ONC and certified by an Authorized Testing and Certification Body via a testing process defined by the National Institute for Standards and Technology. Further, the certified EHR technology had to be used in a "meaningful way," extensively spelled out in published regulations, called "Meaningful Use" (Box 30.7).

Medicare Access and CHIP Reauthorization Act of 2015

By 2015, a decade of the HITECH program had led to the adoption of at least a "Basic EHR with Clinician Notes" by 84% of Non-Federal Acute Care Hospitals (US hospital EMR market share, 2019). However, a substantial number of hospitals failed to meet the deadline for Stage 2 Meaningful Use criteria (Adler-Milstein et al., 2014). Ongoing criticism of the program led to the replacement of Meaningful Use with "Advancing Care Information" Performance Category in Medicare Access and CHIP Reauthorization Act of 2015 (MACRA) as part of the Merit-Based Incentive Payment System (MIPS) (MIPS).

Ongoing legislative updates continue to impact EHR requirements often adding to end-user IT overhead burden. Suffice it to say, hospitals must be prepared to adjust as policymakers seek to drive healthcare in a direction often to suit evolving political ideology (Box 30.8).

Negative Impact of HITECH Due to Rapid Transition to Certified EHRs

While HITECH may have accelerated the development and implementation of some key HIT functions, it also inhibited

others (Botta & Cutler, 2014). In a cruel twist of fate, while not directly focused on EDs, HITECH negatively impacted nearly every ED in the United States (Box 30.9). In the effort to meet Meaningful Use criteria, hospitals were forced to update or replace their EHRs. In most instances, this meant the loss of time-tested stand-alone "Best-in-Breed" ED Information Systems (EDIS), which were rapidly replaced by certified enterprise-EMR/EHR with "ED Modules" (KLAS, 2009). In addition to the disruption caused by the implementation of a new HIT system, the new ED modules had much less functionality than "Best-in-Breed" EDIS that EDs had come to rely on upon (KLAS Performance Report: EDIS, 2013). From an HIT functionality and efficiency standpoint, this set EDIS back at least 10 years.

Patient Safety

With the 1999 IOM report *To Err Is Human*, the age of patient "safety" began. The report estimated up to 98,000 lives were lost annually due to hospital medical errors, which catalyzed a revolution to improve the quality of care (Institute of Medicine, 1999). In 2001, a subsequent report, *Crossing the Quality Chasm* (Institute of Medicine, 2001) outlined necessary changes to effect improvements in healthcare safety, which 10 years later had yet to be achieved. In 2012, the IOM proposed new strategies to advance quality and safety in yet another report, *Best Care at Lower Cost: The Path to Continuously Learning Health Care in America* (Institute of Medicine, 2012). Nevertheless, the challenges of creating a safer healthcare system continue, despite controversy about its magnitude (Rodwin et al., 2020). Of note, each of the IOM reports identified HIT as an effective strategy for safer, more effective care in all settings.

When designed and implemented appropriately, HIT can improve healthcare providers' performance, support better communication between patients and healthcare providers, and enhance patient safety, all of which ultimately leads to better care (Sensmeier, 2015). For example, the number of patients who receive the correct medication in hospitals increases significantly when hospitals implement computerized prescribing and use barcoded medication administration (Wulff et al., 2011). However, poorly designed and implemented EHRs can actually create new hazards in an already overly complex healthcare delivery system. To protect patients, EHRs must be designed and used in ways that maximize patient safety while minimizing the risk of harm. HIT can better help patients if it becomes more usable, more interoperable, and easier to implement and maintain.

Institute of Medicine Report on Health Information Technology and Patient Safety

In collaboration with HHS, the 2011 IOM report, *HIT and Patient Safety* states that "safe use of HIT relies on several factors, including clinicians and patients" (Institute of Medicine, 2011). Safety analyses should not look for a single cause, but consider the system as a whole and the interplay of people, process, and technology. Vendors, administrators, end users, government, and the private sector all have roles to play. The IOM's recommendations include improving transparency in the reporting of HIT safety incidents and enhancing monitoring of HIT products (Box 30.10). The IOM report also examined a broad range of health information technologies, including EHRs, secure patient portals, and Health Information Exchanges (HIEs).

The Health IT Patient Safety Action and Surveillance Plan (2013) (Office of the National Coordinator for Health IT, 2013)

This policy initiative created a new HIT Safety Center Roadmap published by ONC in 2015. This outlined a 5-year plan for creating a federal resource, as a public-private partnership, to focus on aggregating data from HIT-related adverse events. The center has three major tasks: (1) convening groups of stakeholders to learn more about HT-related risks; (2) researching hazards and disseminating information gleaned from these activities, which could include real-world pilot testing and implementation; and (3) evaluating HIT safety solutions (Prepared by RTI, 2021).

Patient Safety and Quality

The government-sponsored Agency for Healthcare Research and Quality (AHRQ) began offering grants in 2004 for planning, implementing, and testing the value of both EHRs and HIEs. As such, "AHRQ supports health services research initiatives that seek to improve the quality of healthcare in America. Its mission is to produce evidence to make healthcare safer, higher quality, more accessible, equitable, and affordable, and to work within HHS and with other partners to make sure that

the evidence is understood and used" (AHRQ, 2021). AHRQ works to fulfill its mission through collaboration with leading academic institutions, hospitals, physician offices, healthcare systems, and many other settings across the nation. The Agency has a broad research portfolio that touches on nearly every aspect of healthcare.

In March 2011, under the auspices of AHRQ, HHS released the *National Quality Strategy* for health improvement, the first effort to create a national framework to help guide local, state, and national efforts to improve the quality of care in the United States (AHRQ National Quality Strategy, 2021). This strategy recognizes HIT as critical to improving the quality of care, improving health outcomes, and reducing costs.

AHRQ has ongoing HIT initiatives (called "Digital Healthcare Research") related to patient care and quality (AHRQ digital healthcare research initiatives, 2021). It remains a driving force for national healthcare policy initiatives and HIT application toward patient safety and quality.

CONCLUSION AND FUTURE DIRECTIONS

This chapter describes *current* health policy initiatives with a focus on HIT and health policy leadership responsibilities of health professionals and informaticians. By understanding informatics-related health policy issues, the role of the professional organizations, the current federal structural support for HIT, and specific approaches for participating in the advocacy process, health and informatics leaders will have a significant impact on this nation's health policy.

At the same time, the future of healthcare is shaping up right in front of our eyes with rapid advances in digital healthcare technologies well beyond mere electronic information (EHR). Artificial and augmented intelligence, machine learning, augmented reality and virtual reality, 3D printing, telehealth, robotics, nanotechnology, and "hyper-automation" (Hyperautomation by hyperscience, 2021) all have promise to dramatically alter the practice of medicine and patient care. We must be diligent to stay abreast of these emerging healthcare innovations to control technology and not the other way around. As in other industries (e.g., driverless vehicles in transportation), we must work together with current technology and embrace emerging healthcare technologies to even stay relevant in the future.

As HIT and related technologies advance, healthcare policy will take on a new and increasingly more important purpose. Healthcare leaders, and particularly informaticists, have a responsibility to be at the forefront of the direction, use, and utility of these emerging and potentially disruptive innovations.

Some might say that "digital transformation" in healthcare began in the late 1990s (Sukhova, 2016). Others will say it is just now beginning. But Winston Churchill put it best, "Now this is not the end. It is not even the beginning of the end. But it is the end of the beginning" (Churchill, 2021).

There is still work to be done. Through strong leadership and active participation, we will be able to organize and complete the challenging work necessary to create policy that will transform healthcare.

> ### BOX 30.10 2011 Institute of Medicine Health Information Technology and Patient Safety Recommendation Summary
>
> - HHS should ensure that vendors support users in freely exchanging information about HIT experiences and issues, including safety.
> - ONC should work with the private sector to make comparative user experiences publicly available.
> - HHS should fund a new Health IT Safety Council within an existing standards organization to evaluate criteria for judging the safety of health IT.
> - HHS should establish a mechanism for vendors and users to report health IT-related deaths, serious injuries, or unsafe conditions.
> - HHS should recommend that Congress establish an independent federal entity, similar to the National Transportation Safety Board, to perform investigations in a transparent, non-punitive manner.

HHS, U.S. Department of Health and Human Services; *HIT,* Health information technology; *IOM,* Institute of Medicine; *ONC,* Office of the National Coordinator for Health Information Technology.

The Medical Futurist: "Our task at the moment is to face our fears about the future with courage; to turn to technologies with an open mind, and to prepare for the changing world with as much knowledge as possible" (10 ways technology, 2021).

ACKNOWLEDGMENT

The authors wish to acknowledge the contributions of Joyce Sensmeier and Judy Murphy to the previous edition of this chapter.

DISCUSSION QUESTIONS

1. Outline the basic healthcare policy competencies for health informatics leaders.
2. Discuss how the Federal Health IT Strategic Plan might impact future HIT policy and, in turn, future projects and programs supporting the use of HIT in the United States.
3. Outline the process (six steps) for developing and implementing effective informatics policy.
4. What future technology has the most potential to change the practice of medicine?

CASE STUDY

Mr. Smith Goes to Washington is a 1939 American film starring James Stewart and Jean Arthur about one man's effect on American politics. Today, health leaders make their own trips to our nation's capital, and while the focus may be different, the experience is no less exciting. Here is a case study illustrating one example.

It started with a phone call requesting an informaticist to testify via written and oral testimony at a Congressional hearing on Standards for HIT related to the HITECH Act, hosted by the House Subcommittee on Technology and Innovation. The organization that was contacted selected the chair of its HIT committee and the preparation began. Written testimony, a biography, *curriculum vitae*, and financial disclosure form needed to be submitted in advance. The team created testimony to address the House Subcommittee's two questions: What progress has ONC made since the enactment of the HITECH Act regarding meeting (1) interoperability needs and (2) information security standards for EHRs and HIT systems?

Preparation leveraged previous testimony, position statements, and background materials. Experts with knowledge of privacy and security standards were interviewed. Multiple rounds of comments were made before the testimony was "final" and ready for submission.

Next, abbreviated oral comments were prepared, for a maximum of 5 minutes, focusing on three key persuasive points. Repeated practice honed the delivery to meet the 5-minute limit.

Then came the "inquisition," a dry run facing a team of experts who drilled questions that might be asked by the subcommittee members. One lesson learned was to get to the point quickly and use follow-up responses as an opportunity to reemphasize the three key points from the testimony. Getting to know the subcommittee members was an important task to recognize faces and understand the implications of their districts, political party, recent activities, and relevant legislation they supported.

On the day of the testimony, the team met in advance of the hearing to calm nerves and review key points. All the panelists then met in the Subcommittee chairman's office for introductions and a prehearing briefing to put the panelists at ease. It was announced that the hearing would be delayed due to critical votes on the House floor and flight reservations had to be rebooked.

At the revised appointed time, panelists entered the hearing room taking their seats at a row of tables facing the dais, where the committee members and staff were seated. Each panelist had a microphone, timer, and stop light that tracked the time limit. During the testimony, the stop light changed from green to yellow, then red when each speaker's 5-minute limit was reached.

The oral testimony was flawless. One member asked if their hospital had ever been hacked, a question that had not been anticipated. But was an opportunity to reiterate a key point about the need for better enforcement against hackers. The hearing was broadcast live on CSPAN and the internet, with a transcript available in the public hearing record, and a video clip of the testimony posted on YouTube.

Overall, it was a positive experience, made easy by proper preparation. An unexpected upgrade to first class on the flight home made it all that better.

While *Mr. Smith Goes to Washington* made James Stewart a major movie star, the objective of this exercise was more pedestrian: influencing national policy to improve patient care, safety, and security of HIT.

Discussion Questions

1. How can healthcare providers leverage their clinical background when offering testimony at a legislative committee hearing?
2. How can personal experience be used to drive home key points in testimony?
3. How should one plan for the unexpected when asked to participate in a legislative hearing?

REFERENCES

10 ways technology is changing healthcare. (2020). The Medical Futurist, https://medicalfuturist.com/ten-ways-technology-changing-healthcare/#. Accessed October 27, 2021.

About the ONC. (2021). https://www.healthit.gov/topic/about-onc Accessed October 27, 2021.

Adler-Milstein, J., DesRoches, C. M., Furukawa, M. F., Worzala, C., Charles, D., Kralovec, P., et al. (2014). More than half of US hospitals have at least a basic EHR, but stage 2 criteria remain challenging for most. *Health Affairs (Millwood)*, *33*(9), 1664–1671.

AHRQ digital healthcare research initiatives. (2021).https://www.ahrq.gov/topics/health-information-technology-hit.html. Accessed October 27, 2021.

AHRQ National Quality Strategy. (2021). https://www.ahrq.gov/workingforquality/about/index.html. Accessed October 27, 2021.

AHRQ Strategic Plan. (2021). https://www.ahrq.gov/cpi/about/mission/strategic-plan/strategic-plan.html. Accessed October 27, 2021.

Alexander, D., & Halley, E. C. (2015). Establishing nursing informatics in public policy. In V. Saba & K. A. McCormick (Eds.), Essentials of nursing informatics (6th ed., pp. 281–291). New York, NY: McGraw-Hill.

American Academy of Nursing. Nurses on boards coalition. (2014). https://campaignforaction.org/resource/national-coalition-launches-effort-place-10000-nurses-governing-boards-2020/. Accessed October 27, 2021.

American Board of Preventive Medicine Subspecialty in Clinical Informatics. (2021). https://www.theabpm.org/become-certified/subspecialties/clinical-informatics/. Accessed October 27, 2021.

American Recovery and Reinvestment Act of 2009, Public Law 111-5, HITECH Act, Sec. 13001 (February 17, 2009).

Andrews, M. (2018). Public policy failure: 'How often?' and 'what is failure, anyway'? A study of world bank project performance. Center for International Development Faculty Working Paper No. 344 at Harvard University, December 2018.

Ash, J. S., Berg, M., & Coiera, E. (2004). Some unintended consequences of information technology in health care: The nature of patient care information system-related errors. *Journal of the American Medical Informatics Association*, *11*(2), 104–112.

Bloomrosen, M., Starren, J., Lorenzi, N. M., Ash, J. S., Patel, V. L., & Shortliffe, E. H. (2011). Anticipating and addressing the unintended consequences of health IT and policy: A report from the AMIA 2009 Health Policy Meeting. *Journal of the American Medical Informatics Association*, *18*(1), 82–90.

Blumenthal, D. (2009 May 1). Stimulating the adoption of health information technology. *West Virginia Medical Journal*, *105*(3), 28–30.

Botta, M. D., & Cutler, D. M. (2014). Meaningful use: Floor or ceiling? *Healthc (Amst)*, *2*(1), 48–52.

Burke, T. (2010). The health information technology provisions in the American Recovery and Reinvestment Act of 2009: implications for public health policy and practice. *Public Health Rep*, *125*(1), 141–145.

Churchill, W.S. (1942). The end of the beginning. London, England. http://www.churchill-society-london.org.uk/EndoBegn.html. Accessed October 27, 2021.

Committee on Quality of Health Care in America. (2001). *Crossing the quality chasm: A new health system for the 21st century*. Washington, DC: National Academy Press.

Consolidated Omnibus Budget Reconciliation Act of 1985 (Passed April 7, 1986-Effective Aug 1, 1986), 42 U.S.C. § 1395dd.

Gillis, C. L. (2011). Developing policy leadership in nursing: Three wishes. *Nursing Outlook*, *59*(4), 179–181.

Healthcare Information and Management Systems Society (HIMSS), (2011). *Position statement on transforming nursing practice through technology and informatics*. Chicago, IL: HIMSS.

Hersh, W. (2006). Who are the informaticians? What we know and should know. *Journal of the American Medical Informatics Association*, *13*(2), 166–170. https://www.ncbi.nlm.nih.gov/pmc/articles/PMC1447543/.

HHS organizational chart. (2021). https://www.hhs.gov/about/agencies/orgchart/index.html. Accessed October 27, 2021.

Hyperautomation by hyperscience. (2021).https://hyperscience.com/what-is-hyperautomation/. Accessed October 27, 2021.

Information technology strategic plan FY 2021–2023: https://www.hhs.gov/sites/default/files/hhs-it-strategic-plan-final-fy2021-2023.pdf. Accessed October 27, 2021.

Institute of Medicine. Assessing progress on the Institute of Medicine report—the future of nursing: Report in brief. (2015). https://www.nap.edu/catalog/21838/assessing-progress-on-the-institute-of-medicine-report-the-future-of-nursing. Accessed October 27, 2021.

Institute of Medicine. (2012). *Best care at lower cost: The path to continuously learning health care in America*. Washington, DC: National Academy Press.

Institute of Medicine. (2001). *Crossing the quality chasm: A new health system for the 21st century*. Washington, DC: National Academy Press.

Institute of Medicine. (2011). *HIT and patient safety: Building safer systems for better care*. Washington, DC: The National Academies Press.

Institute of Medicine. (1999). *To err is human: Building a safer health system*. Washington, DC: National Academy Press.

KFF analysis of National Health Expenditure (NHE) data. (2021). https://www.healthsystemtracker.org/chart-collection/u-s-spending-healthcare-changed-time/#item-usspendingovertime_1. Accessed October 27, 2021.

KLAS Performance Report: EDIS 2013: Revealing the physicians' voice. KLAS Research, Orem, UT. January 2013.

KLAS: Emergency department information systems is best of breed still the best approach? KLAS Research, Orem, UT. December 15, 2009.

Koppel, R., Metlay, J. P., Cohen, A., Abaluck, B., Localio, A. R., Kimmel, S. E., et al. (2005). Role of computerized physician order entry systems in facilitating medication errors. *Journal of the American Medical Association*, *293*(10), 1197–1203.

Law vs policy. What's the difference? (2019, October 13). https://careers.uw.edu/blog/2019/10/13/law-vs-policy-whats-the-difference/. Accessed October 27, 2021.

MIPS Overview. https://qpp.cms.gov/mips/overview.

NEWPORT F. (2019). Americans' mixed views of healthcare and healthcare reform. GALLUP. May 21, 2019. https://news.gallup.com/opinion/polling-matters/257711/americans-mixed-views-healthcare-healthcare-reform.aspx. Accessed October 27, 2021.

Office of the National Coordinator for Health IT. Health IT Patient Safety Action and Surveillance Plan. (2013). https://www.healthit.gov/sites/default/files/safety_plan_master.pdf. Accessed October 27, 2021.

ONC 2020–2025 federal health IT strategic plan. (2021). https://www.healthit.gov/topic/2020-2025-federal-health-it-strategic-plan. Accessed October 27, 2021

Oxford Languages Dictionary. (n.d.).

Patel, R. (2019). Meeting the unfulfilled promises of electronic health records. Forbes Technology Council. August 22, 2019. https://www.forbes.com/sites/forbestechcouncil/2019/08/22/

meeting-the-unfulfilled-promises-of-electronic-health-records/?sh=7109b6811362. Accessed October 27, 2021.

Patient Protection and Affordable Care Act (PPACA), Public Law 111–148 (2010, March 23) and Health Care and Education Reconciliation Act of 2010, Public Law 111–152 (2010, March 30).

Prepared by RTI International for Office of the National Coordinator for Health IT. Health IT safety center roadmap. https://www.healthit.gov/buzz-blog/wp-content/uploads/2015/07/Health-it-safety-center-roadmap.pdf. Accessed October 27, 2021.

Rodwin, B. A., Bilan, V. P., Merchant, N. B., Steffens, C. G., Grimshaw, A. A., Bastian, L. A., et al. (2020). Rate of preventable mortality in hospitalized patients: A systematic review and meta-analysis. *Journal of General Internal Medicine, 35*(7), 2099–2106.

Ross, H., Kieffer, W., & Durst, Z. Industry voices—the 2nd-generation CMIO/CHIO is evolving into a strategic role and team leader. Fierce Healthcare. September 25, 2019. https://www.fiercehealthcare.com/tech/industry-voices-second-generation-cmio-chio-evolving-into-a-strategic-role-and-team-leader. Accessed October 27, 2021.

Saba, V., & McCormick, K. A. (Eds.). (2015). Essentials of nursing informatics (6th ed.). New York, NY: McGraw-Hill.

Sensmeier, J. (2015). Patient safety and IT trends. *Nurs Manag, 46*(11), 24–26.

Stone, D. (2011). *Policy paradox: The art of political decision making* (3rd ed.). W. W. Norton & Company.

Sukhova, M. (2016, December 12). Digital transformation: History, present, and future trends. *Auriga Blog* https://auriga.com/blog/2016/digital-transformation-history-present-and-future-trends/. Accessed October 27, 2021.

Tang, P. C. (2003). Key capabilities of an electronic health record system: a letter report: *Committee on Data Standards for Patient Safety: Institute of Medicine Committee on Data Standards for Patient Safety*. Washington, DC: Institute of Medicine.

The Joint Commission. https://www.jointcommission.org/accreditation-and-certification/become-accredited/what-is-accreditation/.

The Office of the National Coordinator (ONC) for Health Information Technology. (2021). Federal health IT strategic plan 2015–2020. https://www.healthit.gov/sites/default/files/9-5-federalhealthitstratplanfinal_0.pdf. Accessed October 27, 2021.

U.S. Department of Health & Human Services. HHS strategic plan FY 2018–2022. https://www.hhs.gov/about/strategic-plan/index.html.

US hospital EMR market share 2019 report. KLAS, April 30, 2019.

Valenta, A. L., Berner, E. S., Boren, S. A., Deckard, G. J., Eldredge, C., Fridsma, D. B., et al. (2018). AMIA Board White Paper: AMIA 2017 core competencies for applied health informatics education at the master's degree level. *Journal of the American Medical Informatics Association, 25*(12), 1657–1668. https://doi.org/10.1093/jamia/ocy132.

Wang, M. D., Khanna, R., & Najafi, N. (2017). Characterizing the source of text in electronic health record progress notes. *JAMA Internal Medicine, 177*(8), 1212–1213.

World Health Organization health policy definition. (2021). https://www.euro.who.int/en/health-topics/health-policy. Accessed October 27, 2021.

Wulff, K., Cummings, G. G., Marck, P., & Yurtseven, O. (2011). Medication administration technologies and patient safety: A mixed-method systematic review. *Journal of Advanced Nursing, 67*(10), 2080–2095.

31

Health Information Technology Governance

Kensaku Kawamoto, Jim Livingston,
Maia Hightower, and Donna Roach

The constant and complex changes in the US healthcare ecosystem require precision methods and robust oversight. It is critical that healthcare organizations develop a health information technology (health IT) governance structure that allows priorities and direction to be promptly adapted to these ongoing changes.

OBJECTIVES

At the completion of this chapter, the reader will be prepared to:
1. Describe why health IT governance is needed.
2. Describe key considerations for the establishment of health IT governance.
3. Discuss factors to consider when making recommendations for establishing health IT governance.

KEY TERMS

health IT capability maturity assessment, 491

health IT governance, 487

ABSTRACT ❖

Health information technology (health IT)—the leveraging of information systems to improve health and care—represents a critical enabler for healthcare organizations to achieve strategic objectives, operational excellence, and future viability. To optimize the value of health IT resources, a healthcare organization must have in place effective governance to ensure IT's alignment with institutional strategic objectives and the effective prioritization of limited resources. This chapter provides direction and insight into various issues that must be considered in establishing that governance structure. In addition, recommendations are provided for establishing an effective health informatics governance structure that is aligned with institutional strategic objectives, effectively prioritizes competing health IT needs, appropriately manages risks, enables excellence in both operations and innovation, and is tailored to the unique culture and characteristics of the organization.

INTRODUCTION

As an emerging element of our healthcare delivery system, the concept of health IT governance is far from mature in all but the most advanced healthcare facilities. There are some relevant resources on health IT governance available in the literature, such as a book by Kropf and Scalzi published by the Healthcare Information and Management Systems Society (Kropf and Scalzi, 2012). Additionally, the Association for Health Information Management Association (AHIMA) has an Introduction to Information Systems for Health Information Technology, 4th edition, which covers relevant governance discussions (Kavanaugh-Burke & Sayles, 2021). There are also relevant resources on specific aspects of health IT governance, such as data governance (Rosenbaum, 2010) and the application of artificial intelligence in healthcare (Reddy et al., 2020). In this chapter, the authors build on these resources and offer their perspectives on health IT governance based on their extensive experience in providing administrative leadership in organizations ranging from large multihospital systems to academic medical centers (AMCs). These organizations demonstrate varying degrees of sophistication regarding electronic health record (EHR) systems and associated health IT capabilities. Because establishing operational processes (e.g., for proposing and reviewing project proposals) is much more straightforward than establishing an effective governance structure that appropriately owns and uses these processes, this chapter focuses on health IT governance structure rather than on the processes used to operationalize the governance. This chapter focuses on the health IT governance of larger healthcare organizations such as AMCs because of the expertise of the authors. However, we believe the general principles and recommendations provided in this chapter should be equally applicable to other healthcare settings, such as small and medium-sized healthcare organizations and post-acute facilities.

HEALTH INFORMATION TECHNOLOGY GOVERNANCE: NEED AND CORE COMPONENTS

Health IT Governance Needs

Healthcare is an information-intensive endeavor; health IT represents a core pillar that enables and supports a modern healthcare organization's ability to achieve its strategic and operational objectives. Health IT encompasses all aspects of a healthcare organization's clinical and business activities, including clinical care delivery, billing, human resource management, staffing, financial management, population health management, research, education, innovation, and the tracking and improvement of care value, while maintaining secure system access that is always available. Larger organizations may have hundreds of computer systems and applications. Given the broad and deep involvement of health IT in all aspects of an organization's mission and operations, healthcare organizations must ensure their health IT efforts are aligned with their key objectives. Moreover, a healthcare organization's strategic and operational initiatives often require health IT resources to be optimally effective. Whether it is responding to a pandemic, care pathway implementation, population health management, medication safety, or cyber security incidents, it is rare for a key healthcare initiative not to require health IT support. Thus, the need for health IT resources (e.g., analysts and software developers) will often significantly exceed the available capacity of such resources. The critical nature of effective health IT governance then arises from the following fundamental interrelated needs:

1. The need to ensure alignment of health IT resources with institutional priorities
2. The need to effectively prioritize the use of health IT resources in the face of competing demands for these limited resources

Core Components of Health IT Governance

Healthcare enterprises are often recognized as being one of the most complex of all organizational structures. Consequently, when one speaks of "institutional priorities," the list is often long and generated from multiple sources. Historically, beyond priorities established by senior leadership, requests for health IT resources are received from clinicians, researchers, the finance and quality departments, specialists who are refining clinical processes or investigating clinical variances, and so forth. More recently, increasing requests from institutional stakeholders are being submitted as they work on emerging areas of priority in healthcare, such as payment reform, public health emergencies, personalized medicine, and more sophisticated costing methodologies. In summary, the demand for health IT resources

and expertise is growing rapidly, the requests are coming from a broader group of constituencies, and the institutional priorities are becoming much less clear. Without effective governance, key stakeholders—including healthcare providers—will be frustrated by delayed or inadequate IT support and a resource allocation rationale they do not understand. Moreover, the overall resource allocation is likely to be suboptimal for addressing institutional strategic priorities, and organizations may even be supporting conflicting and overlapping projects.

The role of health IT governance is to help to clarify priorities, allocate resources, manage risks, and if necessary, approve the funding to support the expansion of available health IT resources. Health IT governance should also be accountable to track and monitor the benefits of these investments.

Effective health IT governance must include the following components to meet these needs:

- Organizational structures are responsible for clearly defining institutional priorities. Typically, this function is primarily the responsibility of the board of directors and senior leadership of a healthcare organization.
- Organizational structures are responsible for ensuring that health IT efforts are aligned with institutional priorities and used optimally.
- All the while, accompanying processes are needed to operationalize the governance. For example, health IT governance typically incorporates the processes in Box 31.1. Establishing such operational processes is much more straightforward compared to establishing a governance structure that appropriately owns and uses these processes; therefore, the remainder of the chapter will focus on the health IT governance structure rather than on the processes used to operationalize the governance.

A sample health IT governance structure, adapted from recommendations by Hoehn, is provided below:

- Board of directors and executive management, responsible for setting the overall health IT strategy and clear expectations within the context of institutional priorities
- Clinical IT governance committee, including a chief medical officer, chief nursing officer, chief medical informatics officer, chief nursing informatics officer, chief information officer, other relevant operational executives (e.g., chief operating officer, chief financial officer), and appropriate clinical and administrative department chairs, responsible

---

BOX 31.1   Health Information Technology Governance Activities and Processes

- Formal processes for proposing new projects requiring health IT resources (e.g., formal submission templates outlining major aspects of a project such as purpose, scope, estimated timelines, and resources; see Chapter 17 for details about project management)
- Planning future directions and investments
- Evaluating and prioritizing potential projects; evaluating, approving, and prioritizing changes to the EHR system (e.g., the introduction of new clinical decision support alerts and reminders)
- Approving funding
- Monitoring return on investment for projects

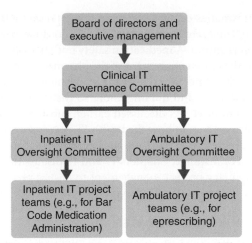

Fig 31.1 Sample health information technology *(IT)* governance structure.

for establishing and overseeing the implementation of the health IT strategic plan

- Various committees reporting to clinical IT governance committee, responsible for overseeing operational execution of clinical IT initiatives consistent with institutional priorities and the health IT strategic plan (Hoehn, 2010).

Fig. 31.1 shows an example of an organizational chart demonstrating this kind of health IT governance structure. The figure shows approaches that an institution may take to create IT governance. Each institution may need to adapt this governance structure to incorporate other committees with overlapping responsibilities. The next section discusses this and other relevant issues that should be considered in establishing any health IT governance.

KEY INSIGHTS

Respect Current Decision-Making Structures

Establishing a health IT governance requires strong consideration and respect for governance structures and decision-making processes already in place within the organization. For example, if the culture is for clinical department chairs to have a strong voice in institutional decisions, then the health IT governance should ensure adequate representation. Furthermore, it is important that strong alignment be demonstrated between the initiatives of the broader organization and the focus of the health IT program. For example, if understanding and improving care value is a key focus of the institution, then supporting the measurement and improvement of value (versus only profit) should be a key priority of the health IT program. If a health IT governance model does not demonstrate this alignment between organizational priorities and the priorities of the health IT program, barriers to effective outcomes and communication could be erected needlessly.

Time invested in determining who "owns" key elements of IT governance is time well spent (Weill & Ross, 2005). Fortunate cases allow existing committees to modify and embrace the requirements for health IT governance. Examples of suboptimal

governance include decision-making dominated by the loudest voice, governance in which IT drives the decisions, the lack of good governance, and vendor-controlled decision-making.

Shift in Organizational Mindset

Healthcare organizations have and continue to be focused on developing IT infrastructure and implementing many applications. The latter have consisted primarily of transaction-based applications that support the revenue cycle, back-office functions such as payroll, and the delivery of clinical care (e.g., EHRs). Under the 2009 American Recovery and Reimbursement Act (ARRA), a funding source was created for EHRs, with the intent to improve physician efficiency and patient care. A greater focus was placed on system interoperability, which has led to improved data standardization. Recently, data warehouses with an array of decision support and analytical tools developed by both vendors and in-house resources have emerged. These allow analysis across specialty systems—for example, powerful queries can be made across clinical, financial, and staffing systems to more accurately understand the value of care delivered (i.e., outcomes achieved in relation to costs incurred) (Kawamoto et al., 2015). The increasing sophistication of the IT environment has enabled both clinical and administrative leaders to leverage data in support of their programs and services while also increasing the expectations that such leaders have of their colleagues in IT. For example, an institution could conduct analyses about a new warfarin clinic and its impact on patient outcomes and its associated operational costs to the institution for staffing, supplies, and management. Litigation avoidance costs could also be considered in these analyses.

The emergence of the Internet in the early 1990s and smartphones in the late 2000s led to customer expectations that information about all topics should be at the fingertips of both clinicians and customers (often with little consideration given to whether the information is accurate or can be trusted). As a result, patients and families have new expectations in terms of both access to and transparency of data from their caregivers, with the expectations of patients, families, and other healthcare consumers often exceeding that of healthcare providers and institutions.

Recently, increased government interest in health reform has brought regulatory mandates and incentives, as well as new market pressures, to the forefront. For example, healthcare is increasingly being reimbursed for the value provided to patients, rather than simply on the volume of services rendered. Another example indicates how federal regulations related to the 21st Century Cures Act of 2016 (Office of the National Coordinator for Health IT, 2021) are enabling third-party digital health innovations to be directly integrated with the EHR and its user interface (Kawamoto et al., 2021). Organizations have had to commit significant resources to health IT to refine clinical care delivery processes and improve outcomes to effectively respond to these changes.

These internal and external forces are causing organizations to rethink their priorities and how capital, operational dollars, and human resources are focused. This requires a change in health IT governance that organizational leaders are unprepared for. Information has become a strategic asset that is essential to survival within the current healthcare context, and the demands on those with health IT expertise are expanding quickly. Prioritization of projects becomes imperative as the demands rapidly outstrip the internal capacity to meet the need. This is the role of IT governance.

The Continual Increase in Demand for Health Information Technology

Due in large part to the successful implementation of core enabling technologies such as EHR systems and computerized provider order entry (CPOE) systems, a continual increase is evident in demand for health IT resources by providers and administrators who increasingly see health IT as a key tool for achieving organizational goals. Indeed, the implementation of core clinical information systems is just the beginning of an institution's health IT road map, as the availability of these core infrastructure components opens the possibility of ever more advanced uses of health IT, whether it be data mining, point-of-care decision support, predictive analytics, or population health management. Moreover, especially within AMCs, a growing demand exists for health IT resources to support innovation and research missions, such as health services research, outcomes research, and personalized healthcare research. Readers are referred to Chapters 13, 14, 23 and 24 as examples of this growing demand for IT support. Again, this continual increase in the demands for health IT resources and the need to prioritize and manage these demands is a core role of health IT governance.

Governance Does Not Depend on Specific Technology Choices

The selection of specific health IT solutions, such as an EHR system, is undoubtedly critical health IT decision for an institution. However, the health IT governance should be independent of any technology choices. Instead, the health IT governance should guide those types of technologies and technology choices. For example, the selection of an EHR system, population health management tool, or business intelligence platform should be within the scope of the expected responsibility of a health IT governance structure. It is imperative that the governance structure has mechanisms in place to obtain the perspectives of all relevant stakeholders and make decisions in a manner that fosters stakeholder buy-in and sustained support for these oftentimes long-term health IT investment decisions. For instance, clinicians, nurses, and pharmacists are obvious key stakeholders in EHR governance structures, while quality improvement and financial analysts are clearly needed for business intelligence initiatives.

Coordination and Collaboration With Diverse Stakeholders

Because of their nature, health IT initiatives require the close coordination and collaboration of various institutional stakeholders. For example, an EHR system implementation will affect virtually every area of a healthcare organization. This need for multi-stakeholder engagement is discussed in detail in Chapters 18 and 20. Thus, a traditional governance structure that is informatics centered by nature may present a barrier to the type of integrated, cross-stakeholder coordination and collaboration required. A medication safety initiative, for example, may need the close engagement of the pharmacy and therapeutics committee and other relevant stakeholders from groups such as pharmacy and nursing, more so than a health IT governance committee. As discussed earlier, substantial consideration must be given to how the health IT governance considers and coordinates with existing governance structures outside health IT. For instance, Chapters 17 and 18 discuss the need for interdisciplinary project management to ensure projects fulfill the needs of diverse stakeholder groups.

Risk Identification and Management

Healthcare is a complex, information-intensive endeavor, and health IT endeavors are accompanied by both benefits and risks. For example, making patient information more easily accessible to patients over the Internet can facilitate patient-centered care and is now federally mandated (Office of the National Coordinator for Health IT, 2021), but this could increase cyber security risks. Another example suggests that increasing the pool of individuals authorized to access the data warehouse can enhance the institution's analytical capabilities, but it also increases the pool of individuals whose access credentials could be compromised through techniques such as phishing. A key role for health IT governance is to identify risks and ensure institutional leaders determine the acceptable risks given the risk mitigation measures in place.

Enabling Excellence in Both Operations and Innovation

A key consideration for health IT governance is how to enable both reliable operations and disruptive innovations. One potential approach suggested by Gartner is to use what they refer to as "bimodal IT," in which predictable operations (Mode 1) and exploratory innovation (Mode 2) are governed as two separate lines of work (Gartner Research, 2014). This approach must consider, however, that there is a continuum and inter-dependence between these lines of work (Bloomberg, 2015). Ultimately, what is desired is a governance approach that enables both highly predictable operations and transformative innovations.

RECOMMENDATIONS

One of the biggest challenges for organizations addressing health IT governance is deciding where to begin. As mentioned, there is very little literature to provide guidance on the effective governance of health IT. The following recommendations are provided with the understanding that this is an evolving area of focus in the industry. Organizations may well need to make course corrections or experiment with different approaches until a more permanent solution emerges.

Assess Current Governance and Investigate Peer Approaches

A good starting point in developing a health IT governance model is obtaining an understanding of the current health IT

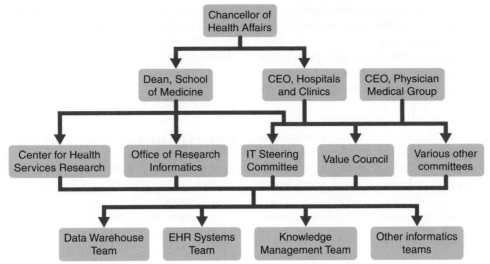

Fig 31.2 Sample informatics governance structure for an academic health system. *CEO,* Chief executive officer; *EHR,* electronic health record; *IT,* information technology

structure and culture. Areas to assess include the degree to which senior leaders view IT and analytics as core to the organization's mission, as well as the structures and processes in place to ensure that IT efforts are aligned with institutional priorities. As a part of this self-assessment, an organization should explicitly identify the current health IT governance structure and processes, including the various channels through which committees and institutional stakeholders currently request informatics resources and how those institutional needs are prioritized. A simple Strengths, Weaknesses, Opportunities, and Threats (SWOT) analysis can assist in this effort and should be performed on a regular basis.

There is no single model for health IT governance, just as there is no single model for other areas of organizational governance. Rather than offering a prescriptive solution, the organization can investigate health IT governance models that are already in place at organizations of comparable size and complexity. Key questions to consider when investigating other organizations' health IT governance include the following:

- How mature is the health IT capability at the organization? What are the potential implications to governance if an organization has a significantly different health IT capability?
- What is the official governance structure and process?
- Are there ad hoc governance processes in place, for example, in terms of individual, institutional leaders requesting health IT governance support and prioritizing informatics activities?
- What works well with the governance? What could be improved?
- Are there aspects of the governance that are dependent on unique characteristics of the organization, such as its culture or specific individuals?

Fig. 31.2 provides a sample health IT governance structure that may be appropriate for a large academic health system. Note that this structure is significantly more complicated than the one in Fig. 31.1, which may be more feasible and appropriate for a smaller healthcare system or a healthcare system

with fewer competing needs related to research and education. In this sample governance structure, there are three primary sources of authority: the dean of the school of medicine, the chief executive officer (CEO) of the hospitals and clinics, and the CEO of the physician medical group, which in this case is independent of the university. In this organizational structure, the primary health IT governance is intended to be the IT steering committee, which oversees the creation and implementation of the health IT strategic governance plan. However, other committees and organizational subunits also make significant demands on health IT resources, including a center for health services research, an office of research informatics, a value council with oversight of initiatives to improve care value, and various other committees as for finance and population health management. The key to enabling effective prioritization in this environment is global prioritization of the various competing initiatives by the senior leadership and, more importantly, determination of what will need to wait until the priority initiatives are completed. Also critical to enabling this sample health IT governance structure to work effectively is empowering the IT steering committee to adjudicate competing demands in terms of large-scale initiatives that require significant capital funding and operational resources.

Design, Implement, and Iteratively Enhance Informatics Governance

Following the baseline assessment of current health IT governance and the evaluation of the benefits and limitations of the governance models in place at peer institutions, the findings should be synthesized, and a small number of candidate governance approaches should be generated for consideration by senior leaders and other key informatics stakeholders. In developing these candidate approaches, the following principles should be considered:

- Balance the sophistication of the health IT governance model with the scope of the organization's health IT capabilities and needs.

- Develop a health IT governance structure that is reflective of the high level of organizational collaboration required for an effective health IT governance program.
- Propose a health IT governance structure that reports to the highest strategic body within the organization, whether that is an executive-level committee or a senior-level executive position.
- Consider and align with the unique characteristics and culture of the institution. For example, consider the viewpoints and preferences of key senior leaders and whether the organization has a centralized culture with top-down decision-making or a decentralized culture with consensus-driven decision-making.
- Ensure that key risks are considered and adjudicated by appropriate leaders.
- Consider establishing innovation groups or programs. For example, we have had significant success with a digital health innovation initiative called ReImagine EHR, which is led by the Associate Chief Medical Information Officer and overseen by a steering committee co-chaired by the Chief Information Officer and Chief Medical Information Officer (Kawamoto et al., 2021).

Following an open discussion of the candidate health IT governance model by senior leaders and other key stakeholders, the candidate approach deemed to be most suitable for the organization should be refined with operational details. Moreover, to the extent possible, consensus regarding the candidate approach should be developed across all stakeholder groups, with groups and individuals that have traditionally had a central role in the use and prioritization of health IT governance resources.

When sufficient institutional consensus has been attained, the new health IT governance model should be implemented. A charter should be developed that provides the guiding principles and overall scope of responsibilities while identifying committee membership, processes, and decision-making. The impact of the new model, including unintended consequences, should be actively evaluated. The health IT governance should then be iteratively assessed and refined as needed, with the goal of ensuring that health IT is fully aligned with the strategic direction of the institution and that limited health IT resources are used optimally.

CONCLUSION AND FUTURE DIRECTIONS

Looking forward, healthcare organizations are likely to face ever more opportunities and challenges that require the effective leveraging of health IT. Given the rapidly changing healthcare environment, it will be critical for healthcare organizations to develop a health IT governance structure that allows priorities and direction to be rapidly adapted to these changes. Moreover, given the increasingly vital role of health IT in a healthcare organization, it is important for health IT governance to incorporate the viewpoints of relevant stakeholders, such as providers, from across the enterprise. The governance approach needs to be balanced and collaborative yet still capable of focusing on strategic priorities without being pulled in a thousand directions by various competing demands. Risks will need to be visible to leaders and appropriately managed, and a thoughtful approach should be taken on enabling excellence in both operations and innovation. In looking toward, the opportunities and challenges ahead for healthcare organizations, a key factor in an organization's ability to survive and thrive will be its ability to implement effective health IT governance.

ACKNOWLEDGMENT

The authors wish to acknowledge the contribution of Jim Turnbull to the previous edition of this chapter.

DISCUSSION QUESTIONS

1. What unique characteristics within the organizational culture at your institution are relevant in terms of their impact on health IT governance?
2. Describe the current state of health IT governance at your organization.
3. How does the current health IT structure at your institution support or hinder the effectiveness of informatics specialists in nursing, medicine, and other disciplines?
4. What opportunities do you see health IT governance to facilitate the achievement of strategic priorities at your institution?
5. Who do you think should make the ultimate decision on whether key IT risks are worth taking at your institution?
6. How do you think IT innovation should be governed and enabled at your institution?

CASE STUDY

Imagine that you have been hired as the chief information officer (CIO) of an academic healthcare system. The healthcare system consists of several large hospitals and several dozen outpatient clinics, all using the same EHR system. There is an affiliated but independent physician practice group as well as a School of Medicine with a strong research focus. The current health IT governance structure is as described in Fig. 31.2, except that the current committee's function independently of one another, and as a result, health IT resources are being overwhelmed by requests coming from a variety of sources, each with its own priority list. As one of your first tasks on the job, you have been asked to lead the formulation and implementation of a new health IT governance structure. The effectiveness of the new governance structure will be critical to your success and the success of your team and the institution.

Discussion Questions

1. How would you go about assessing the current state of health IT governance and your organization's health IT governance capabilities?

2. What issues would you need to consider in recommending improved health IT governance at your institution?

3. How could the informatics governance at your institution be more centralized to allow an enterprise-wide approach to prioritizing informatics efforts?

REFERENCES

Bloomberg, J. (2015, September 26). Bimodal IT: Gartner's recipe for disaster. Forbes.

Gartner Research. (2014). Bimodal IT: How to be digitally agile without making a mess. Available at: https://www.gartner.com/en/documents/2798217.

Hoehn, B. J. (2010). Clinical information technology governance. *Journal of Healthcare Information Management, 24*(2), 13–14.

Kavanaugh-Burke, L., & Sayles, N. B. (2021). *Introduction to information systems for health information technology* (4th Edition). Chicago: American Health Information Management Association.

Kawamoto, K., Kukhareva, P. V., Weir, C., Flynn, M. C., Nanjo, C. J., Martin, D. K., et al. (2021). Establishing a multidisciplinary initiative for interoperable electronic health record innovations at an academic medical center. *JAMIA Open, 4*(3). https://doi.org/10.1093/jamiaopen/ooab041. ooab041.

Kawamoto, K., Martin, C. J., Williams, C., Tu, M. C., Park, C. G., Hunter, C., et al. (2015). Value Driven Outcomes (VDO): a pragmatic, modular, and extensible software framework for understanding and improving health care costs and outcomes. *Journal of the American Medical Informatics Association, 22*(1), 223–235.

Kropf, R., & Scalzi, G. (2012). *IT governance in hospitals and health systems*. Chicago, IL: Healthcare Information and Management Systems Society.

Office of the National Coordinator for Health IT. (2021). 21st Century Cures Act Final Rule. Available from: https://www.healthit.gov/curesrule/.

Reddy, S., Allan, S., Coghlan, S., & Cooper, P. (2020). A governance model for the application of AI in health care. *Journal of the American Medical Informatics Association, 27*(3), 491–497.

Rosenbaum, S. (2010, Oct). Data governance and stewardship: Designing data stewardship entities and advancing data access. *Health Services Research, 45*(5 Pt 2), 1442–1455.

Weill, P., & Ross, J. (2005). A matrixed approach to designing IT governance. *MIT Sloan Management Review, 46*(2), 26–34.

32

Global Health Informatics

Ashish Joshi

OBJECTIVES

At the completion of this chapter, the reader will be prepared to:

1. Explain the role of digital penetration in global health informatics.
2. Identify how digital health strategies influence digital health networks.
3. Describe how emerging technologies and approaches can best contribute to digital health.
4. Examine global usage of applications that support expanded access to healthcare.
5. Describe methods of scaling and sustaining digital health initiatives in low-middle-income countries.

KEY TERMS

artificial intelligence (AI), 498

cloud computing, 498

digital health, 495

digital transformation, 495

Internet of Things (IoT), 498

machine learning (ML), 498

telehealth/telemedicine, 499

wireless technologies, 494

ABSTRACT ❖

This chapter describes a global view of the growth, proliferation, and application of health informatics. It provides an overview of where we have been, the explosion of digital health, and a vision of where we may be headed. There is no crystal ball for a concrete pathway in determining where health informatics will travel, but inferences and predications can be articulated to provide a sense of what lies ahead.

GROWTH AND PROLIFERATION OF INFORMATION AND COMMUNICATIONS TECHNOLOGIES

Trends in Digital Penetration

The growth of the Internet and mobile wireless technologies have assisted in shifting the way healthcare is addressed in many countries. As of 2021, there are almost 4.6 billion active internet users, equivalent to 59% of the global population (ITU, 2021). Ninety-three percent of the world population has access to a mobile-broadband network. The percentage of individuals using the Internet increased from 38.6%in 2017 to 44.5% by the end of 2019 (ITU, 2021). Between 2015 and 2020, 4 G network coverage increased two-fold globally. While almost all urban areas in the world are covered by a mobile broadband network, many gaps persist in rural areas. In the least development countries (LDC),

17% of the rural population has no mobile coverage at all, and 19% of the rural population is only covered by a 2 G network (ITU, 2021). Significant technological gains, including rapid improvement in Internet access, have been emerging in low middle-income countries (LMICs) (Hamill et al., 2015). It has been made possible through the lower cost and greater efficiency of the new technology (Mansell, 2011). It is specifically seen in Africa, where cellular networks are expanding rapidly, facilitating wireless access to the Internet (Hagg et al., 2018). Globally, about 72% of households in urban areas had access to the Internet at home in 2019, almost twice as much as in rural areas (nearly 38%) (Fig. 32.1A). The urban-rural gap was small in developed countries, but in developing countries, urban access to the Internet was 2.3 times as high as rural access (Fig. 32.1B) (ITU, 2021).

According to the International Telecommunication Union (ITU), the total number of mobile-cellular telephone subscriptions declined. In mid-2020, there were an estimated 105 mobile-cellular subscriptions per 100 inhabitants, decreasing from 108 in 2019 (ITU, 2021). This decline was driven by developing countries; the number of subscriptions decreased from 103 in 2019 to 99 in mid-2020 while the trend was still upwards for the developed countries. Recent findings demonstrate that a 10% increase in internet speed can increase economic growth by 1.3% in LMICs (Minges, 2016; Katz, 2012). This rapid growth and potential are now influenced by digital innovations. Governments globally plan to increase coverage of initiatives by reaching remote areas or individuals.

Integration of Digital Technology With Healthcare

Digital transformation of healthcare can be disruptive. Technologies such as the Internet of Things (IoT), virtual care (VC), artificial intelligence (AI), big data (BD), and wearable sensors create a continuum of care to enhance population health outcomes. These technologies influence clinical diagnosis and therapeutics, treatment decisions, self-management, and person-centered care.

It facilitates supporting greater evidence-based knowledge, skills, and competencies for professionals to support health care.

Healthcare services are facing growing challenges, and half the world still lacks access to essential health services. There is a global need to find more efficient ways to deliver healthcare services while reducing costs and improving outcomes. The adoption of digital healthcare tools and services is a vital step toward upgrading the quality and consistency of healthcare services in emerging nations. The integration of technology within health began as electronic health (eHealth). E-health is described as electronic platforms for the provision of health information and services, data collection and management and when used in context to mobile phones, it is called as mobile health (mHealth) (Minges, 2016). **Digital health** expands the concept of eHealth to include digital consumers, with a more comprehensive range of smart and connected devices. The broad scope of digital health includes mHealth, health information technology (IT), wearable devices, telehealth and telemedicine, and personalized medicine. The trajectory of digital health will continue to evolve

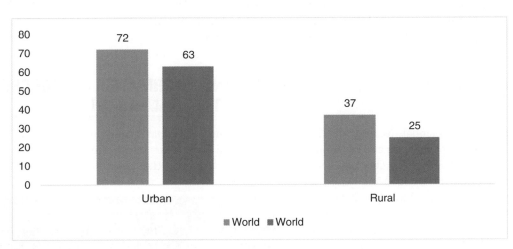

A

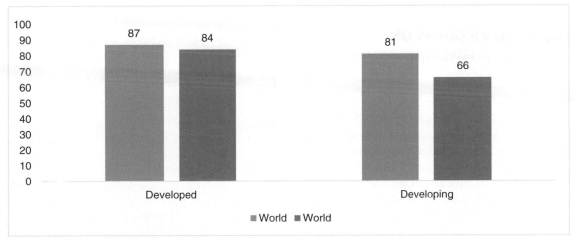

B

Fig. 32.1 (A) Comparing percentage of household internet and computer access across urban and rural settings globally, 2019. (B) Comparing percentage of household internet and computer access across developed and developing countries, 2019.

and accelerate and promises to address access to health services and information (Phua et al., 2015).

Healthcare delivery is a complex effort at both individual and population levels. Inequitable access to health care is one of the major health system concerns for LMICs. Health inequities are caused by complex social, economic, and political factors. Advances in IT infrastructure and mobile computing power in many LMICs have raised confidence that AI might help to address challenges unique to the field of global health and accelerate achievement of the health-related sustainable development goals (Labrique et al., 2018). Global health informatics (GHI) is the informatics discipline focused on empowering people to use appropriate technology to provide information-based solutions with a global perspective that supports healthcare for all (Richards et al., 2013). GHIs aim to share informatics knowledge, skills, and research with an emphasis on low-income, low-resource countries. GHI aims to facilitate local innovations to promote the highest health standards. Individuals in poor and developing countries have the least access to health services due to low financial resources, lack of infrastructure, and other barriers to accessing the needed services. Healthcare challenges in LMICs have been the focus of many digital initiatives intended to enhance access to healthcare and the quality of healthcare delivery.

GLOBAL STRATEGY ON DIGITAL HEALTH

Global Digital Health Strategies

Digital health holds significant potential to provide and improve health services worldwide. Information and communications technologies (ICTs) can enhance the quality and delivery of health care services around the world. Many countries require institutional support to develop national digital health strategies—particularly in LMICs that face staffing and other physical resource constraints. The World Health Assembly, through its resolution WHA58.28 on eHealth in 2005, urged the Member States to consider drawing up a long-term strategic plan for developing and implementing eHealth services to develop the infrastructure for ICTs for health (WHO, 2021). There was an emphasis to create a consistent eHealth vision. It should be aligned with the country's health priorities and resources. Further, there should be a need to create a framework for monitoring and evaluating eHealth implementation and progress.

In 2013, the Health Assembly adopted resolution WHA66.24 on eHealth standardization and interoperability (WHO, 2021). This resolution urged the Member States to consider developing policies and legislative mechanisms linked to an overall national eHealth strategy. The Digital Regional East African Community Health (REACH) initiative was launched in 2017. This digital initiative aims to create an enabling environment for digital health across the East African Community (EAC) region (Digital reach initiative, n.d.). These include the partner states of the Republic of Burundi, the Republic of Kenya, the Republic of Rwanda, the Republic of South Sudan, the United Republic of Tanzania, and the Republic of Uganda (Mahmood et al., 2020). In May 2018, the Health Assembly adopted resolution WHA71.7 on digital

health (World Health Organization [WHO, 2021]). The focus was to develop, in close consultation with the Member States and with inputs from relevant stakeholders, a global strategy on digital health. In 2019, the United Nations (UN) Secretary General's High-Level Panel on Digital Cooperation recommended that by 2030, every adult should have affordable access to digital networks, as well as digitally enabled financial and health services, to make a substantial contribution to achieving the sustainable development goals (SDG) (UN Secretary-General's High-level Panel on Digital Cooperation, 2018). In October 2019, *The Lancet and Financial Times* inaugurated a joint Commission focused on the convergence of digital health, AI, and universal health coverage (Table 32.1) (Kickbusch et al., 2019).

Influence of Global Digital Health Strategy

The global strategy on digital health 2020–2025 was endorsed by the Seventy-third World Health Assembly in decision WHA73 in 2020 (Table 32.2) (WHO, 2021). There is an increasing agreement that strategic and innovative use of ICTs will be an essential enabling factor towards achieving World Health Organization (WHO) triple billion targets (WHO, 2021). The global strategy on digital health enhances and complements the work of existing and newly created digital health networks.

EMERGING INFORMATICS APPROACHES TO SUPPORT DIGITAL HEALTH

A wide range of digital health initiatives have been piloted in response to specific healthcare challenges in LMICs. AI, machine learning (ML), cloud computing (CC), the IoT,

TABLE 32.1   Strategies Facilitating Adoption of Digital Health Across Global Settings

Year	WHO Resolution	Description
2005	WHA58.28	Long-term strategic plan for developing and implementing eHealth services
2013	WHA66.24	Develop policies and legislative mechanisms linked to an overall national eHealth strategy
2017	Regional East African Community Health initiative	Improve health outcomes through digital technologies in the East African Community (EAC) region
2018	WHA71.7	Potential of digital technologies to advance the Sustainable Development Goals
2019	United Nations	Every adult should have affordable access to digitally enabled financial and health services by 2030
2019	Lancet and Financial Times Commission	Focused on the convergence of digital health, artificial intelligence (AI), and universal health coverage (UHC)
2020	WHA73	Endorse global strategy on digital health

eHealth, Electronic health; *WHO*, World Health Organization.

TABLE 32.2 WHO Global Strategy on Digital Health 2020–2025

Strategic Objective	Policy Options and Actions	Outputs
Promote global collaboration and advance the transfer of knowledge on digital health	Co-create global strategy on digital health	Digital health is prioritized and integrated into health systems
	Establish a knowledge management approach	Convene multistakeholder groups and scale up digital health and innovation toward SDGs
	Support countries in establishing information centers for disease surveillance	Establish information centers for disease surveillance
	Mitigate threats associated with the use of digital technologies to improve health and enable universal health coverage	
Advance implementation of national digital health strategies	Stimulate and support every country to adopt or review, own, and strengthen its national digital health strategy	A national digital health strategy is integrated into the national health strategy
	All end-user communities and beneficiary populations are adequately engaged in the design and development phases	A dynamic digital health maturity model assessment to guide the prioritization of national investment in digital health
	Facilitate a systematic engagement of all relevant stakeholders as part of an integrated digital health ecosystem	
	Define a national digital health architecture blueprint or roadmap, adopt open-source health data standards and interoperability of health information systems	
	Adopt legal and ethical frameworks for assuring patient safety, data security, appropriate use and ownership of health data	
	Identify and promote sustainable financing models in support of digital health development	
	Design, implement and monitor a change management plan	
Strengthen governance for digital health at global, regional, and national levels	Strengthen governance of digital health structures, including regulatory frameworks	Agree on the appropriate global use of health data and on concepts such as health data as a global public good
	Coordinate investments in evidence-based approaches	Develop guidelines on global interoperability standards for digital health
	Promote and facilitate digital health competencies in education and training curricula	Global guidance on planning, development, and use of digital hospitals
	Promote capacity-building for leaders of public health authorities	Develop recommendations for pseudonymization and anonymization of health data
Advocate people-centered health systems that are enabled by digital health	Place people at the center of digital health	Improved digital health literacy in using and understanding digital health technologies
	Management of health at the population level through digital health applications	Validate the performance of digital health tools and services
	Monitoring the contribution of digital systems to health system processes	Establish global minimum health data standards for prioritized digital health technologies
	Strengthen gender equality and health equity approaches and accessibility for people with disabilities to promote an inclusive digital society with enhanced digital health skills	Develop global guidance on personalized medicine.
	Effective public participation and transparency in digital health decision-making processes	
	Develop digital health training or Massive Open Online Courses to improve digital health literacy	
	Create an international communication campaign to sensitize people to the benefits of digital health solutions	

WHO, World Health Organization.

and many more evolving technological arenas will shape the world's future.

Artificial Intelligence

In 1956, researchers coined the term **artificial intelligence (AI)**, a branch of computer science that deals with the simulation of intelligent behavior in computers (Russell, 2010). Data generated in large volumes has created a surplus of opportunities for applying AI to enhance individual and population health outcomes. Many AI applications have been deployed in high-income country settings. Similarly, AI has shown evidence of public health change in resource-poor countries. It is mainly due to increased mobile phone penetration, developments in CC, and significant investments in digitizing health information.

However, the use of AI in resource-poor settings remains promising. AI-driven health interventions in LMICs broadly fit into four categories: (Elveren & Yumuşak, 2011) (a) *Diagnosis*, (b) *Mortality and morbidity risk assessment*, (c) *Disease outbreak prediction and surveillance*, and (d) *Health policy and planning*. The majority of AI studies have focused on communicable diseases and other infectious and non-infectious diseases. AI-driven interventions have been shown to enhance clinical decision-making in diagnosing tuberculosis (Elveren & Yumuşak, 2011) and malaria (Andrade et al., 2010). AI research has aimed at improving the performance of health facilities, allocating resources, and other health system issues. AI-driven interventions aim to characterize the risk to predict disease severity in patients with dengue fever (Phakhounthong et al., 2018), malaria (Johnston et al., 2019), and children with acute infections (Kwizera et al., 2019). Researchers have used this approach to predict disease outbreaks and evaluate disease surveillance tools. AI-driven health interventions can also be used to support program policy and planning (Huang and Wu, 2017).

There remain several ethical, regulatory, and practical issues that require guidance before scale-up in LMICs (Wahl et al., 2018). One of the most important challenges facing AI in LMICs relates to the appropriate design and development of interventions driven by local needs, health system constraints, and disease burden. Another major challenge relates to ethnic, socioeconomic, and gender biases during the development of AI applications. New types of data sharing protocols and interoperability, reporting, and methodological standards are needed globally to inform the development and evaluation of AI health interventions in LMIC settings (Schwalbe & Wahl, 2020).

Machine Learning

Most AI-driven health interventions use some form of machine learning or signal processing, or both. **Machine learning (ML)** refers to the process through which computers, models, or algorithms, learn and improve from data and processes (Burkov, 2019). ML can be used in tasks such as classification, clustering or prediction (Rebala et al., 2019). Systematic reviews have explored the accuracy of ML for diagnosis or outcome prediction (de Filippis et al., 2019; Bradley et al., 2019; Shung et al., 2019). Most of the research studies included in these reviews

have come from high-income countries, and the findings may not apply to LMICs. It is primarily due to variability in access to healthcare and the difference in the disease burden.

Cloud Computing

Cloud computing (CC) refers to using a network of remote servers to store, manage, access, and process data rather than a single personal computer or hard drive (Mell & Grance, 2011). Organizations have quickly adopted CC due to increased reliability and considerable cost savings. CC provides three different Web-based service models—software as a service (SaaS), platform as a service (PaaS), and infrastructure as a service (IaaS) (Mell & Grance, 2011). CC can deliver essential IT resources such as processing, storage (IaaS), and platforms with programming languages, tools, and libraries that support users in developing and deploying software (PaaS). CC provides ready-to-use software applications (SaaS) to healthcare organizations. CC can be used with public health and patient data. It aimed to improve interactive voice response (IVR) telephone calls for managing non-communicable diseases (NCDs) despite the lack of adequate IT infrastructure in the country (Piette et al., 2011).

Digital health should become an integral component of health priorities. It should benefit people in a way that is ethical, safe, secure, reliable, equitable and sustainable (WHO, 2021). Sharing health data for the purpose of public interest should be encouraged with the patient's consent. Such sharing is vital to the building of a knowledge base and can contribute to the enhancement of quality of processes, the outcomes of health services, and the continuity of care for patients.

Internet of Things

Internet of Things (IoT) is a system of wireless, interrelated, and connected digital devices. It can collect, send, and store data over a network without requiring human-to-human or human-to-computer interaction (Kelly et al., 2020). IoT can collect health-related data from individuals, including computing devices, mobile phones, smart bands, and wearables (Dang et al., 2019). Health data gets recorded and connected to the Internet resulting in an ability to track and monitor health progress providing quality and low-cost medical care (Yin et al., 2016).

The architecture of IoT in health care delivery consists of three basic layers (Fig. 32.2) (Sethi & Sarangi, 2017):

- *Processed layer*: Sensors are devices that can perceive changes in an environment and include devices such as medical sensors, and smart device sensors. Sensor technologies allow for treatments to be monitored in real time.
- *Network level*: Includes wired and wireless networks. They communicate and store processed information either locally or at a centralized location. Evolving 5 G networks are expected to be a major driver of the growth of IoT applications for healthcare (Li et al., 2018).
- *Application layer*: It interprets and applies data responsible for delivering application-specific services to the user. Some of the most promising healthcare applications that IoT provides are through AI.

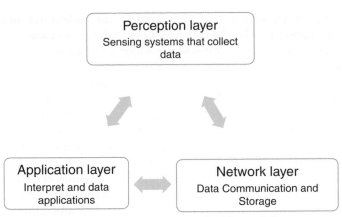

Fig. 32.2 Internet of Things architecture in healthcare delivery.

TABLE 32.3 Barriers to Telemedicine Adoption in Low Middle Income Countries	
Barriers to Adoption of Telemedicine in LMICs	
Scarcity of trained health care workers	Human factors
The difficulty of patient transportation	Fear of change
In-person care costs	Loss of political control
Reluctance to seek a second opinion	Loss of professional control over patients

LMICs, Low middle income countries.

IoT has the potential to improve population health. It helps in early risk factor identification, disease diagnoses, treatment, and remote monitoring. IoT offers the opportunity to link with non-health IoT technologies to monitor daily activities, provide support with information, and promote behavior changes. These data could provide valuable information about population-level surveillance in diseases and accidents, risk factors, and environmental conditions (Pacheco et al., 2019).

Policy support is one of the most important enablers of IoT; many countries already have policies in place for eHealth (Global internet of things policies 2018–2019, 2019). Cyber risk is a major obstacle to the broad adoption of IoT (Jalali et al., 2019). The privacy of patients must be ensured to prevent unauthorized identification and tracking. It is also important for health systems to be aware of the inequities that may eventuate from the widespread implementation of IoT for healthcare.

INFORMATICS APPLICATIONS IN GLOBAL SETTINGS

Telehealth/Telemedicine

Telehealth, a term interchangeably used with telemedicine, is defined as the use of telecommunication devices for remote delivery of medical care (Field, 1996). It is also defined as using medical information that is exchanged from one site to another through electronic communication to improve a patient's health. Increasing internet access, inexpensive personal computers, and more people owing smartphones have made it easier to implement telehealth services. Telemedicine has the potential to address various hurdles to primary healthcare in LMICs (Ngwa et al., 2020; Wootton, 2008; Hsieh et al., 2001; Quintana & Safran, 2015). New telemedicine-promoting policies and global mobile phone access in many LMICs help bridge gaps in care. Telemedicine brings the promise of real-time collaboration, consultation, and supervision with health care providers in understaffed, difficult-to-reach, and remote areas. Several telemedicine interventions have been effectively implemented in LMICs (Delaigue et al., 2018). Some interventions involve improving HbA1c levels, treatment adherence, and self-efficacy (Peimani et al., 2016; Saleh et al., 2018). Telehealth addresses

mental health service access and quality gap worldwide. Telemedicine can help in providing prompts and alerts as per evidence-based protocol checklists.

Telemedicine in LMICs has both barriers and advantages. Barriers are technical, cultural, financial, and regulatory (Jefee-Bahloul & Zayour, 2017). Some of the technological barriers include access to technology, and the Internet, low bandwidth, and scheduling across different time zones (Jefee-Bahloul et al., 2014; Inman et al., 2019). Another concern is that many healthcare providers have not developed a telehealth safety protocol (Table 32.3).

Despite several barriers to telehealth, there are several advantages of telehealth in low-resource settings, including flexibility in scheduling, enhanced access to supervision and consultation, and allowing patients to schedule appointments without difficulty. It further improves communication in real time between the patients and the providers. Prior studies highlight the importance of seven key components required for LMIC health systems to adopt telemedicine. These include:

- Government approvals
- Identification of telemedicine users
- Choosing the tech platform
- Alignment of financial incentives
- Defining workflows
- Training health worker team
- Patient engagement.

The role of healthcare providers, reimbursement, and regulatory compliance should be taken into consideration when designing telemedicine workflows.

Clear government regulations of telemedicine interventions did not exist in many LMICs during the COVID-19 pandemic (Mahmood et al., 2020). The Chinese government released guidelines that increased reimbursement coverage for follow-up online medical consultations and promoted doorstep delivery of prescriptions acquired through "internet hospitals" (State Medical Insurance Bureau State Health Commission, 2020). India's Ministry of Health and Family Welfare also released national telemedicine practice guidelines in March 2020 (Ministry of Health and Family Welfare, 2020). This framework provided instructions for prescribing medications and conducting follow-up care for chronic diseases. Indonesian health platform Halodoc allows to hire or contract telemedicine-dedicated pool of clinicians who provide consultations for healthcare workers in the community or patients at home (Djalante et al., 2020). Low-cost and widely used communication platforms such as WhatsApp or WeChat are a means to rapidly expand telemedicine services in LMICs. In the Philippines, government designed a telemedicine system for both suspected COVID-19 and non-COVID-19 chronic disease patients. Patients are referred to the appropriate health care provider and offered contactless prescription deliveries (Caliwan, 2020). The Resolve to Save Lives global hypertension control initiative recently developed two telemedicine workflows—"hub and spoke" and "direct to patient"—to both maintain continuity of care and address emergency situations for established hypertension patients (Resolve to Save Lives, 2020).

Digital literacy training, access to interpreters or clinicians who speak local languages, and active outreach to high-risk individuals should be employed to promote telemedicine uptake. It is also essential to establish long-term financial value to health systems when implementing new or adapting current telemedicine programs (Bagayoko et al., 2014). Engaging healthcare providers and patients is critical to creating a sustainable telehealth program.

Electronic Health Records

Electronic health records (EHR) digitally store healthcare information about an individual's life with the purpose of supporting continuity of care, education, and research. Health Insurance Portability and Accountability Act (HIPAA) defines EHR as an electronic record of health-related information on an individual that is created, gathered, managed, and consulted by authorized healthcare clinicians and staff (HIPAA, 2021). The terms "electronic medical record" (EMR), computer-based patient record (CPR), electronic patient record (EPR), personal health record (PHR), and computerized medical record (CMR) may also be treated synonymously with EHR (Aminpour et al., 2014). EHRs can enable the collection and use of data for achieving better health both at the patient and population health levels (Kumar et al., 2020). The collected patients' data can be used in research (Menachemi & Collum, 2011; Häyrinen et al., 2008; Lobach & Detmer, 2007; Jensen et al., 2012; Coorevits et al., 2013) to study diseases and extract knowledge from clinical data.

Despite the advantages of EHRs, the majority of developing countries cannot afford expensive proprietary software from big vendors. It is also important to consider other associated expenses such as power supply, Internet connection, staff training, and system support. Thus, the adoption of open-source EHR (OS EHR) is a possible solution for LMICs. One of the biggest open-source software (OSS) communities in health care is the Open Medical Record System (OpenMRS) led by Regenstrief Institute and Partners in Health. Initially, the system was implemented in Kenya and then was rapidly adopted by other healthcare organizations (Akanbi et al., 2012; Mamlin et al., 2006; Mohammed-Rajput et al., 2011; Tierney et al., 2010; Catalani et al., 2014). Currently, OpenMRS has become an EHR platform with developers all over the world. Bahmni, an integrated clinical software, provides a universal solution for healthcare institutions. It combines three

open-source platforms: (a) OpenMRS for patient records, (b) OpenELIS (OpenELIS Foundation) for laboratory management, and (c) OpenERP (Odoo SA) for hospitals' accounting operations. Bahmni has been deployed mainly in low-resource settings such as India, Bangladesh, and Nepal (Bahmni, 2017) and now growing and spreading to other regions (Syzdykova et al., 2017). OpenEMR is an EHR software, medical practice management software (PMS), and ERP software whose goal is to ensure that all people have access to high-quality medical care through its software and services. OpenEMR comes with a great amount of functionality, including modules of Health Information System (HIS), patient records and management, support for billing and claims management, ERP, and information management.

Some of the challenges related to the implementation and adoption of EHR in LMICs include: poor infrastructure (lack of stable electricity, unreliable Internet connectivity, and inadequate computer equipment), inadequate technical support, limited computer skills and training, and limited funding (Odekunle et al., 2017; Ngugi et al., 2018; Khalifa, 2013; Farzianpour et al., 2015; Sood et al., 2008; Jawhari et al., 2016). The use of the EHRs can also be affected by data quality issues, such as completeness, accuracy, and timeliness (Boonstra & Broekhuis, 2010) and EHRs interoperability across healthcare facilities (Kihuba et al., 2016). Clear measures of system availability, use, data quality, and reporting capabilities will ensure that decision-makers have clear and early visibility into the success and challenges facing system use (Ngugi et al., 2021).

The WHO digital health strategy highlights the role of EHRs as a key to achieving better health goals. However, there is a lack of evidence explaining national and sub-national EHR development in limited resource settings. The development and use of modern EHR systems in LMICs are still in an early stage. The development of digital infrastructure requires a significant investment of time and money (Aminpour et al., 2014). The stakeholder engagement is key to the development of EHRs in LMICs. The sustainability of EHRs in developed countries is driven by policy incentives and revenue generation for service delivery; the LMICs continue to rely on external funding to develop disease-specific EMRs. The business model for the development of EHRs in LMICs is largely aimed at public health care services with minimal or no service fees, government funding, and donor grants. Many of the LMIC countries have eHealth policies but only few of them have developed an EHR-related guidance document.

For example, Kenya has developed national guidance documents for EMR, while India has published revised national EHR standards. Tanzania published guidance for the development of integrated electronic management systems. Each country approaches EHR development from its own perspective and is at different stages. Evaluation of EHRs should include quantitative, qualitative, and mixed methods to examine EHR system functionalities, user acceptance and efficiency, and its impact on health outcomes. Patient engagement is minimal or nonexistent in the development of EHRs. Research should focus on identifying appropriate business models for developing national and sub-national EHRs in the healthcare system of LMICs.

There is a need for research to recommend appropriate health information architecture at all levels of the health care system.

Health Information Systems

Reliable, timely, and transparent data on health services is crucial to enhancing the performance of health systems (World Health Organization, 2010, 2012). HIS have been implemented in many LMICs to support these functions. HIS facilitate prioritization of resource allocation, strategy development, and policymaking. Substantial investments have been made in developing and strengthening HISs in many LMICs (Mutale et al., 2013; Warren et al., 2013). Interventions targeting data collection, processing, analysis, and dissemination have increased the accessibility of HIS data (Mutale et al., 2013; Gimbel et al., 2017).

Newer web-based systems have been adopted in many LMICs over the last decade (Kiberu et al., 2014; Hazel et al., 2018). The most common is the District Health Information System 2 (DHIS 2) platform. This platform is the basis for several countries' national health management information systems (HMIS) (Dehnavieh et al., 2018). The District Health Information System (DHIS) records were first introduced by the University of Oslo in 1994 and used for information management and decision making. A significant initiative under the umbrella of DHIS was the introduction of DHIS Version 2 (DHIS2) software. DHIS2 is an integrated, open-source, and web-based platform for health data collection, validation, analysis, and presentation of aggregated and individual data (Manoj, 2013; Gathogo, 2014). DHIS2 collects aggregated data on logistic supplies, procurement, human resources, and health indicators. It improves health service delivery by strengthening the HMIS.

There is evidence that using DHIS2 has improved health reporting in countries including Kenya, South Africa, and Malawi (Kiberu et al., 2014). Evidence from Uganda and Kenya shows that implementation of DHIS2 has improved reporting of immunization coverage, antenatal care (ANC) visits, and facility delivery rate (Kiberu et al., 2014). In Laos, the effective implementation of DHIS2 on maternal and child health (MNCH) surveillance data improved service delivery through identification of service coverage, barriers to access to services, and causes of maternal death (Chu et al., 2017). In Sri Lanka, DHIS2 data for MNCH information management has also improved the quality of care.

Despite its advantages in effectively reporting health indicator data, studies have shown persistent underuse of HIS data for research purposes in LMICs (Ranasinghe et al., 2012; Cresswell et al., 2013). A number of factors contribute to the underuse of HIS data (Chun Tie et al., 2019; Nowell et al., 2017):

- Data timeliness
- Lack of publicly available data for secondary analysis
- Incomplete data
- Data accuracy
- Lack of well-trained technical staff

An improved and harmonized health reporting system is critical for health system strengthening. It can generate timely information for proper planning, monitoring, and evaluation of service delivery at all levels of the health system.

Mobile Health Applications

mHealth is one of the key pillars of ICTs for healthcare. The WHO defined mHealth as covering medical and public health practice supported by mobile devices, such as mobile phones, patient monitoring devices, personal digital assistants (PDAs), and other wireless devices (World Health Organization, 2011). Emergence of mHealth has the potential to play an essential role in the transformation of healthcare on a global scale. This use of mobile technology in healthcare has improved the quality of health care and reduced healthcare costs. mHealth is potentially effective for patient education and awareness solutions. African countries are the most commonly studied settings for mHealth compared to other developing world regions.

The mobile short message service (SMS) has been the most common mHealth technology tool used in several healthcare settings. Despite some technological advances, identifying the most urgent healthcare challenges that can benefit from mHealth systems in a cost-effective way, scalability, technology awareness, user acceptance, and other human interaction factors are some challenges for deploying these in the developing world. MHealth allows individuals to seek health information quickly, conveniently, and confidentially, enabling accurate diagnosis and treatment. The role of mHealth systems in improving the more urgent healthcare needs of the developing world remains important. The quality of evidence suggests that improvements in the implementation fidelity and use of behavior change theories are needed for future mHealth interventions in LMICs. Further research is warranted to identify which mHealth features will lead to better health outcomes and which specific groups and LMIC locations.

Personal Health Records

PHR is described as an electronic application through which individuals can access, manage, and share their health information and that of others for whom they are authorized in a private, secure, and confidential environment (Tang et al., 2006). PHR is also referred to as personally controlled health records (PCHRs) comprising ICTs that can potentially help all types of end users in maintaining health and wellness. PHRs relate to digitally stored health care information about an individual patient under the control of that patient or their caregiver (Genitsaridi et al., 2015; Kern et al., 2009). EMRs and EHRs are typically maintained by healthcare providers or payor organizations (Hoerbst et al., 2010; Tang et al., 2006).

Researchers have classified PHRs into three main categories: *standalone*, *tethered*, and *interconnected* (Detmer et al., 2008). PHRs require users to manually enter data to populate their health information and medical history. The content of these applications is under direct physical control and ownership of the consumer. PHR systems are typically offered as extensions of a healthcare institution's own backend EHR or EMR system. It provides users access to parts of their own EHRs, also referred to as patient portals. It includes additional functionality such as communication tools for email, messaging, appointment scheduling, and prescription renewals (Gaskin et al., 2017). *Interconnected* PHRs described as the preferred type of PHR in terms of data control, record portability, and system interoperability (Barbarito et al., 2015; Johnson et al., 2013). These systems can usually be populated with patient information from a variety of sources, including physician EMRs, hospital EHRs, insurance carriers, health plan sponsors, labs, and pharmacies (Johnson et al., 2013).

PHRs have been demonstrated to improve patient adherence, reduce medical errors, improve patient-provider communication, improve chronic disease management, and promote behavior change. PHRs have been demonstrated several benefits. PHRs have not been widely adopted in low- and middle-income countries. PHR agenda for LMICs include policy, technology, sustainability agenda, and evidence (Mwogi & Were, 2017)

Disease Surveillance

In recent years, a significant increase in the use of informatics solutions in the field of global health. The leading application of IT in global health was collecting data through electronic surveys and data collection forms (Jayatilleke, 2020). Disease surveillance data collected through surveys and forms are transferred and stored in centralized surveillance information systems. These databases are often found on a country level. A more recent trend is the use of graphical information as well as decision support systems to make use of the surveillance data. The application of BD methods to medical data offers the opportunity to transform healthcare.

Increased data sharing of public health data is most beneficial for low- and middle-income countries, as most of the morbidity and mortality burden of infectious diseases lies in them. The 2019/2020 global pandemic of the novel coronavirus (COVID-19) has shown the importance of public health data sharing and its benefits on a worldwide scale, including in high-income countries. In addition to the data-sharing issue, these public health data are rarely used beyond their primary purpose.

Most countries have communicable disease surveillance systems in place (Guide to monitoring and evaluating communicable disease surveillance and response systems, 2006; Comprehensive Assessment of National Surveillance Systems in Sri Lanka, 2004; Integrated Disease Surveillance Program, n.d.). Nepal has a hospital-based sentinel surveillance system. It covers 82 hospitals covering all 75 districts for reporting selected water-borne and food-borne diseases in addition to a Health Management Information System (HIS) (Government of Nepal, n.d.). Similarly, the National Surveillance Program for Communicable Diseases (NSPCD) was launched in India from 1997 to 1998. Integrated Disease Surveillance Project (IDSP), formally launched in 2004, has infectious disease surveillance improved since then. Monitoring and evaluation have been weak, and there is a shortage of human resources (Raut and Bhola, 2014). Integrated Disease Surveillance and Response (IDSR) has been implemented successfully in most countries in Africa (Fall et al., 2019).

Several recommendations were made for the successful implementation of surveillance tools in LMICs (Guide to monitoring and evaluating communicable disease surveillance and response systems, 2006). Some of these recommendations include (a) having legislations and regulations in place to get surveillance done

effectively, (b) different diseases may need different surveillance strategies based on the objective of the surveillance system, and (c) laboratory capacity crucial for communicable disease surveillance, and (d) trained staff. Integrated Surveillance Systems should be implemented in all countries using modern technology to improve the speed of detection and control of outbreaks and to implement infection prevention and control measures in a community setting. Capacity building with an adequate number of trained healthcare workers will be important to improve healthcare surveillance. Improving laboratory capacity with proper quality assurance programs is important to support communicable disease surveillance (Jayatilleke, 2020).

COVID-19 Pandemic

Digital interventions provide many opportunities for strengthening health systems and could be vital resources in the current public health emergency (Mahmood et al., 2020). The coronavirus disease (COVID-19) pandemic has uncovered many areas of public health preparedness that are lacking, especially in LMICs. Digital health interventions can help stakeholders to overcome several health systems challenges. These challenges include an insufficient supply of commodities, poor adherence to guidelines by healthcare professionals, treatment by patients, and a loss of patients to follow-up. *The role of ICTs and digital services and the digital infrastructure to manage COVID-19 pandemic has become central to lessening the pandemic impact.* Digital tools can play a crucial role in monitoring and quality control Infection Prevention and Control practices. WHO has recommended that suspected COVID-19 cases with mild symptoms and no underlying problems can usually be treated at home with careful clinical monitoring (World Health Organization, 2020). Future needs include the addition of AI algorithms to rapidly identify high-risk situations and mitigate them even more quickly (Chen et al., 2020). Many supportive and reliable informatics infrastructures have been developed by various countries during the recent months of the COVID-19 outbreak (Reeves et al., 2020). Digital health tools can support health care systems through surveillance, screening, triage, diagnosis, monitoring, and contact tracing (Dong et al., 2020). Some barriers must be overcome to ensure the benefits of digital health; Internet connectivity may be limited in remote areas and not affordable for many (Hoffer-Hawlik et al., 2020). Sometimes, voice calling may be the most appropriate way to provide telemedicine services. Digital tools can be invaluable in reducing exposure risk for public health personnel.

SCALING DIGITAL HEALTH IN GLOBAL SETTINGS

Critical Factors for Scaling Success

A wide range of digital health initiatives initiated in response to healthcare challenges in LMICs. The emphasis of digital health initiatives is towards scalability, integration, and sustainability. It also aims to enhance both health system processes and health outcomes. Five key focus areas have been identified as being critical for success:

- Intrinsic program characteristics: Initiative must offer tangible benefits to address an unmet need, with end-user input from the outset.
- All stakeholders must be engaged, trained, and motivated to implement a new initiative.
- The technical profile of the initiative should be driven by simplicity, interoperability, and adaptability.
- Presence of an appropriate infrastructure to support the use of digital initiatives at scale.
- Alignment with broader healthcare policy is essential.
- Sustainable funding, including in the private sector, will support long-term growth.

Scaling and Sustaining Digital Health Initiatives in Low-Middle-Income Countries

Scaling and sustaining digital health initiatives in LMICs has emphasized five critical focus areas (8):

- Program characteristics
  - *User-centered design*: An essential principle for successful digital health initiatives. E.g., A Ghana-based telemedicine initiative based on end-user insights enabled the roll of telemedicine services nationwide and benefited the health system (Novartis Foundation, 2010).
  - *Real-time data collection and analysis*: Enabling users to track their own performance in real-time is a major shift from current monthly or annual reporting. E.g., The CommCare platform (CommCare, 2017) enables immediate data entry and real-time monitoring. The Open Smart Register Platform by the Ministry of Health, Bangladesh digitizes paper registries in MNCH (Smart Register, 2017; El Arifeen et al., 2013) allowing local and national level supervisors to use real-time dashboards for supportive supervision and to compare health center performance.
  - *Contextually relevant innovations*
- *Human factors*: It is critical that end-users are interested, trained, and prepared to utilize digital health solutions. Effective, sustainable support systems, as well as clarity on roles and accountability for decision-making are essential components. The importance of human resource capacity cannot be disregarded as programs plan to scale up.
- *Technical factors*: Critical components of scalability and sustainability. One key technical feature to consider is simplicity in function, as simple systems may be easier to scale (Agarwal et al., 2016). Simple solutions tend to be less dependent on the extrinsic environment. They often rely on more robust cellular channels such as SMS, IVR, unstructured supplementary service data (USSD), or voice rather than Internet or data. The *mDiabetes Project* in Senegal (World Health Organization, 2017) and *BBC Mobile Kunji* (BBC Mobile Action, 2015) are some examples of digital health innovations with rapid scale-up with their inherent simplicity. Each of them provides a simple daily SMS with health advice to patients with diabetes, and other helps community health workers in Bihar to counsel families. Interoperability

is another key focal area of a new global partnership known as the Health Data Collaborative (HDC) and the Principles for Digital Development (Principles for digital development, 2014). Interoperable systems can talk to one another and share information. The use of commonly available platforms such as CommCare, OpenSRP, OpenMRS, and OpenDataKitis both encouraging interoperability and providing (Smart Register, 2017; OpenMRS, 2017; OpenDataKit, 2013) a framework for easy adaptation.

- *Healthcare ecosystem*: Human and technical factors is the environment in which the digital health initiative must function at scale. This includes financial support, regulatory standards, and frameworks that ensure compliance with national health guidelines and strategies. In the example of the Uganda mHealth moratorium, the government chose to align the goals of digital health with a broader national health strategy (Huang et al., 2017). The funding plan for a digital health program must be clear from the beginning. Contingency planning is another important factor to consider for scaling digital health programs. The roll-out of the electronic tool to Improve Quality of Health (eTIQH) in Tanzania and Mali benefited from a combined top-down and bottom-up approach for reaching scale (PATH).
- *Broader extrinsic ecosystem*: Reliability and bandwidth of networks and availability of electricity are key extrinsic limiting factors affecting the scaling of digital health projects in LMICs. The availability of high-quality hardware was also identified as a local ecosystem constraint limiting scale-up. Data management and storage, assurance of patient data security, and reliable offline and backup systems to address the needs of the LMICs must all be considered during the design phase of a digital solution. Offline capacity with the ability to store and delay the upload of data is an important feature of digital solutions in LMICs.

Digital health innovators must actively advocate for investments required for scale-up. Gaps in policies and standards or an unstable infrastructure will certainly hinder the scalability of digital health innovations. A close partnership among stakeholders, from inception through to scale-up, is important. The scaling process needs to be dynamic and flexible and allow adaptations for changes in the human or technology needs of the system. The private sector has an important role in initiating and scaling digital health initiatives (International Finance Corporation, 2011). Digital Impact Alliance (DIAL) and Digital Square, and other international agencies, governments, philanthropies, donors and academics aim to improve health data through shared investments in global goods, to accelerate progress and scale-up of successful digital health solutions (Health Data Collaborative, 2017a, 2017b; Digital Impact Alliance DIAL, 2021; PATH, 2017). The different working groups of the HDC will be developing standards, indicators, and other tools recommended for countries to collect, analyze, and use health data.

CONCLUSION AND FUTURE DIRECTIONS

The course of digital health toward scale will certainly continue to evolve and accelerate. Working in GHIs requires an innate understanding of the differences in countries' characteristics, health challenges, and priorities have a direct impact on how information systems should be developed and used. Policies and funding are shaping the course of GHIs. The field seeks to better understand the impact that solutions have on health outcomes. Advances in IT infrastructure and mobile computing power in many LMICs have raised confidence that AI might help to address challenges unique to the field of global health and accelerate achievement of the health-related sustainable development goals (Labrique et al., 2018).

Despite advancements in digital technology, significant gaps remain in our understanding of which interventions are effective and what is necessary to ensure effective deployment. Future research should examine the long-term effects of equity in access to and cost-effectiveness and efficiency of digital demand generation interventions. There is an urgent need to invest in efforts to engage and access new digital health technologies. Future research should include experimental and well-designed quasi-experimental studies to examine features of digital use for health in LMICS. The appropriate use of digital health takes the following dimensions into consideration: health promotion and disease prevention, patient safety, ethics, interoperability, intellectual property, data security, privacy, cost-effectiveness, patient engagement, and affordability. It should be people-centered, trust-based, evidence-based, effective, efficient, sustainable, inclusive, equitable, and contextualized.

Digital health will be valued and adopted if it is accessible and supports equitable and universal access to quality health services; enhances the efficiency and sustainability of health systems in delivering quality, affordable and equitable care; and strengthens and scales up health promotion, disease prevention, diagnosis, management, rehabilitation, and palliative care. Digital health needs to be supported by adequate investment in governance, institutional and workforce capacity, and data use training, planning, and management that is required as health systems and services are increasingly digitized.

ACKNOWLEDGMENT

The author would like to acknowledge the contributions of Hyeoun-Ae Park and Nicholas R. Hardiker to the previous edition of this chapter.

DISCUSSION QUESTIONS

1. Discuss two examples of implementation of global health informatics interventions in LMICs?
2. Compare and contrast the challenges and opportunities toward the design and development of health informatics interventions in global settings?
3. What are the different government programs and policies that have been outlined to support the adoption of health informatics solutions in global settings?
4. What skills, knowledge, and competencies are needed to prepare the 21st-century workforce in global health informatics?
5. List some of the limitations of scaling global health informatics innovations in LMICs?

CASE STUDY

Imagine you have been tasked to design, develop and implement a public health dashboard to track the progress of Sustainable Development Goals across LMICs. You have been provided with the list of broad outcomes that you should achieve through the implementation of this population health dashboard. The proposed dashboard should take into consideration technological, human factors, and other data elements into consideration

Discussion Questions

1. Describe the approach that you will take before you plan the design and development of the proposed dashboard tracking sustainable development goals.
2. What are the factors that you would take into consideration before planning the implementation and evaluation of the proposed dashboard platform?

REFERENCES

Agarwal, S., Rosenblum, L., Goldschmidt, T., Carras, M., Goal, N., & Labrique, A. B. (2016). *Mobile technology in support of frontline health workers* (86). Johns Hopkins University Global mHealth Initiative 2016.

Akanbi, M. O., Ocheke, A. N., Agaba, P. A., Daniyam, C. A., Agaba, E. I., Okeke, E. N., et al. (2012). Use of electronic health records in sub-Saharan Africa: Progress and challenges. *Journal of Medicine in the Tropics, 14*(1), 1–6.

Aminpour, F., Sadoughi, F., & Ahamdi, M. (2014). Utilization of open source electronic health record around the world: A systematic review. *Journal of Research in Medical Sciences: The Official Journal of Isfahan University of Medical Sciences, 19*(1), 57–64.

Andrade, B. B., Reis-Filho, A., Barros, A. M., Souza-Neto, S. M., Nogueira, L. L., Fukutani, K. F., et al. (2010). Towards a precise test for malaria diagnosis in the Brazilian Amazon: comparison among field microscopy, a rapid diagnostic test, nested PCR, and a computational expert system based on artificial neural networks. *Malaria Journal, 9*, 117.

Bagayoko, C. O., Traoré, D., Thevoz, L., Diabaté, S., Pecoul, D., Niang, M., et al. (2014). Medical and economic benefits of telehealth in low- and middle-income countries: Results of a study in four district hospitals in Mali. *BMC Health Services Research, 14*(Suppl 1), S9.

Bahmni. (2017, November1). Implementations. https://www.bahmni. org/implementations.

Barbarito, F., Pinciroli, F., Barone, A., Pizzo, F., Ranza, R., Mason, J., et al. (2015). Implementing the lifelong personal health record in a regionalised health information system: The case of Lombardy, Italy. *Computers in Biology and Medicine, 59*, 164–174.

BBC Mobile Action. (2015). *How does the Mobile Kunji audio visual job aid support engagement between front line health workers and their beneficiaries in Bihar, India?* http://downloads.bbc.co.uk/ mediaaction/pdf/research-summaries/mobile-kunji-india-december-2015.pdf.

Boonstra, A., & Broekhuis, M. (2010). Barriers to the acceptance of electronic medical records by physicians from systematic review to taxonomy and interventions. *BMC Health Services Research, 10*, 231. https://doi.org/10.1186/1472-6963-10-231.

Bradley, A., van der Meer, R., & McKay, C. (2019). Personalized pancreatic cancer management: A systematic review of how machine learning is supporting decision-making. *Pancreas, 48*, 598–604.

Burkov, A. (2019). *The Hundred-page machine learning book.*

Caliwan, C. L. (2020). *Taguig launches 'telemedicine' program amid Covid-19.* Philippine News Agency. Available from. https://www. pna.gov.ph/articles/1098024.

Catalani, C., Green, E., Owiti, P., Keny, A., Diero, L., Yeung, A., Israelski, D., & Biondich, P. (2014, Aug 29). A clinical decision support system for integrating tuberculosis and HIV care in Kenya: A human-centered design approach. *PLoS One, 9*(8), e103205.

Chen, X., Tian, J., Li, G., & Li, G. (2020, Apr). Initiation of a new infection control system for the COVID-19 outbreak. *The Lancet Infectious Diseases, 20*(4), 397–398.

Chu, A., Phommavong, C., Lewis, J., Braa, J., & Senyoni, W. (2017). Applying ICT to health information systems (HIS) in low resource settings: Implementing DHIS2 as an integrated health information platform in Lao PDR: *International conference on social implications of computers in developing countries.* Springer.

Chun Tie, Y., Birks, M., & Francis, K. (2019). Grounded theory research: A design framework for novice researchers. *SAGE Open Medicine, 7* 2050312118822927.

CommCare. (2017). *Introducing CommCare Solutions.* 1–3. https:// www.commcarehq.org/solutions/.

Comprehensive Assessment of National Surveillance Systems in Sri Lanka; Joint Assessment Report 4–13 March 2003, World Health Organization Regional Office for South-East Asia New Delhi February 2004.

Coorevits, P., Sundgren, M., Klein, G. O., Bahr, A., Claerhout, B., Daniel, C., et al. (2013). Electronic health records: New opportunities for clinical research. *Journal of Internal Medicine, 274*(6), 547–560.

Cresswell, K. M., Bates, D. W., & Sheikh, A. (2013). Ten key considerations for the successful implementation and adoption of large-scale health information technology. *Journal of the American Medical Informatics Association, 20*(e1), e9–e13.

Dang, L. M., Piran, M. J., Han, D., Min, K., & Moon, H. (2019). A survey on Internet of things and cloud computing for healthcare. *Electronics., 8*(7), 768.

de Filippis, R., Carbone, E. A., Gaetano, R., Bruni, A., Pugliese, V., Segura-Garcia, C., et al. (2019). Machine learning techniques in a structural and functional MRI diagnostic approach in schizophrenia: A systematic review. *Neuropsychiatric Disease and Treatment, 15*, 1605–1627.

Dehnavieh, R., Haghdoost, A., Khosravi, A., Hoseinabadi, F., Rahimi, H., Poursheikhali, A., et al. (June 2018). The district health information system (DHIS2): A literature review and meta-synthesis of its strengths and operational challenges based on the experiences of 11 countries. *Health Information Management Journal*, 1833358318777713.

Delaigue, S., Bonnardot, L., Steichen, O., Garcia, D. M., Venugopal, R., Saint-Sauveur, J. F., et al. (2018). Seven years of telemedicine in Médecins Sans Frontières demonstrate that offering direct specialist expertise in the frontline brings clinical and educational value. *Journal of Global Health, 8*(2), 020414.

Detmer, D., Bloomrosen, M., Raymond, B., & Tang, P. (2008). Integrated personal health records: Transformative tools for consumer-centric care. *BMC Medical Informatics and Decision making, 8*, 45.

Digital Impact Alliance (DIAL). *What we do.* 2017. https:// digitalimpactalliance.org/. Accessed August 30, 2021.

Digital reach initiative. (n.d.). https://www.eahealth.org/sites/www. eahealth.org/files/content/attachments/2019-08-06/Digital-REACH-Initiative-Compendium_20181009_custom.pdf

Djalante, R., Lassa, J., Setiamarga, D., Sudjatma, A., Indrawan, M., Haryanto, B., et al. (2020). Review and analysis of current responses to COVID-19 in Indonesia: Period of January to March 2020. *Progress in Disaster Science, 6*, 100091.

Dong, E., Du, H., & Gardner, L. (2020). An interactive web-based dashboard to track COVID-19 in real time. *The Lancet. Infectious Diseases, 20*(5), 533–534.

El Arifeen, S., Christou, A., Reichenbach, L., Osman, F. A., Azad, K., Islam, K. S., et al. (2013). Community-based approaches and partnerships: Innovations in health-service delivery in Bangladesh. *Lancet, 382*, 2012–2026.

Elveren, E., & Yumuşak, N. (2011). Tuberculosis disease diagnosis using artificial neural network trained with genetic algorithm. *Journal of Medical Systems, 35*, 329–332.

Fall, I. S., Rajatonirina, S., Yahaya, A. A., Zabulon, Y., Nsubuga, P., Nanyunja, M., et al. (2019). Integrated disease surveillance and response (IDSR) strategy: Current status, challenges and perspectives for the future in Africa. *BMJ Global Health, 4*(4), e001427.

Farzianpour, F., Amirian, S., & Byravan, R. (2015). An investigation on the barriers and facilitators of the implementation of electronic health records (EHR). *Health, 7*(12), 1665–1670.

Field, M. J. (Ed.), (1996). *Telemedicine: A guide to assessing telecommunications in health care.* Washington, DC: National Academies Press. Institute of Medicine (US) Committee on Evaluating Clinical Applications of Telemedicine.

Gaskin, G. L., Longhurst, C. A., Slayton, R., & Das, A. K. (2017, Dec 16). Sociotechnical challenges of developing an interoperable personal health record: Lessons learned. *Applied Clinical Informatics, 02*(04), 406–419.

Gathogo, J. K. (2014). *A model for post-implementation valuation of health information systems: The case of the DHIS 2 in Kenya.* University of Nairobi.

Genitsaridi, I., Kondylakis, H., Koumakis, L., Marias, K., & Tsiknakis, M. (2015, Apr). Evaluation of personal health record systems through the lenses of EC research projects. *Computers in Biology and Medicine, 59*, 175–185.

Gimbel, S., Mwanza, M., Nisingizwe, M. P., Michel, C., Hirschhorn, L., & PHIT, A. H. I. (2017). Partnership Collaborative. Improving data quality across 3 sub-Saharan African countries using the consolidated framework for implementation research (CFIR): Results from the African health initiative. *BMC Health Services Research, 17*(Suppl 3), 828.

Global Internet of things policies 2018–2019. *Research and Markets*. 2019. Accessed June 4, 2020. https://www.globenewswire.com/news-release/2019/05/30/1859482/0/en/Global-Internet-of-Things-Policies-2018-2019.html

Government of Nepal. (n.d.). Ministry of Health and Population, Department of Health Services, Epidemiology and Disease Control Division Kathmandu, Nepal. http://www.edcd.gov.np/section/surveillance-of-communicable-disease-program.

Hagg, E., Dahinten, V. S., & Currie, L. M. (2018). The emerging use of social media for health-related purposes in low and middle-income countries: A scoping review. *International Journal of Medical Informatics*, 115, 92–105. https://doi.org/10.1016/j.ijmedinf.2018.04.010.

Hamill, S., Turk, T., Murukutla, N., Ghamrawy, M., & Mullin, S. (2015). I "like" MPOWER: using facebook, online ads and new media to mobilise tobacco control communities in low-income and middle-income countries. *Tob Control*, 24(3), 306–312. https://doi.org/10.1136/tobaccocontrol-2012-050946.

Häyrinen, K., Saranto, K., & Nykänen, P. (2008). Definition, structure, content, use and impacts of electronic health records: A review of the research literature. *International Journal of Medical Informatics*, 77(5), 291–304.

Hazel, E., Wilson, E., Anifalaje, A., Sawadogo-Lewis, T., & Heidkamp, R. (2018). Building integrated data systems for health and nutrition program evaluations: Lessons learned from a multi-country implementation of a DHIS 2-based system. *Journal of Global Health*, 8(2), 20307.

Health Data Collaborative. (2017a). Health data collaborative: Better data, better health. 1–4. https://www.healthdatacollaborative.org/what-we-do/.

Health Data Collaborative. (2017b). *Health data collaborative: Operational workplan 2016–2017*. https://www.healthdatacollaborative.org/fileadmin/uploads/hdc/Documents/HDC_Operational_Workplan.pdf.

HIPAA. (2021). *The definition of electronic health record*. Accessed on 2021 August 30. Available from: http://www.hipaa.com/2009/05/the-definition-of-electronic-health-record.

Hoerbst, A., Kohl, C. D., Knaup, P., & Ammenwerth, E. (2010). Attitudes and behaviors related to the introduction of electronic health records among Austrian and German citizens. *International Journal of Medical Informatics*, 79(2), 81–89.

Hoffer-Hawlik, M. A., Moran, A. E., Burka, D., Kaur, P., Cai, J., Frieden, T. R., et al. (2020). Leveraging telemedicine for chronic disease management in low- and middle-income countries during Covid-19. *Global Heart.*, 15(1), 63.

Hsieh, R. K., Hjelm, N. M., Lee, J. C., & Aldis, J. W. (2001). Telemedicine in China. *International Journal of Medical Informatics*, 61, 139–146.

Huang, D., & Wu, Z. (2017). Forecasting outpatient visits using empirical mode decomposition coupled with back-propagation artificial neural networks optimized by particle swarm optimization. *PLoS One*, 12(2), e0172539.

Huang, F., Blaschke, S., & Lucas, H. (2017). Beyond pilotitis: Taking digital health interventions to the national level in China and Uganda. *Global Health*, 13, 49.

Inman, A. G., Soheilian, S. S., & Luu, L. P. (2019). Telesupervision: Building bridges in a digital era. *Journal of Clinical Psychology*, 75(2), 292–301.

Integrated Disease Surveillance Program. (n.d.). Ministry of Health & Family Welfare, Government of India. https://idsp.nic.in/.

International Finance Corporation. (2011). The business of health in Africa: Partnering with the private sector to improve people's lives. https://doi.org/10.1080/03056248608703687.

ITU. (2021). https://www.itu.int/en/ITU-D/Statistics/Documents/facts/FactsFigures2020.pdf. Accessed August 30, 2021.

Jalali, M. S., Kaiser, J. P., Siegel, M., & Madnick, S. (2019). The internet of things promises new benefits and risks: a systematic analysis of adoption dynamics of IoT products. *IEEE Security and Privacy*, 17(2), 39–48.

Jawhari, B., Ludwick, D., Keenan, L., Zakus, D., & Hayward, R. (2016). Benefits and challenges of EMR implementations in low resource settings: A state-of-the-art review. *BMC Medical Informatics and Decision Making*, 16(1), 1–12. https://doi.org/10.1186/s12911-016-0354-8. Available from.

Jayatilleke, K. (2020). Challenges in Implementing Surveillance Tools of High-Income Countries (HICs) in Low Middle Income Countries (LMICs). *Current Treatment Options in Infectious Diseases*, 12(3), 191–201.

Jefee-Bahloul, H., Moustafa, M. K., Shebl, F. M., & Barkil-Oteo, A. (2014). Pilot assessment and survey of Syrian refugees' psychological stress and openness to referral for telepsychiatry (PASSPORT Study). *Telemedicine Journal and e-Health: The Official Journal of the American Telemedicine Association*, 20(10), 977–979.

Jefee-Bahloul, H., & Zayour, Z. (2017). Telemental health in the Middle East. In H. Jefee-Bahloul, A. Barkil-Oteo, & E. F. Augusterfer (Eds.), *Telemental health in resource-limited global settings*. New York, NY: Oxford University Press.

Jensen, P. B., Jensen, L. J., & Brunak, S. (2012 May 2). Mining electronic health records: Towards better research applications and clinical care. *Nature Reviews. Genetics.*, 13(6), 395–405.

Johnson, K., Jimison, H. B., & Mandl, K. D. (2013). Consumer health informatics personal health records: *Biomedical informatics* (pp. 517–539). London: Springer.

Johnston, I. G., Hoffmann, T., Greenbury, S. F., Cominetti, O., Jallow, M., Kwiatkowski, D., et al. (2019). Precision identification of high-risk phenotypes and progression pathways in severe malaria without requiring longitudinal data. *NPJ Digital Medicine*, 2, 63.

Katz, R. (2012). *Impact of broadband on the economy: Research to date and policy issues*. ITU: Committed to Connecting the World. URL: https://www.itu.int/ITU-D/treg/broadband/ITU-BB-Reports_Impact-of-Broadband-on-the-Economy.pdf. Accessed April 25, 2018.

Kelly, J. T., Campbell, K. L., Gong, E., & Scuffham, P. (2020). The internet of things: Impact and implications for health care delivery. *Journal of Medical Internet Research*, 22(11), e20135.

Kern, J., Fister, K., & Polasek, O. (2009). Active patient role in recording health data: *Encyclopedia of information science and technology* (pp. 14–19) (2nd ed.). Hershey, Pennsylvania, United States: IGI Global.

Khalifa, M. (2013). Barriers to health information systems and electronic medical records implementation. A field study of Saudi Arabian hospitals. *Procedia Computer Science*, 21, 335–342.

Kiberu, V. M., Matovu, J. K., Makumbi, F., Kyozira, C., Mukooyo, E., & Wanyenze, R. K. (2014). Strengthening district-based health reporting through the district health management information software system: The Ugandan experience. *BMC Medical Informatics and Decision Making*, 14(1), 40.

Kiberu, V. M., Matovu, J. K. B., Makumbi, F., Kyozira, C., Mukooyo, E., & Wanyenze, R. K. (2014a). Strengthening district-based health reporting through the district health management information software system: The Ugandan experience. *BMC Medical Informatics and Decision Making*, 14, 40.

Kickbusch, I., Agrawal, A., Jack, A., Lee, N., & Horton, R. (2019). Governing health futures 2030: Growing up in a digital world-a joint The Lancet and Financial Times Commission. *Lancet*, 394(10206), 1309.

Kihuba, E., Gheorghe, A., Bozzani, F., English, M., & Griffiths, U. K. (2016). Opportunities and challenges for implementing cost accounting systems in the Kenyan health system. *Global Health Action, 9*(1), 30621.

Kwizera, A., Kissoon, N., Musa, N., Urayeneza, O., Mujyarugamba, P., & Patterson, A. J. (2019). A machine learning-based triage tool for children with acute infection in a low resource setting. *Pediatric Critical Care Medicine: A Journal of the Society of Critical Care Medicine and the World Federation of Pediatric Intensive and Critical Care Societies, 20*, e524–e530.

Labrique, A. B., Wadhwani, C., Williams, K. A., Lamptey, P., Hesp, C., Luk, R., & Aerts, A. (2018). Best practices in scaling digital health in low and middle income countries. *Global Health, 14*, 103. https://globalizationandhealth.biomedcentral.com/articles/10.1186/s12992-018-0424-z.

Li, S., Xu, L. D., & Zhao, S. (2018). 5G internet of things: A survey. *Journal of Industrial Information Integration, 10*, 1–9.

Lobach, D. F., & Detmer, D. E. (2007). Research challenges for electronic health records. *American Journal of Preventive Medicine, 32*(5 Suppl), S104–S111.

Mahmood, S., Hasan, K., Colder Carras, M., & Labrique, A. (2020). Global preparedness against COVID-19: We must leverage the power of digital health. *JMIR Public Health and Surveillance, 6*(2), e18980,

Mahmood, S., Hasan, K., Colder Carras, M., & Labrique, A. (2020). Global preparedness against COVID-19: We must leverage the power of digital health. *JMIR Public Health Surveillance, 6*(2), e18980. https://doi.org/10.2196/18980.

Mahmood, S., Hasan, K., Colder Carras, M., & Labrique, A. (2020). Global preparedness against COVID-19: We must leverage the power of digital health. *JMIR Public Health and Surveillance, 6*(2), e18980.

Mamlin, B. W., Biondich, P. G., Wolfe, B. A., Fraser, H., Jazayeri, D., Allen, C., et al. (2006). Cooking up an open source EMR for developing countries: OpenMRS—a recipe for successful collaboration. *AMIA. Annual Symposium Proceedings/AMIA Symposium, 2006*, 529–533.

Manoj, M. (2013). Customising DHIS2 for maternal and child health information management in Sri Lanka. *Sri Lanka Journal of Bio-Medical Informatics, 3*(2).

Mansell, R. (2011). Digital opportunities and the missing link for developing countries. *Oxford Review of Economic Policy, 17*(2), 282–295.

Mell, P., & Grance, T. (2011). *NIST definition of cloud computing.* National Institute of Standards and Technology.

Menachemi, N., & Collum, T. H. (2011). Benefits and drawbacks of electronic health record systems. *Risk Management and Healthcare Policy, 4*, 47–55.

Minges, M. (2016). *Exploring the relationship between broadband and economic growth.* The World Bank. http://documents.worldbank.org/curated/en/178701467988875888/pdf/102955-WP-Box394845B-PUBLIC-WDR16-BP-Exploring-the-Relationship-between-Broadband-and-Economic-Growth-Minges.pdf.

Ministry of Health and Family Welfare, Government of India. *Telemedicine Practice Guidelines.* 2020. Available from https://www.mohfw.gov.in/pdf/Telemedicine.pdf. Accessed September 1, 2021.

Mohammed-Rajput, N. A., Smith, D. C., Mamlin, B., Biondich, P., Doebbeling, B. N., & Open, M. R. S. (2011). Collaborative Investigators. OpenMRS, a global medical records system collaborative: Factors influencing successful implementation. *AMIA. Annual Symposium Proceedings/AMIA Symposium, 2011*, 960–968.

Mutale, W., Chintu, N., Amoroso, C., Awoonor-Williams, K., Phillips, J., Baynes, C., et al. (2013). Improving health information systems for decision making across five sub-Saharan African countries: Implementation strategies from the African health initiative. *BMC Health Services Research, 13*(Suppl 2), 1–12.

Mwogi, T., & Were, M. C. (2017). Setting the agenda for personal health records in low- and middle-income countries. *Studies in Health Technology and Informatics, 245*, 1234.

Ngugi, P., Babic, A., Kariuki, J., Santas, X., Naanyu, V., & Were, M. C. (2021). Development of standard indicators to assess use of electronic health record systems implemented in low-and medium-income countries. *PLoS One, 16*(1), e0244917.

Ngugi, P., Were, M. C., & Babic, A. (2018). Facilitators and barriers of electronic medical records systems implementation in low resource settings: A holistic view. *Studies in Health Technology and Informatics, 251*, 187–190.

Ngwa, W., Olver, I., & Schmeler, K. M. (2020). The use of health-related technology to reduce the gap between developed and undeveloped regions around the globe. *American Society of Clinical Oncology Educational Book, 40*, 1–10.

Novartis Foundation. (2010). *Telemedicine project in Ghana Healthcare.* 2010. http://www.novartisfoundation.org/_file/133/telemed-en.pdf.

Nowell, L. S., Norris, J. M., White, D. E., & Moules, N. J. (2017). Thematic analysis: Striving to meet the trustworthiness criteria. *International Journal of Qualitative Methods, 16*(1). 1609406917733847.

Odekunle, F. F., Odekunle, R. O., & Shankar, S. (2017). Why sub-Saharan Africa lags in electronic health record adoption and possible strategies to increase its adoption in this region. *International Journal of Health Sciences (Qassim) [Internet], 11*(4), 59–64.

OpenDataKit. *About OpenDataKit.* 2013. 1–2. https://opendatakit.org/.

OpenMRS. (2017). *About OpenMRS.* 1–5. http://openmrs.org/about/.

Pacheco, R., Dias, S., & Rodrigues, Q. (2019). Rodrigues smart cities and healthcare: A systematic review. *Technologies, 7*(3), 58.

PATH. (2017). *Digital Square: New global initiative will connect the world for better health through digital technology.* 1–7. http://www.path.org/news/press-room/846/. Accessed August 25, 2021.

PATH. *The journey to better data for better health in Tanzania.* http://www.path.org/publications/files/DHS_health_tanzania_rpt1.pdf.

Peimani, M., Rambod, C., Omidvar, M., Larijani, B., Ghodssi-Ghassemabadi, R., Tootee, A., et al. (2016). Effectiveness of short message service-based intervention (SMS) on self-care in type 2 diabetes: a feasibility study. *Primary Care Diabetes, 10*(4), 251–258. https://doi.org/10.1016/j.pcd.2015.11.001.

Phakhounthong, K., Chaovalit, P., & Jittamala, P. (2018). Predicting the severity of dengue fever in children on admission based on clinical features and laboratory indicators: Application of classification tree analysis. *BMC Pediatrics, 18*, 109.

Phua, K. H., Sheikh, K., Tang, S., & Lin, V. (2015 Novv). Editorial—health systems of Asia: Equity, governance and social impact. *Social Science & Medicine, 145*, 141–144.

Piette, J. D., Mendoza-Avelares, M. O., Ganser, M., Mohamed, M., Marinec, N., & Krishnan, S. (2011). A preliminary study of a cloud-computing model for chronic illness self-care support in an underdeveloped country. *American Journal of Preventive Medicine, 40*, 629–632.

Principles for digital development. (2014). https://digitalprinciples.org. Accessed August 30, 2021.

Quintana, Y., & Safran, C. (2015). Global challenges in people-centered e-health. *Studies in Health Technology and Informatics, 216,* 97.

Ranasinghe, K. I., Chan, T., & Yaralagadda, P. (2012). Information support for health information management in regional Sri Lanka: Health managers' perspectives. *Health Information Management Journal, 41*(3), 20–26.

Raut, D. K., & Bhola, A. (2014). Integrated disease surveillance in India: Way forward. *Global Journal of Public Health Medicine (GJMEDPH), 3*(4), 1–10.

Rebala, G., Ravi, A., & Churiwala, S. (2019). *An introduction to machine learning.* Springer International Publishing.

Reeves, J. J., Hollandsworth, H. M., Torriani, F. J., Taplitz, R., Abeles, S., Tai-Seale, M., et al. (2020). Rapid response to COVID-19: Health informatics support for outbreak management in an academic health system. *Journal of the American Medical Informatics Association, 27*(6), 853–859.

Resolve to Save Lives. (2020). *Leveraging technology to improve health care during the COVID-19 pandemic and beyond 2020.* Available from https://linkscommunity.org/assets/PDFs/cov039_telemedicine_v3_14may2020.pdf.

Richards, J., Douglas, G., & Fraser, H. S. F. (2013). Perspectives on global public health informatics. In *Public health informatics and information systems,* 619–644.

Russell, S. J. (2010). *Artificial intelligence: A modern approach.* Upper Saddle River, NJ: Prentice Hall.

Saleh, S., Farah, A., Dimassi, H., El Arnaout, N., Constantin, J., Osman, M., et al. (2018). Using mobile health to enhance outcomes of non-communicable diseases care in rural settings and refugee camps: randomized controlled trial. *JMIR mHealth and uHealth, 6*(7), e137. https://doi.org/10.2196/mhealth.8146.

Schwalbe, N., & Wahl, B. (2020). Artificial intelligence and the future of global health. *Lancet, 395*(10236), 1579–1586.

Sethi, P., & Sarangi, S. (2017). Internet of things: Architectures, protocols, and applications. *Journal of Electrical and Computer Engineering*

Shung, D., Simonov, M., Gentry, M., Au, B., & Laine, L. (2019). Machine learning to predict outcomes in patients with acute gastrointestinal bleeding: A systematic review. *Digestive Diseases and Sciences, 64,* 2078–2087.

Smart Register. (2017). *About OpenSRP.* http://smartregister.org/about-about-opensrp.html.

Smart Register. (2017). *THRIVE Bangladesh: Health focus and application use.* 2017. http://smartregister.org/implementations-bangladesh.html.

Sood S.P., Nwabueze S.N., Mbarika V.W.A., Prakash N., Chatterjee S., Ray P., et al. (2008). Electronic medical records: A review comparing the challenges in developed and developing countries. In: *Proceedings of the Annual Hawaii International Conference on System Sciences.*

State Medical Insurance Bureau State Health Commission. (2020). *Guiding Opinions of the National Health Insurance Commission of the National Medical Insurance Bureau on Promoting the "Internet +" Medical Insurance Service during the Prevention and Control of the New Coronary Pneumonia Outbreak.* Available from http://www.nhsa.gov.cn/art/2020/3/2/art_37_2750.html. Accessed August 30, 2021.

Syzdykova, A., Zolfo, M., Malta, A., Diro, E., & Oliveira, J. L. (2017). Customization of OpenMRS for leishmaniasis research and treatment center in Ethiopia. *Journal of the International Society for Telemedicine and eHealth, 5,* e65.

Tang, P. C., Ash, J. S., Bates, D. W., Overhage, J. M., & Sands, D. Z. (2006). Personal health records: definitions, benefits, and strategies for overcoming barriers to adoption. *Journal of the American Medical Informatics Association, 13*(2), 121–126.

Tang, P. C., Ash, J. S., Bates, D. W., Overhage, J. M., & Sands, D. Z. (2006 Marr). Personal health records: Definitions, benefits, and strategies for overcoming barriers to adoption. *Journal of the American Medical Informatics Association, 13*(2), 121–126.

Tierney, W. M., Achieng, M., Baker, E., Bell, A., Biondich, P., Braitstein, P., et al. (2010). Experience implementing electronic health records in three East African countries. *Studies in Health Technology and Informatics, 160*(Pt 1), 371–375.

UN Secretary-General's High-level Panel on Digital Cooperation. (2018). *The age of digital interdependence.* 2018. https://www.un.org/en/pdfs/DigitalCooperation-report-for%20web.pdf. Accessed August 25, 2021.

Update: *Integrated diseases surveillance and response implementation in Ethiopia.* https://www.who.int/countries/eth/areas/surveillance/en/idsr_implementation.pdf.

Wahl, B., Cossy-Gantner, A., Germann, S., & Schwalbe, N. R. (2018). Artificial intelligence (AI) and global health: how can AI contribute to health in resource-poor settings? *BMJ Global Health, 3*(4), e000798.

Warren, A. E., Wyss, K., Shakarishvili, G., Atun, R., & de Savigny, D. (2013). Global health initiative investments and health systems strengthening: A content analysis of global fund investments. *Globalization and Health, 9*(1), 30.

Wootton, R. (2008). Telemedicine support for the developing world. *Journal of Telemedicine and Telecare, 14,* 109–114.

World Health Organization (WHO). https://apps.who.int/gb/ebwha/pdf_files/WHA58-REC1/english/A58_2005_REC1-en.pdf. Accessed August 29, 2021.

World Health Organization (WHO). https://apps.who.int/iris/bitstream/handle/10665/344249/9789240020924-eng.pdf. Accessed August 29, 2021.

World Health Organization. (2006). Guide to monitoring and evaluating communicable disease surveillance and response systems. WHO/CDS/EPR/LYO/2006.2. https://www.who.int/csr/resources/publications/surveillance/WHO_CDS_EPR_LYO_2006_2.pdf

World Health Organization. (2010). *Monitoring the building blocks of health systems: a handbook of indicators and their measurement strategies.* Geneva. http://www.who.int/healthinfo/systems/WHO_MBHSS_2010_full_web.pdf?ua=1.

World Health Organization. (2011). *mHealth: New horizons for health through mobile technologies.* Geneva, Switzerland: World Health Organization.

World Health Organization. (2012). *Framework and standards for country health information systems* (2nd ed.), Geneva. http://www.who.int/healthinfo/country_monitoring_evaluation/who-hmn-framework-standards-chi.pdf.

World Health Organization. (2017). *mDiabetes, an innovative programme to improve the health of people with diabetes in Senegal.* http://www.afro.who.int/news/mdiabetes-innovative-programme-improve-health-people-diabetes-senegal.

World Health Organization. (2020, March 17). *Home care for patients with COVID-19 presenting with mild symptoms and management of their contacts.* https://tinyurl.com/t5nenma

Yin, Y., Zeng, Y., Chen, X., & Fan, Y. (2016). The internet of things in healthcare: An overview. *Journal of Industrial Information Integration, 1,* 3–13.

33

Informatics and the Future of Healthcare

Timothy Tsai, John D. Manning, and Michael Wang

*Health informatics can be described as an interprofessional discipline
that is grounded in the present while planning for the future.*

OBJECTIVES

At the completion of this chapter, the reader will be prepared to:
1. Describe the trends in EHR and personal health informatics.
2. Describe trends in the broader healthcare technology ecosystem.

KEY TERMS

extrapolation, 513

futures research, 510

human factors engineering, 519

learning healthcare systems, 518

optimization, 516

predictive analytics, 517

social determinants of health, 515

trend analysis, 512

ABSTRACT ❖

This chapter expands on the future directions sections included
in the individual chapters and provides broad guidance about the
future of health informatics. First, healthcare trends in society are
outlined. Second, futures studies or futurology (methods to analyze probable future directions in any field) is discussed. Third,
an overview of future directions in healthcare and informatics is
given: (1) person-centered health, the fusion of health information
technology (health IT) into healthcare and concomitant implications for health informatics; (2) technical trends in health IT, such
as the internet of things (IoT) and cybersecurity issues; and (3)
clinical informatics trends, including analytics, data visualization, and improving the user experience (UX). The last topics are
discussed in more detail because of their profound impacts on
society, healthcare, and health informatics in the future.

INTRODUCTION

Health informatics can be described as an interprofessional discipline grounded in the present while planning for the future.
Health professionals and informatics specialists are implementing today's health information technology (health IT) while
simultaneously creating the foundation for the technology of
tomorrow. By reviewing current trends and predictions, as well
as employing tools for predicting and managing the future,
health professionals and informatics specialists can prepare for
their leadership roles in planning effective and innovative future
healthcare information systems.

Health IT and informatics will play integral roles in the
future of all aspects of healthcare. Precisely which informatics
trends will prevail is not completely clear; however, emerging
areas can be seen. In each of the chapters in this book, authors
outlined evolving areas of influence, as well as material on
healthcare trends in society, trends in EHR and personal health
informatics, and trends in the broader healthcare technology
system.

To understand the future of health informatics, healthcare providers and informaticians need to be aware of societal
trends. Examples of trends in society include *healthcare costs*.
Current projected annual growth is 5.4% for 2019–2028 and
may reach up to $6.2 trillion dollars by 2028 (Chantrill, 2016;
Centers for Medicare and Medicaid Services, 2021). Although
costs are still predicted to rise over time, current spending projections are now $2.5 trillion less due to the Affordable Care Act
in the United States and the economic recession that occurred
in the late 2000s (Holahan & McMorrow, 2015).

1. *Aging populations.* From 2000 to 2050, the global population
   of those aged 60 years or older will rise from 600 million to
   more than 2 billion (World Health Organization WHO, 2011).
2. *Increasing numbers of patients with chronic diseases.* According to the World Health Organization (WHO), chronic
   diseases such as ischemic heart disease, stroke, and chronic
   obstructive pulmonary disease represent the leading causes
   of death worldwide, with ischemic heart disease now representing 16% of global deaths annually (World Health

Organization [WHO], 2021). The rate for diabetes alone across the globe is predicted to increase from 382 million in 2013 to 592 million by 2035 (Guariguata et al., 2014).

3. *Predicted shortage of healthcare providers.* By 2030, the number of U.S. seniors is expected to increase by 55% compared to 2015 (Kirch & Petelle, 2017). Registered nurses who had joined the healthcare workforce in unprecedented numbers beginning in the 1970s are also slated to retire, to which an estimated 1 million nurses will likely have retired between the years of 2017–2030 alone (Buerhaus et al., 2017). In addition to this, a national shortage of 40,800 to 104,900 physicians is expected by 2030, seen mostly in primary care and surgical specialties, and with significant variation across states and regions (Kirch & Petelle, 2017; Zhang et al., 2020; Markit, 2017).

These trends clearly have implications for the future practice of health informatics. However, how does one determine and plan for these implications? Futures research, or futurology, the method used to determine future directions and trends in any field, can help answer this question.

Futures Research (Futurology)

This section introduces readers to levels of change that can be anticipated in future trends. By analyzing methodologies and tools for predicting, planning for, and managing the future, health professionals and informatics specialists can prepare for the leadership roles they will play in planning future healthcare information systems. With a better understanding of the potential future, healthcare providers and informatics professionals can make better decisions today.

Defining Futures Research (Futurology)

Futures research is the rational and systematic study of the future, with the goal of identifying possible, probable, and preferable futures. The focus can be anywhere from 5 to 50 years in the future. The formal study of the future goes by several names, including *foresight and futures studies*, *strategic foresight*, *prospective studies*, *prognostic studies*, and *futurology*. Using a research approach to study the future formally began after World War II. Initially this field of study aroused skepticism. Since that time, institutes, foundations, and professional associations have been established supporting the field of futures studies. Examples of these are included in Box 33.1. In addition, educational programs related to futures studies now use the various futurology terms to describe their programs. Box 33.2 includes examples of university programs in futures studies. Researchers and corporate strategists are also

using concepts, theories, principles, and methods based on the field of futures research. Despite the initial skepticism today, futures studies techniques are accepted, educational programs are available, and these methods can be very useful for healthcare providers and informaticians.

Health and informatics professionals can use traditional forecasting and planning methods in combination with futures studies methods. Strategic planning in health informatics typically focuses on projects 1 to 3 years in the future. Institutional long-range planning tends to focus on 5 to 10 years in the future. Vendor contracts for major healthcare informatics systems often cover a 10-year period, spanning both strategic and long-range planning.

There are differences between forecasting and futures studies. First, forecasters focus on incremental changes from existing trends, while futurists focus on systemic, transformational change. Second, futurists do not offer a single prediction. Rather, they describe alternative, possible, and preferable futures, keeping in mind that the future will be created, in most part, by decisions made today. The technical, political, and sociocultural infrastructure being built today will have a major impact on the choices of tomorrow. Both traditional forecasting and futures studies methods are key to planning health informatics projects (Nordlund, 2012). Understanding the impact of future trends and using this information for planning begins by understanding the degree and scope of change that occurs over time.

Future Directions and Scope of Change

Degrees or the scope of change can be divided into three levels (Nelson & Englebardt, 2002). First-level change does not really change the process being used or the goal one might want to achieve. This level of change makes the process in use more effective and efficient. Replacing a typewriter with a word processor is an example of a first-level change. The user is still producing a document, but the technology makes the process more effective and efficient. Within the levels of change, first-level change is the least disruptive and the most comfortable. In many ways, requests that new technology be designed to fit the workflow of healthcare providers is, in reality, a request, or perhaps a demand, for first-level change only. In fact, if the equipment and related procedures do not support the current roles and responsibilities of the healthcare providers, they quickly develop workarounds to meet their requirement that the degree of change be limited to a first-level change.

A second-level change involves changing how a specific outcome is achieved. For example, the peer review process tradi-

---

BOX 33.1 Futures Studies

- Selected Associations, Institutes, and FoundationsAcceleration Studies Foundation, http://accelerating.org/index.html
- Copenhagen Institute for Future Studies, http://cifs.dk/about-us/
- Foresight Canada, http://www.foresightcanada.ca
- Fullerton and Cypress Colleges, and School of Continuing Education: Center for the Future, http://fcfutures.fullcoll.edu
- The Arlington Institute, http://www.arlingtoninstitute.org
- Association of Professional Futurists, http://www.profuturists.org

- The Institute for Alternative Futures (IAF) http://www.altfutures.org/home
- The Club of Rome, http://www.clubofrome.org
- *The Futurist*, http://www.wfs.org/futurist/about-futurist
- Institute for the Future, http://www.iftf.org/home
- The Millennium Project, http://www.millennium-project.org
- World Future Society, http://www.wfs.org/node/920
- World Futures Studies Federation (WFSF), http://www.wfsf.org

IAF, Institute for Alternative Futures; *WFSF,* World Futures Studies Federation.

tionally used by professional journals involved sending a submitted manuscript to a limited number of selected experts for anonymous opinions. The goal was to ensure that only the highest quality articles were published. The process of review and revision could take weeks or months. In addition, with a limited number of experts screening what was published, a degree of professional censorship existed. Articles representing a paradigm shift in thinking risked being rejected by this limited set of reviewers. Today, professional online journals and journals that have prepublished online versions of an article usually offer their readers the opportunity to comment. Introducing the opportunity for readers to comment is now changing who is involved in peer review and how the peer review process is completed.

Another example of second-level change is demonstrated by patient groups within social media applications. These are changing what and how patients learn about their health problems. Groups of patients help each other read and interpret the latest research to create a new level of health literacy within these groups. Social media interactions not only change the process for achieving an outcome but also change the relationships between the participants. As patients become organized and more health literate, they take a more active role in their own care and move from the role of patients needing education about their diseases into more of a collegial role, even sharing new and innovative findings with healthcare providers.

The scope of change at this level creates both excitement and anxiety within professional groups and among individual healthcare providers. The scope of practice, policies, procedures, and established professional customs, such as professional boundaries, are challenged, and resistance to this challenge can be expected. For example, in healthcare, the goals of improved health for individuals, families, groups, and communities have not changed, but technology is changing the roles and responsibilities related to how these goals might be achieved.

A third-level change alters the process and can also refocus the goal. For example, a hyperlinked multimedia journal, with a process for adding reader comments and linking to related publications, may change not only the definition of an expert but also the historical gold standard for review of new information and knowledge.

Another example is the use of knowledge discovery and data mining in the research process. In the traditional approach to scientific research, the researcher begins with a theory and a theoretically based hypothesis. This foundation is used to determine what variables or data are collected and how those data are analyzed. With knowledge discovery and data mining, the goal is to discover clusters and relationships among existing data with no preconceived concept of theories, data collection, or how these data are related, redefining (or at least expanding) the concept of the research process.

Third-level change involves changes at the societal and institutional level, typically occurring over extended periods of time. For instance, the evolving role of the nurse from a handmaiden for the physician to a leader in healthcare delivery can be seen as a third-level change. Both the goal of nursing, from an efficient and effective handmaiden to a leader, is changing, as well as the activities that make up the nursing process.

Today, innovations in healthcare and computer technology are interactively creating first-, second-, and third-level changes, creating the future of healthcare within a society that is also undergoing change in most other society-based institutions. Informatics experts are among the key leaders managing and guiding these change processes within healthcare. However, they face challenges in achieving these goals.

The Challenge of Anticipating Future Directions

Over 50 years ago, in 1970, Toffler published the book *Future Shock* (Toffler, 1970). One of the themes in the book was "what happens to people when they are overwhelmed by change. It is about how we adapt or fail to adapt to the future" (Toffler, 1970). Interestingly, *Future Shock* was written long before the widespread use of personal computers or the internet. As Toffler identified decades ago in a slower-paced world, the degree and speed of change may be overwhelming. Today, this includes both providers and consumers of healthcare who are amid exponential knowledge growth and must adapt to the overwhelming changes in healthcare.

While there are no research methods for predicting the future with absolute certainty, techniques can be used to rationally predict future directions and trends. A historical example of this is the publication of the book *Megatrends* by Naisbitt (1982) well before the general population was aware of the internet or the potential of owning a computer. Megatrends are trends that affect all aspects of society. The 10 trends identified by Naisbitt are listed in Box 33.3. These trends, identified years ago, continue to have a major influence on health informatics today.

While health providers and health informatics specialists clearly recognize the importance of planning and the long-term implications of building today's healthcare information

BOX 33.3   Naisbitt's Megatrends for the 1980s

- Industrial society → Information society
- Forced technology → High tech/High touch
- National economy → World economy
- Short term → Long term
- Centralized → Decentralized

- Institutional help → Self-help
- Representative democracy → Participatory democracy
- Hierarchies → Networking
- North → South
- Either/Or → Multiple options

systems, immediate challenges exist in thinking about the future. First, present issues are often more pressing and take a higher priority over tasks that can wait for another day. This type of thinking is sometimes referred to as "putting out fires." For example, a health informatics specialist may spend an afternoon answering users' questions, but as the number of communications increases, the notes documenting these calls can become increasingly sparse. Trends and patterns that could be used as a basis for a new education and training program, or for upgrading functions in the current healthcare informatics system, can be lost in the pressing demands of the moment.

Second, small rates of growth often seem insignificant. However, major trends start from small, persistent rates of growth. This is especially true when dealing with exponential growth. Previously, few patients asked for copies of their health reports, and a very small percentage of those patients would have considered accessing their healthcare data via the internet. As of October 2015, the Office of the National Coordinator (ONC) reported that over 90% of hospitals provide patients the option of viewing their health data online. See Table 33.1 for additional details about how hospitals and providers are engaging patients in their own healthcare via the internet and personal health records (PHRs).

Third, there are intellectual, imaginative, and emotional limits to the amount of change that individuals and organizations can anticipate. The imagined future is built on assumptions developed in the past and therefore includes gaps and misinterpretations. Future predictions can seem vague, and the further one investigates the future, the more disconnects exist between the present and the significance of the future. For example, nurses educated in small diploma schools in the 1950s and 1960s usually called a physician to restart an intravenous (IV). If nurses from that era were asked to predict the future of nursing, they would have struggled to anticipate the high levels of responsibility common in today's staff nurse role, where starting an IV is a common task.

Approaches for Predicting

Qualitative and quantitative methods are used in traditional forecasting and planning as well as by futurists to foresee, manage, and create the future. The use of established research methods separates these researchers from soothsayers. Multiple methods used in concert are needed to identify and address future challenges. Selected examples of methods used in the conduction of futures research are presented here. In addition, Box 33.4 includes resources for exploring other methodologies used in this field of study.

Trend Analysis and Extrapolation

Trend analysis involves looking at historical data to identify trends over time. For example, a log of help desk calls demonstrates that over the past 2 months, there has been an increasing number of calls from clinical managers and department heads

TABLE 33.1   Extent of Patient Engagement Functions in Hospitals

Online Patient Engagement Functionality	Percent of Hospitals with Capability			
	2012	2013	2014	2015
Online Capabilities Incentivized by Federal Policy				
View information from health/medical record	24	39.8	90.8	95.1
Download information from health/medical record	14.3	27.8	82.2	86.8
Transmit care/referral summaries to a third party	N/A[a]	11.6	66.4	71.5
View, download, and transmit health information	N/A[a]	10	64	68.8
Secure messaging with health care provider[b]	N/A[a]	N/A[a]	51.3	63
Online Capabilities Not Incentivized by Federal Policy				
Request to update health/medical record	30.9	32.8	72.4	77.1
Pay bills	49.3	55.4	66.9	74.1
Schedule appointments	21.6	29.8	41.4	43.6
Request prescription refills	19.3	27	39.4	42.1
Submit patient-generated data	7.3	12.5	32.5	37.1

[a]Measure was not collected in survey year.
[b]Secure messaging was added to survey in 2014.
From Office of the National Coordinator for Health Information Technology. (2016, September). *U.S. hospital adoption of patient engagement functionalities: Health IT Quick-Stat #24.* dashboard.healthit.gov/quickstats/pages/FIG-Hospital-Adoption-of-Patient-Engagement-Functionalities.php.

BOX 33.4   Futures Studies Methodologies Resources

- The Institute for Ethics and Emerging Technologies, http://ieet.org/index.php/IEET/more/brin20150909
- Methods and Approaches of Futures Studies, http://crab.rutgers.edu/~goertzel/futuristmethods.htm
- World Future Society:
- Methods, http://www.wfs.org/methods

- Methodologies Forum, http://www.wfs.org/method.htm
- Futures Research Methodology Version 3.0, http://www.millennium-project.org/millennium/FRM-V3.html
- Five Views of the Future: A Strategic Analysis Framework, http://www.tfi.com/pubs/w/pdf/5views_wp.pdf

concerning the institution's newly introduced budget software. This new software offers options and levels of analysis that are more robust and complex than the software that was used in the past. Initially, calls occurred from three managers who work in the same division. However, these managers are now making very few calls. Instead, the calls are coming from a different division. Extrapolation consists of extending these historical data into the future. For example, if the trend line is sloping upward, one would continue this line at the same degree of slope into future time periods. This historical upward trend line will not continue forever. Eventually the growth will start to slow, and an S curve will develop. With an S curve, the growth is initially slow but then becomes very rapid. Once the event begins to reach its natural limit, the rate of growth slows again, creating an S-shaped curve.

A potential example of this pattern is the general public's potential use of PHRs and increasing access to their own data. Government organizations including the Centers for Medicare and Medicaid Services (CMS) and the Office of the National Coordinator for Health Information Technology (ONC) have created new guidelines and policies on interoperability, on patient access of their own medical data, and on improved health information exchange using established technical standards such as Fast Healthcare Interoperability Resources (FHIR) and the United States Core Data for Interoperability (USCDI) (CMS, 2021). The expected patterns of growth can be used to plan the future directions of health systems and their technological adoption. The need for these services can be expected to grow and then level off.

Application of Futures Research

Health and informatics professionals can use methodologies and strategies from futures studies in two primary ways. First, is foreseeing or predicting future trends and directions. For example, in the 1970s and 1980s, healthcare was financed via fee-for-service funding approaches. Health information systems were designed to capture charges but not to measure the cost of care. Items, including nursing and other services, are included in the patient's charge for a hospital room. In a fee-for-service approach, the contribution of nursing and other services to the total cost was irrelevant. Cost and charges did not need to correlate. The charge could be whatever the market would bear.

The introduction of the prospective payment system in the 1980s and managed care in the 1990s is now followed by the current value-based approach, Merit-Based Incentive Payment System (MIPS), included with the Medicare Access and CHIP Reauthorization Act (MACRA) of 2015. These initiatives require that healthcare institutions capture costs and quality rather than just charges. Existing information systems were never designed to facilitate capturing discrete costs (versus charges). The ability to predict these kinds of major changes in healthcare delivery could be a significant advantage to vendors and healthcare institutions alike. By predicting the potential costs and benefits, one is better prepared to manage these events. Cost-benefit analysis is an example of using futures studies for management.

Creating the future is the second way in which health informatics specialists use futures studies methods. By thinking of future scenarios, health and informatics professionals can work toward creating the environment in which these futures might be possible. By using the work of futurists, as well as applying the methods and tools of futures studies, it is feasible to imagine potential future trends and directions, and thereby work to create preferable future directions.

THE FUTURE OF HEALTH INFORMATICS

Health informatics is and will remain a dynamic and complex field. We aim to provide an overview and insight into trends that we believe will make a significant impact in how care is delivered. A list of current promising trends, as well as potential future trends, are outlined in the following discussions:

1 Looking further into the future can influence thinking about near-term trends. Outside the field of healthcare, contemporary issues of *The Futurist* (http://www.wfs.org/futurist) list annual outlooks. A sampling of trends pertinent to healthcare include the following: *tiny chips.* Computer chips will shrink to the size of dust and be ubiquitous (Yonck, 2013).

2 *Vast amounts of transmitted personal health data.* Embedded or swallowed sensors will collect and transmit an array of personal data (Meskó, 2014).

3 *New leader skills.* These will be shaped by those with social networking, content management, data mining, and innovation skills. New job titles include but are not limited to Chief Clinical Informatics Officer, (Kannry & Fridsma, 2016) Chief Innovation Officer, (Stevenson & Euchner, 2013) Chief Digital Officer, (Tumbas et al., 2018) Chief Content Officer, and Chief Data Scientist (Bisk, 2012).

4 *Nanotechnology products.* Buckypaper is composed of industrial-grade carbon nanotubes and is 100 times stronger than steel per unit of weight. It conducts electricity like copper and disperses heat like steel or brass (Bisk, 2012).

5 *Nanorobots or nanobots.* These carry molecule-sized elements, can detect cancer, and are being developed by researchers at Harvard University (Yonck, 2012).

6 *Evolving models of care.* With payers emphasizing value-based care, there is an opportunity to leverage social determinants of health (SDOH) data as well as patient generated health data.

7 *Improving user experience.* This is the opportunity to align multiple facets of healthcare delivery to have continuous improvement and innovation that leverages engaged patients and the community (Committee on the Learning Health Care System in America and Institute of Medicine, 2014).

These more futuristic trends are important to monitor and may inform near-term trends. Near-term future trends are (1) person-centered health and concomitant implications for health informatics; (2) technical trends in health IT such as the internet of things (IoT) and cybersecurity issues; and (3) clinical informatics trends, including what is beyond traditional EHRs, improving the user experience (UX), predictive analytics, and data visualization.

Person-Centered Health and Informatics

An obvious shift has occurred away from provider-centric healthcare toward person-centered health (Moreau-Gaudry & Voros, 2015; Kogan et al., 2016). The importance of this shift is underscored in a number of chapters of this book: The Evolving ePatient; mHealth: The intersection of mobile technology and Health; PHRs; and Social Media Tools for Health Informatics. This direction will continue to accelerate over time, although healthcare and informatics will see the fusion of these separate areas in the future.

The term person-centered health is used as a generic term to encompass ideas about the various terms in use today: person-centered care, patient-centered care, precision medicine, and consumer-centered care. Person-centered care embodies personal choice and autonomy in healthcare decision making (Kogan et al., 2016). More specifically, this newer term most frequently includes these six principles: (1) whole-person care, (2) respect and value, (3) choice, (4) dignity, (5) self-determination, and (6) purposeful living. They are being applied to the care of older adults in particular (Kogan et al., 2016). Precision (or personalized) medicine includes a central premise that health interventions are tailored to specific individual differences such as genome, environments, and lifestyle (Office of the Press Secretary, 2015). For example, therapeutics would be tailored specifically to individuals' genetic tumor compositions and their responses to previous interventions. No matter the current term, the shift is toward tailoring care to and improved support of health decision making for individuals. This shift has substantial implications for informatics because these areas are highly data-centric. Demiris and Kneale (2015) outlined initial informatics support for the move toward person- and patient-centric care (e.g., improvements in clinical decision support, e-tools to support care transitions, PHRs, and telehealth). Two other near-term informatics trends are outlined in support of person-centered health in the future: (1) increasing access to care and (2) personal data integration.

Increasing Access to Care

EHRs by design are organization- and provider-focused. The movement toward person-centered health requires rethinking the design of disparate health data into a person-centric format. Aspects of traditional care settings, supported by EHRs, and to a lesser extent by PHRs, are evolving into remote, on-demand services for non-emergent services. In recent years this has only accelerated as complex, chronic care disease management shifts make waves in the consumer-facing technology space while the COVID-19 pandemic has widened adoption of telehealth. Through informatics tools, consumers are supported as they assume more responsibility for their own care, especially consumers with chronic diseases. Informatics support via apps is expanding at an enormous rate. The global mHealth apps market was valued at $40 billion dollars in 2020 and has an expected growth rate of over 17% from 2021 to 2028 (Grand View Research, 2021). Although the care models of the future are not precisely clear, the move is toward care anytime, anywhere for areas such as primary care and chronic care.

1 The design of tailored, person-centered applications provides a wealth of opportunities for research and development, including the following: Theory-based studies on the impact of person-centered health IT products;

2 The effectiveness of changing care models on care collaboration for individuals focused on person-centered health.

Evolving Models of Care

As technology continues to rapidly evolve, opportunities exist to update and revise how care is delivered. Large, external pressures (including sequelae from the strain faced on US and international healthcare systems seen due to global pressures from a pandemic response) have exemplified both the need for change across traditional care paradigms and the opportunity for technology to assist in areas where they previously played only a minor role.

Telemedicine has become increasingly popular and more widely adopted across care areas and service lines. Much of this growth may be directly attributed to the need for remote care delivery following the COVID-19 pandemic, (Leiman et al., 2021; Fiks et al., 2021; James et al., 2021; Cinar et al., 2020; Royce et al., 2020; Katz et al., 2020) though a trend towards increasing use of telemedicine can be seen prior to COVID-19's impact. One such example is the Center for Medicare and Medicaid Innovation's (CMMI's) support of a new Emergency Triage, Treat, and Transport (ET3) model, wherein Emergency Medicine Services (EMS) to provide on-scene care, often in conjunction with real time virtual medical control (Munjal et al., 2019). This ET3 model allows for paramedics to care for patients at the home or a care area where they called for assistance, potentially without the need for transport to a nearby hospital or Emergency Department. Similar virtual care models that allow for the ordering of lab or imaging tests prior to in-person evaluation at an urgent care, Emergency Department, or primary care physician's office exist, thus saving time prior to an in-person clinical visit.

Healthcare models have already begun a transition towards value-based care (McCarthy, 2015) on treating and supporting patients with multiple chronic conditions (Savitz & Bayliss, 2021) and on reducing administrative waste (Kocher, 2021). An increasing focus is being placed on unmet health-related social needs and the need for increased access to care delivery services to help address them (Ruiz Escobar et al., 2021).

Social Determinants of Health

As we discuss evolving models of care, it is important to discuss how SDOH have played a role, and will continue to do so, in how we think about healthcare. The WHO defines SDOH as the non-medical factors that influence health outcomes (WHO, 2017). These factors include education, food insecurity, access to health services. These are growing health considerations and have a parallel growth in the data that is generated related to SDOH. Recommendation from the US Office of the National Coordinator for Health Information Technology recommends improving infrastructure to support the use of SDOH data and a clinical application (The National Coordinator for Health Information Technology, 2015). This means that health systems will have the opportunity to leverage different data to make an impact in the lives of their patients. This will also spotlight challenges that must be addressed, namely logistical concerns, interoperability, and challenges with data standards.

Community-based organizations (CBOs) have been able to help their communities by linking their residents with key resources for things like transportation and food. By bringing on a new partner such as a large healthcare organization, CBOs may potentially become overwhelmed, given their limited resources and capacity. There will be a need for these CBO networks to communicate with EHRs to have significant integration with the health system (Health Affairs, 2021). The solution will also need to harness data standards that are widely accepted in order to maximize interoperability.

The aggregation of SDOH data combined with the extensive health data provides a unique opportunity to address more contributors of health. This will also come with ethical questions that must be considered. Could use of these data promote biases and further exacerbate healthcare inequalities? How are SDOH data generated, and what measures are in place to ensure security of these data? Will they be accessible to payers, and might that impact coverage? There is a tremendous opportunity bridging the intersection of health informatics and SDOH to make an impact in the lives of patients. This must be done with careful consideration to overcome challenges.

Personal Data Integration

Simple personal monitoring tools such as electronic scales and remote blood glucose monitors are already expanding into a suite of robust biometric sensor technologies. There has been significant adoption in smart home technology, with revenue projected to reach $28 billion by 2021 and a projected growth of 12% (Smart Home, 2021). No doubt, many people will be actively monitoring and interpreting their own data from these devices with further expansion of its capabilities.

The increase in personal data mandates an amalgamation of pertinent health data beyond a casual level and away from informal personal records or users keeping data in their heads. Instead, these will need to include data integration across disparate sources for an interpretable individual view. Today, mHealth apps and online services result in stand-alone data viewed primarily by patients and families. Thus, the challenge will be to effect data integration across diverse sources and to provide monitoring with appropriate interventions for any acute changes. Future research and evaluation might include the following:

1. Evaluating the impact of role changes from provider-centric to patient-centric data
2. Exploring outcomes of the new digital divide among individuals who cannot or choose not to be "quantified" by personal data.

Technical Trends

Technical aspects of health informatics are trending toward cloud computing and remote application services. Two other important technical trends are especially relevant for the near future: the IoT and increased cybersecurity threats.

The Internet of Things

Simply put, the IoT refers to a network of connected devices (Morgan, 2014). Currently, the IoT might be used to remotely monitor a patient after discharge (Harpham, 2015) or to track equipment or people inside health facilities. In the future, the IoT has broader applications. With multiple devices and people connected via the internet, new applications are possible. A simple application might involve improved remote physiologic monitoring using sensors. For example, flexible and wearable sensors, which adhere to skin better, and silicon-based materials, which conduct signals better, can combine with the IoT to allow improved, remote physiologic monitoring for patients (Khan et al., 2016). More complex IoT applications in a facility might include a suite of interacting devices and applications, including:

1. Physiologic monitoring across hospital units and areas without equipment changes
2. Inpatient assignments coordinated with nurses' experience levels due to the integration of smart staffing and scheduling applications with patient conditions
3. Consumable supplies and medications automatically creating their own charges on patients' bills
4. Consumable supplies automatically reordering themselves when supplies run low
5. Durable medical equipment that automatically appears on units when a discharge order is written
6. Changes in provider and patient treatment adherence and monitoring with the IoT data

Note that with expanded connectivity, the available health data increases, but so too do the risks of health data privacy and cybersecurity issues increase.

Cybersecurity Threats and Mitigation

One of the most ominous risks in health informatics now and in the future is the increase in cybersecurity threats. With the proliferation of devices, their connectivity to the IoT, the increased use of mHealth apps, and the increase in health data posted on social media, cybersecurity threats will increase in volume and severity. New threats are emerging. For example, the University of Vermont (UVM) Medical Center employees were locked out of the EHR and other vital programs for nearly a month (Weiner, 2021). The impact of this ransomware attack was estimated to be nearly $50 million in lost revenue, not to mention the impact it had on patients. According to a survey of healthcare organizations globally, over a third have reported being targeted by ransomware in 2020 (Sophos, 2021). Without proper large-scale prevention and mitigation approaches, these incidents will likely continue to remain prevalent.

The informatics future will surely include more emphasis on health IT security, improved security using thorough risk assessments, and increased fiscal allocations for cybersecurity. A particular emphasis will be on improving the cybersecurity of personal health devices and preparing for the IoT connections. Policies, procedures, and code will be developed to prevent hacking and to avert paying ransoms in the future. Future research might include the following:

1. The impact of threats on patients' willingness to share private data such as mental health concerns
2. National efforts to combat cybersecurity threats

CLINICAL INFORMATICS

Beyond EHRs 2.0

With EHR adoption rates rising, especially for ambulatory practices (Jamoom et al., 2016), leaders and informaticians are shifting the focus away from basic implementations to other issues such as system optimization and data science. One of the most common foci is system optimization. The term *optimization* is used for both initial and post-implementation efforts. Users can benefit from applying known principles for project management and systems implementation, as well as by using available guides such as Strategies for Optimizing an EHR System (Health Information Technology Research Center [HITRC], 2018) from the ONC for Health IT. **Optimization,** more importantly, includes post-implementation evaluations, ongoing training, and system re-tailoring where needed. Installations obviously do not end with go-live. Institutions consider EHR installations as continual transformation instead.

In an editorial for *The New England Journal of Medicine*, Mandl and Kohane argue that vendors propagated a myth of complexity that precludes innovation and that EHRs are different than more flexible and robust consumer technology (Mandl & Kohane, 2012). EHR usability is now known to be linked to provider burnout for physicians and nurses alike (Melnick et al., 2020, 2021).

These growing concerns about EHR usability have led to speculation of a future where patients' data live in external, shared, universal data store, invoking ideas about an optimal data system previously described by Celi et al., (Celi et al., 2014; Rowley, 2017) Health information organizations were initially thought to meet this need, but have thus far had mixed success (Adler-Milstein et al., 2021; Everson et al., 2021). Meanwhile, some larger EHR vendors have created application stores where third parties can develop software to supplement core EHR experiences though metrics on their adoption remain sparse.

Newer infrastructures, such as cloud computing, middleware, and mobile applications, could also allow more robust integration efforts at the healthcare provider and consumer end of computing. Facilities are already incorporating mHealth apps into their suite of applications, although current statistics indicate that only about 2% of patients are currently using them (Accenture, 2015). Previous authors indicated that disruptive technologies for EHRs are needed to displace the current model of EHRs (Mandl & Kohane, 2012).

EHR interoperability efforts will continue, especially in the United States, where the diversity of products and components has caused the nation to lag behind others in creating integrated, person-centered, and longitudinal EHRs. Regional integration efforts have helped in the effort to share data, although interoperability beyond regions will be a continuous, costly future direction for the US informatics research, and operational efforts on ontologies will continue to facilitate this work. In the short term, a decision about the use of one or two specific ontologies, versus an endorsement of a suite of competing ontologies, especially for nursing, is urgently needed. A more long-term solution may be found in the current research on natural language processing and semantic mapping, where the process of mapping concepts can be automated.

From a policy perspective, there has been increasing enthusiasm for interoperability in recent years, with significant technical and policy advancements in the United States. The 21st Century Cures Act specifically addresses both information blocking and semantic interoperability. From the information blocking perspective, the 21st Century Cures Act specifically defines information blocking and penalties associated with the process (Posnack, 2020). Meanwhile, to assist with semantic normalization and interoperability, the legislation integrates technical standards such as FHIR and data-specific code systems such as LOINC, ICD, and SNOMED into national policy and is increasing the control patients have over how their data is shared between clinical services (HL7, 2021; Redox, 2020). Furthermore, with the USCDI, there is now a data standard that all EHR vendors are required to expose via an Application Programming Interface (API), which will become the catalyst for new models of care that are decoupled from the traditional healthcare system-centered approaches (Jones et al., 2021).

Potential areas for future research include the following:

1. Impacts of integrative views of patient-centered data across traditional EHR modules and disciplines
2. Cost-effectiveness research and comparative effectiveness for EHR designs

Improving the user experience for health information technology

Efforts to improve the UX for health IT have now begun after years of relative neglect. More efforts are needed. Leaders are recognizing that UX issues can affect patient safety as well as user efficiency and satisfaction. Healthcare providers deplore the poor usability of today's EHRs. Improving the UX for health IT is an obvious future trend. Institutions such as Hawaii Pacific

Health have created systems that receive EHR end-user feedback to quickly triage and make necessary changes (Forward, 2020).

On a more hopeful note, large health IT vendors have hired UX professionals and are employing user-centered design techniques. These efforts were incentivized by Meaningful Use requirements. Whether these efforts continue as robustly remains to be seen. At this writing, UX improvements are occurring more slowly for nurses and allied health professionals than for physicians.

In the future, repositories for excellent designs and solutions to current UX issues will be needed. Typically, each site grapples with problems *de novo*, meaning wasted effort across the nation. Excellent, generic designs should be constructed and shared for common applications such as assessments, eMARs, and the like.

1. Due to current complaints by users, federal UX requirements will expand (beyond medical devices regulated by the US Food and Drug Administration), and vendors will have to respond to the need for improved products. Organizations will need to increase their knowledge about and skills for improving the UX. Excellent resources for meeting this challenge are the Healthcare Information and Management Systems Society (HIMSS) Usability Maturity Model (Staggers & Rodney, 2012), the ONC's SAFER (Safety Assurance Factors for EHR Resilience) guides (HealthIT. gov, 2018), and documents from the National Institute for Standards and Technology (NIST) (Lowry et al., 2015). There are multiple research directions for improving the UX. Examples include the following: Comparative effectiveness research on EHR and device designs, especially for complex patient views, such as clinical summaries, care transitions, and eMARs.

2. Developing and implementing best design practices agnostic of vendors. Decoupling user views from underlying code could occur so that optimal designs could be downloaded by healthcare providers and layered onto their local data.

3. Determining outcomes for varying application designs. For instance, improved displays can positively affect clinicians' situation awareness and performance in intensive care units (ICUs) (Koch et al., 2012; Görges & Staggers, 2008; Drews & Westenskow, 2006). Similar studies for other applications could be completed.

Analytics (Big Data) and Data Visualization

The world is generating massive amounts of data. IBM estimates that 2.5 quintillion bytes of information are generated each day (Perez, 2020). In the life sciences, genomic data have created large datasets for analyses. Bioinformatics efforts are underway to integrate data across disparate fields. For example, the National Center for Integrative Biomedical Informatics from the National Institutes of Health is developing interactive, integrated, analytic, and modeling technologies from molecular biology, experimental data, and the published literature (Athey et al., 2012).

Within healthcare, data warehouses combine longitudinal, administration, and financial data into a searchable database,

although typically at the local or healthcare enterprise level. Now, the boundaries are blurring among personal health data sources: mHealth, social media, wearable, and sensor devices, and PHRs, (Fernández-Luque & Bau, 2015) so opportunities for increased data collection are manifest. Thus, data from personal devices such as sensor data and mobile and remote technologies could be integrated with EHR data soon. Personalized medicine efforts, including genomic data and nanotechnology, promise the expansion of these kinds of databases even further.

With these super-sized datasets, an unparalleled opportunity exists to examine data and issues across thousands of data points integrated across fields (population data, genomics). The challenge is that the ability *to collect* these types of data has outstripped the ability *to analyze* them (Holland et al., 2015). Within data science, data analytics help in sense making by revealing patterns in datasets. The future of big data in healthcare should see rapid progress in the normalization and mobilization of healthcare data for clinically actionable insights, which will rely on machine learning to process such vast amounts of data at scale.

Machine Learning/Artificial Intelligence

Machine learning has been discussed at length in other chapters of this text. Here, we will discuss current trends and future directions for machine learning in healthcare. Five specific trends will be explored: (1) predictive analytics; (2) how machine learning empowers the learning healthcare system; (3) how machine learning supplements clinical care; (4) risks involved in how machine learning interacts with SDOH; and (5) the importance of interpretability in machine learning.

Predictive analytics

According to current national and regional presentations, Chief Information Officers (CIOs) and health IT leaders are moving their foci to predictive analytics, the use of past data to predict future trends. The goal is to present data to decision makers as close to real time as possible. A common operational example might be the real-time analysis of vital sign trends in a patient on a medical-surgical unit to predict a patient's level of care to anticipate hospital bed needs. On a more complex level, healthcare systems may amass near real-time data from traditional sources like physiologic monitoring and less traditional sources including patient-generated or reported health data, analyzing them, and displaying data in near real time for care decisions across complex datasets.

From an analytics tool's perspective, Shameer et al. (2017) depict a model for data integration and subsequent analyses at the individual level (Fig. 33.1). Here, data from various sources would be integrated for uses in person-centered health and precision medicine to provide individualized predictive analytics. This type of real-time analysis is a marriage of EHRs and decision support, and it is now being implemented both as bespoke solutions at the healthcare-system level and more broadly by larger EHR vendors (Shameer et al., 2017; Manz et al., 2020; EHRIntelligence, 2020). As this type of real time analysis becomes available at the individual level, healthcare providers

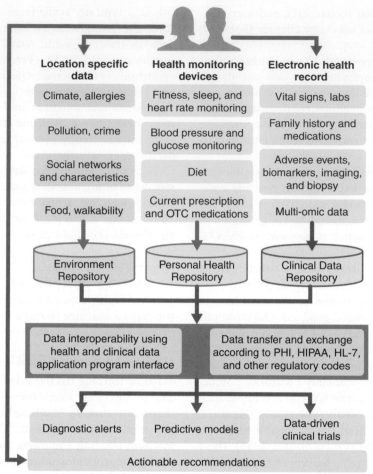

Fig 33.1 Healthcare and wellcare data model. (From Shameer, K., Badgeley, M. A., Glicksberg, B. S., Morgan, J. W., & Dudley, J. T. (2016). Translational bioinformatics in the era of real-time biomedical health care and wellness data streams. *Briefings in Bioinformatics*, 18(1):105–124. pii: bbv118. Reprinted with permission from Oxford University Press.)

will be challenged to integrate yet more information into their cognitive processes and workflow.

In other examples, predictive analytics could be useful at the population level in detecting global diseases such as the Zika virus or even in real-time fraud detection for someone attempting to use information to cheat on insurance coverage, like credit card fraud detection is done today. These kinds of advanced applications are predicated on having quality source data, standards for integration and appropriate integrated data, and a capability of being able to interpret data using tools like data visualization.

How Machine Learning Empowers the Learning Healthcare System

The idea of a **Learning Healthcare System** was first introduced to healthcare in 2007 by the United States Institute of Medicine (IoM, now the National Academy of Medicine) (IOM, 2007), which later defined it as a system in which "science, informatics, incentives, and culture are aligned for continuous improvement and innovation, with best practices seamlessly embedded in the delivery process, [with] patients and families being active participants in all elements, and new

knowledge captured as an integral by-product of the delivery experience" (Committee on the Learning Health Care System in America and Institute of Medicine, 2014). Since its introduction, measuring the impact of learning healthcare system efforts have been difficult despite researcher interest (Budrionis & Bellika, 2016). Much of the work remains proof of concept/proposed. This was most recently exposed at scale during the COVID-19 pandemic (Romanelli et al. 2021). Machine learning has a particular use case in addressing data infrastructure issues with particular use cases identifying care improvement targets (Romanelli et al., 2021) and harnessing large data sets to deliver actionable insights to the point of care (Manz et al. 2020).

Looking to the future, we anticipate that machine learning will be empowered by significant investments now being made into data normalization, especially within the United States (Jones et al. 2021; HL7 International, 2021). Once data are better normalized and more seamlessly able to flow across healthcare systems to researchers, machine learning should rapidly be able to scale operational solutions that are already in process now while also creating a flywheel of clinical applications that will kickstart the learning healthcare system.

Supplementing Clinical Care

What clinical applications will be targeted by machine learning in the next decade or so? To date, challenges in gaining access to data at scale has led to a first wave of machine learning applications targeting operational inefficiencies in the healthcare system. This has included applications such as deploying Natural Language Processing (NLP) to extract billing codes from free text notes, predicting lengths of stay to help with hospital staffing, and predicting no-show rates to optimize clinic efficiency. Consumer facing Machine Learning (ML) applications are now gaining popularity as well.

Machine learning applications will also play a crucial role supporting next-generation clinical care delivery models. Triaging patients to telehealth, in-person, or even inpatient health care settings will increase healthcare system efficiency. Meanwhile, care navigation applications act as "digital advocates" for patients with complex health care problems such as cancer or heart failure. As care delivery models become more specialized, technology-enabled, and varied, machine learning will be critical in matching patients to the right clinical resources.

Systemizing Bias, Worsening Disparities

As machine learning models get deployed at scale, caution will need to be taken with regard to how ML algorithms impact the equity of care delivery that they allocate/enable. Several papers published in the late 2010s have identified how ML models can result in greater inequity in healthcare resource allocation. As such, techniques and best practices will be needed to protect vulnerable populations from being further marginalized. In the current state of healthcare, techniques that can reduce the bias of ML algorithms are being developed (Obermeyer et al., 2019). Meanwhile, best practices around the deployment of ML can also prevent their unintentional widening of healthcare disparities (Discrimination by artificial intelligence in a commercial electronic health record—a case study, 2021).

Interpretability

Aside from tuning machine learning models themselves and deploying them in ways that reduce disparity, building interpretable machine learning models is another strategy to mitigate ML worsening healthcare disparities. Defined in (citation), machine learning interpretability is defined as any method of machine learning that can explain its predictions in a way that a human can understand. For example, in logistic regressions, weights are provided to each of the variables that go into a model. As a result, users of logistic regressions can understand what variables are most important in predicting an outcome. This is commonly seen in popular logistic regression predictors such as the PERC score (Kline). Though interpretable models historically have not been as performant as "black box" models such as CNNs and random forests, the ability for a clinician to "validate" the rules driving predictions builds trust in the model while also enabling clinicians to know when to clinically override them (John Chen's paper). Newer trends have demonstrated an increased enthusiasm for interpretable machine learning models, and it is anticipated that the performance of this flavor of machine learning model will continue to improve.

Data Visualization

In 2017, a systematic literature review was conducted on the prevalence, type, and setting of the data visualization articles present in healthcare (Wu et al., 2019). A total of 78 studies were evaluated across a number of target audiences (including healthcare providers, patients, and administrators), evaluation settings (including clinical settings, lab settings, and partial rollouts), and deployment targets (early prototype to operational deployment). The authors provided a summary of common evaluation practices as well as opportunities for future work within the visual analytics space. Note that data visualization types exist from a taxonomy published in 1996, (Shneiderman, 1996) though the field of data visualization has continued to evolve and progress. One example of a newer data visualization approach is the UpSet plot (Fig. 33.2), which focuses on visualizing multiple data sets across aggregation and intersection thresholds (Lex et al., 2014).

An Increasing Role for Human Factors Engineering

Human factors engineering (HFE) is the scientific discipline that focuses on the interaction between humans and the other elements of a system that they are using, with a specific focus on human well-being and overall system performance (Human Factors and Ergonomics Society, 2021). HFE has roots in system design dating back to the mid-1900s, particularly with regard to aviation and military system design, though its impact has continued to expand

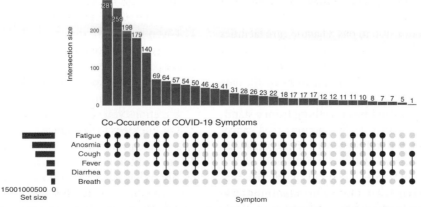

Fig 33.2 Example of an upset plot visualization used to observe the co-occurrence of reported COVID-19 Symptoms. (From Healy, K. [2020]. "Upset plots." Kieran Healy (blog). April 16, 2020. https://kieranhealy.org/blog/archives/2020/04/16/upset-plots/.)

within healthcare (Cafazzo & St-Cyr, 2012). HFE practices may draw from a number of scientific disciplines and principles, including but not limited to those stemming from psychology, sociology, engineering, UX, design, informatics, etc (Human Factors and Ergonomics Society, 2021). One popular sociotechnical model in healthcare includes the Systems Engineering Initiative for Patient Safety 2.0 (SEIPS 2.0) model, which provides a holistic approach to the various factors within healthcare, including people, organizations, tools and technology, internal environment, external environment, and tasks (Holden et al., 2013). HFE approaches have continued opportunity to improve on the overall safety and efficacy of system design across a myriad of informatics, mobile app/mHealth, IoT, wearables, and similar domains (Turner et al., 2017). Human factors may also be embedded into organizational learning processes to help optimize patient safety and improve clinician outcomes (Carayon, 2019). Studies focusing on task load (Harry et al., 2021; Shanafelt et al., 2016), on EHR usage (Arndt et al., 2017; Hill et al., 2013; Sinsky et al., 2016), and on burnout (Shanafelt et al., 2016; Han et al., 2019; Shanafelt et al., 2017) may harness principles extending from or overlapping with the human factors space. HFE principles may also be applied to patient safety learning laboratory settings (Businger et al., 2020) or may be directly embedded into clinical practice. These principles, including those arising from the realms of usability and biomedical informatics, may serve as continued means with which to help implement and study the impact of change as health systems continue to adopt and implement a Learning Health System approach (Taylor et al., 2021; Kohn et al., 2019).

CONCLUSION AND FUTURE DIRECTIONS

Health professionals, informatics specialists, and leaders cannot afford to leave the future to chance. They must proactively and systematically identify future trends and directions in society, healthcare, technology, and informatics. This information and knowledge can provide the foundation for designing and building health information systems of the future. The methods and trends discussed in this chapter provide tools and ideas for health professional informaticians to use in identifying important future trends locally, regionally, and nationally.

As the rate of change continues to expand, it is expected that healthcare providers and informaticians will increase their use of e-tools and methods of futures research to predict and plan for an informatics-supported future in healthcare.

ACKNOWLEDGMENT

The authors wish to acknowledge the contributions of Nancy Staggers, Ramona Nelson, and David E. Jones to the previous edition of this chapter.

DISCUSSION QUESTIONS

1. In your work setting, which future trend(s) are likely to have the largest effect on patient care and related information systems?
2. Select one of the chapter topics in this book. For example, you might select mHealth or personal health records. Use the three levels of change to describe how your selected area of informatics might evolve over the next several years.
3. Use Box 33.4 to access and explore a futures research methodology that was not discussed in this chapter. Describe the methodology and how it could be used in health informatics.
4. Compare and contrast the trends of EHR directions and personal healthcare informatics. Where do they overlap and where do they differ?
5. How do you see the described clinical informatics trends evolving, and what challenges do you see?
6. What are the upcoming legislative opportunities and barriers regarding the future of health informatics?
7. How do you see pandemics such as COVID-19 either negatively or positively affecting health informatics trends?

CASE STUDY

You have just been hired as a clinical informatics leader for a new health system. The health system has 23 acute care facilities and 36 outpatient clinics. It serves as a regional referral center for three states in the Midwest. Your installed base includes a vendor supplied EHR from a national vendor. Work on the data warehouse is being rethought. Your site has more than 300 varying applications across sites, including everything from a stand-alone pharmacy application for drug interactions to a cancer registry. Your goal is to provide IT support for the organizational vision of being the premier health organization in patient safety for the region. Your goal is also to provide predictive analytics for patient care for your ICUs. One of the first things you want to do is to plan for the future of IT.

Discussion Questions

1. Given the future directions discussed in this chapter, select the two directions you want to emphasize. Provide rationale for your choices.
2. Discuss how you can use methodologies from futures research to plan for your preferred future with the future directions you selected in Question 1.
3. Outline steps to introduce the chief executive officer to nanotechnology and its potential impact on the organization.
4. You want to increase collaborative work with a local university. What future directions for education do you think are most important as CIO?

REFERENCES

Accenture. (2015). Losing patience: Why healthcare providers need to up their mobile game. https://www.accenture.com/_acnmedia/Accenture/Conversion-Assets/DotCom/Documents/Global/PDF/Dualpub_24/Accenture-Chart-Fewer-Downloads-Lower-Ratings.pdf

Adler-Milstein, J., Garg, A., Zhao, W., & Patel, V. (2021). A survey of health information exchange organizations in advance of a nationwide connectivity framework. *Health Affairs, 40*(5), 736–744. https://doi.org/10.1377/hlthaff.2020.01497.

Arndt, B. G., Beasley, J. W., Watkinson, M. D., et al. (2017). Tethered to the EHR: Primary care physician workload assessment using EHR event log data and time-motion observations. *Annals of Family Medicine, 15*(5), 419–426. https://doi.org/10.1370/afm.2121.

Athey, B. D., Cavalcoli, J. D., Jagadish, H. V., et al. (2012). The NIH National Center for Integrative Biomedical Informatics (NCIBI). *Journal of the American Medical Informatics Association, 19*(2), 166–170. https://doi.org/10.1136/amiajnl-2011-000552.

Bisk, T. (2012). Unlimiting energy's growth. *The Futurist, 46*(3), 29–31. https://search.proquest.com/openview/51cf5701b5a8c809a9a480f0c095c80c/1?pq-origsite=gscholar&cbl=47758

Budrionis, A., & Bellika, J. G. (2016). The learning healthcare system: where are we now? A systematic review. *Journal of Biomedical Informatics, 64*, 87–92. https://doi.org/10.1016/j.jbi.2016.09.018.

Buerhaus, P. I., Skinner, L. E., Auerbach, D. I., & Staiger, D. O. (2017). Four challenges facing the nursing workforce in the United States. *Journal of Nursing Regulation, 8*(2), 40–46. https://doi.org/10.1016/S2155-8256(17)30097-2.

Businger, A. C., Fuller, T. E., Schnipper, J. L., Rossetti, S. C., Schnock, K. O., Rozenblum, R., et al. (2020). Lessons learned implementing a complex and innovative patient safety learning laboratory project in a large academic medical center. *Journal of the American Medical Informatics Association, 27*(2), 301–307. https://doi.org/10.1093/jamia/ocz193.

Cafazzo, J. A., & St-Cyr, O. (2012). From discovery to design: the evolution of human factors in healthcare. *Healthc Q, 15*, 24–29. https://doi.org/10.12927/hcq.2012.22845.

Carayon, P. (2019). Human factors in health(care) informatics: toward continuous sociotechnical system design. *Studies in Health Technology and Informatics, 265*, 22–27. https://doi.org/10.3233/SHTI190131.

Celi, L. A., Csete, M., & Stone, D. (2014). Optimal data systems. *Current Opinion in Critical Care, 20*(5), 573–580. https://doi.org/10.1097/mcc.0000000000000137.

Centers for Medicare and Medicaid Services. National Health Expenditures Projections 2019–2028. Accessed August 27, 2021. https://www.cms.gov/Research-Statistics-Data-and-Systems/Statistics-Trends-and-Reports/NationalHealthExpendData/NHE-Fact-Sheet.

Centers for Medicare and Medicaid Services (CMS). (2021). Policies and Technology for Interoperability and burden reduction. Accessed August 30, 2021. https://www.cms.gov/Regulations-and-Guidance/Guidance/Interoperability/index

Chantrill C. US Government healthcare spending history with charts. Accessed February 11, 2016. http://www.usgovernmentspending.com/healthcare_spending

Cinar, P., Kubal, T., Freifeld, A., et al. (2020). Safety at the time of the COVID-19 pandemic: How to keep our oncology patients and healthcare workers safe. *Journal of the National Comprehensive Cancer Network*, 1–6. https://doi.org/10.6004/jnccn.2020.7572. Published online April 15.

Committee on the Learning Health Care System in America, & Institute of Medicine. (2014). In M. Smith, R. Saunders, L. Stuckhardt, & J. M. McGinnis (Eds.), *Best care at lower cost: The path to continuously learning health care in America*. National Academies Press (US). http://doi.org/10.17226/13444.

Demiris, G., & Kneale, L. (2015). Informatics systems and tools to facilitate patient-centered care coordination. *Yearbook of Medical Informatics, 10*(1), 15–21. https://doi.org/10.15265/IY-2015-003.

Discrimination by artificial intelligence in a commercial electronic health record—a case study. Accessed August 31, 2021. https://www.healthaffairs.org/do/10.1377/hblog20200128.626576/full/

Drews, F. A., & Westenskow, D. R. (2006). The right picture is worth a thousand numbers: data displays in anesthesia. *Hum Factors, 48*(1), 59–71. https://doi.org/10.1518/001872006776412270.

EHRIntelligence. (2020). Epic Systems, Cerner lead EHR vendors in AI development. Accessed August 31, 2021. https://ehrintelligence.com/news/epic-systems-cerner-lead-ehr-vendors-in-ai-development

Everson, J., Patel, V., & Adler-Milstein, J. (2021). Information blocking remains prevalent at the start of 21st Century Cures Act: Results from a survey of health information exchange organizations. *Journal of the American Medical Informatics Association, 28*(4), 727–732. https://doi.org/10.1093/jamia/ocaa323.

Fernández-Luque, L., & Bau, T. (2015). Health and social media: Perfect storm of information. *Healthcare Informatics Research, 21*(2), 67. https://doi.org/10.4258/hir.2015.21.2.67.

Fiks, A. G., Jenssen, B. P., & Ray, K. N. (2021). A defining moment for pediatric primary care telehealth. *JAMA Pediatrics, 175*(1), 9–10. https://doi.org/10.1001/jamapediatrics.2020.1881.

Forward, A. S. (2020). Getting rid of stupid stuff: The original launch. AMA Ed Hub. Accessed September 1, 2021. https://edhub.ama-assn.org/steps-forward/module/2758834

Görges, M., & Staggers, N. (2008). Evaluations of physiological monitoring displays: A systematic review. *Journal of Clinical Monitoring and Computing, 22*(1), 45–66. https://doi.org/10.1007/s10877-007-9106-8.

Grand View Research. (2021). mHealth Apps Market Size _ Industry Report, 2021-2028. Published online February 2021. https://www.grandviewresearch.com/industry-analysis/mhealth-app-market

Guariguata, L., Whiting, D. R., Hambleton, I., Beagley, J., Linnenkamp, U., & Shaw, J. E. (2014). Global estimates of diabetes prevalence for 2013 and projections for 2035. *Diabetes Research and Clinical Practice, 103*(2), 137–149. https://doi.org/10.1016/j.diabres.2013.11.002.

Han, S., Shanafelt, T. D., Sinsky, C. A., et al. (2019). Estimating the attributable cost of physician burnout in the United States. *Annals of Internal Medicine, 170*(11), 784–790. https://doi.org/10.7326/M18-1422.

Harpham B. (2015). How the Internet of Things is changing healthcare and transportation. Accessed July 2, 2016. https://www.cio.com/article/2981481/how-the-internet-of-things-is-changing-healthcare-and-transportation.html

Harry, E., Sinsky, C., Dyrbye, L. N., et al. (2021). Physician task load and the risk of burnout among US physicians in a national survey. *Joint Commission Journal on Quality and Patient Safety, 47*(2), 76–85. https://doi.org/10.1016/j.jcjq.2020.09.011.

Health Affairs. (2021). Addressing social determinants: Scaling up partnerships with community-based organization networks. Accessed August 30, 2021. https://www.healthaffairs.org/do/10.1377/hblog20200221.672385/full/

Q